RADIATION
— AND —
THYROID CANCER

RADIATION
—— AND ——
THYROID CANCER

Editors

G. Thomas
A. Karaoglou
E. D. Williams

Europeon Commission (EC)
US Department of Energy (US DOE OHER and OIHP)
National Cancer Institute (NCI)
University of Cambridge

EUR 18552 EN

World Scientific
Singapore • New Jersey • London • Hong Kong

Published by

World Scientific Publishing Co. Pte. Ltd.

P O Box 128, Farrer Road, Singapore 912805

USA office: Suite 1B, 1060 Main Street, River Edge, NJ 07661

UK office: 57 Shelton Street, Covent Garden, London WC2H 9HE

British Library Cataloguing-in-Publication Data
A catalogue record for this book is available from the British Library.

ACKNOWLEDGEMENTS

The Organising Committee wishes to express its thanks to the European Commission, the U.S. Department of Energy -OHER and OIHP-, The US National Cancer Institute and the University of Cambridge for the support they gave to this meeting. We also thank the members of the Programme Committee who were always there to help, the invited speakers, the session chairpersons, the referees, all the speakers and all of the participants for the lively discussions. Special thanks to the Cambridge team without whom the whole organisation of the meeting would not have been so successful. Their help has been invaluable.

Proceedings of an International Seminar on
RADIATION AND THYROID CANCER

ISBN 981-02-3814-2

This book is printed on acid-free paper.

Printed in Singapore by Uto-Print

Contents

RADIATION AND THE INCIDENCE OF THYROID CANCER IN MAN II

SYMPOSIUM ON CHERNOBYL AND THYROID CANCER (invited papers)

Proffered Papers

Proffered Papers

Posters

Posters

ASCERTAINING AND PREDICTING THE CONSEQUENCES OF A
NUCLEAR ACCIDENT

FUTURE PROSPECTS

RADIATION AND THYROID CANCER

Proceedings Editors

G. Thomas	University of Cambridge, UK
A. Karaoglou	European Commission, B
E.D. Williams	University of Cambridge, UK

Organising Committee

A. Karaoglou	European Commission, B
R. Neta	Department Of Energy, OIHP, USA
G. Thomas	University of Cambridge, UK
B. Wachholz	National Cancer Institute, USA
E.D. Williams	University of Cambridge, UK

Programme Committee

D. Becker	NY Hospital-Cornell Med Center, USA
K.H. Chadwick	European Commission, B
E. Demidchik	Minsk State Medical Institute, BEL
L.E. Holm	Swedish Radiation Protection Inst., SE
A. Kellerer	University of Munich, D
S. Nagataki	RERF, J
A. Pinchera	University of Pisa, I
Ch. Reiners	University of Würzburg, D
M. Schlumberger	Inst. Gustave-Roussy, FR
N. Tronko	Inst.Endocrinol. & Metabol., UKR
A. Tsyb	Academy of Medical Sciences, RUS
E.D. Williams	University of Cambridge, UK

Local Organisation

G. Thomas	University of Cambridge, UK
L. Fothergill	University of Cambridge, UK

Scientific Secretariat

A. Karaoglou	European Commission, B

Session Chairmen

D. Becker	NY Hospital-Cornell Med Center, USA
A. Bouville	NCI, USA
G. Burrow	Yale Univ School of Medicine, USA
E. Cardis	IARC, FR
K.H. Chadwick	European Commission? B
E.P. Demidchik	Minsk State Medical Institute, BEL
F. Hawkins	DOE, OIHP, USA
L.E. Holm	Swedish Radiation Protection Inst., S
A. Karaoglou	European Commission, B
S. Nagataki	RERF, J
R. Neta	DOE, OIHP, USA
A. Pinchera	University of Pisa, I
Ch. Reiners	University of Würzburg, D
J. Robbins	NIH, USA
J. Sinnaeve	European Commission, B
V. Stepanenko	Med Rad Res Center, RUS
G. Thomas	University of Cambridge, UK
N.D. Tronko	Inst.Endocrinol. & Metabol., UKR
A.F. Tsyb	Academy of Medical Sciences, RUS
B. Wachholz	NCI, USA
E.D. Williams	University of Cambridge, UK

Young Scientist Awards

Abrosimov A.	RUS
Abylkassimova Z.	Kazakhstan
Berkovski V.	UKR
Pozharskaya V	BEL
Troshina K	RUS
Zaitsev E.V.	RUS
Zurnagdhy L.	UKR
Nascimento Achn	BRA
Schoemaker M.J.	NL

EDITORIAL

Radiation and Thyroid cancer

This is the first International Conference in this very important area. The occurrence of a considerable increase in incidence of thyroid cancer in children in areas exposed to fallout from the Chernobyl nuclear reactor accident has drawn attention to the need for a better understanding of the relationship between radiation exposure, especially from the radionuclides of iodine, and the risk of thyroid cancer. An increase in thyroid cancer has been reported both in patients exposed to therapeutic and diagnostic external radiation, and in the population exposed to radiation from the Hiroshima and Nagasaki atomic bombs. While there is no evidence of a significant increase of this cancer in patients treated with radioactive iodine, an increase in thyroid cancer incidence was found in the Marshall islands population after exposure to fallout from a thermonuclear explosion, and now an increase has been observed in children exposed to fallout from Chernobyl. The principal aims of this meeting were to address the relationship between radiation and thyroid cancer, to explore the many factors influencing the interactions between radiation and the thyroid cell that together determine the likelihood of a cancer and to examine the most recent evidence derived from studies of the effects of Chernobyl within the broader context of other experience of radiation induced thyroid carcinoma. In summary, a comprehensive assessment of our understanding of radiation and thyroid cancer was reviewed, with particular emphasis upon the extensive information from the Chernobyl experience and the practical importance of this knowledge in relation to public exposure to radiation in general, and reactor accidents in particular, was discussed.

The Conference was held at the University of Cambridge, St. John's College, 20-23rd July 1998. There were 120 participants from different parts of the world, including nine young scientists (3 from Russia, 2 from the Ukraine, 1 from Belarus, 1 from Kazakhstan, 1 from Brazil and 1 from The Netherlands). We were pleased to note that the scientists involved in this field are seeking increased international collaboration, including the exchange of results, materials and ideas. Another important outcome was made possible by the presence and cooperation of these scientists; it became clear during the meeting that efforts to establish Chernobyl-related thyroid tissue, nucleic acid and data banks in Belarus, Russia and the Ukraine, soon will be initiated. This will be a first step to standardise the histological material and clinical data in the three countries and to establish a resource available to the scientific community for future studies.

It is with great pleasure that we thank all of the participants who contributed to the scientific quality of the meeting and to the climate of international friendship, and we share the belief that this Conference gives new perspectives for future research in Radiation and Thyroid Cancer.

The Organising Committee

Introduction

Radiation and Thyroid Cancer

J. Sinnaeve, Head of Unit, Radiation Protection Research, European Commission, Directorate General for Science Research and Development; *F. Hawkins*, Director of the Office of International Health Programmes, US Department of Energy, *B. Wachholz*, National Cancer Institute, US, opened the meeting.

J. Sinnaeve welcomed all participants on behalf of the European Commission to this Conference and expressed his gratefulness to the University of Cambridge, who invited the EC to hold the Conference in Cambridge and in particular to Professor Dillwyn Williams and to Dr Gerry Thomas for their enthusiasm and efforts in co-organising the Conference. The US Department of Energy's and the US National Cancer Institute's involvement in the organisation of the meeting documents the continued intensive and rewarding co-operation in many areas of radiation protection.

He pointed out that the aim of the meeting is to describe the link between radiation and thyroid cancer, to explore the many factors influencing the interaction between radiation and the thyroid cell and to place the post-Chernobyl observed thyroid effects in the wider context of other experience on radiation induced thyroid carcinoma.

In his opening comments, *J. Sinnaeve* reminded us that the Radiation Protection Research has supported studies on post-Chernobyl childhood thyroid cancer since 1992, following the reported increase in this cancer in children living near Chernobyl. An International Panel of Experts were put together to arrive to a consensus on these reportings; a report describing the needs and the recommendations for action was published by this panel under the auspices of the EC. This was a starting point to interest the decision-takers to grant technical assistance and humanitarian aid for the treatment of these children in the heavily affected areas in the former Soviet Union. The results of the period 92-96 were presented at the International Conference "Radiological consequences of the Chernobyl accident", Minsk, Belarus, in March 1996. Today, in the fourth framework programme of the EC, there are 10 research contracts on Radiation and Thyroid Cancer. They cover the whole spectrum of this disease: prevention, diagnosis, characterisation and treatment. Most importantly the creation of a thyroid tissue and data bank in the three States of the former Soviet Union is the biggest success and guarantee to preserve and further study this disease. *J. Sinnaeve* stressed the importance of this work and added that thyroid cancer in children will continue to be a priority for the 5th framework programme of the EC, covering the period 1998-2002.

J. Sinnaeve concluded by noting that this Conference will hopefully give new perspectives and identify focused needs for future research in this field and open doors for closer International co-operation.

F. Hawkins welcomed all participants on behalf of the DOE on the occasion of this First International Conference on Radiation and Thyroid Cancer. He congratulated the programme and organising committees who have done a first rate job putting together an interesting and thought provoking three days of presentations and discussions.

This meeting holds great promise for all of us who share a desire to better understand the relationship between radiation and thyroid cancer due to radiation exposure, the mechanisms of radiation carcinogenesis, and the prevention and treatment of thyroid cancer. He expressed his hope that this meeting will spur new insights and initiatives to answer the questions that will inevitably remain unanswered for now.

F. Hawkins added that he is optimistic about the future. We have before us the opportunity to strengthen International radiation health studies. The OIHP's work with the Radiation Effects Research Foundation in Japan, the joint co-ordinating committee for radiation effects research in Russia, and the work in the Republic of the Marshall Islands proves that international co-operation and scientific collaboration are the keys to our success.. *F. Hawkins* concluded by mentioning this meeting could be a catalyst to earnestly begin that process. He wished all a successful and rewarding meeting

B. Wachholz welcomed the participants to a week of exciting and informative science. In his opening remarks, he stated that the National Cancer Institute (a major component within the US National Institutes of Health) is pleased to have the opportunity to be a co-sponsor of this timely international gathering of many of the world's experts on the subject of "Radiation and Thyroid Cancer". It has been more than 2 years since the several 10th anniversary meetings associated with the Chernobyl accident, and much has occurred since then, both in the affected countries and in related studies elsewhere in the world; consequently, it is appropriate that this meeting include other studies in addition to the Chernobyl experience. In the US, for example, there is renewed interest in and concern over the exposure of segments of the US population to radioactive iodine produced by atmospheric nuclear weapons tests that took place primarily in the 1950s, and also to iodine-131 resulting from atmospheric releases from nuclear weapons facilities. More broadly, the US is co-operating with scientists, physicians and international organizations in a number of countries to study the relationships between radiation and the thyroid. It is indicative of the importance of the subject matter that there is co-operation also among the several US agencies that individually or jointly fund these studies in the US and elsewhere

B. Wachholz pointed out that it is well worth noting the increased collegial cooperation among scientists and governments in recent years, especially in comparison to the uncertainties sometimes apparent in earlier years. Only in this way can we leverage and maximise our collective resources for the work yet to be done, which in some cases is expected to continue for quite some years.

Finally, *B. Wachholz* acknowledged the NCI's appreciation to the organisers of this meeting, particularly Dr. Gerry Thomas, Sir Dillwyn Williams and their colleagues, for both the sientific content of the program and the amenities in this historic setting in Cambridge, to the co-sponsors at the European Commission and at the Department of Energy, and to all of those who have the interest and have taken the time to attend this meeting.

J. Sinnaeve
F. Hawkins
B. Wachholz

EXTERNAL RADIATION AND THE THYROID CANCER RISK IN HUMANS

ELAINE RON

Radiation Epidemiology Branch, National Cancer Institute, NIH, Bethesda, MD 20895,
USA
E-mail: rone@epndce.nci.nih.gov

ARTHUR B. SCHNEIDER

Department of Medicine, Section of Endocrinology, University of Illinois at Chicago,
Chicago, IL 60612, USA
E-mail: abschnei@vic.edu

Numerous epidemiologic studies have clearly demonstrated that acute, external radiation exposure increases the frequency of thyroid neoplasia in humans, particularly when the exposure occurs during early childhood. Studies of the survivors of the atomic bombings in Hiroshima and Nagasaki, as well as of populations receiving radiotherapy for benign or malignant diseases have been the major sources of information about radiation-induced thyroid cancer. Although the studies were conducted in several countries using different methodologies, the risk estimates for childhood exposure are fairly consistent and a linear dose-response relationship describe the data well. In contrast, adult exposure to external radiation has not been linked to thyroid cancers.

The clinical course of radiation-associated thyroid cancers depends on whether they are detected during routine care or during early-detection screening. Thyroid cancer incidence increases markedly when irradiated populations are screened; however, the slope of the dose-response relationship does not appear to change significantly. With screening, the fraction of patients diagnosed with cancers <15 mm is significantly higher than when thyroid cancer s are diagnosed during routine medical care.

1   INTRODUCTION

The thyroid gland in children is particularly vulnerable to the tumorigenic effects of ionizing radiation (1-3). A linear dose-response relationship has been demonstrated in most studies of persons exposed to x- or gamma radiation during childhood or adolescence, and the excess risk appears to persist for decades. Less is known about adult exposure, but current data indicate that the adult thyroid gland is relatively insensitive to the tumorigenic effects of radiation. During the last ten years, several new or updated studies on radiation and thyroid cancer have been published. The data from these studies suggested that a pooled analysis could help answer some of the remaining important questions concerning the shape of the dose-response relationship, the effect of gender and age at exposure, the pattern of risk by attained age and time since exposure, and the influence of fractionated exposure on risk.

2 EVIDENCE OF AN ASSOCIATION BETWEEN RADIATION AND THYROID CANCER

The major single source of data on thyroid cancer and external radiation is the Life Span Study (LSS) of the atomic bomb survivors in Hiroshima and Nagasaki, Japan (4), but knowledge about radiation-associated thyroid tumors also comes from a variety of studies of medical (diagnostic, radiotherapy for benign and malignant disease), occupational (medical workers, nuclear workers) and environmental (persons exposed to fallout from bomb testing, naturally high background areas) areas (1). Until the 1960s, radiotherapy was used frequently to treat a wide variety of benign diseases. Studies of these medically irradiated populations have provided a great deal of information, but most concern childhood exposure. Studies of environmental and occupational exposures have been much less informative, partly because the doses are very low and, therefore, huge numbers of subjects are needed for adequate statistical power. In addition, occupational studies frequently are based on mortality data, which are not very useful for a relatively non-lethal disease such as thyroid cancer.

A pooled analysis of seven major studies of acute, external radiation exposure (with individual doses to the thyroid gland) was performed (5). The studies were conducted in several countries. Combined they included almost 120,000 people (about half were exposed), nearly 700 thyroid cancers and 3,000,000 person years of follow-up (4, 6-11). More women than men were in the total study population. Exposed children (less than 15 years old) were included in all but the study of cervical cancer patients, whereas data on adult exposures were available only from the studies of atomic bomb survivors and cervical cancer patients.

The data from each of the individual studies were consistent with a linear dose-response relationship, although there was a suggestion from the study of childhood cancer that the excess relative risk may level off at very high doses (>10 Gy). The pooled ERR_{1Gy} was 7.7 (95% CI =2.1, 28.7) and the $EAR/10^4$ PYGy was 4.4 (95% CI =1.9, 10.1) (Table 1). Risk estimates for three cohorts that are not included in the pooled analysis are consistent with those observed in the pooled analysis (12-14). In the pooled analysis, the excess relative risk decreased with increasing age at exposure; persons exposed between the ages of 10-14 years had one-fifth the risk of those exposed before age five years. The pooled analysis indicated that for persons whose thyroid gland was exposed to 1 Gy before age 15 years of age, about 88% of the cancers could be attributed to radiation exposure. The excess relative risk was highest 15-19 years after exposure, but remained elevated even after 40 years. Although the ERR per Gy was about two times higher for women than for men, this difference was neither statistically significant nor consistent across studies. There was weak evidence that fractionated exposure might have been somewhat less carcinogenic than acute exposure.

Table 1. Excess relative risk per Gy (ERR/Gy) and
excess absolute risk per 10^4PY-Gy (EAR/10^4PY-Gy)

	Excess relative risk model		Excess absolute risk model	
	ERR/Gy (95% CI)	P-value for linearity	EAR/ 10^4PY-Gy (95% CI)	P-value for linearity
Exposure <15 years old				
Thymus	9.1 (3.6,28.8)	0.41	2.6 (1.7,3.6)	0.67
A-bomb (<15 ATB)	4.7 (1.7,10.9)	0.41	2.7 (1.2,4.6)	0.98
Tinea capitis	32.5 (14.0,57.1)	0.45	7.6 (2.7,13.0)	0.77
Tonsils (MRH)	2.5 (0.6,26.0)	0.24	3.0[a] (0.5,17.1)	0.02
Childhood cancer[b]	1.1 (0.4,29.4)	0.09		
Exposure 15 years old				
Cervical cancer[c]	34.9 (-2.2,)	0.81		
A-bomb (15 ATB)	0.4 (-0.1,1.2)	0.38	0.4 (-0.1,1.4)	0.70

[a] This is the average excess absolute risk, however, the EAR/10^4PY-Gy was 2.4 (95% CI = undetermined,10.4) for follow-up until 1974 and 45.2 (95% CI = -3.2,89.0) for followup after 1974. The EAR/10^4PY-Gy estimates in this study are subject to large variability because of the influence of extreme dose points. These points, however, appeared to have little influence on the ERR/Gy.
[b] ERR/Gy estimates based on setting doses under 2 Gy to the mean dose of 0.74 Gy.
[c] ERR/Gy estimates based on regression of category-specific mean doses. It can be seen that the point estimate is not significant and the confidence interval is extremely large.

The broad range of ages at the time of the bombings makes the LSS the only study that allows a complete assessment of age at exposure effects. The risk of thyroid cancer decreased rapidly with age at the time of the bombings (p <0.001) (4). The excess relative risk for individuals under age 10 at exposure was significantly elevated (ERR$_{1Sv}$=9.5, 95% CI= 0.11-18) and was over three times higher than for those who were 10-19 ATB. Among individuals over 20 years at exposure, there was no significant excess of thyroid cancer (ERR$_{1Sv}$=0.10; 95% CI=< 0.23, 0.75). A similar pattern was observed when an absolute risk model was used.

Microcarcinomas (i.e. small papillary carcinomas which are not clinically evident) are quite common at autopsy. The relationship between radiation exposure and these tumors has been studied in a series of autopsies among atomic bomb survivors (15). The risk of microcarcinomas increased with increasing dose among persons exposed to the bombings. The elevated risk continued for at least 40 years after exposure.

Since diagnostic x-rays are the largest man-made source of exposure to ionizing radiation for the general public, evaluating the role of fractionated exposure is particularly relevant for public health. An association between diagnostic x-rays and thyroid cancer has been reported in two case-control studies from Sweden (16,17), but results from case-control studies can be complicated by the problem of recall bias. To prevent this potential bias, a study conducted in Sweden was designed to obtain information on diagnostic radiation exposure by linking radiology records of diagnostic x-rays to thyroid cancer cases and controls identified through the Swedish cancer or population registries (18). Among 484 cases and an equal number of controls, there was no difference in the number of recorded medical x-rays. Furthermore, when estimated doses were calculated for each diagnostic procedure, no dose-response relationship was observed.

Early studies of radiation workers provided no evidence for an elevated risk of thyroid cancer. More recently, there have been a few positive reports. Since adult, acute exposures have not been linked to thyroid cancer, negative findings following protracted exposure are not surprising, however, the limitations of these occupational studies should be noted: individual doses were available only in the nuclear worker studies; multiple comparisons were made so probability of an increased risk occurring by chance is rather large; the number of thyroid cancer cases in each individual study was small resulting in unstable risk estimates; several of the investigations were based on mortality data and, thus, are not very informative for a disease with an overall 5-year survival rate of over 95%; and finally ascertainment may be better in a medically insured worker population than in the general public.

While most studies of fractionated exposure do not demonstrate in raised risks of thyroid cancer, it should be noted that many of the diagnostic x-ray and occupational exposures occurred among adults. Given the large difference in the sensitivity of the child and adult thyroid gland, it is not clear how fractionated or protracted radiation would affect young children.

3   CLINICAL COURSE OF RADIATION-ASSOCIATED THYROID
     CANCERS

The clinical course of radiation-associated thyroid cancers depends on whether they are detected during routine care or during early-detection screening. Routine screening has a very large effect on the estimated incidence of thyroid nodules and thyroid cancer in exposed populations. The magnitude of the effect depends on how screening is performed. For the thyroid, the least sensitive method of screening is by palpation. A study from Boston compared questionnaire data with palpation findings for subjects irradiated during childhood and non-irradiated comparison subjects (11).

Clinically, the value of screening by palpation is limited. With the development of improved methods to image the thyroid, the large false negative rate of palpation, even for nodules 1.0 cm which are generally considered to be "clinically significant", has become apparent (19,20). More recently, the substantial rate of false positive findings (i.e., apparently palpable nodules that are not confirmed by thyroid ultrasound) has been emphasized (21).

Screening the thyroid with high sensitivity imaging, by isotopic scanning or ultrasonography, increases the observed rate of thyroid tumors even further. The magnitude of the increase depends on the size of the nodule used to define a positive endpoint. In the Michael Reese cohort of patients irradiated for enlarged tonsils, screening, predominantly with thyroid scans, began in 1974. By comparing incidence rates before and after 1974, it was found that the incidence of thyroid cancer increased by about 10-fold as a result of screening. However, the increase in detected tumors did not affect the ERR because it did not vary by dose (22). Thyroid ultrasound was studied in 54 representative subjects from the same cohort. Only seven subjects did not have nodules detected. Among the 47 screenees with nodules, 154 nodules were found, i.e. an average of 3.3 nodules per person (20).

Detection of radiation-related thyroid cancers during screening has a major impact on their clinical characteristics. This is illustrated by comparing the thyroid cancers diagnosed before and after the initiation of screening in the Chicago study (Table 2). The average size of the thyroid cancers discovered by screening was about half that of the cancers found during routine care. Before 1974, more cancers were diagnosed with lymph node metastases, but this is likely due to the younger age at discovery. The remainder of the clinical characteristics did not differ significantly.

The clinical behavior of the radiation-related thyroid cancers in the Chicago study was studied by correlating the presenting clinical features with the frequency of recurrence (6). In this cohort, it was concluded that radiation-related thyroid cancer is not unusually aggressive. In contrast, the recent findings from the Chernobyl-related thyroid cancer cases indicate that they may be more aggressive than expected. The Chernobyl results are largely based on the presenting histological characteristics of the thyroid cancers compared with thyroid cancers in non-irradiated children (24).

Table 2. Clinical characteristics of thyroid cancers detected during routine care compared with those detected during screening.

Characteristic:	Year of surgery for thyroid cancer	
	< 1974 (N = 126[a])	1974 (N = 262[a])
Average size (cm.)	1.89	0.95
Size 1.5 cm	52.3%	16.3%
Lymph node positive	54.3%	23.4%
Multicentric	62.2%	53.3%
Bilobar	30.6%	28.6%
Minor/major invasion	33.6%	24.8%
Major invasion	12.1%	9.6%

[a] Clinical characteristics are unknown for some cancers, so the number of cancers included in each category is not always equal to the total number of cancers.

Despite the wealth of existing knowledge about radiation-associated thyroid cancer, many issues remain unresolved because of insufficient data in individual studies. Future research on radiation-related thyroid cancer should be directed at quantifying lifetime risks, evaluating the long-term clinical course, ascertaining whether there are particularly susceptible individuals or groups that can be identified, and learning more about the carcinogenic effects of ^{131}I exposure, especially during childhood.

References

1. UNSCEAR (United Nations Scientific Committee on the Effects of Atomic Radiation): Sources and effects of ionizing radiation. Publ E94.IX.11, New York, United Nations, 1994.
2. NCRP (National Council on Radiation Protection and measurements). Induction of thyroid cancer by ionizing radiation. Report No. 80, Bethesda, NCRP, 1985.
3. Schneider AB, Ron E. Radiation and thyroid cancer. Lessons from 46 years of study. In: Braverman LE, ed. Diseases of the thyroid. Humana Press, 1997;265-86.
4. Thompson DE, Mabuchi K, Ron E, Soda M, Tokunaga M, Ochikubo S, Sugimoto S, Ikeda T, Terasaki M, Izumi S, Preston DL. Cancer incidence in atomic bomb survivors. Part II: Solid tumors, 1958-87. RERF TR 5-92, *Radiat Res* 1994;**137**:S17-S67.
5. Ron E, Lubin JH, Shore RE, Mabuchi K, Modan B, Pottern LM, Schneider AB, Tucker MA, Boice JD Jr. Thyroid cancer following exposure to external radiation: a pooled analysis of seven studies. *Radiat Res* 1995;**141**:259-77.
6. Shore RE, Woodward E, Hildreth N, et al: Thyroid tumors following thymus irradiation. *JNCI* 1985;**74**:1177-84.
7. Ron E, Modan B, Preston D, Alfandary E, Stovall M, Boice JD Jr. Thyroid neoplasia following low-dose radiation in childhood. *Radiat Res* 1989;**120**:516-31.
8. Schneider AB, Ron E, Lubin JH, Stovall M, Gierlowski TC. Dose-response relationships for radiation-induced thyroid neoplasia: evidence for the prolonged effects of radiation on the thyroid. *J Clin Endocrinol Metab* 1993;**77**:362-9.
9. Tucker MA, Morris Jones PH, Boice JD Jr, et al. Therapeutic radiation at a young age is linked to secondary thyroid cancer. Cancer Res 1991;51:2885-8.
10. Boice JD Jr, Engholm G, Kleinerman RA, et al. Radiation dose and second cancer risk in patients treated for cancer of the cervix. *Radiat Res* 1988;**116**:3-55.
11. Pottern LM, Kaplan MM, Larsen PR, Silva JE, Koenig RJ, Lubin JH, Stovall M, Boice JD Jr. Thyroid Nodularity After Childhood Irradiation for Lymphoid Hyperplasia - A Comparison of Questionnaire and Clinical Findings. *J Clin Epidemiol* 1990;**43**:449-60.
12. Lindberg S, Karlsson P, Arvidsson B, et al. Cancer incidence after radiotherapy for skin haemangioma during infancy. *Acta Oncol* 1995;**34**:735-40.
13. Lundell M, Hakulinen T, Holm L-E. Thyroid cancer after radiotherapy for skin hemangioma in infancy. *Radiat Res* 1994;**140**:334-9.

14. Shore RE, Albert RE, Pasternack BS. Follow-up study of patients treated by x-ray epilation for tinea capitis. *Arch Environ Health* 1976;**31**:17-24.
15. Yoshimoto Y, Ezaki H, Etoh R, Hiraoka T, Akiba S. Prevalence rate of thyroid disease among autopsy cases of the atomic bomb survivors in hiroshima, 1951-1985. *Radiat Res* 1995;**141**:278-286.
16. Wingren G, Hatschek T, Axelson O. Determinants of papillary cancer of the thyroid. *Amer J Epidemiol* 1993;**138**:482-91.
17. Hallquist A, Hardell L, Degerman A, Wingren G, Boquist L. Medical diagnostic and therapeutic ionising radiation and the risk for thyroid cancer: a case-control study. *Eur J Cancer Prev* 1994;**3**:259-67.
18. Inskip PD, Ekbom A, Galanti MR, et al. Medical diagnostic x rays and thyroid cancer. *J Natl Cancer Inst* 1995;**87**:1613-21.
19. Ryo UY, Arnold J, Colman M, Arnold M, Favus M, Frohman L, Schneider A., Stachura M, Pinsky S. Thyroid Scintigram. Sensitivity with Sodium Pertechnetate Tc 99m and Gamma Camera with Pinhole Collimator. *JAMA* 1976;**235**:1235-8.
20. Schneider AB, Bekerman C, Leland J, Rosengarten J, Hyun H, Collins B, Shore-Freedman E, Gierlowski TC. Thyroid nodules in the follow-up of irradiated individuals: Comparison of thyroid ultrasound with scanning and palpation. *J Clin Endocrinol Metab* 1997;**82**:4020-7.
21. Wiest PW, Hartshorne MF, Inskip PD, Crooks LA., Vela BS, Telepak RJ, Williamson M R, Blumhardt R, Bauman JM, Tekkel M. Thyroid palpation versus high-resolution thyroid ultrasonography in the detection of nodules. *J Ultrasound Med* 1998;**17**:487-96.
22. Ron E, Lubin JH, Schneider A.. Thyroid Cancer Incidence. *Nature* 1992;**360**:113.
23. Schneider A.B, Recant W, Pinsky S, Ryo UY, C Bekerman, Shore-Freedman E. Radiation-Induced Thyroid Carcinoma: Clinical Course and results of Therapy in 296 Patients. *Ann Intern Med* 1986;**105**:405-12.
24. Williams ED, Tronko ND, editors. Molecular, Cellular, Biological Characterization of Childhood Thyroid Cancer. International Scientific Collaboration on Consequences of Chernobyl Accident. Luxembourg. European Commission. 1996.

THYROID CANCER AFTER DIAGNOSTIC AND THERAPEUTIC USE OF RADIONUCLIDES; A REVIEW OF THE ASSOCIATION

L.-E. HOLM

Swedish Radiation Protection Institute, S-171 16 Stockholm, Sweden

Radioiodine, mainly ^{131}I, is used in various diagnostic procedures and for treating patients with hyperthyroidism or differentiated thyroid cancer. Relatively little is still known about the carcinogenic hazard of [131]I. Epidemiological studies of patients exposed to ^{131}I cover almost exclusively adult exposures and include about 48,000 patients exposed to diagnostic ^{131}I activities, 5,900 of whom were adolescents or children at the time of exposure; nearly 39,000 patients treated for hyperthyroidism and about 2,800 thyroid cancer patients. These cohorts have had good statistical power to detect effects among adults, but limited power among adolescents and children. Any increased risk for thyroid cancer, other solid cancers or leukaemias that can be convincingly attributed to the radiation from ^{131}I has not yet been observed. The dose delivered to tissues other than thyroid is relatively low, and significant excesses of cancers have only been demonstrated after high ^{131}I activities (> 1,000 MBq). Quantifying the risk of medical ^{131}I exposures in children is an important future task. Studies of populations exposed to fallout from the Chernobyl accident are difficult to interpret, due to the unknown contribution to the effects from short-lived radioiodines and the lack of individual doses. The Chernobyl experience is therefore not likely to contribute as much information concerning the carcinogenic hazards of ^{131}I as we might hope. Exposure to external radiation in childhood is associated with a considerable risk for thyroid cancer. It is unlikely that ^{131}I should carry a greater risk, and available data from medical exposures rather suggests that the risk is lower than that following exposure to external gamma or x rays. The risk for childhood exposure to ^{131}I, however, has yet to be quantified. Identification of new cohorts as well as extended follow-up and pooled analyses of existing cohorts may help us understand why children are so vulnerable and what role underlying host factors might play in thyroid carcinogenesis.

1   INTRODUCTION

The thyroid gland is a unique model in experimental studies for several reasons: the gland concentrates iodine, cell proliferation can be manipulated, and thyroid hormones can be measured. These characteristics have frequently been exploited in the experimental induction of thyroid tumours in animals by iodine deficiency, chemical carcinogens, and goitrogens.[14]

Ionising radiation is still the only established etiologic factor for thyroid cancer in humans, and the thyroid is one of the most radiosensitive organs of the body. Most of the present knowledge on radiation-associated thyroid cancer stems from studies of the A-bomb survivors and of patients exposed to external radiotherapy. An excess of radiation-induced thyroid cancer is generally restricted to young people, with adults showing little excess risk.[19] In a pooled analysis of radiation-associated thyroid cancer after radiation exposure in childhood, including 58,000 exposed children and 700 thyroid cancers, Ron et al.[17] calculated the excess relative risk (ERR) at 1 Sv to 7.7 [95% confidence interval (CI) 2.1-28.7]. A linear model best described the dose-response relationship down to doses of 0.1 Gy, and the risk decreased with increasing age at exposure. Only 2 cancers were found within the first 5 years of exposure.

2   RADIOIODINES

Relatively little is still known about the carcinogenic hazard of ^{131}I, although some experimental studies   suggest that ^{131}I is less effective in inducing cancer than external gamma rays.[14] Radioiodines have been, and are still being used in medicine to diagnose and treat thyroid diseases as well as extra-thyroidal diseases. Three iodine isotopes are at present available for diagnostic and therapeutic purposes.

Iodine −131 is the most commonly used radionuclide to treat hyperthyroidism and thyroid cancer. It is also used in other medical diagnostic procedures. It has a half-life of 8 days and emits β rays with a maximum energy of 0.81 MeV, and γ rays of 0.36 and 0.64 MeV. The radiation dose to the thyroid per becquerel (Bq) [131]I administered is high as compared to that from other radioiodines or [99m]Tc.

Iodine-123 emits γ radiation by electron capture with an energy of 0.16 MeV. It has a half-life of about 13 hours and the thyroid dose per Bq administered is lower than that from [131]I. Because ^{123}I is cyclotron-produced, it is expensive and less available than [131]I.

Iodine-125 has a half-life of 60 days and emits γ rays by electron capture with an energy of 0.04 MeV. Its microdosimetric dose distribution differs greatly from that of ^{131}I, and ^{125}I has been used in attempts to reduce the incidence of hypothyroidism in patients treated for hyperthyroidism.

The epidemiological data available on thyroid cancer risk following exposure to radioiodines deal only with exposure to [131]I.

3   THYROID CANCER IN HUMANS AFTER EXPOSURE TO [131]I

3.1   Patients examined with diagnostic activities of [131]I

Data on cancer risks after diagnostic exposure is at present available from studies of three cohorts. In Sweden, Hall et al.[9] studied 34,104 mostly adult patients examined with diagnostic ^{131}I activities in 1950-69. The mean age at the time of examination was 44 years, 2,408 patients were exposed before 20 years of age and 316 before the age of 10 years. Mean 24-h thyroid uptake was 40%, and the mean administered ^{131}I activity was 1.9 MBq. Patients were followed for an average of 24 years and matched with the Swedish Cancer Register for the period 1958-90. Individual thyroid doses were calculated using administered ^{131}I activity and individual uptake. Thyroid weight was estimated for 48% of the patients and was based on information from the patient records. The estimated average thyroid dose was 1.1 Gy and after correction for thyroid weight 0.8 Gy. A total of 67 cancers were found (SIR=1.4; 95% CI 1.1-1.7). Excess cancers were apparent only among those referred because of a suspected thyroid tumour (SIR=2.9; 95% CI 2.1-3.9), with no increased risk among other patients (SIR=0.8; 95% CI 0.5-1.1). Risk was not related to thyroid dose, time since exposure or age at exposure. Among the 2,408 patients less than 20 years of age, 3 thyroid cancers developed in individuals exposed during the age of 15-19 years (SIR=1.7; 95% CI 0.4-4.9). Two of the cancers developed in subjects not referred under the suspicion of thyroid tumour (SIR=1.4; 95% CI 0.2-5.0). The computed ERR was 0.25 per Gy, compared to an ERR of 4.5 per Gy among A-bomb survivors aged 10-19 at exposure.[19]

Hall et al.[7] also studied palpable thyroid nodules in a sample of women (N=1,005) exposed to diagnostic ^{131}I, and in a comparison group of 248 women attending a mammography screening clinic. The mean thyroid dose from ^{131}I was 0.5 Gy, the average age at exposure was 26 years and 52 years at the clinical examination. Only 17 % were younger than 20 years at the time of exposure. The prevalence of thyroid nodules was 10.6 % in exposed women and 11.7 % among the non-exposed women [relative risk (RR)=0.9; 95% CI 0.6-1.4]. When analysis was restricted to exposed women, the prevalence of nodules was positively associated with thyroid dose (ERR=0.9 per Gy; 95% CI 0.2-1.9). This was due to the association for single nodules. Nodules were nearly twice as common among non-exposed women as among those who received very small doses from [131]I. The ERR was similar for women exposed before age 20 years and those exposed after age 20. No evidence of effect modification by age at exposure was thus seen in this study.

In the United States, Hamilton et al.[10] studied 3,503 children who received ^{131}I for diagnostic purposes during childhood and adolescence and 2,594 matched controls recruited from the same hospitals. The median thyroid dose was about 0.4 Gy and most received less than 1 Gy. Four thyroid cancers occurred 5 years or more after exposure in the ^{131}I-exposed group and 1 cancer among controls (RR=2.9; 95% CI 0.3-70). Based on population-based thyroid cancer incidence rates, 4 thyroid cancers would have been expected in the exposed group if no radiation effect were present (SIR=1.1; 95% CI 0.3-2.8).

Glöbel[5] have conducted a study in Germany of about 14,000 mostly adult patients given ^{131}I for uptake examinations and having an average follow-up of 17 years. From the limited results available, Shore[18] performed a dose-response analysis and found it to be non-significant.

3.2 Patients treated for hyperthyroidism

Iodine-131 is used to treat hyperthyroidism with the aim to deliver a thyroid dose of 60-120 Gy. Several epidemiological studies have analysed cancer risks in patients treated with [131]I. The Co-operative Thyrotoxicosis Therapy Follow-up Study[2] in the United States included about 19,200 patients who received ^{131}I therapy and were followed for a mean of 8 years. No increase of thyroid cancer was seen. After an extended follow-up (average 15 years) for 1,005 patients from the Mayo Clinic,[11] no increased cancer incidence or mortality was observed, with the exception of a significantly elevated thyroid cancer incidence in the ^{131}I-treated group (SIR=3.8; 95% CI 0.8-11.0; n=3). The SIR for thyroid cancer was 0.5 (95% CI 0.0-2.5; n=1) for the 2,141 surgically treated women, and this low risk was likely to be due to the removal of much of the thyroid tissue.

Holm et al.[12] studied cancer risks in about 10,500 Swedish patients receiving ^{131}I in 1950-75. Mean total activity was about 500 MBq. Average doses to organs other than the thyroid were relatively low, with the highest doses to the salivary glands (0.20 Gy) and to the stomach (0.25 Gy). Follow-up was on average 15 years. SIR for thyroid cancers was 1.3 (95% CI 0.8-2.0; n=18) and did not differ for the 10-year survivors. SIR for all cancers combined was 1.1 (95% CI 1.0-1.1; n=1543). Among 10-year survivors, significantly elevated risks were seen for cancers of the stomach, kidney, and brain. Only the risk for stomach cancer (SIR=1.3; 95% CI 1.0-1.7) increased over time (p<0.05) and it tended to increase with increasing activity administered, but this was not statistically significant.

Shore[18] studied some 600 children and adolescents given ^{131}I for hyperthyroidism by pooling data from several small series from the US. The mean follow-up was 10 years and the ERR per Gy for thyroid cancer was estimated at 0.3 (90% CI 0-0.9) and the EAR at 0.1 (90% CI 0-0.2) 10^{-4}PYGy^{-1}.

3.3 Patients treated for thyroid cancer

Follow-up of patients treated for thyroid cancer has been reported from several countries. In such patients the thyroid gland is usually removed surgically, and therefore other cancers than thyroid cancer are the relevant end points to study after ^{131}I therapy. In the United Kingdom, Edmonds and Smith[4] studied 258 patients who received an ablation treatment of 2,900 MBq of ^{131}I, sometimes followed by one or more treatments with 5,500 MBq. The mean follow-up was 10 years and a total of 20 cancers was observed (RR=1.5; 95% CI 0.9-2.3). There were significant excesses for leukaemia (RR=12.0; 95% CI 2.5-35.1; n=3) and bladder cancer (RR=6.5; 95% CI 1.3-19.1; n=3). The estimated mean organ dose was 3.5 Gy to the bone marrow for patients developing leukaemias and 22.9 Gy to the bladder for patients with bladder carcinomas.

In Sweden, Hall et al[8] studied cancer risks in 834 thyroid cancer patients given ^{131}I and in 1,121 patients treated by other means in 1950-75. Mean administered activity was 4,550 MBq and mean follow-up was 14 years. A total of 99 new cancers were observed after ^{131}I therapy (SIR =1.4; 95% CI 1.2-1.8) and 122 new cancers (SIR =1.2, 95% CI 0.9-1.4) in patients not receiving [131]I. Organs receiving <0.1 Gy had a SIR of 1.6 (95% CI 1.1-2.2), compared to SIR = 1.2 (95% CI 0.9-1.6) for organs receiving 0.1-0.6 Gy. The highest SIR was observed for organs receiving at least 1 Gy, i.e. salivary glands, stomach, small intestine and bladder (SIR = 2.6; 95% CI 1.5-4.1). The radiation dose to the stomach and bladder was on average 2.1 Gy, and the salivary glands and small intestine 1.9 and 1.3 Gy, respectively. The bone marrow and the breast received doses between 0.1 and 0.6 Gy. No elevated risk of leukaemia or breast cancer was noted.

Hall et al.[6] also analysed leukaemia incidence among nearly 47,000 mostly adult patients in Sweden given ^{131}I for thyroid cancer, hyperthyroidism or diagnostic purposes. Bone marrow doses were estimated for individual patients based on administered ^{131}I activity and 24-hour thyroid uptake. SIR for all leukaemia, excluding CLL, was 1.1 (95% CI 0.9-1.3). For patients receiving >0.1 Gy to the bone marrow (mean 0.2 Gy) SIR was 1.0 (95% CI 0.3-2.7). No clear association of leukaemia induction by radiation from ^{131}I was thus evident in this study.

In France, de Vathaire[1] studied cancer risks in 1771 patients with thyroid cancer, 1497 of whom received [131]I. Average administered activity was 8,200 MBq and the average bone marrow dose was 0.3 Gy and 0.8 Gy to the whole body. Mean follow-up was 10 years. A total of 80 patients developed a second cancer but no leukaemia was observed.. The risk of colon cancer was related to the administered ^{131}I activity with the highest risk for patients receiving more than 7,500 MBq of [131]I (RR=4.9 (90% CI 1.2-18.5). The ERR for colon cancer was estimated at 0.5 per 1,000 MBq, p=0.02).

4 DISCUSSION

Radiation from internally deposited ^{131}I has yet to be shown convincingly to increase the risk of thyroid cancer in humans, suggesting that perhaps ^{131}I is less effective than external radiation in causing thyroid cancer.[15,19] Additional information is needed, especially in the light of the wide use of ^{131}I in medical diagnosis and therapy, and public concerns about fallout from nuclear weapons tests and releases from reactor accidents, such as that at Chernobyl, which resulted in the exposure of large areas to radioactive iodines.

Epidemiological studies of the medical use of ^{131}I covers almost exclusively adult exposures and include about 48,000 patients exposed to diagnostic ^{131}I activities, 5900 of whom were children or adolescents; nearly 39,000 patients treated for hyperthyroidism and about 2,800 thyroid cancer patients. These cohorts have had good statistical power to detect effects among adults, but limited power among adolescents and children. Any increased risk for thyroid cancer, any other solid cancer or leukaemia that can be convincingly attributed to the radiation from ^{131}I has not yet been observed. The dose delivered to tissues other than thyroid is relatively low, and significant excesses of cancers have only been demonstrated after high ^{131}I activities (> 1000 MBq).

The reasons for a lower carcinogenic effect can be several: the thyroid gland could receive either very high cell-killing doses, or low doses from ^{131}I due to the non-uniformity of ^{131}I dose distribution within the thyroid gland (especially in hyperthyroid patients), the uncertainties in dose estimation is a greater problem for internal than external exposures and the low dose-rate of ^{131}I might allow DNA repair.[15] Because of the cell-killing effect following large ^{131}I activities, risk estimates for thyroid exposure from this radionuclide must depend heavily on assessment of any excess of thyroid cancer after the relatively small activities used for diagnosis.

Age is a strong modifier of risk in thyroid cancer. Epidemiological data on brief external exposure is limited to children and on protracted low-dose exposure to adults. Few studies include a sufficiently large number of children exposed to ^{131}I for medical reasons to draw any firm conclusions. A pooling of data from the Swedish and US studies would result in a SIR of 1.3 (95% CI 0.5-2.6) among the 5,911 ^{131}I-exposed children and adolescents having a mean follow-up of more than 22 years.

Excess risks of thyroid neoplasia and thyroid dysfunction were observed among children on the Marshall Islands people after radioactive fallout in 1954. Only a small proportion of the dose was from [131]I.[16] In an extended follow-up of 2,473 children exposed to fallout from nuclear devices at the Nevada Test Site, a small but non-significant excess of thyroid cancer was reported after a mean thyroid dose of 0.17 Gy.[13] Biases related to selection and dietary recall could, however, not be discounted.

The drastic increase of thyroid cancer in Belarus, Ukraine, and to some extent in parts of Russia affected by the radioactive fallout from the Chernobyl accident in 1986, point to the possible etiologic role of [131]I. Today very few question that the thyroid cancers of children in the Chernobyl area are associated with radiation, but the role of ^{131}I is unclear. Available studies of populations exposed to the fallout are difficult to interpret, since the contribution to the effects from short-lived radioiodines are not known, individual doses are lacking and there are considerable uncertainties in the dosimetry.

The risk for childhood exposure to ^{131}I therefore still has to be quantified. Identification of new cohorts as well as extended follow-up and pooled analyses of existing cohorts may help us understand why children are so vulnerable and what role, if any, underlying host factors might play in thyroid carcinogenesis.

References

1. De Vathaire F, Schlumberger M, Delisle MJ et al. Leukaemias and cancers following iodine-131 administration for thyroid cancer. *Br J Cancer* 1997; **75**: 734–739.
2. Dobyns BM, Sheline GE, Workman JB et al. Malignant and benign neoplasms of the thyroid in patients treated for hyperthyroidism: a report of the Co-operative Thyrotoxicosis Therapy Follow-up Study. *J Clin Endocrinol Metab* 1974; **38**: 976–998.
3. Edmonds CJ, Smith T. The long-term hazards of the treatment of thyroid cancer with radioiodine. *Br J Radiol* 1986; **59**: 45–51.
4. Franklyn JA, Maisonneuve P, Sheppard MC, et al. Mortality after the treatment of hyperthyroidism with radioactive iodine. *N Engl J Med* 1998; **338**: 712–718.
5. Glöbel B, Glöbel H, Oberhausen E. Epidemiologic studies on patients with iodine-131 diagnostic and therapy. In: Kaul A, Neider R, and Pensko J ,eds. *Radiation Risk Protection. Vol II.* International Radiation Protection Association. Köln, 1984: 565–568.
6. Hall P, Boice JD Jr, Berg G et al. Leukaemia incidence after iodine-131 exposure. *Lancet* 1992; **340**: 1–4.
7. Hall P, Fürst CJ, Holm L-E, et al. Thyroid Nodularity after Diagnostic Administration of Iodine-131. *Radiat Res* 1996; **146**, 673–682.
8. Hall P, Holm L-E, Lundell G et al. Cancer risk in thyroid cancer patients. *Br J Cancer* 1991; **64**: 159–163.
9. Hall P, Mattsson A, Boice JD, Jr. Thyroid cancer after diagnostic administration iodine-131. *Radiat Res* 1996; **145**: 86–92.
10. Hamilton PM, Chiacchierini RP, Kaczmarek RG. A Follow-Up Study of Persons Who Had Iodine-131 and Other Diagnostic Procedures During Childhood. US Department of Health and Human Services, Public Health, Food and Drug Administration, Publication FDA 89–8276, 1989.
11. Hoffman DA. Late effects of I-131 therapy in the United States. In: Boice JD Jr. and Fraumeni JF Jr, eds. *Radiation carcinogenesis: Epidemiology and Biological Significance.* Raven Press, New York, 1984: 273–280.
12. Holm L-E, Hall P. Wiklund KE, et al. Cancer risk after iodine-131 therapy for hyperthyroidism. *J Natl Cancer Inst* 1991; **83**: 1072–1077.
13. Kerber RA, Till JE, Simon SL, Lyon JL, Thomas DC, Preston-Martin S, et al. A cohort study of thyroid disease in relation to fallout from nuclear weapons testing. *JAMA* 1993; **270**: 2076–2082.
14. Malone JF. The radiation biology of the thyroid. *Curr Top Radiat Res* 1975; **10**: 263–368.
15. NCRP, Induction of Thyroid Cancer by Ionizing Radiation. Report No. 80, National Council on Radiation Protection and Measurements, Bethesda, MD, 1985.

16. Robbins J, Adams WH. Radiation effects in the Marshall Islands. In: Nagataki S, ed. *Radiation and the thyroid*. Tokyo: Exerpta Medica, 1989: 11–24.
17. Ron E, Lubin JH, Shore RE, et al. Thyroid cancer after exposure to external radiation: a pooled analysis of seven studies. *Radiat Res* 1995; **141**: 259–277.
18. Shore RE. Issues and epidemiological evidence regarding radiation-induced thyroid cancer. *Radiat Res* 1992; **131**: 98–111.
19. United Nations Scientific Committee on the Effects of Atomic Radiation. Sources and effects of ionizing radiation. UNSCEAR 1994 Report to the General Assembly, with scientific annexes. New York: United Nations, 1994.

NEVADA ATMOSPHERIC NUCLEAR BOMB TESTS: ESTIMATION OF THE THYROID DOSES AND HEALTH EFFECTS RESULTING FROM THE IODINE-131 RELEASES

ANDRE BOUVILLE

National Cancer Institute, Bethesda, Maryland 20892, USA

E-mail: ab76o@nih.gov

BRUCE W. WACHHOLZ

National Cancer Institute, Bethesda, Maryland 20892, USA

E-mail: bw36i@nih.gov

ELAINE RON

National Cancer Institute, Bethesda, Maryland 20892, USA

E-mail: rone@epndce.nci.nih.gov

In October 1997, the National Cancer Institute (NCI) released a report containing results of a study to assess the exposures of Americans to iodine-131 fallout from atmospheric nuclear bomb tests carried out at the Nevada Test Site in the 1950s and 1960s, and the radiation doses to the thyroid resulting therefrom. In that report, thyroid dose estimates are presented for the populations of each county of the contiguous United States for each of the 90 nuclear tests that were considered, for 14 age and gender categories, and for 4 milk consumption scenarios.

The collective thyroid dose to the population of the contiguous United States from all atmospheric bomb tests detonated at the Nevada Test Site is estimated to be about 4 x 106 person Gy, corresponding to a per capita thyroid dose of about 20 mGy. The greatest contributions to the collective thyroid dose are estimated to have been due to the Plumbbob test series in 1957, the Tumbler-Snapper test series in 1952, and the Upshot-Knothole test series in 1953. Thyroid doses to representative individuals vary mainly according to age, origin and consumption rate of milk, and place of residence at the time of the tests.

Because little is known about thyroid cancer risk associated with exposure to iodine-131, especially in childhood, the expected number of excess cases had to be predicted based on what is known about childhood exposure to external radiation. The predicted number of lifetime excess thyroid cancer cases associated with the exposure from testing is dependent on the relative biological effectiveness of iodine-131, the effects of gender and age at exposure on radiation risk, the risk coefficient, and the statistical model used. The estimated number of cases range from 7,500 to 75,000 with a 95% uncertainty interval of 1,700-324,000 using one method, and 8,000 to 208,000 using another. It is estimated that over 1/3 of the predicted cases have already been diagnosed.

1   BACKGROUND

In response to a Congressional mandate, the National Cancer Institute published in 1997 a substantial report,6 in which estimates of human exposure to and thyroid radiation doses from iodine-131 resulting from individual nuclear tests conducted at the Nevada Test Site (NTS) are provided. The report is available in printed form and on the world wide web (http://rex.nci.nih.gov; click on "What's New", then on "About Radiation Fallout"). The legislation also called for the assessment of the risk of thyroid cancer associated with radiation thyroid doses due to iodine-131: other studies address this requirement.

Low-yield nuclear tests were conducted at the NTS between 1951 and 1992. From January 1951 through October 1958, 119 tests were conducted, most of them above ground. Nuclear testing was discontinued between November 1958 and September 1961, but from September 1961 until September 1992 more than 800 tests were conducted; with very few exceptions, these tests were detonated underground, under conditions that were designed for containment of radioactive debris. Only 38 of these underground tests resulted in the detection off-site of radioactive materials; the last occurrence of substantial radioactive contamination of the environment took place in December 1970. On October 2, 1992, the United States entered into another moratorium on nuclear weapons testing.

Ninety of the nuclear tests released almost 99% of the total iodine-131 entering the atmosphere from all bomb tests conducted at the NTS. These ninety tests released about 6 EBq of iodine-131, mainly in the years 1952, 1953, and 1957. Some radioiodine was deposited everywhere in the United States; highest deposition densities were immediately downwind of the NTS and lowest deposition densities were on the west coast. In the eastern part of the country, most of the deposited iodine-131 was associated with rain, while in the more arid west, dry deposition prevailed. Because iodine-131 decays with an 8-day half-life, exposure from the released iodine-131 occurred primarily during the first month following a test.

2 ESTIMATING EXPOSURES AND THYROID DOSES

For most people, the major exposure route was the ingestion of cows' milk contaminated as the result of iodine-131 deposited on pasture grasses; other exposure routes such as the inhalation of contaminated air and the ingestion of contaminated leafy vegetables, goats' milk, cottage cheese, and eggs also were considered. Historical measurements of the amounts of radioactivity deposited and of daily rainfall were used as the basis for the dose calculations whenever feasible. Nationwide deposition data were available for all but nine of the ninety tests that were studied in detail; for those nine tests, a mathematical model was used to estimate the atmospheric transport and ground deposition of the iodine-131.

Data on the transfer to milk of iodine-131 deposited on pasture and on regional pasture consumption by cows were used to estimate concentrations of iodine-131 in milk fresh from cows. These concentrations, together with milk distribution patterns in the 1950s, were used to estimate local concentrations of iodine-131 in the cows' milk available for human consumption throughout the country. The categories of fresh cows' milk that were considered include the milk obtained directly from dairy farms, milk purchased in stores, either provided from local or from distant farms, and milk obtained from family cows. Finally, cows' milk consumption rates, based upon diet surveys, were used to estimate the amounts of iodine-131 ingested by humans by age group and by gender. The transfer of iodine-131 to people through other exposure routes (ingestion of leafy vegetables, goats' milk, mother's milk, eggs, and cottage cheese contaminated by iodine-131, as well as inhalation of air contaminated by iodine-131) was similarly analyzed.

Thyroid doses from iodine-131 were estimated for 13 age groups, including the fetus, and adults of both genders, in each county of the contiguous United States and for all periods of exposure. The overall average thyroid dose to the approximately 160 million people in the country during the 1950s was 20 mGy. The uncertainty in this per capita dose is estimated to be a factor of 2, that is, the overall average thyroid dose may have been as small as 10 mGy or as large as 40 mGy, but 20 mGy is the best estimate. The study also demonstrated that there were large variations in thyroid dose from one individual to another. The primary factors contributing to this variation are county of residence, age at the time of exposure, and milk consumption patterns.

2.1   Geography

The geographical location where people lived is very important. In counties east of the NTS in Nevada and Utah, and in some counties in Idaho, Montana, New Mexico, Colorado, and Missouri, the estimated per capita thyroid doses from all tests were highest, in the range of 50 to 160 mGy. In many counties on or near the west coast, the border with Mexico, and parts of Texas and Florida, the estimated per capita thyroid doses were lowest, in the range of 0.01 to 5 mGy. Intermediate values were obtained in the remainder of the country.

2.2   Age

The thyroid doses to individuals at a particular location were strongly dependent upon age at the time of exposure. Thyroid dose estimates resulting from milk consumption were uniformly higher for young children than for adults, assuming that individuals consumed milk at average rates for each age group from the same source. At any particular time, the average thyroid doses resulting from milk consumption for children between 3 months and 5 years of age exceeded the thyroid doses received by adults by at least a factor of ten.

The date of birth and geographic residence of individuals also are strong determinants of the cumulative dose received from all tests (from 1951 to 1970). The variation in cumulative thyroid doses to individuals born at different times, each of whom lived in a single county and consumed cows' milk from local sources at average rates, is illustrated in Table 1. This can be considered a dose table for six typical families located in the identified cities throughout the testing period. The factors affecting the doses to parents are approximately independent of birth dates up to 1930; doses to adult men and women born prior to this time were nearly the same. Thyroid doses to children born about six months prior to the three major test series (1952, 1953, and 1957) were substantially higher than the adult doses, as shown in the three central columns. The last column shows doses to children born in 1958, which is the year when the last test series in the atmosphere took place at the NTS. Cumulative thyroid doses to most of the children born in later years are estimated to be less than 1 mGy.

Table 1. Example calculations showing the variation of the thyroid dose according to date of birth and place of residence of the individual considered

Place of residence	Thyroid dose estimates (mGy)					
	Father, born 9.15.27	Mother, born 10.10.29	Child, born 10.1.51	Child, born 9.15.52	Child, born 11.28.56	Child, born 9.5.58
Los Angeles, CA	0.3	0.4	3	0.8	0.2	0
Salt Lake City, UT	17	18	130	96	56	1
Denver, CO	15	16	120	100	65	2
Chicago, IL	6	7	76	62	20	0.3
Tampa, FL	3	4	18	19	22	0.03
New York, NY	8	9	73	49	21	0.1

2.3   Diet, particularly milk consumption

For individuals within a particular age range, milk consumption can vary substantially. For example, surveys have shown that 10-20% of children between ages 1 and 5 do not consume cows' milk. Their doses were only about one tenth of those received by children who consumed milk at average rates for their age. Conversely, the milk consumption of 5 to 10% of individuals in the same age range was 2-3 times greater than the average and their thyroid doses were therefore proportionally larger. The type of milk consumed also is important. It is estimated that about 20,000 individuals in the U.S. population consumed goats' milk during the time of the bomb tests. Thyroid doses to those individuals could have been 10 to 20 times greater than those to other residents of the same county who were the same age and sex and drank the same amount of cows' milk. On the other hand, thyroid doses received during infancy (0 to 1 y) were much smaller for the infants who consumed mother's milk or formula than for the infants who consumed cows' milk.

2.4   Estimating thyroid doses for specific individuals

The foregoing examples illustrate that the thyroid dose received by any particular individual depends on his/her source of milk and dietary habits and thus may differ considerably from the group dose estimates. Furthermore, the person's total thyroid dose from all tests depends upon place of residence and age at the time of each test. Because of the very large number of variations in residence location, age, and dietary habits, it is not feasible to provide estimates of cumulative doses for specific individuals. However, detailed instructions and examples are provided in the report to permit individuals to estimate their cumulative dose using personal residence and dietary data. In addition, the information available on the world wide web enables the reader to enter a date and county of birth, as well as gender, in order to obtain estimates of thyroid dose applicable to the individuals with those characteristics for each test series and for all tests for a range of milk consumption rates and for various types of milk (including mother's milk, cow's milk, and goat's milk). In these calculations, it is assumed that the individuals did not change their dietary habits or their county of residence during the time period when atmospheric weapons testing took place at the Nevada Test Site.

2.5   Uncertainties and model validation

There are large uncertainties in the estimated thyroid doses given in the report because it is impossible to know all the information needed to determine exact doses.   These uncertainties were assessed in two ways.   First, calculated concentrations of iodine-131 were compared with historical measurements of iodine-131 in man and the environment. Second, the uncertainties in the historical measurements and in each of the factors used to estimate the transfer of iodine-131 to people's thyroids through the various exposure routes yielded an estimate of the total uncertainty. The uncertainty in the thyroid dose estimated for an individual is greater than the uncertainty in the overall average thyroid to the entire United States population. Under the best circumstances, the uncertainty of an individual's thyroid dose from NTS iodine-131 is about a factor of 3, e.g., if the thyroid dose estimate for an individual is 30 mGy, it will likely lie between 10 and 90 mGy, compared with a factor of 2 for the entire U.S. population.

3   ESTIMATING RISKS

Thyroid cancer risk associated with external irradiation by gamma rays and x rays is well quantified. However, information is limited regarding the risk associated with thyroid exposure from ingested or inhaled iodine-131 and precise dose-response estimates are not available. To estimate the thyroid cancer risk from the iodine-131 exposure, it was necessary to extrapolate from what is known about external radiation, taking into account an appropriate value for the relative biological effectiveness (RBE) of iodine-131 compared to gamma rays or x rays. RBE values ranging from 0.1 to 1.0 have been suggested based on experimental data4,7,10 or a comparison of animal and human data.

The risk of induction of thyroid cancer following external irradiation by gamma rays or x rays is derived from studies of the Hiroshima-Nagasaki survivors and of several medically exposed populations. Findings are summarized in a pooled analysis of seven studies.8 The evidence for a radiation-related risk is strong for childhood exposure, and weak or non-existent for adult exposure. The pooled analysis also demonstrated a linear dose-response relationship with no significant difference in risk by gender. The excess relative risk (ERR) decreased sharply with increasing age at exposure. The age-specific excess relative risks are shown in Table 2. Ron et al.8 estimated an ERR of 7.7 per Gy (95% confidence interval = 2.1-28.7), for childhood exposure at ages younger than 15. The radiation-associated risk persisted for at least four decades and although there was evidence of variation in radiation-related relative risk over time following exposure, there was no evidence of a trend.

Table 2. Excess relative risk by age at exposure[1]

Age at exposure, y	ERR at 1 Gy
0 – 4	9.0
5 – 9	5.4
10 - 14	1.8

Land[3] estimated the lifetime excess thyroid cancer cases based on the following assumptions: (a) there is a significant excess risk following exposure before age 20 years, but no risk after age 20 years; (b) there is a linear dose response with age-specific risk co-efficients estimated from modifying factors provided in Ron et al (1995); (c) ERR remains constant over lifetime; (d) ERR is the same for males and females; (e) RBE could range from 0.1 to 1.0; and (f) 0.25% (men) and 0.64% (women) estimated lifetime thyroid cancer rates (SEER 1973-92). Land's estimates and 95% uncertainty intervals are given in Table 3 for various assumed values of RBE. Assuming that the RBE is 0.66, an estimate of 49,000 lifetime excess cases is predicted, with a 95% uncertainty interval ranging from 11,300 to 212,000. This calculation does not take into account the uncertainty of the Ron et al 8 risk estimates.

Table 3. Estimated numbers of lifetime excess thyroid cancer cases for a range of RBE values[3]

Assumed RBE	Estimated number of lifetime excess cancer cases	95% uncertainty interval
1.0	75,000	17,000 – 324,000
0.66	49,000	11,300 – 212,000
0.3	22,000	5,100 – 95,000
0.1	7,500	1,700 – 32,000

Hoffman[1] used a somewhat different method to predict lifetime risk. A probabilistic distribution of RBE values was selected, with discrete values of 1.0, 0.66, 0.5, 0.33, and 0.2 assigned with probabilities of 35%, 40%, 15%, 7%, and 3%, respectively. The uncertainty associated with the Ron et al 8 risk coefficient was also taken into account. A central estimate of 46,000 lifetime excess thyroid cancer cases, with 95% uncertainty limits from 8,000 to 208,000, was obtained by means of a Monte-Carlo simulation analysis (Table 4).

Table 4. Predicted numbers of excess thyroid cancer cases, by gender[1]. The lower and upper limits correspond to a subjective 95% confidence interval

Sex	Lower limit	Central value	Upper limit
Females	6,700	37,000	184,000
Males	1,200	7,400	38,000
TOTAL	8,000	46,000	208,000

4 SUBSEQUENT ACTIVITIES

In order to ensure that the results presented in the NCI report are credible, that the predicted lifetime excess thyroid cancer cases are reasonable, and that their public health implications are understood, the NCI requested the National Academy of Sciences – Institute of Medicine (IOM) to assess the soundness of the dose reconstruction, to provide a preliminary assessment of the public health implications, and to provide guidance to the Department of Health and Human Services for educating and informing members of the public and the medical profession about public health issues related to the thyroid dose estimated presented in the NCI report. It is expected that the IOM report will be available before the end of 1998.

28

References

1. Hoffman FO. Calculation of the Estimated Lifetime Risk of Radiation-Related Thyroid Cancer in the United States from Nevada Test Site Fallout. Report prepared for NAS/IOM committee 1997.

2. Laird NM. (1987) Thyroid Cancer Risk from Exposure to Ionizing Radiation: A Case Study in the Comparative Potency Model. Risk Analysis 1987; 7: 299-309.

3. Land, C. Calculation of the Estimated Lifetime Risk of Radiation-Related Thyroid Cancer in the United States from Nevada Test Site Fallout. Report prepared for NCI 1997.

4. Lee W, Chiacchierini RP, Shleien B, Telles NC (1982), Thyroid tumors following I-131 or localized X-irradiation to the thyroid and pituitary glands in rats. Radiat. Res. 1982; 92: 307.

5. Lubin JH, Ron E. Excess Relative Risk and Excess Absolute Risk Estimates for Pooled Analysis of Thyroid Cancer Following Exposure to External Radiation. Report prepared for NAS/IOM committee 1998.

6. National Cancer Institute. Estimated Exposures and Thyroid Doses Received by the American People from Iodine-131 in Fallout Following Nevada Atmospheric Nuclear Bomb Tests. U.S. Department of Health and Human Services, National Institutes of Health, National Cancer Institute, 1997.

7. NCRP (National Council on Radiation Protection and Measurements). Induction of Thyroid Cancer by Ionizing Radiation. Report No.80. Bethesda, NCRP, 1985.

8. Ron E, Lubin JH, Shore RE, Mabuchi K, Modan B, Pottern LM, Schneider AB, Tucker MA, Boice JD, Jr. Thyroid cancer following exposure to external radiation: a pooled analysis of seven studies. Radiat Res 1995; 141: 255-273.

9. U.S. Department of Energy. United States Nuclear Tests, July 1945 through September 1992. Report DOE/NV-209 (rev. 14); 1994

10. Walinder G. Late effects of irradiation on the thyroid gland in mice. I. Irradiation of adult mice. Acta Radiol. Ther. Phys. Biol. 1972; 11: 433.

STUDIES IN UTAH OF THYROID TUMORS FOLLOWING
NEVADA TEST SITE FALLOUT

ROY E. SHORE

Dept. of Environmental Medicine, New York University Medical
School, 550 First Ave., New York NY 10016, USA
E-mail: shorer01@gcrc.med.nyu.edu

Thyroid cancer prevalence was analyzed among about 2,500 children who lived in southwestern Utah in 1951-58, downwind from the Nevada Test Site (NTS), or in southeastern Arizona which was believed to have little NTS exposure, and who were given thyroid examinations in both 1965-70 and 1985-86. A thyroid dose estimate was made for each person based on residence history, age at exposure and reported milk consumption. The mean estimated thyroid dose from NTS fallout in southwestern Utah was 170 mGy; about 170 subjects receiving ≥ 0.4 Gy and 10 received ≥ 1 Gy. Eight thyroid cancers were detected in the study population compared to 5.4 expected. The risk estimate was similar to that obtained from studies of external irradiation, but the result was also statistically compatible with no excess risk. The scientific value of the study was limited by the small number of cancers detected combined with the relatively low doses. Perhaps the study's greatest contribution was in developing a method to reconstruct individual thyroid doses from limited historical area measurements plus residential and milk-drinking histories.

1 BACKGROUND AND DOSE ESTIMATION

Because of concerns over the amount of ^{131}I fallout in southwestern Utah from the Nevada atomic bomb tests during the 1950's, two thyroid screening programs approximately 20 years apart were conducted to evaluate thyroid nodularity and neoplasia among those who were children at the time of the fallout. The screened cohort consisted of 2,679 students in grades 5-12 in southwestern Utah and nearby Nevada in 1965-67.[5, 8] Many of these were residents in 1953 at the time of test shot HARRY which gave about 75% of the total ^{131}I dose in southern Utah. For comparison, 2,123 students were studied from a county in southeastern Arizona that was thought to be relatively unexposed.

More data were available on which to base dose estimates for southwestern Utah than for most of the remainder of the country, including numerous measurements of external exposure rates and several gummed film collectors which were assayed for total beta activity.[7] Soil measurements of radionuclides also supplemented the original exposure data.[1] Nevertheless, there were still considerable uncertainties in thyroid dose estimates because of micro-meteorological factors, uncertainties in deposition on grasses and in grass ingestion by cows, variations in ^{131}I concentrations in cows' milk and amount of milk consumed, and variations in thyroid uptake and retention.

The estimated thyroid doses in the cohort under study ranged from 0 to 4.6 Gy, with a mean of 13 mGy in Arizona, 50 mGy in Nevada and 170 mGy in southwestern Utah.[7] Only 170 subjects had estimated doses over 0.4 Gy and only 10 over 1 Gy. *In utero* exposures were received by 480 subjects; the *in utero* doses were typically about 25% of the total thyroid doses they received. Till et al [7] estimated the uncertainties in the individual childhood thyroid doses; the majority of the geometric standard deviations of uncertainties on individual dose estimates were between 2 and 4 and averaged about 2.7.

2   PHASE I THYROID SCREENING STUDY IN 1965-70

The original thyroid screening study of 4,818 children in 1965-70 did not have any dosimetry but divided the subjects into those considered exposed and unexposed by virtue of geographic location and time of birth. In this study there was no clear difference in the prevalence of thyroid nodules in the exposed group vs. the unexposed group (RR= 1.2, 95% CI= 0.7-2.0 for total nodular thyroids; RR= 1.9, 95% CI= 0.9-4.0 for thyroid nodules without other pathological findings).[5, 8] Only two thyroid cancers were found, both among those considered to be unexposed.[4, 8]

3   PHASE II THYROID SCREENING STUDY IN 1985-87 AND DOSE-ESTIMATION

In 1985-86 an attempt was made to examine all non-Hispanic whites who still resided in the tri-state area and who had never received radiation treatments of any kind to the head or neck.[2] The study attrition was relatively low for an examination program; 87% of the subjects were located and 78% of the located who were eligible were examined in 1985-86. The number of eligible subjects from phase I (1965-70) was 3,180, of whom 2,473 were screened in phase II (1985-86). The thyroid glands of subjects were examined by palpation by specially trained screeners. Those with suspected pathology were recalled and examined by a thyroidologist. The study preceded the era of ultrasound screening which could have provided an additional degree of objectivity to the thyroid examinations. Thyroid tumors that occurred between the times of the two screening programs were also included if they were pathologically verifiable.

The subjects' mothers (or a surrogate) were interviewed in 1987 to determine the subjects' childhood diets during the 1950's, with a particular focus on milk and vegetable consumption, including sources of milk. Individual dose estimates were calculated for these subjects.

The cumulative number of benign thyroid neoplasms between 1965 and 1986 was 11.[2] As shown in Table 1, 8 thyroid cancers were detected when about 5.4 would have been expected absent radiation exposure. The dose-response analyses were conducted with stratification by state. They reported a relative risk at 1 Gy of 8.9, almost identical to the value of 8.7 derived from the pooled thyroid cancer analysis by Ron et al,[6] although the risk estimate was also compatible with no excess risk (i.e., the lower 90% confidence bound was < 1). Land[3] re-analyzed the data and reported that the risk estimate was sensitive to the specific choices made in the analysis-- e.g., the risk estimate was substantially lower if the analysis was not stratified on state.

Table 1. Dose-response analyses of thyroid nodules and neoplasms (1965-86).[2]

Endpoint	No. of lesions	RR at 1 Gy (90% Confidence Interval)	p-value (one-sided)
All nodules	56	2.2 (< 1, ?)	0.16
All neoplasms	19	8.0 (1.7, ?)	0.02
Cancer	8	8.9 (< 1, ?)	0.10

The greatest limitations of the study were the low doses, dose uncertainties and small number of thyroid cancers (8 observed). There was a concern that the thyroid examiners were not blinded to the geographic location and therefore to the probable dose range of many of the subjects they were examining. A further concern was that the interviews with the mothers concerning the child's milk and leafy vegetable intake were not conducted until after the results of the thyroid examination were known to the subjects. There is unknown as to whether these features of the study may have introduced bias into the results.

In conclusion, this was a groundbreaking dosimetric study of ^{131}I exposure that integrated models of ^{131}I deposition, movement of ^{131}I through the food chain, individual consumption patterns, and age-specific ^{131}I uptake and retention estimates, along with uncertainty estimates on the individual doses. The study was carefully implemented, although not without some methodologic flaws. The study data were competently analyzed, including probably the first set of analyses of radiation epidemiologic data that incorporated the effects of individualized uncertainties in dose estimates.

32

In retrospect, the study probably was necessary to undertake because of widespread public perceptions of risk associated with the fallout. However, the study proved not to be very informative scientifically because of the small number of predicted thyroid cancers based on the dose distribution of the study subjects-- albeit this dose distribution was not well known in advance of the study. Important ingredients to evaluate in allocating support for present and future studies are having a large population with a wide range of doses and having a careful study design and implementation that reduce the potential for study biases to cause erroneous results.

Acknowledgments

This work was supported in part by the Kaplan Comprehensive Cancer Center NCI Grant CA16087 and the NIEHS Center Grant ES-00260 to New York University.

References

1. Beck H, Krey P. Radiation exposures in Utah from Nevada nuclear tests. *Science* 1983; **220**: 18-24.
2. Kerber RA, Till J, Simon S *et al.* A cohort study of thyroid disease in relation to fallout from nuclear weapons testing. *J Am Med Assoc* 1993; **270**: 2076-2082.
3. Land CE. Epidemiological studies of downwinders. **In**: Till JE (ed.), *Environmental Dose Reconstruction and Risk Implications (Proceedings No. 17)*, Bethesda, MD: National Council on Radiation Protection and Measurements, 1996; 311-328.
4. Rallison ML, Dobyns B, Keating F, Rall J, Tyler F. Thyroid disease in children. A survey of subjects potentially exposed to fallout radiation. *Am J Med* 1974; **56**: 457-463.
5. Rallison ML, Dobyns B, Keating F, Rall J, Tyler F. Thyroid nodularity in children. *J Am Med Assoc* 1975; **233**: 1069-1072.
6. Ron E, Lubin J, Shore R *et al.* Thyroid cancer after exposure to external radiation: a pooled analysis of seven studies. *Radiat Res* 1995; **141**: 259-277.
7. Till JE, Simon SL, Kerber R *et al.* The Utah thyroid cohort study: analysis of the dosimetry results. *Health Phys* 1995; **68**: 472-483.
8. Weiss ES, Rallison M, London WT, Thompson GDC. Thyroid nodularity in southwestern Utah school children exposed to fallout radiation. *Am J Pub Health* 1971; **61**: 241-249.

ATOMIC BOMB SURVIVORS POPULATION

SHIGENOBU NAGATAKI

Radiation Effects Research Foundation
5-2 Hijiyama Park, Minami-ku, Hiroshima 732-0815, Japan
E-mail: nagataki@rerf.or.jp

The Atomic Bomb Casualty Commission (ABCC), the predecessor of the Radiation Effects Research Foundation (RERF), was established in 1947 to conduct long-term comprehensive epidemiological and genetic studies of the atomic-bomb survivors. An in-depth follow-up study of mortality in the population of 120,000 persons has continued since 1950. The study of tumor incidence was initiated through record linkage with a tumor registry system in Hiroshima and Nagasaki in 1958. In the same year, biennial medical examinations of 20,000 individuals began. On the basis of these studies, we know that the occurrence of leukemia and cancers associated with atomic bomb radiation is higher than among the non-exposed. Radiation cataracts, benign thyroid tumor, autoimmune thyroid diseases, hyperparathyroidism, cardiovascular disease, chronic liver disease also occur more often. Further studies are necessary to elucidate the mechanisms of radiation related diseases.

1. INTRODUCTION AND BACKGROUND

In August 1945 atomic bombs were detonated over Hiroshima and Nagasaki. Damage in the two cities was caused by a combination of heat, blast, and fire. The energy of the Nagasaki bomb exceeded that of the Hiroshima bomb, but the burned-out areas of Hiroshima were greater because of differences in topography and in the distribution of buildings. Because of the chaotic conditions after the bombings, the precise number of casualties will never be known. Estimates of death range from 90,000 to 140,000 persons in Hiroshima and from 60,000 to 80,000 persons in Nagasaki. Various estimates of the number of casualties have been made; however, the errors associated with the estimates may be quite large.[1,2]

In November 1946, US President Harry Truman approved a directive to the National Academy of Sciences-National Research Council (NAS-NRC) to initiate a long-term investigation of the health effects associated with exposure to radiation from the atomic bombs. With funding provided by the Atomic Energy Commission (AEC), now the Department of Energy (DOE), the NAS-NRC established the Atomic Bomb Casualty Commission (ABCC) in March 1947, and investigations began in 1948. The Government of Japan, through the Japanese National Institute of Health, became a partner in this endeavor.[1,2] In 1975, the Radiation Effects Research Foundation (RERF) was established and assumed the responsibilities of ABCC.[1,2]

2. LONG-TERM COHORT STUDY OF THE ATOMIC BOMB SURVIVORS

Long-term follow-up of this unique radiation-exposed population has provided important information on the early and late health effects of radiation exposure. The goals of RERF are (1) to determine the somatic and genetic late health effects produced in humans resulting from exposure to ionizing radiation, and (2) to obtain information on the temporal pattern of cancer expression. In order to achieve these goals, the longterm follow-up of fixed cohort populations has been underway during the past 5 decades.

The largest and most important of these cohorts is the Life Span Study sample (LSS). The 1950 Japanese National Census identified 284,000 survivors including about 159,000 Hiroshima survivors and 125,000 Nagasaki survivors. This group was used as the basis for the constructing the LSS sample. The original LSS cohort, which included about 99,400 persons, was extended in the late 1960s and again in 1980. The current size of the LSS is 120,000 persons representing a wide range of ages and both sexes. The LSS data are characterized primarily by acute exposure to low LET gamma radiation, with a non-negligible neutron component in Hiroshima. However, there are about 37,000 subjects in the dose range of 0.005 - 0.20 Gy, thus providing substantial information on low-dose effects. Mortality follow-up in the LSS and other RERF cohorts is carried out through access to the records of the mandatory family registration (koseki) system. The ability to access the koseki records guarantees virtually complete mortality ascertainment for persons who have not emigrated out of Japan. Copies of death certificates are obtained for all deceased persons. [1]

In addition to the death certificate-based mortality follow-up, cancer incidence data have recently become available for the LSS cohort through linkage to the Hiroshima and Nagasaki tumor registries. With the cooperation of the local medical associations, population-based tumor registries were established in 1957 in Hiroshima and 1958 in Nagasaki. The Hiroshima and Nagasaki registries are unique among Japanese cancer registries because they use active case ascertainment methods (i.e., trained abstractors visit hospitals and clinics to review records) rather than relying on voluntary reporting by physicians. The Hiroshima and Nagasaki registries are generally regarded as the best tumor registries in Japan. The availability of cancer incidence data is critical for the risk assessment for relatively less fatal cancers, including thyroid, breast and skin cancers. [1]

Another important RERF cohort study is the Adult Health Study (AHS). The AHS sample, a subset of the LSS cohort sample, includes over 20,000 person. Regular biennial clinical examinations of the AHS sample, which began in 1958, are provided in a two-year cycle and are now in the 19th cycle. These examinations serve as the only point of direct contact between RERF and the survivors. Blood and other biological specimens obtained at the time of biennial examination are used for genetics and radiobiology research. Longitudinal data on various clinical endpoints provide unique opportunity for studying the effects of radiation exposure at clinical and sub-clinical levels. In particular, the importance of the AHS data in studies on non-cancer diseases, including cardiovascular diseases and certain benign tumors, has increased as there is emerging evidence on non-cancer disease risks associated with radiation[1].

The LSS provides the most comprehensive data on the risk of cancer associated with whole-body exposure to low linear energy transfer (LET) radiation. Statistically significant excess risks have been demonstrated for leukemia and many of the most common types of solid cancer, including stomach, lung, liver, colon, esophagus, female breast, ovary, and bladder as well as a group of cancers at sites not considered in site-specific analyses. [3, 4] The latest LSS mortality data show that about 335 of some 4,500 solid cancer deaths among those exposed >0.005 Sv are attributable to radiation exposure and that about 90 of 250 leukemia deaths in the same group of survivors are due to radiation exposure.

Table 1. Observed and Expected Deaths (1950-1990)

Dose (Sv)	Subjects	Solid Cancer			Leukemia		
		Observed	Expected	Excess (%)	bserved	Expecte d	Excess (%)
<.005	36,459	3,013	3055	-42(-1.4)	73	64	9(12.3)
.005-.1	32,849	2,795	2710	84 (3.0)	59	62	-3(-5.1)
.10-.20	5,467	504	486	19 (3.8)	11	11	0
.20-.50	6,308	632	555	77(12.2)	27	12	15(55.5)
.50-1	3,202	336	263	73(21.7)	23	7	16(69.5)
1-2	1,608	215	131	84(39.1)	26	4	22(84.6)
2+	679	83	44	39(47.0)	30	2	28(93.3)
Total	86,572	7,578	7244	335 (4.4)	249	162	87(34.9)

(Pierce DA et al: Rdiat. Res., 146:1-27, 1996)

Compared to the malignant tumors, little is known about the radiation effects on benign tumors. This is because benign tumors are rarely fatal and their symptoms are relatively mild, often leading to their not being reported. At present, benign tumors of thyroid and the parathyroid, uterine myoma and autoimmune thyroid disease are known to be related to radiation exposure. [5-9]

38

Figure 1

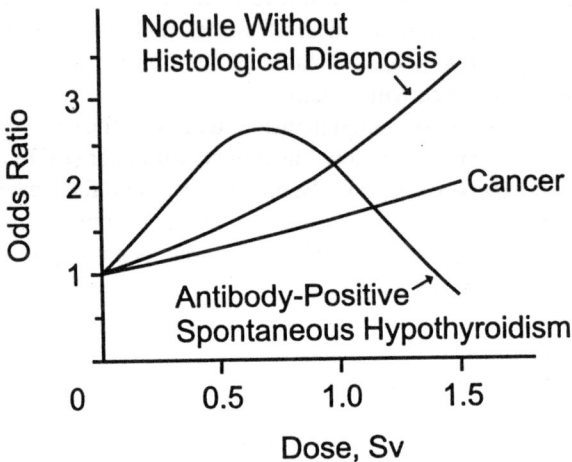

Figure 1. Odds ratios of the prevalence of nodule without histological diagnosis (women only), cancer, and antibody-positive spontaneous hypothyroidism where the prevalence is adjusted for sex and age at the time of bombing (cancer) and for age at the time of bombing (antibody-positive spontaneous hypothyroidism).

Recent analysis of data from LSS have revealed statistically significant dose response for death from diseases other than cancer. [10] By the end of 1990, among the 50,113 LSS survivors with significant exposures, 15,633 noncancer deaths have occurred. Cardiovascular diseases account for nearly half of these deaths with digestive diseases accounting for about 10 % of the total. The death rate following exposure to 0.2 Sv is increased by about 1 % over normal rates. This is less than the death rate for solid cancer, for which the corresponding increases are 7 % for men and 15 % for women following radiation exposure at age 30. [10] In addition, studies of the incidence of myocardial infarction and chronic liver disease in the AHS have shown radiation effect that are consistent with the mortality data. [5, 6]

3. FUTURE

The association of radiation exposure and with leukemia and cancer has been established during 5 decades of data collection among atomic bomb survivors, leading to understanding of the nature and magnitude of risk associated with radiation. However, much more can be learned from further follow-up of the survivors and their children. Although lifetime follow-up is complete for those exposed when older than age 50, more than half of the LSS cohort and over 90% of those exposed as children are alive now. Thus the cancer risk among the young survivors presents one of the most important uncertainties in cancer risk among the atomic bomb survivors. Furthermore, mechanisms of radiation carcinogenesis must be clarified hopefully by molecular biological studies. In addition, analyses of the mortality and incidence study data have recently shown an apparent excess in diseases other than cancer, such as cardiovascular disease among the survivors.

In addition to atomic bombs and accidents of nuclear plants, radiation may come from many social devices and affects the health of human beings, and scientific results on the radiation effects are being utilized in many social groups whose requests to the science are very different. It is the responsibility of scientists of the time to identify, from the diversified social needs, the study themes that would be necessary as the knowledge of human beings in the future and promote studies on such themes.

Acknowledgements

The author gratefully acknowledge the helpful assistance of Dr. Kazunori Kodama in the preparation of this manuscript.

40

References

1. Kodama K, Mabuchi K, Shigematsu I. A Long-Term Cohort Study of the Atomic Bomb Survivors. J Epidemiol, 1996;6:S95-S105.
2. Putnam FW. Hiroshima and Nagasaki revisited: the Atomic Bomb Casualty Commission and the Radiation Effects Research Foundation. Perspect Bio Med, 1994;37:515-545.
3. Pierce DA, Shimizu Y, Preston DL, Vaeth M, Mabuchi K. Studies of the Mortality of Atomic Bomb Survivors. Report 12, Part 1. Cancer: 1950-1990. Radiat Res, 1996;146:1-27.
4. Thompson DE, Mabuchi K, Ron E, Soda M, Tokunaga M, Ochikubo S, Sugimoto S, Ikeda T, Terasaki M, Izumi S, Preston DL. Cancer Incidence in Atomic Bomb Survivors. Part 2: Solid Tumors, 1957-1987. Radiat Res, 1994;137:S17-S67.
5. Kodama K, Fujiwara S, Yamada M, Kasagi F, Shimizu Y, Shigematsu I. Profiles of non-cancer diseases in atomic bomb survivors. Wld Hlth Statist Quart, 1996;49:7-16.
6. Wong FL, Yamada M, Sasaki H, Kodama K, Akiba S, Shimaoka K, Hosoda Y. Noncancer Disease Incidence in the Atomic Bomb Survivors: 1958-1986. Radiat Res, 1993;135:418-430.
7. Nagataki S, Shibata Y, Inoue S, Yokoyama N, Izumi M, Shimaoka K. Thyroid diseases among atomic bomb survivors in Nagasaki. JAMA, 1994;272:364-370.
8. Fujiwara S, Sposto R, Ezaki H. Hyperparathyroidism among atomic bomb survivors in Hiroshima. Radiat Res, 1992;130:372-378.
9. Kawamura S, Kasagi F, Kodama K, Fujiwara S, Yamada M, Ohma K, Ito K. Prevalence of Uterine Myoma Detected by Ultrasound Examination in the Atomic Bomb Survivors. Radiat Res, 1997;147:753-758.
10. Shimizu Y, Kato H, Schull WJ, Hoel D. Studies of the mortality of A-bomb survivors, 9. Mortality, 1950-85: Part 3. Noncancer mortality based on the revised doses (DS86). Radiat Res, 1992;130:249-266.

THYROID CANCER AND THYROID NODULES IN THE PEOPLE OF THE MARSHALL ISLANDS POTENTIALLY EXPOSED TO FALLOUT FROM NUCLEAR WEAPONS TESTING

K.R. TROTT

Department of Radiation Biology, St. Bartholomew's and the Royal London School of Medicine and Dentistry, Charterhouse Square, London, UK

M. J. SCHOEMAKER

Department of Epidemiology and Population Health, London School of Hygiene and Tropical Medicine, London, UK

T. TAKAHASHI

Department of Preventive Medicine and Health Promotion, Nagasaki University School of Medicine, Nagasaki, Japan

K. FUJIMORI, N. NAKASHIMA, H. OHTOMO, M. WATANABE AND S. SATOMI

Second Department of Surgery, Tohoku University School of Medicine, Sendai, Japan

S. L. SIMON

Board on Radiation Effects Research, National Academy of Sciences, Washington DC, USA

The US atomic weapons testing programme in the Pacific conducted between 1946 and 1958 resulted in radioactive contamination of a number of atolls in the Marshall Islands to various degrees. Between 1993 and 1997, as part of the Nationwide Radiological Study of the Republic of the Marshall Islands we studied the prevalence of thyroid nodules and thyroid cancer in 4766 Marshallese potentially exposed to radioiodines from bomb test fallout which is more than 60% of the population at risk. Methods included clinical examination, ultrasound, fine needle aspiration biopsy of all palpable nodules, thyroid function tests on a large sub-sample, and histopathology of surgical specimens of 43 people operated by our team. We diagnosed 41 thyroid cancers and 1430 benign thyroid nodules. Twenty study participants had been operated for thyroid cancer before. Benign thyroid nodules were not related with potential radioiodine exposure. There was a trend of increased cumulative thyroid cancer incidence with increased ^{137}Cs deposition on the atoll of residence in 1954.

1 INTRODUCTION

The nuclear weapons testing progamme conducted between 1946 and 1958 on Bikini atoll and Eniwetak atoll resulted in radioactive contamination of a number of atolls in the Marshall Islands to various degrees. The most serious radiation exposures were caused by early fallout from the test Castle Bravo, a hydrogen bomb detonated on Bikini atoll on 1 March 1954. The radioactive fallout was intense on the inhabited islands of Rongelap atoll resulting in thyroid exposures between 50 and 200 Gy for a one year old child and one tenth of that in Utrik.[1] The exposed communities were evacuated, treated for acute radiation illness and provided with follow-up medical care over the decades since.[2] The most frequent long-term health effect in the exposed population appeared to be an increased frequency of nodular thyroid disease including thyroid cancer.[3]

There is evidence to indicate that residents of other atolls may also have been exposed to radioactive fallout from the Bravo test as well as from some of the other 65 atmospheric explosions. The radioactive contamination on all atolls, consisting mainly of ^{137}Cs, has recently been assessed by the Marshall Islands Nationwide Radiological Study. The data indicate that ten of the 23 inhabited atolls or reef islands have environmental levels of ^{137}Cs enhanced over the level of global fallout received in the mid-Pacific region.[4] However, the extent of exposure of the Marshall Islands population to radioiodines during the testing years has never been assessed. Moreover, little information exists about health consequences among residents of the many atolls other than Rongelap and Utrik except for the study of nodular thyroid disease by Hamilton.[5] Therefore, a nationwide thyroid disease screening programme was initiated to gather data useful for such an evaluation and to advise the Marshallese government on the public health impact of thyroid diseases and on their possible relationship with the radioactive fallout from the nuclear weapons tests.[6]

2 METHODS AND STUDY SUBJECTS

The aim of the study was to investigate as large a proportion as possible of all Marshallese who lived anywhere in the Marshall Islands in 1958 and thus were potentially exposed to fallout from the nuclear weapons tests. From national census data we estimated that this study population would be between 7,000 and 8,000 people living on 23 different atolls. Three study populations were defined, those born before the Bravo test (BRAVO cohort), those born between 1954 and the end of the bomb test period (end of tests cohort), and those born within 5 years after the end of the bomb tests (after testing cohort) to serve as unexposed control.

The thyroid screening programme was composed of two components: a personal interview and a clinical examination. The methods have been described in detail by Takahashi et al.[6] The most important data collected in the interviews was a complete residence history from birth until the examination date as this was to be used to estimate potential exposure to radioiodines. Each study subject was examined sequentially by two endocrine surgeons from Tohoku University School of Medicine first by palpation of the neck and then by the other surgeon who was blinded to the findings of the physical examination, by high resolution ultrasound. Physicians alternated in their assignment to perform ultrasound examination or palpation. Our definition of a nodule as imaged by ultrasound included all focal abnormalities of the echo pattern which was larger than 4 mm. Except for a few who refused, each participant who had a palpable nodule had a fine needle aspiration biopsy during the same examination session. All slides were stained immediately in the Marshall Islands and examined by one pathologist in Tohoku University, Sendai.

Large subgroups of the study population were also examined for thyroid function. Methods have been described in detail by Takahashi et al.[7] 1050 consecutive study participants in Ebeye were examined for the presence of hypothyroidism using a blood spot technique for TSH. In Majuro, a venous blood sample was taken from 3000 consecutive study participants and examined for TSH, T_3, T_4 and anti-thyroid antibodies. In addition, we measured iodine concentration in random urine samples from 363 adults and 163 children.[7]

The statistical analysis was carried out on the BRAVO cohort defined as all people born before March 1, 1954. Two sets of predictor variable were used: 1) ^{137}Cs deposition, and 2) distance and angle from Bikini atoll. Both sets refer to the atolls of residence in 1954. Logistic regression analysis was used to model the probability of having thyroid cancer or benign thyroid nodules. The multivariate models were obtained by backwards stepwise elimination of predictor variables with a p-value greater than 0.10. Age was divided into 5 years age bands, and distance and angle were split up on the basis of the 20, 40, 60, and 80th quantile. The data of ^{137}Cs deposition were log transformed and divided into 5 groups.

3   RESULTS

Between 1993 and 1997, we investigated 7221 Marshallese people. There were 4766 potentially exposed study subjects which is 60-69% of the entire population at risk (Table 1 and 2).

Table 1. Number of study participants by birth cohort

Study Cohort	Number of Subjects
BRAVO[a]	3,712
End of Tests[b]	1,054
After Tests[c]	1,059
Total number of study members=	5,825

[a]born before 1 March 1954
[b]born between 1 March 1954 and 1 March 1959
[c]born between 1 March 1959 and 1 January 1965

Table 2. Clinical methods and number of subjects

Method	Number of Subjects
Clinical examination of the neck and ultrasound	7,221
Fine needle aspiration biopsy	699
Definitive surgery of suspected cancer	
Performed by our team	43
Performed by other surgeons	17
TSH determination	4,050
T_3/T_4 and antithyroid antibodies determination	3,000
Iodine excretion	526

Hypothyroidism was defined as a TSH value of twice the modal value for the blot spot test. This was found in 30/1050 (3%) of the study participants in Ebeye. In the venous blood samples in Majuro, biochemical hypothyroidism was defined as a TSH value of >3.1 µU/ml which was observed in 33/3000 (1.5%). We concluded that hypothyroidism is very rare in the investigated Marshallese population, mild biochemical hypothyroidism was diagnosed in approximately 2%. Also autoimmune thyroiditis is very rare in the Marshall Islands with a prevalence of 33/3000 (1.1%).

The prevalence of thyroid nodules is very high in the adult population of the Marshall Islands (Table 3). Prevalence is higher in females than in males and increases with age. It is similar to that in some central European populations which have been investigated in a similar way with ultrasound screening and individual iodine excretion measurements and found to be moderately deficient in dietary iodine supply. For this reason, we measured iodine excretion (iodine/creatinine ratio) in 526 random urine samples and found that 21% of the adult Marshallese population suffered from moderate iodine deficiency according to the WHO criteria and 1% was severely iodine deficient. Only 25% had an adequate iodine supply. In children, however, the prevalence of iodine deficiency was only half that in adults. The observed iodine deficiency could be regarded as a cause of the high prevalence of nodular thyroid disease. The results are in accordance with those of Gutekunst et al.[8] who studied German and Swedish male adults with a very similar study design comparing ultrasound screening of the thyroid with individual measurements of the iodine/creatinine ratio in random urine samples. Whereas in the population with adequate dietary supply of iodine, the prevalence of thyroid nodules was only 2%, it was 13% in German males which had a 25% frequency of moderate iodine deficiency.

Table 3. Prevalence of Benign Nodules

Cohort	Male	Nodules	%	Female	Nodules	%
BRAVO cohort	1787	379	21.2	1925	726	37.7
End of testing cohort	444	44	9.9	610	144	23.6
After testing cohort	443	33	7.4	616	74	12.0

In the 3712 people of the Bravo cohort we diagnosed 1105 people with thyroid nodules. There were 31 thyroid cancers, 24 of which were papillary carcinomas, 4 micropapillary carcinomas and 3 follicular carcinomas. In addition, we found 99 study participants who had typical scars which indicated previous surgery in the neck region. In 20 of these the histology report stated the diagnosis of thyroid cancer. The analysis of cumulative incidence of thyroid cancer in the Bravo cohort is based on these 51 histologically confirmed cases of thyroid cancer.

The cumulative incidence rate of thyroid cancer in the BRAVO cohort is 1.4% which is higher than found in most screened populations such as Takaya et al.[9] (Table 4). In younger study participants, the cumulative thyroid cancer incidence is still as high as 0.5%. There is a 50% higher cumulative cancer incidence in females than in males. Although the largest number of thyroid cancers was diagnosed in the group of women who were young at the time of the Bravo test, the summary statistics does not suggest any pronounced influence of age at exposure on cumulative thyroid cancer incidence. Moreover, age at exposure and age at diagnosis are closely linked at least in those patients who were diagnosed in our study. In other populations, incidence rates of thyroid cancer tend to peak in the same age groups for which we observed the highest cumulative frequency.[10] We observed a prevalence of 0.5% thyroid cancer in people of only thirty years of age, who could not have been exposed to any radioiodines from the local bomb test fallout. This suggests that Marshallese are different from other populations with regard to thyroid cancer.

Table 4. Cumulative incidence of thyroid cancer

Birth cohort	Male (%)	Female (%)	Total (%)
BRAVO cohort			
Before 1936	6/556	11/561	17/1117
(Adults in 1954)	(1.1%)	(2.0%)	(1.5%)
1936-1945	7/397	6/469	13/866
(Teenagers in 1954)	(1.8%)	(1.3%)	(1.5%)
1945-1953	4/834	17/895	21/1729
(Children in 1954)	(0.5%)	(1.8%)	(1.2%)
End of testing cohort			
1954-1959	4/426	1/592	5/1018
	(0.9%)	(0.3%)	(0.6%)
After testing cohort			
1959-1964	1/461	4/634	5/1095
	(0.2%)	(0.9%)	(0.5%)
Total	22/2674	39/3154	61/5825
	(0.8%)	(1.2%)	(1.0%)

In order to study the relationship between thyroid cancer with potential radioiodine exposure we related cases and controls to the place of residence at the time of the different bomb tests and thus to the level of potential exposure to radioiodines. There was some indication of a trend of decreasing cumulative cancer incidence in the BRAVO cohort with increasing distance from Bikini (Figure 1).

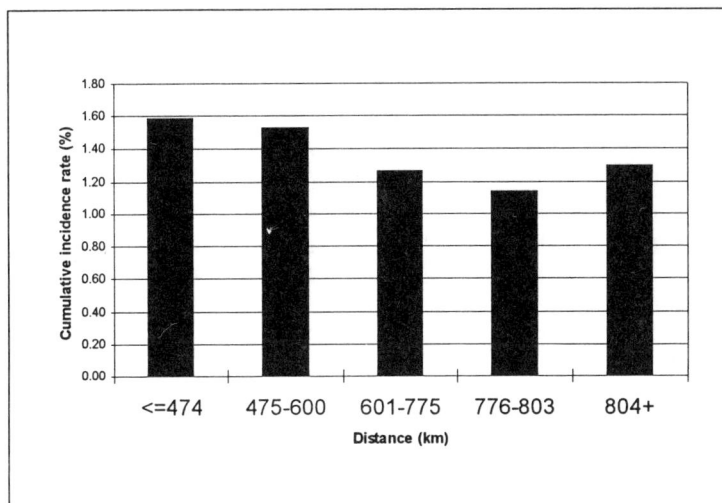

Fig. 1. Cumulative incidence of thyroid cancer against distance from Bikini Atoll

Caesium deposition may be a better indicator of potential exposure to radioiodines than distance. With increasing ^{137}Cs deposition on the atoll of residence in 1954 we observed an increase of cumulative cancer incidence rate (Figure 2).

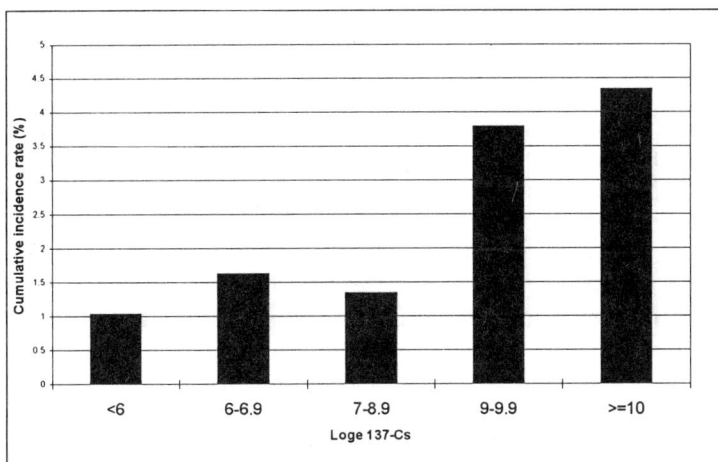

Fig. 2. Cumulative incidence of thyroid cancer against Cs-137 deposition $(\log_e[Bq/m^2])$.

The multivariate analysis of risk factors for thyroid cancer and thyroid nodules suggests that there was little association of benign nodules with potential radioiodine exposure but there was evidence for thyroid cancer being associated with potential radioiodine exposure (Table 5).

Table 5. Results of multivariate analyses

Characteristic	No. of cases (% total)	No. of people	Adjusted OR	95% CI	P-value
Sex					
Male	17 (1.0)	1787	1.00	Reference group	
Female	34 (1.8)	1925	2.29	1.22-4.29	p=0.010
Cs-137 deposition					
<6	20 (1.0)	1920	1.00	Reference group	p=0.081
6	15 (1.6)	921	1.59	0.81-3.12	
7-8	8 (1.3)	598	1.30	0.57-2.97	
>=9	5 (4.0)	125	4.19	1.54-11.41	
			χ^2 trend=4.2, p=0.040		

4   CONCLUSION

We conclude that the prevalence of thyroid nodules and the cumulative incidence rate of thyroid cancer are high in the Marshall Islands. We did not find any indication that benign thyroid nodules are related to potential radiation exposure. On the other hand, there is a trend of increased cumulative thyroid cancer incidence with increasing potential radioiodine exposure as suggested by the two proxy measures of exposure, i.e. distance and caesium deposition. In view of these data, individual thyroid dose reconstruction becomes an essential task for future work. This is by no means a simple undertaking since it has to consider pathways as described by Simon and Graham[11] which are very different from those modelled elsewhere, e.g. in the reconstruction of thyroid doses from the Chernobyl accident.

References

1. Lessard E, Miltenberger R, Conard R, Musolino S, Naidu J, Moorthy A, Schopfer C. Thyroid absorbed dose for people at Rongelap, Utirik and Sifo on March1, 1954. *Brookhaven National Laboratory Report*. BNL-51882, 19852.

2. Conard RA and 9 others. Review of medical findings in a Marshallese population twenty-six years after accidental exposure to radioactive fallout. *Brookhaven National Laboratory Report*. BNL-51261, 19803.

3. Dobyns BM, Hyrmer BA. The surgical management of benign and malignant thyroid neoplasms in Marshall Islanders exposed to hydrogen bomb fallout. *World J Surg* 1992; **16**:126-1404.

4. Simon SL, Graham JC. Findings of the first comprehensive radiological monitoring program of the Republic of the Marshall Islands. *Health Phys* 1997; **73**: 66-855.

5. Hamilton TE, van Belle G, LoGerlo JP. Thyroid neoplasia in Marshall Islanders exposed to nuclear fallout. *JAMA* 1987; **258**: 629-6366.

6. Takahashi T, Trott KR, Fujimori K, Simon SL, Ohtomo H, Nakashima N, Takaya K, Kimura N, Satomi S, Schoemaker MJ. An investigation into the prevalence of thyroid disease on Kwajalein atoll, Marshall Islands. *Health Phys* 1997; **73**: 199-2137.

7. Takahashi T, Bechtner G, Fujimori K, Simon SL, Edwards R, Trott KR. Thyroid nodules, thyroid function and dietary iodine in the Marshall Islands. *Int J Epidemiol* (submitted 1998).

8. Gutekunst R, Smolarek H, Hasenpusch U, Stubbe P, Friedrich HJ, Wood WG, Scriba PC. Goitre epidemiology: thyroid volume, iodine excretion, thyroglobulin and thyrotropin in Germany and Sweden. *Acta Endocrin* 1986; **112**: 494-5019.

9. Takaya K, Taguchi Y, Sasaki T, Miura K, Kaneda I, Nakano Y, Jimbo M, Satomi S, Tanimura S, Wagatsuma M. Evaluation of mass screening for thyroid disease in Kamaishi City, Japan. *Tohoku Med J* 1982; **96**: 22-27 10.

10. McConahey WM, Hay ID, Woolner LB, van Heerden JA, Taylor WF. Papillary thyroid cancer treated at the Mayo Clinic, 1946 through 1970 Initial manifestations, pathological findings, therapy, and outcome. *Mayo Clin Proc* 1986; **61**: 978-996

11. Simon SL, Graham JC. Dose assessment activities in the Republic of the Marshall Islands. *Health Phys* 1996; **71**: 438-456

THYROID CANCER PROMOTED BY RADIATION IN YOUNG PEOPLE OF BELARUS (CLINICAL AND EPIDEMIOLOGICAL FEATURES)

E.DEMIDCHIK[1], A.MROCHEK[1], Yu.DEMIDCHIK[2], T.VORONTSOVA[1],
E.CHERSTVOY[2], J.KENIGSBERG[1], V.REBEKO[1], A.SUGENOYA[1]

[1]*Thyroid Cancer Center of The Institute for Radiation Medicine and Endocrinology,
Scorina av.,64, 220013, Minsk, Belarus*
[2]*Minsk State Medical Institute, Dzerzhinsky av., 220116, Minsk, Belarus*
E-mail: demidchik@msmi.minsk.by

Chernobyl disaster caused a high incidence of thyroid cancer in young population of Belarus. For the period of twelve years standard incidence in adults reached 7.9 : 100 000 and in children 3-4 : 100 000. Since 1996 the incidence rates in children gradually decreasing and the incidence in adults continues to increase.

The problem of high incidence for thyroid carcinomas will remain actual for many years may be for the whole life duration of the population who underwent irradiation by radioactive iodine.

Thyroid cancer promoted by radiation has a highly aggressive nature. Even small carcinomas from 3 to 9 mm in largest measurement can extend into surrounding tissues of the neck and form multiple metastases in lymph nodes and lungs, mostly in cases of extrathyroidal spread.

There is no doubt that a high incidence of thyroid cancer in children and adolescents of Belarus is caused by Chernobyl Nuclear Power Plant disaster. No other environmental failure could originate that tumor. This conclusion was made many times by different groups of scientists [1], WHO experts [2] and IAEA [3].

Earlier we reported the trends in incidence rates for pediatric thyroid carcinomas and some features of the course of the disease and its therapy. It was shown that thyroid carcinomas developed mostly in children who lived in southern regions of Belarus [4,5]. We also noted a highly aggressive potential of pediatric thyroid carcinomas [6].

Since than the situation has become different. The purpose of this study is to demonstrate the current trends in incidence as well as to emphasize the clinical features for thyroid carcinomas in children, adolescents and young adults.

For the period of 12 years after the Chernobyl disaster the incidence for thyroid carcinoma increased on 4057 cases as compared with the same period of time before. Since 1974 to1985 thyroid carcinomas developed in 1392 patients, but from 1986 up to the July,1998 5449 new cases were diagnosed. The standard index of incidence reached 7.9 per 100 000 in population above 18 years old and 3-4: 100 000 in children (Fig.1).

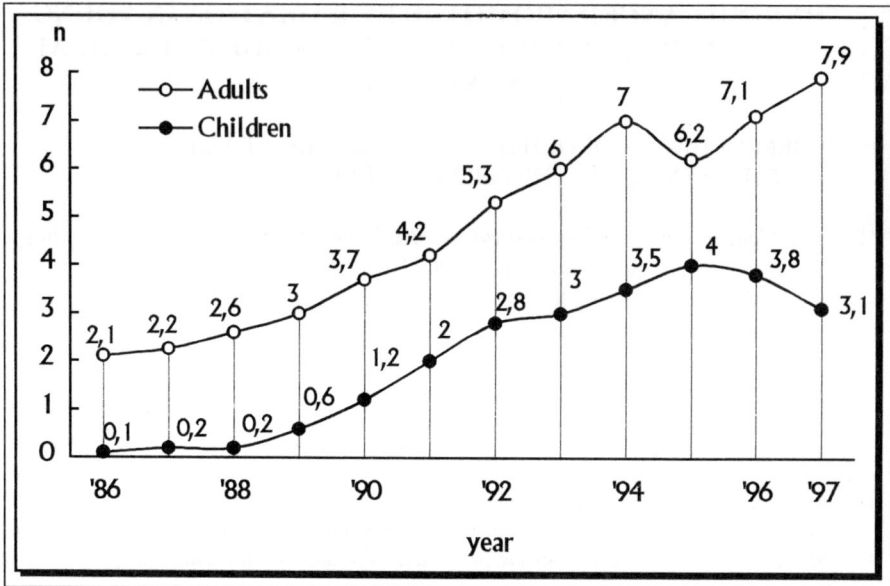

Fig.1 Index of incidence per 100 000

The significant increase of incidence for thyroid carcinoma was observed in children, teenagers and adults under 30 (Table 1).

Table 1 Thyroid cancer in young people before and after Chernobyl

Age	1974-1985	1986-1998*
3-14	8	600
15-18	13	132
19-29	117	438
Total	138	1170

Note: * 6 months of 1998

Thyroid carcinomas were mainly diagnosed in children born before the accident. After iodine-131 disintegration spontaneous carcinomas were diagnosed only in six children patients born in 1987 and 1988.

Of 5449 patients with thyroid cancer 1012 (18.6%) at the time of the accident were at the age from 0 to 18 years old. The high risk was detected in patients who were under five at the accident (Fig.2).

Incidence rates in children have permanently been rising till the recent time. Since 1996 a number of children patients have gradually been decreasing and the incidence rates in adults continue to increase (Fig.3 and 4).

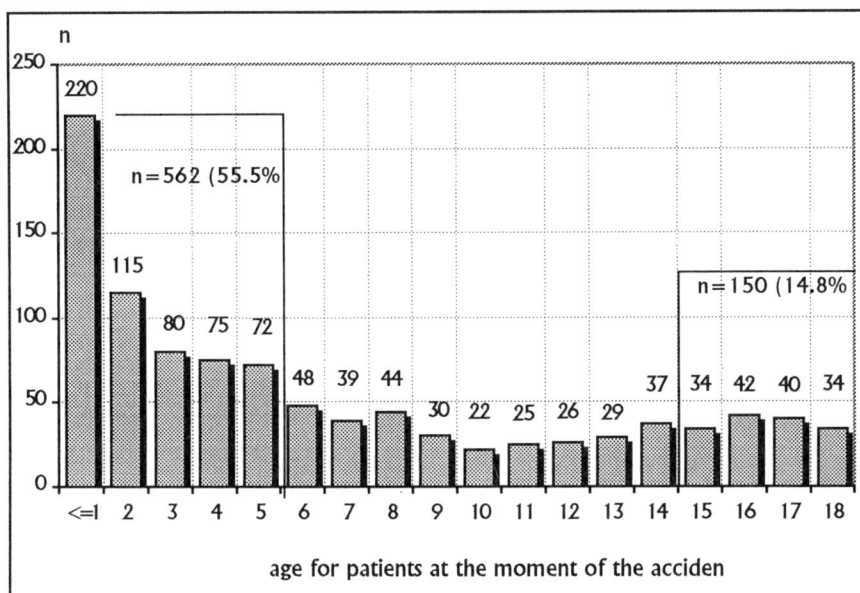

Fig.2 Patient's age at the time of the Chernobyl accident

Thyroid cancer promoted by radiation has a highly aggressive nature. Even small carcinomas from 3 to 9 mm in the largest measurement can extend into surrounding tissues of the neck and form multiple metastases in lymph nodes and lungs, mostly in cases of extrathyroidal spread (Table 5 and 6).

Table 5 Cancer less than 1 cm in largest measurement in children and its extent

Tumor size (mm)	Cases	pT1b	pT4	Metastases	
				pN1	M1
3	5	1	0	1	0
4	8	2	1	1	1
5	16	4	1	8	1
6	17	4	2	4	0
7	30	6	5	16	1
8	39	11	9	21	1
9	27	8	5	17	1
Total	142 (100%)	36 (25.4%)	23 (16.2%)	68 (47.9%)	5 (3.5%)

Table 6 Thyroid cancer metastases in children patients

Tumor size (mm)	Cases	pT1b (%)	Metastases (%) pN1	M1
pT1-3	342	21.9	56.1	6.7
pT4				
	252	33.5	84.1	32.1
Total	594*	28.9%	68.3%	17.5%

Note: *6 patients underwent surgery in other countries

Conclusion

The feature of the first decade after Chernobyl accident was in a high incidence level for thyroid carcinoma in pediatric patients. There is a good reason to consider that during the second decade we will observe the peek of incidence for young people in the age group from 15 to 34.

We emphasize that thyroid carcinomas in young population have an aggressive nature with high potential for metastatic disease and tumor spread into surrounding tissues.

References

1. Nagasaki Symposium on Chernobyl: Update and Future, ed. *Nagataki S.* Amsterdam, Elsevier, 1994.
2. Медицинские последствия Чернобыльской аварии. Научный отчёт. *ВОЗ,* Женева, 1996.
3. One decade after Chernobyl: Summing up the consequences of the accident. *IAEA,* Vienna, 1997
4. Kazakov V.S., Demidchik E.P., Astakhova L.N. Thyroid cancer after Chernobyl. *Nature* 1992; **359**, 21
5. Demidchik E.P., Kazakov V.S., Astakhova L.N. et al. Thyroid cancer in children after the Chernobyl accident: clinical and epidemiological evaluation of 251 cases in the Republic of Belarus. In: Nagasaki Symposium on Chernobyl: Update and Future, ed. *Nagataki S.* Amsterdam, Elsevier, 1994.
6. Демидчик Е.П., Цыб А.Ф., Лушников Е.Ф. *Рак щитовидной железы у детей.* Москва: Медицина, 1996

THE PATHOMORPHOLOGY OF CHILDHOOD PAPILLARY THYROID CARCINOMA IN BELARUS IN DIFFERENT PERIODS AFTER THE CHERNOBYL ACCIDENT (1991-1997)

E.CHERSTVOY, V.POZHARSKAYA, A.NEROVNYA

Department of Pathology, Minsk State Medical Institute, Dzerzhinski av. 83, 220116 Minsk, Belarus

Histological slides from 458 childhood thyroid carcinomas from Belarus (1991-1997) were examined. Papillary thyroid carcinoma was diagnosed in 96,5%. All papillary carcinomas were subdivided in accordance with predominant histological structures in tumor node - "pure" follicular, papillary, solid variants, "mixed" variants with prevailing follicular, solid and papillary structures and diffuse sclerosing variant. According to study clinicomorphological features of papillary thyroid carcinoma in relation to latent period were picked out two groups of patients. The first goup consisted of 108 children, operated on in 1991-1992 years, hypothetic latent period was 5-6 years. The second group consisted of 149 children, operated on in 1996-1997 years, hypothetic latent period was 10-11 years. A significant (p<0,05) increasing of papillary carcinoma cases with follicular structures was defined with increasing of latent period. The number of papillary carcinoma cases with solid structures was invariable in two groups of the patients. These changes were not related to the age distinctions in two groups. The decreasing (p<0,05) of expression and extrathyroid spreading and intrathyroid lymphogenic dissemination of papillary thyroid carcinoma was revealed with the increasing of latent period.There was no significant difference in frequency of blood vessel invasion in two groups of patients with papillary cancer.

1. Introduction

Twelve years have passed after the accident at the Chernobyl Nuclear station, however, at present the patients, who were 3-4 years old at the moment of the accidentá are continued to operate on at the Centre for Thyroid Tumours. Now they are 13-14 years old. The purpose of present research is to define clinicomorphological features of papillary thyroid carcinoma (PTC) in children of Belarus, operated on in different years after Chernobyl accident and, accordingly, with different latent period of tumour.

2. Pathomorphology

Histological specimens of thyroid carcinoma from 458 children 5-14 years, who underwent surgery at the Centre for Thyroid Tumours in Minsk from 1991 till 1997 were examined.

A size and histoarchitecture of predominant tumor node, intra- and extrathyroid lymphogenic dissemination, blood vessel and thyroid anatomical capsule invasion were estimated morphologically.

A number of clinical data - age of the patients at the moment of operation and at the moment of the Chernobyl accident, sex, residence of patients at the moment of Chernobyl accident and presence of distant metastases of PTC (primary discovered and relapses) were evaluated too.

At the time of Chernobyl Nuclear accident 76,5% of the patients were living in the mostly affected regions of Belarus Republic. The mean age of the patients at the moment of surgery was 10,9±0,1 years, it changed from 8,8±0,4 years in 1991 till 12,7±0,1 years in 1997. The mean age of the patients at the accident was 3,0±0,1 years. 71% of children underwent surgery before 4 years old. Five children were born after Chernobyl accident. Thyroid carcinomas were diagnosed in 303 girls and 155 boys. Sex ratio (F:M) in all examined cases was 1,95:1.

Papillary thyroid carcinoma was diagnosed in 96,5%, follicular in 2,6%, medullary thyroid carcinoma in 0,9%. Only cases of PTC were analysed in present research, as great prevailing of PTC was registered. According to the purpose of research, two groups of patients, operated on in 1991-1992 and in 1996-1997 were compared. The first goup consisted of 108 children. The mean age of the patients at the moment of operation was 8,8±0,4 years, sex ratio (F:M) was 1,6:1, hypothetic latent period was 5-6 years. The second group consisted of 149 children. The mean age of the patients at the moment of operation was 12,3±0,1 years, sex ratio (F:M) was 1,9:1, hypothetic latent period was 10-11 years [1].

Gross characteristic showed significant decreasing of the cases with diffuse growth of PTC, when on the section of thyroid gland were defined a lot of small tumour foci without predominant tumour node. In 1991-1992 years the percentage of such cases was 25,0, in 1996-1997 years - 2,0. At the same time there was no significant difference in the frequency of microcarcinomas - 45,2% and 34,9% accordingly in two groups of patients. The mean diameter of tumor node was 1,3+0,1 sm. It was not considerably changed in different years after the Chernobyl accident.

All papillary carcinomas were subdivided in accordance with predominant histological structures in tumor node for microscopic characteristic. "Pure" follicular, papillary, solid variants and "mixed" variants with prevailing follicular, solid and papillary structures and diffuse sclerosing variant (DSV) were picked out [4]. Diagnosis of DSV and follicular variant was made in accordance with criteria of Second Edition of Histological Typing of Thyroid Tumours (WHO) [2]. Papillary variant was classified if there were exclusively papillary structures in tumor node, solid variant - if solid component consisted of 70% of tumor. The frequency of different PTC variants presents in table 1.

Table 1
The frequency of papillary thyroid carcinoma variants

Variant	Number (%)
"Pure"follicular	68 (15,4%)
"Mixed" follicular	143 (32,5%)
"Pure" papillary	29 (6,5%)
"Mixed" papillary	103 (23,3%)
"Pure" solid	36 (8,1%)
"Mixed" solid	48 (10,8%)
Diffuse sclerosing	15 (3,4%)

In relation to duration of the latent period there were definite significant (p<0,05) changes of the structure of the different histological variants of papillary carcinoma. The part of variants with papillary structures ("pure" and "mixed") was decreased from 41,7% in 1991-1992 years till 20,8% in 1996-1997 years and DSV - from 7,4% till 0,7% accordingly in the course of time. The frequency of variants with follicular structures ("pure" and "mixed" follicular) was increased from 31,5% in 1991-1992 years till 57,7% in 1996-1997 years. These changes did not concern to the variants with solid structures ("pure" and "mixed" solid). In 1991-1992 and 1996-1997 years theirs frequencies were 19,5% and 19,4%.

Statistical analysis did not find any significant correlation between a patient's age and histological variant of PTC. Significant (p<0,05) decreasing of extrathyroid tumour growth frequency was registered in 1996-1997 years in comparison with 1991-1992 years - 42,4% and 74,1% accordingly. It can relate to different reasons and to the measures of timely diagnosis of thyroid tumors in children of Belarus Republic too. The same tendency is following in regard to the frequency of lymphogenic dissemination of carcinoma in thyroid gland in dependence on duration of latent period. It significantly (p<0,05) was decreased in 1996-1997 years in comparison with 1991-1992 years from 84,3% till 63,8%. However the frequency of PTC metastases to region lymph nodes was remaining quite high and invariable (72,2% and 69,8%).

Reverse correlation (p<0,05) between a patient's age at the moment of operation and frequency of thyroid anatomical capsule invasion, frequency and spreading of intra- and extrathyroid tumour dissemination was found. Another important property of PTC, blood vessel invasion, was defined in 34% of all cases. Table 2 shows its distribution in dependence on tumour histological features.

Table 2
The frequency of vascular invasion with different variants of PTC (1991-1997)

Variant	Number (%)
"Mixed" solid	20 (42,6%)
"Pure" solid	15 (41,7%)
"Mixed" papillary	35 (35,0%)
"Pure" papillary	10 (34,5%)
"Mixed" follicular	49 (34,5%)
Diffuse sclerosing	5 (33,3%)
"Pure" follicular	15 (22,1%)

There were clinical data about distant metastases in 375 patients. They were revealed in 52 children (13,9%). Table 3 shows distribution of cases with distant metastases according to histological variant of PTC.

Table 3
The frequency of blood metastases in patient with different variants of PTC (1991-1996)

Variant	Number (%)
Diffuse sclerosing	5 (33,3%)
"Mixed" solid	8 (21,0%)
"Mixed" papillary	14 (15,9%)
"Mixed" follicular	14 (11,9%)
"Pure" follicular	7 (11,3%)
"Pure" solid	3 (10,0%)
"Pure" papillary	1 (4,4%)

It is very interesting that blood vessel invasion of the papillary carcinoma was not found in half part of the histological slides in such patients. It was received data about dependence of distant metastases' frequency on patient's age - the younger child, the more often blood metastases were revealed ($p < 0,05$).

3. Immunohistochemical and Molecular Biology studies

Synthesis and storage of thyroglobulin in tumour cells identified by immunohistochemistry and hybridization in situ were analysed in 57 cases of PTC.

Comparative evaluation of immunohistochemistry and hybridization in situ data has not established any correlation between synthesis and storage of thyroglobulin by tumour cells. However, examination of thyroglobulin expression in solid, follicular and papillary structures of PTC permitted to define some features. Data of immunohistochemistry and hybridization in situ pointed to decreasing ($p<0,05$) of the level of thyroglobulin synthesis and storage in solid structures of papillary carcinoma. It is interesting with the relation to high frequency of blood vessel invasion and therefore risk of distant metastases in patients with predominant solid structures of PTC[3].

Also, analysis of hybridization in situ data has shown a certain dependence on the sex: boys have ($p<0,05$) thyroglobulin synthesis of tumour cells decreased without any bond with morphological types of PTC [5]. Decrease of thyroglobulin synthesis of tumour cells may witness about decrease of tumour grade differentiation. Alongside with other histological features, such correlation permits to expect a more severe follow-up of the disease. It is known that PTC is more rare in male than in female, but the prognosis of disease is less favorable in male. However, we cannot extrapolate received results to adults, as additional research will be required.

4. Conclusions

1. A significant ($p<0,05$) increasing of PTC cases with follicular structures and decreasing of PTC cases with papillary structures and diffuse sclerosing variant was defined with increasing of latent period. The number of PTC cases with solid structures was invariable in two groups of the patients.
2. The frequency of PTC metastases to regional lymph nodes was quite high and invariable in two groups of patients.
3. The decreasing ($p<0,05$) of expression and extrathyroid spreading and intrathyroid lymphogenic dissemination of PTC was revealed with the increasing of latent period.
4. There was no significant difference in frequency of blood vessel invasion in two groups of patients with PTC.
5. Reverse correlation ($p<0,05$) between a patient's age and the frequency of thyroid capsule invasion, extra- and intrathyroid tumour dissemination, blood metastases was found.

Acknowledgements

The authors wish to acknowledge the help of ECP8 and Copernicus partners from Western Europe in the preparation and conduct immunohistochemical and molucular biological studies.

60

References

1. Falk SA. Thyroid disease: Endocrinology, Surgery, Nuclear Medicine and Radiotherapy. New York: Raven Press, 1990: 401-471.
2. Hedinger C, Williams ED, Sobin LH. Histological Typing of Thyroid Tumours. Second Edition. London: Springer-Verlag, 1988.
3. Неровня АМ, Солдатенко ПП. Солидный вариант папиллярного рака щитовидной железы. Материалы первого конгресса морфологов Беларуси 26-27 сентября 1996 года. Минск, 1996: 67.
4. Черствой ЕД, Неровня АМ, Анищенко СЛ. Рак щитовидной железы у детей (морфологическая характеристика 142 случаев). Охрана материанства и детства в условиях воздействия последствий катастрофы на Чернобыльской АЭС. Материалы научных исследований 1993 года. Минск, 1993: 193-198.
5. Черствой ЕД, Неровня АМ, Пожарская ВП. Некоторые аспекты иммуногистохимической и молекулярно-биологической характеристики папиллярного рака щитовидной железы у детей. Архив патологии 1998; 2: 8-12.

THE POST-CHERNOBYL INCIDENCE OF CHILDHOOD THYROID CANCER IN UKRAINE

M. TRONKO, T. BOGDANOVA, I. KOMISARENKO, S. RYBAKOV,
A. KOVALENKO, O. EPSHTEIN, V. OLIYNYK AND V. TERESHCHENKO
*Institute of Endocrinology and Metabolism of the Academy of Medical Sciences,
Vyshgorodska Str.,69, Kyiv 254114, Ukraine
E-mail: tb@viaduk.net*

I. LIKHTAREV, I. KAIRO AND M. CHEPURNOY
*Research Centre of Radiation Medicine of the Academy of Medical Sciences,
Melnikov Str., 52, Kyiv 252050, Ukraine
E-mail: vil@rpi.kiev.ua*

An analysis of thyroid cancer incidence in children and adolescents of Ukraine (0-18 years of age at the time of surgery) showed that for the period 1986 to 1997 577 cases have been registered. Among 358 cases in children (0-14 years of age at the time of surgery) the incidence per 100000 children's population for the whole of Ukraine has increased from 0.05 (before the Chernobyl accident) to 0.11 in 1986-1990, 0.39 in 1991-1995, and 0.44 in 1996-1997. The increase of incidence takes place mainly at the expense of children who were aged in 1986 up to 5 years. In children aged up to 15 years, beginning from 1990, an increase of additional incidence has been noted with increase of thyroid exposure dose. In 290 patients who were operated at the Institute of Endocrinology, a majority of cases (>90%) represented papillary carcinomas. 53% of carcinomas belong to T_4 category according to TNM Classification. In 56.9% of cases regional metastases, and in 16.5% distant metastases in lungs have been revealed. Thus, the data presented concerning geographical, age distribution of thyroid cancer cases, their relationship with thyroid exposure dose, clinical and morphological characteristics, support the radiation genesis of these tumors.

Numerous investigations have demonstrated that the problem of thyroid diseases, in particular, of childhood thyroid cancer, is the most topical problem arisen after the Chernobyl accident.[1-5] Investigations carried out in the framework of national and international programmes at the V.P.Komisarenko Institute of Endocrinology and Metabolism of the Academy of Medical Sciences of Ukraine, led to creation of a clinical-morphological register, which includes all the cases of thyroid cancer in patients who were aged at the time of the accident up to 18 years. This register contains data on the age, sex, place of residence of the patient at the period of the Chernobyl accident and during the operation, duration of disease, results of clinical examinations, extent of surgery, data on thyroid exposure doses received, results of morphological studies of tumor.[6] The material accumulated covers thyroid cancer cases revealed in Ukraine in 1981 - 1997. This register is continually supplemented with information about new cancer cases, and available data are being corrected, what allows to analyse the up-to-date status of this disease in Ukraine in the above age groups.

When estimating the register's data depending on the age of patients with thyroid carcinoma at the moment of the accident, it should be noted that for the post-Chernobyl period (1986 to 1997) it has been registered in Ukraine 1109 cases of thyroid cancer in patients born in 1968 and later (0 to 18 years at the time of the accident). Among them 751 persons were children aged up to 15 years during the accident (0 to 14 years at the moment of the accident), and 358 were adolescents aged 15 to 18 years. 11 cases of thyroid carcinoma in children born after the Chernobyl accident were additionally included in the register. Thus, at present, the register includes 1120 cases of post-Chernobyl thyroid carcinomas.

According to their age at the time of surgery, the above patients were distributed as follows: 358 were children aged up to 15 years (0 to 14 years at the time of surgery); 219 were adolescents aged 15 to 18 years at the moment of surgery; and 543 were young adults aged 19 to 29 years, who were children and adolescents during the accident.

The rate of increase of the incidence is the highest in children operated at the age up to 15 years (Table 1). So, if for the period 1981 to 1985 25 cases of cancer in children (average: 5.0 a year) were registered, for 1986- 1990 their number was equal to 60 (average: 12 a year), and in 1991-1995 there were 206 cases (average: 41 a year). 56 cases in 1996 and 36 cases in 1997 (preliminary data) have been revealed. It should be noted that among 358 cases, 343 ones have been registered in children born before the accident; 4 cases in children born in the first months after the accident (radiation exposure of thyroid gland occurred during the last trimester of the mother's pregnancy); and only 11 cases were revealed in children who were born after the Chernobyl accident (1 case in 1992; 1 case in 1993; 1 case in 1994; 2 cases in 1995; 4 cases in 1996, and 2 cases in 1997).

Table 1. Number of thyroid cancer cases and incidence per 10^5 person-years for children aged 0–14 at the time of surgery in Ukraine.

	1986	1987	1988	1989	1990	1991	1992	1993	1994	1995	1996	1997
Num	8	7	8	11	26	22	49	44	44	47	56	36
Inc.	0.07	0.06	0.07	0.10	0.24	0.20	0.45	0.41	0.42	0.46	0.55	0.35

The incidence per 100,000 children's population for the whole of Ukraine for 1981-1985 fluctuated within 0.04 to 0.06, 0.05 on the average. In 1986-1990 this index increased by 2.2 times (0.11), in 1991-1995 by 7.8 times (0.39), and in 1996 by 11.2 times (0.56) as compared to the average rate before the Chernobyl accident. In 1997 the average incidence for the whole of Ukraine made 0.35 case per 100 thousand children (Table 1).

This increase of incidence took place mainly at the expense of 6 northern regions of Ukraine: Kyiv, Chernihiv, Zhytomir, Cherkasy, Rivne oblasts and city of Kyiv, where the highest contamination with iodine radioisotopes as a result of the accident was noted (Table 2).

Table 2. Incidence of thyroid cancers per 10^5 person-years for children aged 0–14 at the time of surgery in 6 northern regions and other regions of Ukraine.

	1986	1987	1988	1989	1990	1991	1992	1993	1994	1995	1996	1997
6 reg	0.13	0	0.09	0.18	0.51	0.61	1.60	1.30	1.30	1.60	1.90	1.40
Oth.	0.06	0.08	0.07	0.08	0.17	0.10	0.17	0.18	0.21	0.19	0.23	0.11

In these 6 regions the average annual incidence for 1981-1985 made only 0.009 (one case of cancer in a child from Cherkasy oblast). In 1986-1990 the incidence rate increased in the mentioned regions until 0.18, what is twice as high as the total rate for the other 21 regions (0.09). In 1991-1995 the incidence already made 1.28 and was 7.5 times as high as in other regions. In 1996-1997 the incidence per 100 thousand children for the 6 mentioned regions (1.6) already exceeded by 9.4 times the average rate for the rest of Ukraine.

A special attention should be paid to the data on the incidence among children evacuated from the towns of Pripyat, Chernobyl, and the settlements of the Chernobyl district. Last years, the highest rates have been registered in this group. The first case of thyroid cancer among children who have been evacuated from the above regions has been revealed in 1990. During the period 1991 to 1997, their number reached 17, and, as a whole, for all the period analysed their number makes 17. The age, at the time of the accident, of all the children operated did not exceed 9 years, and the average annual incidence for the above period reached 27.0 per 100 thousand evacuated children of this age group.

An analysis of the incidence of malignant thyroid tumors in adolescents who have been operated at the age of 15 to 18, showed that in 1981-1985 34 cases, and in 1986-1997 219 cases of cancer have been revealed. The average number of cases in this group of patients before the Chernobyl accident made 7 cases a year; in the first years after the accident - 10; in 1991-1995 - 22; in 1996 - 29; and in 1997 - 26 cases a year (Table 3). A trustworthy increase in the incidence of malignant thyroid tumors in adolescents has been reported later than in children, beginning from 1994, and, as appears from the above data, it had a less pronounced character as compared to the same rate in children.

Table 3. Number of thyroid cancer cases and incidence per 10^5 person-years for adolescents aged 15–18 at the time of surgery in Ukraine.

	1986	1987	1988	1989	1990	1991	1992	1993	1994	1995	1996	1997
Num	7	8	8	15	14	21	18	18	27	28	29	26
Inc.	0.24	0.27	0.27	0.50	0.47	0.71	0.61	0.61	0.93	0.96	0.99	0.89

This fact is also confirmed by recounting the number of cancer cases per 100 thousand adolescent's population (Table 3), what is evidence that during the period analysed the incidence among adolescents in Ukraine exceeded the rate before Chernobyl (0.24 on the average for the period 1981-1985) in 1986-1990 by 1.5 time (average: 0.35); in 1991-1995 by 3.2 times (average 0.77); in 1996 by 4.1 times (0.99), and in 1997 (preliminary data) by 3.7 times (0.89 per 100 thousand adolescents).

In these 6 most affected regions thyroid cancer incidence in adolescents also exceeded the same rate for the rest of Ukraine for the period of the noted increase (1990 to 1997) to a less extent than in children: by 3.1 times (Table 4).

Table 4. Incidence of thyroid cancers per 10^5 person-years for adolescents aged 15–18 at the time of surgery in 6 northern regions and other regions of Ukraine.

	1986	1987	1988	1989	1990	1991	1992	1993	1994	1995	1996	1997
6 reg	0	0.68	0.17	0.51	0.85	1.40	1.20	1.60	3.00	1.60	1.70	2.30
Oth.	0.30	0.17	0.30	0.50	0.38	0.55	0.46	0.38	0.43	0.81	0.81	0.55

An analysis of the distribution of all the 566 children and adolescents (except 11 post-Chernobyl cases) depending on their age at the time of the accident, showed that in 1986-1990 the proportion of children who were aged, during the accident, up to 5 years made 13.4%, and of those aged from 5 to 9 years - 23.2% (in all 36,6%). In 1991-1995 the proportion of children aged, during the accident, 0 to 4 years increased by 3 times (until 40.8%), and of those aged 5 to 9 years by 1.9 time (until 43.1%). The total rate was 2.3 times as high as the previous one, reaching 83.9%.

In 1996-1997 the proportion of children aged 0 to 4 years during the accident among the patients furtherly affected by thyroid cancer, already made 66.2%, while the part of children 5-9 years decreased until 33.8%. It should be stressed that the proportion of children aged 10 to 14 years during the accident and of adolescents aged 15 to 18 years is, on the contrary, gradually decreasing from 43.8% (children aged 10-14) and 19.6% (adolescents aged 15-18) in 1986-1990 until 16.1% and 0%, respectively, in 1991-1995. In 1996-1997 these age groups were absent (Table 5).

Table 5. Age distribution of children and adolescents operated on for a thyroid cancer
in 1986-1997 (at the time of the accident).

Age group	1986	1987	1988	1989	1990	1991	1992	1993	1994	1995	1996	1997
in utero	0	0	0	0	0	0	1	1	0	0	1	1
0-4	0	0	0	1	14	7	29	24	31	36	51	41
5-9	2	2	6	5	11	15	22	26	34	37	29	18
10-14	6	6	5	17	15	21	14	10	5	0	0	0
15-18	7	7	5	3	0	0	0	0	0	0	0	0
Total	15	15	16	26	40	43	66	61	70	73	81	60

It follows from the above that, despite an increase in time interval after the accident and in spite of an increase, from year to year, of the mean age of the subjects operated on, the most marked increase of incidence mainly took place at the expense of children who were aged in 1986 up to 5 years and whose thyroid gland was the most sensitive to the radioactive iodine effect.

Characterizing 290 cases of thyroid carcinomas which were removed in children and adolescents at the Clinic of the Institute of Endocrinology and Metabolism during the period 1986-1997 according to TNM system, it should be noted that 53.1% of tumors belonged to T_4 category in case of infiltrative tumor growth out of the thyroid capsule. There were only 6 tumors measuring less than 1 cm, i.e. microcarcinomas, and they made 2.1% from the total number of the cases observed. Lymph node dissection was performed in 57.3% of cases in children and adolescents. Microscopicaly unilateral metastases in regional lymph nodes were noted in 29.3%, bilateral ones in 27.6% of patients. As a whole, metastases in regional lymph nodes were revealed in 56.9% of children and adolescents having been operated on at our Institute. Distant metastases in lungs at preoperative period were reported in 3.8% of patients by radiological investigations (Table 6). Furthermly, at different terms after thyroidectomy, using radioiodine diagnosis, lung metastases were revealed in 48 from 290 children and adolescents having been operated on at our Institute in post-Chernobyl years, what made 16.5% from the total number of cases, distant metastases being reported in children much more often (in 18.7%) than in adolescents (6.1%).

Table 6. Thyroid cancer for TNM-system (1986–1997).

Category		Number of patients	%
T_1	tumor less than 1 cm	6	2,1
T_2	tumor from 1 to 4 cm	88	30,3
T_3	tumor more than 4 cm	42	14,5
T_4	tumor of any size with growth out of thyroid capsule	154	53,1
N_1	one side regional metastases	85	29,3
N_2	both side regional metastases	80	27,6
M_1	distant metastases	11	3,8

When choosing the surgical tactics for thyroid cancer in children and adolescents, thyroidectomy was the treatment of choice. Total or near-total thyroidectomy was performed in 83.1% of cases. In 17 cases a final thyroidectomy was performed after organ-preserving surgery performed in other clinics.

Among possible postoperative complications, an unilateral paresis of recurrent nerve took place in 5.5% of cases and a bilateral paresis in 8.6%. A persistent postoperative hypoparathyroidism was noted in 6.5% of patients.

In June 1996, the Department for radioiodine diagnosis and radioiodine therapy for patients who have been operated for a thyroid cancer, has begun functioning at the Institute of Endocrinology and Metabolism. Formerly, children and adolescents were treated in other medical establishments of Ukraine.

249 children and adolescents operated on for a thyroid cancer, in which scintigraphy revealed residual thyroid tissue, regional and distant metastases, are followed up in the above Department. In 145 from them (58.2%) metastases in regional lymph nodes, and in 60 patients (24.1%) distant metastases in lungs were noted. Therapy with radioactive iodine was successful in 44.1% of patients with regional metastases and in 31.7% of patients with distant metastases. The rest of patients are being followed up and they continue to receive courses of radioiodine therapy.

An analysis of the relationship between the incidence rate of thyroid cancer and thyroid exposure dose received has been performed for five northern regions of Ukraine where the highest contamination following the Chernobyl accident took place: Kyiv (including the city of Kyiv) oblast, Chernihiv, Zhytomir, Cherkasy and Rivne oblasts. An estimate of the average age-related thyroid exposure dose was made taking into account the place of residence of the child or adolescent with thyroid carcinoma at the time of the accident. [2,5]

For the children operated at the age of 0 to 14 years at the moment of surgery, a constant increase of additional incidence was noted, beginning from 1990, practically in all dose zones. The most important increase was noted for the zone with the highest mean exposure rate: more than 1 Gy (Table 7). The importance of this fact becomes more evident if we take into account that the cohort of subjects aged 0 to 14 years at the moment of surgery decreases in number with each period of observation, and this cohort consists of more and more young age groups at the moment of exposure.

Table 7. Thyroid cancer incidence per 10^5 person-years and excess incidence for children aged 0–14 at the time of operation in the dose zones of the five northern regions of Ukraine.

Thyroid dose, Gy	1986–1987		1988–1989		1990–1991		1992–1993		1994–1995		1996-1997	
	Incidence	Excess Incidence[1]	Incidence	Excess Incidence[1]	Incidence	Excess Incidence[1]	Incidence	Excess Incidence[1]	Incidence	Excess Incidence[1]	Incidence	Excess Incidence[1]
0.01+	0	0	0.21	0.10	0.26	0.13	0.31	0.16	0.82	0.64	0.58	0.37
0.05+	0.13	0.04	0.25	0.14	0.72	0.59	1.69	1.54	2.46	2.28	2.56	2.35
0.1+	0	0	0	0	0.26	0.13	2.28	2.13	4.14	3.96	4.66	4.45
0.3+	0	0	0	0	2.13	2.00	3.37	3.22	5.23	5.05	13.67	13.46
0.5+	0	0	0	0	2.91	2.78	10.86	10.71	0.94	0.76	13.40	13.19
1.0+	0	0	0	0	0	0	22.66	22.50	22.42	22.24	42.57	42.36

[1] - excess incidence = incidence – baseline incidence; baseline incidence for children aged 0–14 is estimated for age distribution of Ukraine in 1989 (Census data) as varied from 0.095 cases per 10^5 person-years in 1986–1987 up to 0.2101 cases per 10^5 person-years in 1996-1997.

In adolescents aged 15-18 years there was no significant relationship between excess incidence and thyroid dose (Table 8).

Table 8. Thyroid cancer incidence per 10^5 person-years and excess incidence for adolescents aged 15–18 at the time of operation in the dose zones of the five northern regions of Ukraine.

Thyroid dose, Gy	1986–1987		1988–1989		1990–1991		1992–1993		1994–1995		1996-1997	
	Incidence	Excess Incidence[1]	Incidence	Excess Incidence[1]	Incidence	Excess Incidence[1]	Incidence	Excess Incidence[1]	Incidence	Excess Incidence[1]	Incidence	Excess Incidence[1]
0.01+	0	0	0	0	0.67	0.29	1.37	0.99	1.44	1.06	0	0
0.05+	0.32	0	0.15	0	0.91	0.53	1.88	1.49	2.36	1.98	2.38	1.99
0.1+	0	0	0.36	0	1.38	1.00	0	0	2.57	2.19	1.09	0.71
0.3+	3.21	2.83	1.51	1.12	3.00	2.62	1.54	1.16	0	0	5.93	5.55
0.5+	0	0	0	0	0	0	1.59	1.20	3.19	2.81	1.58	1.20
1.0+	0	0	0	0	0	0	0	0	0	0	12.67	12.28

[1] - excess incidence = incidence – baseline incidence; baseline incidence for adolescents aged 15-18 is estimated for age distribution of Ukraine in 1989 (Census data) as 0.385 cases per 10^5 person-years every period of observation.

A morphological analysis of thyroid carcinomas removed in children and adolescents at the Clinic of the Institute of Endocrinology and Metabolism of the Academy of Medical Sciences of Ukraine in 1986-1997 showed that an overwhelming majority of tumors were represented by papillary carcinomas (93% in children and 91% in adolescents).

Papillary carcinomas were subdivided into the following histological subtypes: typical papillary variant, solid-follicular variant, and diffuse-sclerotic variant. Typical papillary variant was revealed in 10.7% of cases in children and in 26.0% of cases in adolescents; solid-follicular variant in 79.8% of cases in children and in 69.6% of cases in adolescents; diffuse-sclerotic variant in 7.5% of cases in children and in 2.2% of cases in adolescents. Therefore, thyroid carcinomas removed in children and adolescents after the Chernobyl accident were represented in a majority of cases by papillary forms, mainly with solid-follicular structure. Solid-follicular variants of tumors, as our previous studies showed, manifested high invasive properties, showing signs of intraglandular and extrathyroid spreading, lymphatic and blood invasion. [7-9]

Moreover, it has been demonstrated an increase in the incidence and risk of development of the above histological variant of papillary carcinoma with increase of thyroid exposure dose of radioactive iodine during the Chernobyl accident, what is an additional evidence of the radiation origin of the carcinomas studied. [9]

Thus, the data presented concerning geographical, age distribution of thyroid cancer cases, their relationship with thyroid exposure dose, clinical and morphological characteristics, support the radiation genesis of these tumors.

References

1. Kazakov V, Demidchik E, Astakhova L. Thyroid cancer after Chernobyl. *Nature* 1992; **359:** 21-23.
2. Likhtarev IA, Sobolev BG, Kairo IA, Tronko ND, Bogdanova TI, Oleinic VA, Epshtein EV, Beral V. Thyroid cancer in the Ukraine. *Nature* 1995; **375:** 365.
3. *The radiological consequences of the Chernobyl accident.* Brussels-Luxemburg: ECSC-EC-EAEC, 1996: 1192 p.
4. *The Chernobyl Accident. Thyroid Abnormalities in children, Congenital Abnormalities and other radiation related information. The First Ten Years.* Takeichi N, Satow Y, Masterson RH, ed. Hiroshima: Nakamoto Sogo Printing, 1996: 271 a.
5. Jacob P, Goulko G, Heidenreich WF, Likhtarev I, Kairo I, Tronko ND, Bogdanova TI, Kenigsberg J, Buglova E, Drozdovitch V, Golovneva A, Demidchik EP, Beral V. Thyroid cancer risk to children calculated. *Nature* 1998; **392:** 31-32.
6. Tronko N, Epstein Ye, Oleinik V, Bogdanova TI, Likhtarev I, Gulko G, Kairo I, Sobolev B. Thyroid gland in children after Chernobyl accident (yersterday and today). In: Sh Nagataki, ed. *Nagasaki Symposium on Chernobyl: Update and Future,* Excerpta Medica, Intern. Congress Series 1074: Elsevier, 1994:31-46.
7. Bogdanova T, Bragarnik M, Tronko ND, Harach YR, Thomas GA, E.D.Williams. Childhood thyroid cancer after Chernobyl. *J Endocrinol* 1995; **144:** 25.
8. *Molecular, cellular, biological characterization of childhood thyroid cancer.* ED Williams and ND Tronko, ed. Brussels-Luxemburg: ECSC-EC-EAEC, 1996: 105 p.
9. Tronko M, Bogdanova T. *Thyroid cancer in children of Ukraine (Consequences of the Chernobyl accident).* Kyiv: Chornobylinterniform, 1997: 200 p (in Russian).

of the study area and less in the ... ...
thyroid cancer cases. For the study area in Belarus and for the whole study area the
cumulative distributions of the collective thyroid dose and the number of thyroid cancer
cases are similar, indicating ... ... quantities ... Belarus and
Russia the situation is less uniform. In the study area about 75% of the population
has thyroid doses below 0.4 Gy, ... and the collective thyroid
dose and the number of ... ... of the Chernobyl ... population has thyroid
doses above or equal to 0.4 Gy ... ...
In the study area ... ...

Table 1: Observed number of thyroid cancer cases and expected number for development of thyroid cancer.

1976-1979		
1980-1985		
1986		

4. Discussion

Although studies of thyroid cancer ... ...
longer time of follow-up than the observation since after the Chernobyl accident
and ... the observation ... ... it is interesting to
compare the results.

The EAR/PD for ages at exposure of 5-15 years found in this study for
exposures after the Chernobyl accident is comparable to the risk observed ...

THYROID RETROSPECTIVE DOSIMETRY PROBLEMS IN UKRAINE. ACHIEVEMENTS AND DELUSIONS

I.LIKHTAREV, I.KAYRO, V.SHPAK, N.TALERKO

Radiation Protection Institute, 53 Melnikova Street, Kiev-50, Ukraine
E-mail: rpi@public.ua.net, vlad@rpi.kiev.ua

In this report we consider questions on history of thyroid retrospective dosimetry in Ukraine, arguments for revision of dose assessments, methodology and some results of modern revision of dose assessments, and problem of uncertainty of assessments. Modern retrospection in Ukraine is conducted in order to include the real dynamics of territories' contamination into the system of retrospective dosimetry of thyroid exposure. This new system utilizes results obtained using the Atmospheric transport model (LEDI), Multicomponent thyroid intake function model (MIM) and Age average dose model (ADM). Revision of doses for those measured has led to correction (decrease) of dose estimates in average by factor ranging from $0.54 - 0.83$ with 90% quantile from 0.23 to 1.12 for the territories with different dynamics of air contamination with ^{131}I.

1 History of retrospective thyroid dosimetry in Ukraine

Researches on thyroid retrospective dosimetry in Ukraine have been conducted for 12 years. *During the first years* after the Chernobyl accident the aims of retrospective dosimetry had been the following: instant damage assessment and prediction of possible consequences. On this early stage a certain conservatism of obtained estimates proved to be unavoidable. Therefore, during the first post-accident year dose estimates had been based on results of thyroid activity measurements without taking into account the quality of these measurements and using the simple single intake model. This latter approximation only contained 1.5-2 divisible conservatism level [1].

During the consequent years the main aim of retrospective dosimetry had been, first of all, the revealing of those territories where the thyroid doses in the population had been the highest. The additional incentive for retrospective-dosimetry studies was the state legislation of Ukraine. In the Ukrainian legislation all decisions on granting privileges and compensations and provision of social compensations' policies to the suffered contingents depended on thyroid doses' values. On this stage the model of prolonged intake of thyroid activity was used for dose calculations with *assumption of a single release* as of 26 April 1986. This led to specification (decrease) of the initial dose estimates by 30-50% [1]. All the studies in the area of retrospective dosimetry had been conducted with the final aim of average age dose estimation in each settlement of Ukraine. Retrospection became the main matter of a special national program "Thyrodosimetric passportization of Ukraine". The method of retrospection was based on assessing regressional dependence among doses obtained through direct measurements and a series of important indirect data.

72

These data contains most of all levels of radiocaesium contamination in a settlement for further extrapolation of established dependencies on territories without thyroid activity measurements. Extrapolation was conducted within selected sectors and segments with uniform dynamics of radioiodine contamination considering the motion direction of radioactive clouds of accident's release origin [2].

Besides to the above-mentioned aims of retrospective dosimetry the more important role has been given to dosimetry support of epidemiological studies and obtaining specified estimates of risk of thyroid exposure's stochastic effects. This led to an increase in demands for accuracy of definition of all the epidemiological process' components, namely: quantity of cancer cases, number of human-years under observation and thyroid exposure. Exactly on this stage there is also a sharp increase in demands for quality of dose estimates' retrospection, reliability and, finally, the demands increase for narrowing of the uncertainties interval.

Even though the method described above had been used for reconstruction of average age doses in 20865 settlements in 17 oblasts' of Ukraine from 1992 till 1996, by 1997 enough reasons have been accumulated for improvement of calculation-methodical background and for conduction of the next dose estimates' revision

2 Arguments for revision of dose assessments

Since 1997 there has been commenced development of a new strategy for retrospective dosimetry and preparation for the next revision of thyroid exposure dose estimates. The reasons for this revision were as follows:

- Significance of registration of contamination dynamics and especially of the commencement and the finishing of fallout in assessing doses for those measured;

- Revision of calibration coefficients;

- Insufficiency of information on local ^{137}Cs fallout;

- New sources of information (meteorology, questionnaires);

- Expansion of knowledge due to utilization of methods, models, technologies from adjacent areas (model of atmospheric transport, GIS technologies, modeling of dynamic systems);

- Improvement of intake function model in order to utilize individual questionnaires' information.

3 Main features of modern dose retrospection

Informational background for creation of new models and, finally, for revision of previous dose estimates were the following geocoded databases (DB):

- DB of settlements;

- DB of environment monitoring, Cs, γ-dose rate, meteorological data, fallout;

- DB of thyroid activity measurements;

- DB of questionnaires.

Utilization of the above-mentioned sources of information allowed developing and parameterizing the three models as a main set of instruments on the following stages of dose revision:

a) development, adjustment, testing and verification of models – Atmospheric transport model (LEDI), Multicomponent thyroid intake function model (MIM) and Age average thyroid dose model (ADM);

b) calculation of ^{131}I concentration field in the air above Ukraine and spatial – time GIS-quires for reconstruction of dynamics of daily ^{131}I concentration in each settlement;

c) calculation of individual doses for those measured under the MIM model;

d) calculation of average age doses using the LEDI and MIM for areas with no measurements.

3.1 Atmospheric transport model

In order to recreate picture of atmospheric spreading of radionuclides released in the initial period of the Chernobyl accident there has been used a regional model of atmospheric transport LEDI [3]. For the Chernobyl accident the model has been verified on the data of radioactive contamination's measurements of the Ukrainian territory with [137]Cs [4, 5]. The calculations conducted have enabled to explain formation of the major large-scale spots of radioactive contamination on the territory of Ukraine.

The Langrangian-Eulerian diffusion model of admixture transport in the atmosphere considers:

- unstationarity (daily movement of characteristics of the frontier atmospheric layer or weather changes) and spatial heterogeneity of atmospheric meteorological characteristics;

- different types of source by the length of release (instantaneous, prolonged, stationary), by the phase composition (gas, aerosol), by the isotope composition;

For the studies on thyrodosimetric passportization there are used the results in forms of *volumetric concentration of radioactivity in the frontier layer*.

The model utilizes the following input information:

- meteorological information (three-dimensional wind fields and temperatures in the lowest atmospheric layer, data on the quantity of rainfall on the meteorological watch network);

- data on the parameters of release (power of release, its phase-nuclide composition etc.).

As the input meteorological information there have been used data from atmospheric radio-sounding conducted by the system of aerological stations of Goscomgidromet (State committee for hydro-meteorology) of the former USSR. It included the measured vertical temperature's profiles, speeds and directions of wind, pressures in 9 points of sounding located in Ukraine and also in Gomel (Belorussia) and Kursk (Russia) from 26 April 1986 till 7 May 1986. The soundings were conducted 4 times a day every 6 hours.

In order to calculate wet disposition of admixture with atmospheric rainfall in the process model there has been used information from rainfall-measurement network of Goscomgidromet of Ukraine on 103 meteostations and 411 meteoposts in Ukraine (including 22 meteostations and 47 meteoposts on the territories of Kiev, Zhitomir and Chernigiv oblasts).

Data on the time motion of ^{131}I release intensity during the first 10 days after the accident were taken from [6]. It is known that in the accidental release's radioiodine was in three different physical-chemical forms, namely: aerosol, molecular and organic, for which speeds of precipitation differ. In model calculations we included the "affective" speed of dry precipitation of radioiodine. The value of this parameter was set at 0.7 cm s^{-1}.

3.2 Multicomponent thyroid intake function model

In order to model the function of ^{131}I intake into thyroid there is used a multicomponent model describing the dynamics of radioiodine intake into major pathways: air, leafy vegetables and milk. Mathematical description of the model is a system of equations describing the dynamics of activity as stated below.

$$V(t,s,q_0)=q_0\times\sum_J \int_0^\infty V_{js}\, e^{-\lambda_a t}\, dt\,, \quad j\in\left\{1,...,n_s\right\}$$ 　　Air

$$dy_1(t)/dt=-\lambda_g\, y_1(t)+b_1 V(t,s,q_0),\quad y_1(0)=0;$$ 　　Grass, leafy vegetables

$$dy_2(t)/dt=-\lambda_m\, y_2(t)+b_2\, y_1,\quad y_2(0)=0);$$ 　　Milk

$$U(t,age)=w_{Th}\times(w_{inh}(age)\,V(t,s,q_0)+$$ 　　Intake function

$$+\,w_1(age)\,y_1(t)\,+\,w_m(age)\,y_2(t))$$

$$dA(t;age)/dt = -\lambda(age)\,A(t;age)+U(t,age),\quad a(0)=0$$ 　　Thyroid

The following parameters are used in the model:

$\lambda a, \lambda g, \lambda m, \lambda(age)$ - effective loss constants for air, leafy vegetables, milk and thyroid, reference data [7,8];

b_1 and b_2 - coefficients of effectiveness of transition from air into pasture grass and from grass into milk [7];

w_{th}, $w_{inh}(age)$, $w_l(age)$, $w_m(age)$ - parameters of capture of ^{131}I from blood by thyroid, effectiveness of activity's transition into blood through inhalations multiplied by the age level of ventilation, age levels of leafy vegetables and milk consumption, values of parameters are taken from literature sources [9] and DB questionnaires;

V_{js}, - average daily specific ^{131}I concentration in the near-soil air layer on the days (j) of arrival of radioactive clouds to a settlement s, there are used the results of calculations under the LEDI model;

q_0 - factor of model activity values' correction under results of individual measurements.

3.3 Age average dose model

Transition from individual doses under direct measurements to retrospective reconstruction of age average doses by settlements is accomplished under the Age average dose model (ADM). Statistical model represents logarithms of individual doses for persons of age a in a settlement k (ε_{aik}) as a sum of logarithm of a dose normalized by all the ages at a given settlement (m_k) and a logarithm of age correction factor ξ_{ai}, which reflects age and individual mutability of dose:

$$\varepsilon_{aik} = m_k + \xi_{ai},$$

where ξ_{ai} – has normal distribution with parameters

$$\xi_{ai} \cong N\left(\mu_a, \delta_a^2\right).$$

Numerical methods of solving the equation of maximum likelihood function in samples of measurements in urban and rural settlements in each oblast' define estimates of unknown parameters:

- vector of parameters' estimates $\{m_k^*\}$ with dimension K, where K – is the number of settlements in a sample;

- vector of age parameters' estimates $\{\mu_a^*\}$ with dimension A, where A – is the number of considered age groups (usually equaling to 19);

- vector of age parameters' estimates $\{\delta_a^{2*}\}$ (with dimension A).

Average dose for age a in a settlement k is calculated as follows:

$$\overline{D}_{ak}^* = exp\left(m_k^* + \mu_a^* + 0.5\delta_a^{2*}\right).$$

4 Results

The result of dose estimates' revision for those measured was analyzed using the ψ-correction factor, which is the ratio of individual dose calculated under the model of real duration of fallouts D_i^{pf} to the previous dose estimate under the model of single fallouts D_i^{sf}:

$$\psi = \frac{D_i^{pf}}{D_i^{sf}}.$$

Distribution of ψ-factor in oblasts with measurements bears multi-modal character, which reflects the complicated picture of dynamics of formation of air contamination with ^{131}I. The average value of the ψ-factor in oblasts with measurements and the 90% quantile of its distribution are shown in table 1 below.

Table 1. Spatial distribution of ψ correction factor

Oblast'	Children aged 0-7 y			Children aged 8-18 y		
	n	Mean ψ	90% quantile	n	Mean ψ	90% quantile
Kiev	3127	0.54	[0.23; 0.80]	23059	0.57	[0.31; 0.79]
Zhitomir	9492	0.66	[0.36; 0.92]	20818	0.64	[0.34; 0.97]
Chernigiv	15822	0.83	[0.55; 1.09]	20958	0.83	[0.58; 1.12]
30 –km zone	691	0.61	[0.25; 0.89]	2196	0.72	[0.30; 0.97]
Pripyat' town	622	0.75	[0.31; 0.93]	2132	0.82	[0.47; 1.00]

5 Conclusions

Retrospective reconstruction of the real dynamics of radioiodine contamination of territory and utilization of a new calculation-method base has led to correction (decrease) of dose estimates for those measured in average by factor ranging from 0.54 – 0.83 with 90% quantile from 0.23 to 1.12 for the territories with different dynamics of air contamination with ^{131}I.

The preliminary results of the latest dose revision based on specified retrospective-dosimetry models inevitably lead to revision of the previously calculated and published estimates of risk of radio-induced thyroid cancer cases for Ukrainian children.

Analysis of correlations between the average age thyroid activity over a settlement with its modal value obtained under the LEDI and MIM evidences that together with rayons in which there is observed a high (with correlation coefficient up to 0.88) functional dependence between the considered values, there stand out territories where such dependence is not established. This evidences that further development of the LEDI model is required.

The authors have dedicated this article to the *problems* of retrospective dosimetry. What are the delusions? Our almost 12-year experience indicates that the naïve hopes of epidemiologists for obtaining the "final" dose estimates are nothing but delusions. We are not the pioneers of discovering this conclusion because half-a-century history of dose support of epidemiological researches on victims of atomic bombings proves this conclusion.

6 Acknowledgements

This study was supported by the INCO-COPERNICUS project IC15CT960306 of the European Commission, and by Ministry of emergency situations of Ukraine. We want to thank our collaborators from GSF-Institut für Strahlenschutz: P.Jacob, W.F.Heidenreich and G.Goulko for the constant friendly cooperation and help in work performed.

References

1. Likhtarev IA, Shandala NK, Gulko GM, Kairo IA, Chepurny NI (1993) Ukrainian thyroid doses after the Chernobyl accident. *Health Physics* **64**:594-599.

2. Likhtarev I, Sobolev B. Kairo I, Tabachny L, Jacob P, Pröhl G, Goulko (1996) Results of large scale thyroid dose reconstruction in Ukraine. In *The radiological consequences of the Chernobyl accident*, Karaoglou A, Desmet G, Kelly GN, Menzel HG (eds) pp 1021-1034. EUR 16544 EN.

3. Buikov M. V., Garger E. K. and Talerko N. N. (1992) Research into the formation of spotted pattern of radioactive fallout with the Lagrangian-Eulerian model. *Meteorologiya i gidrologiya*, **12**: 33 - 45 (in Russian).

4. Buikov MV, Garger EK, Talerko NN (1995) The application of Lagrangian-Eulerian model of aerosol transfer to the interpretation of the spot pattern of the field of radioactive contamination due to Chernobyl NPP accident. In *Extended Synopses of an International Symposium on Environmental Impact of Radioactive Releases*, pp 143-144. IAEA, Vienna.

5. Talerko NN, Kuzmenko AG, Likhtarev IA (1997) Modeling of consequences of a severe radiation accident for different meteorological conditions of radioactive release transport in the atmosphere. In *Collection of reports from scientific-practical conference "Science. Chernobyl-96"*, pp 28-36. Kiev, Ukraine (in Russian)

6. Izrael YA (Ed) (1990) Chernobyl: Radiation Contamination of Environment, pp 87-90. Gidrometeizdat Leningrad (in Russian).

7. Müller H, Pröhl G. (1993) ECOSYS-87: A Dynamic model for assessing radiological consequences of nuclear accidents. *Health Physics* **64**: 232-252.

8. Arephjeva ZS, Badjin VI, Gavrilin YI, Gordeev KI, Ilyin LA, Krjuchkov VP, Margulis UY, Osanov DP, Krusch VT **(1988)**. Guidance on thyroid dose estimation during the intake of iodine radioisotopes into the human organism. Energoatomizdat, Moscow (in Russian)

9. International Commission on Radiological Protection (1989) Age-dependent doses to members of the public from intakes of radionuclides (part 1). Oxford: Pergamon Press; ICRP Publication 56.

DEVELOPMENT OF CANCER AND NON-CANCER THYROID DISEASES IN CHILDREN AND ADOLESCENTS AFTER THE CHERNOBYL ACCIDENT

A.F. TSYB, V.V .SHAKHTARIN, E.F. LUSHNIKOV, V.F. STEPANENKO, V.P. SNYKOV, E.M. PARSHKOV, S.F. TROFIMOVA,

Medical Radiological Research Center of Russian Academy of Medical Sciences, Koroliov str. 4, Obninsk, 249020, Russia

Findings of the study show that iodine deficiency in combination with radiation make effect on frequency of occurrence of thyroid abnormalities. Effect of radiation on occurrence of non-cancer thyroid disorders, in particular diffuse euthyroid goitre and nodules, is manifested if radiation dose to the target is above 100 cGy against the background of iodine deficiency (renal iodine excretion is less than 7.5 µg/dl). Iodine deficiency is a factor increasing ERR/Dm of thyroid cancer. The results of the study allow one to suggest that the effect of radiation on the thyroid can be reduced by minimising iodine deficiency in the affected territories.

The effect of radiation on induction of thyroid abnormalities is widely discussed in scientific literature. Nowadays the effect of radiation on development of malignant and benign thyroid tumors is recognized[1,7,9,10,12]. Radiation-induced thyroiditis is suggested to be developed if radiation dose to the thyroid is higher than certain threshold [8]. Change of functional activity of hypophysial-thyroid system in children exposed to radiation due to the Chernobyl accident is observed in 1986-1987[2,5].

At the same time it is commonly recognized that iodine deficiency influences the development of all thyroid abnormalities including thyroid cancer [3].

It is known that almost all the most affected territories of Belorus, Russia and the Ukraine are zones of goitre endemy[4]. Until middle sixties iodine prophylactics was conducted there]. Therefore association of thyroid abnormalities with radiation due to the Chernobyl accident should be examined with consideration for existing iodine deficiency.

In Russia the most affected territories are in the following 7 south-western raions of Bryansk oblast: Gordeevsky, Klintsovsky, Zlynkovsky, Klimovsky, Krasnogorsky, Novozybkovsky and Starodubsky. The level of soil contamination with ^{137}Cs ranges from 1 to more than 40 Ci/km^2. The size of population of the most affected areas is about 500 thousand persons.

Nonuniform contamination of limited territory with radionuclides, the large size of the affected population as well as existence of goitre endemy are the basis for the study of combined effect of radiation and iodine deficiency on development of thyroid abnormalities.

Materials and methods

1. Iodine deficiency was estimated by renal excretion of iodine. Seven affected and three "clean" (<1 Ci/km^2) raions of Bryansk oblast were taken in the study. Concentration of iodine in urine was measured by arcenid-cerium method. Iodine deficiency was estimated by the concentration of iodine in urine according to recommendations of WHO/UNICEF, 1992. 3070 residents of 75 settlements of the raions in the study were examined. A settlement was selected with consideration for the following terms: regular iodine prophylactics was not undertaken in the previous calendar year; distribution of settlements over the territory of a raion is homogenous. Those who got iodine-containing and thyroid pharmaceuticals during the last 6 months were excluded from the study wherever possible.

2. Demographic information for every settlement under the study was reproduced from census of 1989. In April 1986 119,785 persons born from 1968 to 1986 were living in the studied areas.

3. Reconstruction of dose from ^{131}I to every age group in every settlement was performed. Estimation of the effective radiation dose to the thyroid of those residing in the affected areas is very complicated task. It is still topical problem. The experts have arrived at the conclusion that existing models for thyroid dose reconstruction are appropriate and can be used in practice[6]. Models described in the article of Stepanenko et al.[11] were employed in the study.

4. Clinical examination of the thyroid was performed for 37,042 persons born in 1968 and later. The examined persons resided in the areas under the study. The diagnostic workup included examination by endocrinologist, ultrasound scanning and morphometry of the thyroid, laboratory tests (determination of thyroid hormones and antibodies to the thyroid), fine needle biopsy if necessary. Tissue samples taken off at the time of surgery were reviewed and results were taken into consideration as well.

5. Diagnosis for thyroid cancer was reviewed by panel of pathologists. For the period from 1986 to June 1998 34 thyroid cancer cases in those who were born from 1968 to 1986 and resided in the affected areas in May-July 1986 were registered.

Results

The map of iodine provision in Bryansk oblast was made up on the basis of 3070 measurements of concentration of iodine in urine. Areas in which renal iodine excretion is >10 μg/dl, 10.0-7.5 μg/dl, 7.5-5.0 μg/dl and less than 5.0 μg/dl are marked. In order to obtain more detailed data, the territory of slight degree of iodine deficiency was divided into two zones: 10.0-7.5 μg/dl and 7.5 -5.0 mg/dl.

In table 1 data on renal excretion of iodine within bounders of marked territories are given. Magnitude of median is very close to mean standard deviation. It means that distribution of the concentration of iodine in urine is symmetric within limits of each zone. Variations of the level of iodine in urine between the data attributed to each zone are confident, p<0.001. The results show that slight iodine deficiency (renal excretion of iodine 10.0-5.0 μg/dl) is in the major part of the studied territory, in the less area the iodine deficiency is moderate (<5.0 μg/dl) or iodine provision is normal (>10 mg/dl). However, town of Klimovo and large settlement Gordeevka are in the zone of moderate iodine deficiency, and towns of Surazh, Mglin, Unecha are in the zone of normal iodine provision.

Table1. Iodine concentration in urine of residents of south-western areas of Bryansk oblast

Iodine deficiency (μg/dl)	Number of the examined	Number of settlements	Mean value (μg/dl)	Standard deviation (μg/dl)	Median (μg/dl)
<5	441	8	3.51	1.02	3.64
5.0 - 7.5	920	26	6.41	0.90	6.42
7.5 - 10	862	23	8.56	0.85	8.72
>10	847	18	12.88	2.53	12.94
TOTAL	3070	75			

In May 1986 the size of population born 1968-1986 been living in territories of moderate (<5.0 μg/dl), slight (5.0-7.5 μg/dl; 7.5-10.0 μg/dl) and normal (>10.0 μg/dl) level of iodine deficiency was 8 325, 60 442, 18 178 and 32 840 persons respectively.

In figure 1 the map of iodine deficiency and radiation dose to the thyroid of adults is presented. Various combinations of thyroid dose and iodine deficiency occur. In children the relationship of two factors (radiation and concentration of iodine in urine) is more complicated because thyroid dose depends on the age at the time of exposure, Thyroid dose from radioiodines to children and adolescents residing in the studied areas fluctuates from several to 240 cGy, the mean dose is 75 cGy.

Results of clinical examination of 37 042 persons show that frequency of occurrence of thyroid abnormalities depends on age. Diffuse euthyroid goitre rarely occurs in children under 3 years of age, it is detected in 16-19% children at the age 7-8 years. Increase in occurrence of diffuse euthyroid goitre to 25-26% of children at the age of puberty is observed. Certain decrease in the frequency of the disease occurrence is observed in adolescents. The second increase is observed in young adults at the age of 20 years. Occurrence of diffuse euthyroid goitre among females is higher than among males.

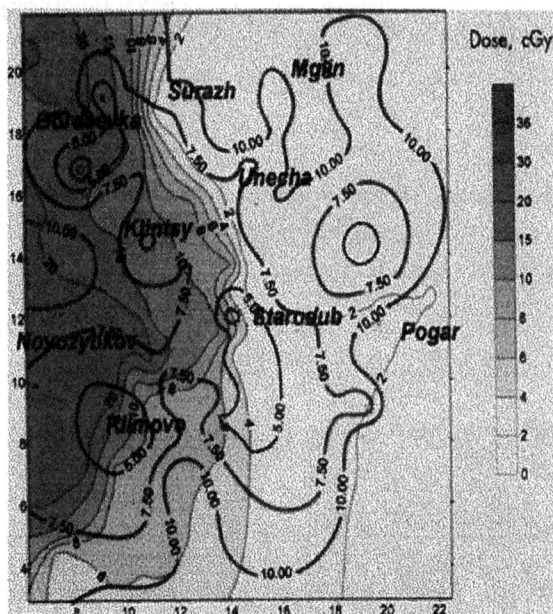

Fig1. Map of iodine deficiency and mean radiation dose to thyroid gland of adults

Frequency of occurrence of nodular abnormalities (adenomas, nodular goitre, cysts, focal thyroiditis) and its relation to the age is much more pronounced.

Nodular thyroid abnormalities are detected in children of 4 years of age, at the age of 8-13 years nodular abnormalities are detected in 1-2% of the examined. The number of cases increases with age. In persons older than 18 years nodular abnormalities are detected in 4-7% of examined patients. The occurrence of diseases of concern is two times higher in females than in males.

In accordance with criteria of ICCIDD the observed frequency of occurrence of diffuse euthyroid goitre and nodular thyroid abnormalities is characteristic of areas of slight iodine deficiency (10.0-7.5 µg/dl; 7.5-5.0 mg/dl). The results of clinical examination of the thyroid gland are in line with data on renal excretion of iodine.

To study the effect of radiation and iodine deficiency on the development of thyroid abnormalities we selected group of children of 7-14 years of age at the time of clinical examination from 37 042 of examined persons. The children are residents of territories with renal excretion of iodine 10.0-7.5 µg/dl and 7.5-5.0 µg/dl. The size of subgroups is 4 795 and 15 046 respectively. Restriction of the selection by the age of 7-14 years was made for minimisation of effect of age in the development of thyroid diseases.

Iodine deficiency expressed as renal excretion of 10-7.5 µg/dl does not cause any confident changes of frequency of thyroid abnormalities in the range of thyroid dose between 0-240 cGy.

In Table 2 data on thyroid diseases in children with the same thyroid dose residing in territories with renal excretion 7.5-5.0 µg/dl are given. In contrast to the above subgroup the frequency of occurrence of diffuse euthyroid goitre and nodular abnormalities increases confidently among boys and girls with thyroid dose higher than 100 cGy, who have lived in territories with iodine deficiency of 7.5-5.0µg/dl. Frequency of occurrence of the goitre in boys within thyroid dose ranges 0-50 cGy and 50-100 cGy is 16.8 and 17.7% respectively. If the dose is above 100 cGy the frequency of occurrence increases to 29.2% (p<0.001). Frequency of occurrence of goitre in girls with dose ranged 0-50 cGy and 50-100 cGy is 23.6 and 18.8 % respectively. If the dose is above 100 cGy, the frequency of occurrence is 32.9% (p<0.001).

Table 2. Frequency of occurrence (%) of thyroid abnormalities in children of 7-14 years of age. renal excretion of iodine in the territory of residence - 5.0 - 7.5 µg/dl

Sex	Number of subjects	Abnormality	Radiation dose, cGy		
			0 - 50	>50 - 100	>100
Boys	7639	Euthyroid goitre	16.8 (15.5 - 18.1)	17.7 (16.3 - 19.1)	29.2* (25.3 - 33.6)
		Nodules	0.6 (0.3 - 0.9)	0.7 (0.4 - 1.0)	2.5* (1.5 - 4.0)
Girls	7407	Euthyroid goitre	23.6 (21.8 - 25.3)	18.8 (17.3 - 20.3)	32.9* (28.6 - 37.8)
		Nodules	1.1 (0.8 - 1.5)	1.2 (0.9 - 1.6)	3.9* (2.5 - 5.7)

95% confidence interval is given in brackets
* - p<0.001

Frequency of occurrence of nodular abnormalities changes by the same way. The frequency of occurrence of abnormalities in boys with thyroid doses 0-100 cGy is 0.6-0.7% (p<0.01) and 2.5% if the dose is above 100 cGy. In girls with dose less than 100 cGy the abnormalities occur in 1.1-1.2% of the examined, if the dose is above 100 cGy the frequency of abnormalities is 3.9% (p<0.001).

So, it is evident that thyroid dose and iodine deficiency effect on the frequency of occurrence of thyroid disorders.

In children residing at the top interval limit of slight degree of iodine deficiency (10.0-7.5 µg/dl of iodine in urine) thyroid dose of 0-240 cGy does not influence the frequency of occurrence of thyroid abnormalities. In children residing at the low interval limit of slight iodine deficiency (7.5 -5.0 µg/dl of iodine in urine) thyroid dose above 100 cGy influences the development of goitre and nodular thyroid abnormalities.

The panel of pathologists verified diagnosis of thyroid cancer in persons born from 1968 to 1986 been residing in Bryansk oblast. Of 105 cases reviewed the diagnosis was confirmed for 62 cases. In 43 cases conclusions of panel members were not ambiguous. The consideration of these cases in epidemiological analysis seems to be questionable.

Confirmed thyroid cancer cases only were taken in epidemiological analysis of thyroid cancer incidence among residents of Bryansk oblast who were born within the period from 1968-1986. Epidemiological estimation of the desease incidence among residents of Bryansk oblast with account for verified cases is given below.

Absolute number of thyroid cancer cases in girls is 1.5 times higher than that in boys. Relative risk (RR), however, is higher in boys than in girls (5.00 and 2.44 respectively, p<0.9), because of higher baseline incidence. There is a trend for decreasing RR with increasing the age at the time of exposure. In the group of 0-4 years of age RR is 12.9 and 34.28 for boys and girls respectively.

Qualitative and quantitative distinction between the incidence of thyroid cancer among children and adolescents of contaminated south-western and "clean" raions of Bryansk oblast is observed. For the period from 1986 to 1997 RR of thyroid cancer in the two sub-groups is 8.13 and 1.78 respectively (p<0.05). The biggest distinction between RRs is in the age group of 0-4 years at the time of exposure (67.74 and 4.72 respectively (p<0.05). In other age groups distinction between RRs in two sub-groups is not confident.

In the areas in which iodine deficiency has been studied for 12 years 34 thyroid cancer cases were diagnosed. 3 cases were detected in areas with iodine deficiency less than 5μg/dl; 24 cases were in territories with iodine deficiency of 5.0-7.5 μg/dl, 4 cases were in territories with iodine deficiency of 7.5-10.0 μg/dl and 3 cases were in territories with iodine deficiency above 10.0 μg/dl. In figure 2 relationship between excess relative risk (ERR) of thyroid cancer among children and adolescents and iodine deficiency is presented. ERR is normalised to dose of 1Gy. The magnitude of ERR is seen to be confident, it considerably depends on the level of iodine provision in the area under the study. So, ERR of thyroid cancer in patients with mean thyroid dose of 1 Gy residing in territory of normal level of iodine deficiency (>10μg/dl) is 15, and the ERR for those living under high iodine deficiency (<2.0 μg/dl) is 26.0.

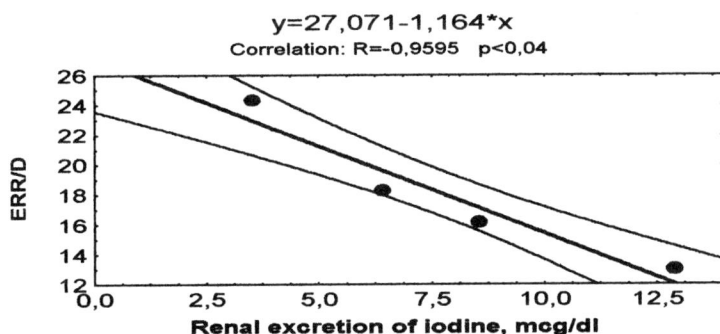

$$y = 27,071 - 1,164 * x$$
Correlation: R=-0,9595 p<0,04

Fig. 2. Relationship of ERR to the level of iodine deficiency, ERR is normalised to thyroid dose of 1 Gy

Conclusions

Results of the study show that there is combined effect of radiation and iodine endemy on development of thyroid abnormalities. Radiation effects on development of thyroid abnormalities, in particular, euthyroid goitre and nodular disorders, if iodine deficiency is less than 7.5 µg/dl. Iodine deficiency increases coefficient of ERR of thyroid cancer normalised to dose of 1 Gy. The results obtained allow one to suggest that minimisation of iodine deficiency in the affected territories due to the Chernobyl accident can contribute to mitigation of radiation effect on the thyroid.

Acknowledgements

Authors are very grateful to:
Prof. S. DAVIS, Fred Hutchinson Cancer Research Center, Seattle, Washington, USA, for very useful discussion and comments to the content of this paper.

This work has been supported in part by Grant N N00014-94-1-0049 issued to Georgetown University from the Office of Naval Research in support of the International Consortium for Research on the Health Effects of Radiation. The contents are solely the responsibility of the authors and do not necessarily reflect the views of the Office of Naval Research or Georgetown University.

References

1. Abelin T., Averkin J., Egger M. et al. Thyroid cancer in Belarus post-Chernobyl: improved detection or increased incidence. *Soz Praventivmed* 1994; **39**: 189-197.
2. Astachova L.N., Polyanskaya O.N., Drozd V.M., et al. Functional status of hypophysial-thyroid system in children and adolescents. *Zdravoohranenie in Belarus* 1993; **N1**:4-7. (In Russian)
3. Delange F. *Iodine nutrition and risk of thyroid irradiation from nuclear accidents. Iodine prophylaxis following nuclear accidents.* Oxford, New-York, Frankfurt, Sao Paulo, Sidney, Tokyo, Toronto, 1988.
4. *Endemic goitre.* Geneva: WHO, 1963. Ed. by F.U.Klemens, De Merlous.
5. Epstein E.V., Olejnik V.A., Tronko N.D. Possible lesions of the thyroid gland in children exposed to radionuclides of iodine following the accident at the Chernobyl NPP. *Problemy endocrinologii* 1992; **N4**: 21-22
6. Jacob P. and Likhtarev I. *Pathway analysis and dose distributions.* EUR 16541, Luxembourg: European Commission, 1996.
7. Nagataki S., Hirayu H., Izumi M. et al. High prevalence of thyroid nodule in area of radioactive fallout. *Lancet* 1989; **v.2**: p.375.

8. Pinchera A., Fenzi G.F., Mariotti S. et al. Iodine and autoimmune thyroid disease. In:"Iodine prophylaxis following nuclear accidents". Oxford, New York, Frankfurt, Sao Paulo, Sidney, Tokyo, Toronto, 1988; p.39.

9. Ron E., Moden B. Benign and malignant thyroid neoplasms after childhood irradiation for tinea capitis. *J.Nat.Cancer Ins.* 1980, **v.65**: p.7.

10. Shore R.E. Human thyroid cancer induction by ionizing radiation: summary of studies based on external irradiation and radioactive iodines. *The radiological consequences of the Chernobyl accident,* EUR 16544 EN, 669-676, Luxembourg, 1996.

11. Stepanenko V.F., Tsyb A.F., Parshkov E.M. et al. Retrospective thyroid absorbed doses estimation in Russia following the Chernobyl accident: progress and application to dosimetrical evaluation of childhood thyroid cancer morbidity. *Effects of low-level radiation for residents near Semipalatinsk nuclear test site,* Edited by M.Hoshi, J.Takada, R.Kim and Y.Nitta, 1996.

12. Tsyb A.F., Parshkov E.M., Shakhtarin V.V. et al. Thyroid cancer in children and adolescents of Bryansk and Kaluga region. *The radiological consequences of the Chernobyl accident,* EUR 16544 EN, 691-698, Luxembourg, 1996.

RISK OF RADIOGENIC THYROID CANCER IN RUSSIA FOLLOWING THE CHERNOBYL ACCIDENT

V. K. IVANOV, A. I. GORSKI, V. A. PITKEVITCH, A. F. TSYB

Medical Radiological Research Centre,
Russian Academy of Medical Sciences, Obninsk, Russia
E-mail: mrrc@obninsk.ru

E. CARDIS

International Agency for Research on Cancer, Lyon, France
E-mail: cardis@iarc.fr

H. STORM

Institute of Cancer Epidemiology, Danish Cancer Society, Copenhagen, Denmark
E-mail: Hans@epi.cancer.dk

Results of analysis of thyroid cancer incidence in the territories of Russia most contaminated after the Chernobyl accident are given. In the work data on incidence in the Bryansk, Kaluga, Orel and Tula regions (5240 thousand persons) are used.

For the analysis 3082 (age of 0-60 years) cases of thyroid cancer are considered from 1982 to 1996. Of them, 78 cases were among children and adolescents and 178 among the population who were children and adolescents at the time of the accident in 1986.

Excess absolute risk (EAR) was assessed with the use of reconstructed doses to the thyroid of exposed children and adolescents (age of 0-17 years) of Bryansk region. Cases detected over the period 1991 to 1996 were taken in the study. Dose-risk linear relationship was obtained. EAR is 2.21 (95% CI: 0.74, 3.68) per 10^4PYGy for girls and 1.62 (95% CI: -0.04, 3.23) per 10^4PYGy for boys.

A dependence of risk of cancer on age at exposure has been derived. For children of 0-4 years at exposure the risk of induction of radiogenic thyroid cancer is 14 times higher than in adults. On the average, the risk coefficient in children and adolescents at the time of exposure is about 2.3 times higher that in adults.

1 INTRODUCTION

According to the results of studies performed in Russia, the Ukraine and Belorus after the Chernobyl accident essential increase in thyroid cancer incidence in the contaminated with radionuclides areas has occurred. One of potential causes of the growth is exposure of thyroid in the residents of the contaminated areas to incorporated iodine-131 (^{131}I). This problem is particularly urgent for those residents of the contaminated areas who were children and adolescents during the exposure, as the risk of developing cancer (as well as dose) is strongly dependent on the age at the exposure.

Reconstructed ^{131}I depositions in the territory of Russia is available.[1] As of to-day, reconstruction of dose to the thyroid has been performed to the population of Bryansk region only.

Therefore the population of Russia as a whole was used as a control (zero-dose) in analysis of the incidence in the territories of the above mentioned regions. One of the major limitations of the used approach is a possible bias in the derived values of radiation risk due to changing intensity of screening of thyroid cancers in the post-Chernobyl period and in determination of "controls". For this reason, the work places particular emphasis to these matters. At the same time, an advantage of the approach is taking into account of all detected cases of thyroid cancer (it is very essential point for that rare disease thyroid cancer) in the four most contaminated regions of Russia to estimate indicators of incidence in different age groups prior to the Chernobyl accident and after it.

The purpose of the present work is to analyse the dynamics of thyroid cancer incidence in four regions of Russia with the population of 4330 thousand people at the age of 0-60 years (the number of children and adolescents is 1217 thousand persons) in 1982-1996.

2   MATERIALS AND METHODS

2.1   General Description of Medical and Demographic Data

The primary source of demographic information was data of federal state statistic bodies and regional statistic committees.

Detected thyroid cancer cases (among the population of 0-60 years of age) are official data of oncological dispensaries in Bryansk, Kaluga, Tula and Orel regions in charge of registration of cancer patients in accordance with regulations of Ministry of Health of Russia. A total of 3082 cases were detected from 1982 to 1996. Among them 2618 cases are among females (50 cases among girls of 0-17 years of age) and 464 cases among males (28 cases among boys of 0-17 years of age). There were 178 cases among persons born in 1969-1986, who were children and adolescents at the time of exposure (46 boys an 132 girls).

Among the children born after the accident from 1987 to 1996 2 cases of thyroid cancer was reported (the beginning of the period is chosen to include foetal exposure).

The dynamics of thyroid cancer incidence in the study regions in comparison with Russia is presented in Figure 1. Figure 1 presents a standardised incidence ratio (SIR) with 95% confidence intervals (SIR = observed number of cases/expected number of cases) for all four regions altogether. The confidence levels are calculated according to.[2] The dynamics of SIR in 1982-1996 in the four regions reveals an interesting feature. Indeed, in 1982-1986 the thyroid cancer incidence, both in males and females, was lower than in Russia (Russia as a whole is taken as control). In 1982-1986 SIR less than 1. In the second period 1987-1991 SIR, on the average, is more than 1 (1.6 times higher), i.e. the incidence in the four regions becomes higher than in Russia as a whole. As the period 1987-1991 is a latent period in radiation induction of thyroid cancer, the growth of incidence in this period can be attributed to introduction of a specialised examination system in these regions (the screening effect). After 1991 a certain growth of thyroid cancer incidence in the four regions of Russia under the study is observed.

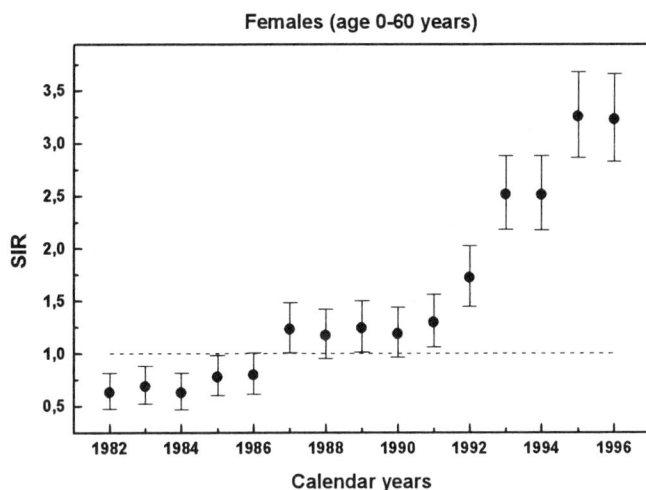

Fig. 1. Dynamics of standardised thyroid cancer incidence ratio in the four regions under consideration together (control - Russia).

2.2 Estimation of Relationship between Risk and the Age at Exposure

The risks of development of radiation-induced cancer at the same thyroid dose is known to depend on age at exposure.[3] For malignant neoplasms of most sites, the decrease in age at exposure leads to an increase in the risk of cancer. This equally applies to radiation-induced thyroid cancer.[4-5] So, induction of radiation-induced cancers should be maximum for those who were children and adolescents at exposure time.

To prove this statement two time intervals were considered: the first period from 1982 to 1990 included a pre-accident time period from 1982 to 1986 and the latent period of 5 years from 1986 to 1990 inclusive. This was assumed to be the period of spontaneous cancers. The second (postlatent) period covered from 1991 to 1996 when radiation-induced thyroid cancer could be developed. The correctness of dividing into the above time intervals is confirmed by the dynamics of SIR of thyroid cancer in the regions under study as compared to Russia (Figure 1).

Let us consider the ratio of observed (over 4 regions) and expected (in Russia in general) incidence in the considered time intervals among individuals of age i at the beginning of each time interval:

$$RR_i = \frac{observed_i}{exp\,ected_i} = \frac{\sum_k c_{i,i+k}}{\sum_k \lambda_{i+k,k} \times n_{i,i+k}},$$

$k=0,1,...,m$ for the first examination, $k=0,1,...,n$ for the second examination, and $(i+k)$ is age at diagnosis;

$c_{i,i+k}$ - number of cases among individuals at the age of i by the early of considered time interval, in k years, at the age of $i+k$;

$\lambda_{i+k,k}$ - thyroid cancer incidence rate in Russia as a whole. The second index k takes into account changes of the rate with time;

$n_{i,i+k}$ - number of individuals been at the age of i by the early of the considered time interval in k years, at the age of $i+k$.

The quantity of RR_i for individuals of age i in 1986 is an estimate of relative risk of development of radiation-induced cancer and age at exposure.

The 95% confidence intervals have been calculated according to.[2] To compare the distribution of RR for children and adolescents with that for adults over considered time intervals and to eliminate possible screening effect, the distributions have been normalised as average weighted RR for adults. The size of age groups has been taken into account.

2.3 Doses of Internal Exposure to the Thyroid of Residents of Bryansk Region due to Incorporated [131]I. Calculation of Dose-Response Relationship and Risk Coefficients

To estimate dose to the thyroid by incorporated ^{131}I the results of individual radiometry of the thyroid of 1864 persons residing in 96 settlements of Bryansk region were used. For calculation of doses due to internal exposure we used the model[6], paths of intake of ^{131}I via inhalation and feeding were taken into account in the model. Using linkage procedure the thyroid dose was estimated for residents of the Bryansk region. Age ratio of the population has been taken into account. The estimated collective dose to the thyroid is 34200 person Gy, average dose is 23 mGy. Thyroid dose to the exposed children and adolescents is 56 mGy.

Model for absolute risk was used for calculation of coefficients of relationship between the dose and incidence rate:

$$\lambda(u, D, a) = \lambda_0(u) + EAR(u, a) \times D(a),$$

λ_0 is rate of baseline incidence at the age u;
D - dose to the thyroid;
a - age at exposure.

For calculation of model parameters we used the method of maximal likelihood with suggestion that Poisson distribution of cases with time exists.

3   RESULTS

Figure 2 presents results of calculating risk of radiation-related thyroid cancer in children and adolescents with respect to adults with 95% confidence intervals. It can be seen that the relations for girls in the period of spontaneous cancers are close to unity and differ significantly from unity in the assumed period of development of radiation-induced cancers (1991-1996) for children and adolescents.

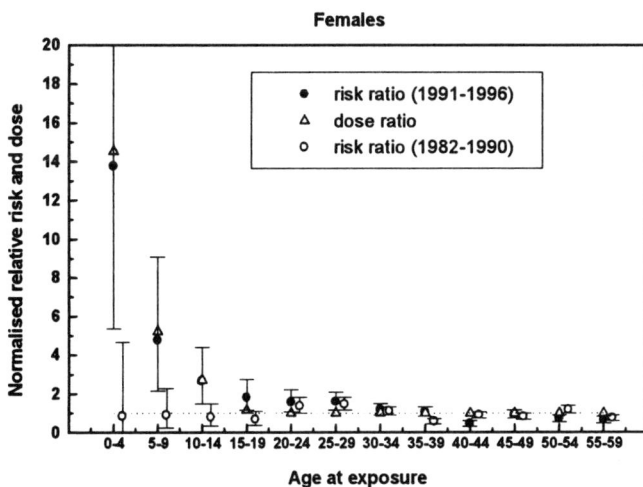

Fig. 2. Ratios of risks (RR) and doses (D) as a function of age at exposure and calendar period.

The points on the plot are shifted to reveal the bias in the values. As is seen from Figure 2, the relative risk of development of radiation-induced cancer for girls of 0-4 years of age at exposure is 14 times and for those of 5-9 years - 5 times higher than the risk for adults in the considered period 1991-1996. On the average, the risk coefficient in children and adolescents at the time of exposure is about 2.3 times higher that in adults. In[3,6] the relation of thyroid dose **D** and unit activity of incorporated ^{131}I has been derived as a function of age at the time of the Chernobyl accident. It has been shown that the difference in absorbed doses to the younger age groups can occur earlier than at the age of 20-24 years at exposure. The distribution of dose **D** is also shown in Figure 2. The dose is normalised to unity at age at exposure 20-24 years. The shape of the curve of relative risk in postlatent period is in good agreement with the thyroid dose. Reconstruction of doses to the thyroid in Bryansk region allowed us to estimate relationship between dose and radiation risk for the disease.

Figure 3 shows relationship between incidence rate of thyroid cancer among girls exposed to radiation at the age of 0-17 years and the thyroid dose. 48 cases diagnosed over 1991-1996 were analysed. All doses were divided into 8 dose intervals, the width of the interval was matched by criteria of homogenous distribution of number of persons and cases. Median interval dose is calculated with the account for the weigh of the size of age group of the population laying in a dose interval.

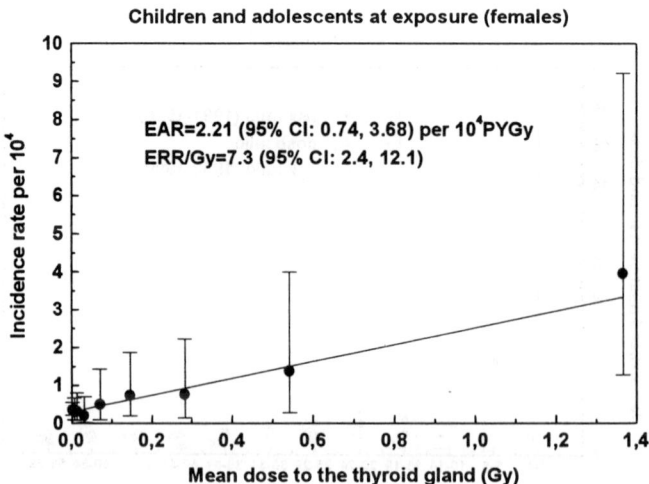

Fig. 3. Relationship between dose and thyroid cancer incidence rate among children and adolescents at the age of exposure (females) over the period of observation 1991 to1996.

From the Figure it is seen that dose-effect curve is close to line. It fits up-to-date ideas on existence of relationship between dose and thyroid cancer. Excess absolute risk EAR (angular coefficient of the relationship) is 2.21 (95% CI: 0.74, 3.68) per 10^4PYGy. Relative risk (ratio of EAR to the incidence rate at zero dose) is 7.3 (95% CI: 2.4, 12.1). The obtained value of EAR within confidence limits corresponds to the value of risk for children and adolescents (girls) due to exposure to incorporated ^{131}I given in[7] - $2.5\times(4/3)\times(1/3)=1.1$ $[10^{-4}$PYGy$]^{-1}$. EAR is 1.62 (95% CI: -0.04, 3.23) per 10^4PYGy for boys, however it is not statistically significant, may be, because of less number of thyroid cancer cases (25).

4 CONCLUSION

In conclusion, let us formulate again the main results:

- the highest risk of developing thyroid cancer has been found in children up to 4 years at exposure (for them the risk is 14 times higher that for adults). On the average, the risk coefficient in children and adolescents at the time of exposure is about 2.3 times higher that in adults;

- coefficients for excess absolute risk (EAR) of development of radiation-induced thyroid cancer in exposed children and adolescents of Bryansk region is 2.21 (95% CI: 0.74, 3.68) per 10^4PYGy for girls and 1.62 (95% CI: -0.04, 3.23) per 10^4PYGy for boys;

- the risk for children born prior to the Chernobyl accident is in good agreement with the age dependence of thyroid doses from incorporated ^{131}I.

Thus, the analysis of thyroid cancer incidence in the territories of Russia significantly contaminated due to the Chernobyl accident indicates convincingly the radiation nature of the detected increasing incidence cancers in children and adolescents.

96

References

1. Pitkevitch VA, Duba VV, Ivanov VK et al. Reconstruction of the composition of the Chernobyl radionuclide fallout and external radiation absorbed doses to the population in areas of Russia. *Radiat Prot Dosimetry* 1996; **64**: 69-92.
2. Breslow NE and Day N. *Statistical methods in cancer epidemiology. Vol.II - The design and analysis of cohort studies.* Lyon: International agency for research on cancer, 1987; **82**: 69-75.
3. Age dependent doses to members of the public from intake of radionuclides. *ICRP publication* 1989; **56**: 45-51.
4. Shore RE. Issues and epidemiological evidence regarding radiation-induced thyroid cancer. *Radiation Research* 1992; **131**: 98-117.
5. Ron E, Lubin JY, Shore RE, Mabuchi K, Modan B, Pottern LM, Shneider A, Tucker M and Boice JD. Thyroid cancer after exposure to external radiation: a pooled analysis of seven studies. *Radiation Research* 1995; **141**: 259-277.
6. Zvonova IA, Balonov MI. Radioiodine dosimetry and prediction of consequences of the thyroid exposure of the Russian population following the Chernobyl accident. In: The Chernobyl papers, ed. Mervin SE and Balonov MI. Washington: REPS, 1993: 71-126.
7. Health effects on populations of exposure to low levels of ionising radiation. National Academy of Sciences Committee on the Biological Effects of Ionizing Radiation. BEIR V Reports. Washington DC: US National Academy of sciences 1990.

THYROID EXPOSURES OF CHILDREN AND ADOLESCENTS DUE TO THE CHERNOBYL ACCIDENT: THE RESULTING CANCER RISK

P. JACOB, G. GOULKO AND W.F. HEIDENREICH

GSF - Institut für Strahlenschutz, D-85764 Neuherberg, Deutschland
E-mail :jacob@gsf.de

I. KAIRO AND I. LIKHTAREV

Radiation Protection Institute, 252050 Kiev, Ukraine
E-mail: likh@rpi.ua

J. KENIGSBERG AND E. BUGLOVA

Scientific Research and Clinical Institute of Radiatiation *Medicine and Endocrinology,*
220600 Minsk, Belarus
E-mail: dcc@belamir1.belpak.minsk.by

I. ZVONOVA AND M. BALONOV

Research and Technical Center Protection, 197101 St. Petersburg, Russia
E-mail:ira@katia.stud.pu.ru

T.I. BOGDANOVA AND N.D. TRONKO

Ukrainian Research Institute of Endocrinology and Metabolism, 254114 Kiev, Ukraine
E-mail:tb@viaduk.net

E.P. DEMIDCHIK

Thyroid Cancer Center, 220600 Minsk, Belarus

Thyroid cancer cases in the period 1991 to 1995 among the birth cohort 1968 to end of May 1986 in 5821 settlements (villages or towns) in Ukraine, Belarus and Russia were analysed. Average thyroid doses in several age groups in each of the settlements were estimated. Excess incidence was estimated by using the thyroid cancer incidence in southern Ukraine as background incidence. The excess absolute risk per unit dose (EARDPD) was found to be comparable to that after external exposures. No age-at-exposure effect was detected. The EARPD of females is by about a factor of 2 higher than that for males.

1   Introduction

The current knowledge on thyroid cancer risk due to ^{131}I incorporations during childhood or adolescence is limited. Results of three studies have been published for thyroid doses below 10 Gy [1-3]. Higher doses have a large potential of cell killing and are not considered here. The three studies had low statistical power due to small collective thyroid doses in the cohorts (below $4 \cdot 10^3$ person·Gy), and small numbers of expected (below six) and observed (below or equal to eight) thyroid cancer cases.

After the Chernobyl accident there was a large increase of the thyroid cancer incidence among those who were exposed during childhood or adolescence. More than 70% of the internal thyroid doses of the population in the contaminated area was due to ^{131}I [4], external exposures added a negligible amount. Therefore the thyroid cancer incidence after Chernobyl has a large potential for deriving new information on the ^{131}I induced risk.

In an aggregate study [5] average thyroid doses to children in 5821 settlements (villages and towns) in Ukraine, Belarus and Russia and the related cancer risk were assessed. It is the purpose of the this paper to present additional data and results.

2 Method

Register data were analysed for the thyroid cancer incidence in the period 1991 to 1995 among the birth cohort 1968 to end of May 1986. The data sets in the register contain name, birth date, gender, and date of surgery, so the group considered had ages of 4.6 to 28 years at the time of operation. The data sets were extended by the place of residence at the time of the accident. The study was performed for 5821 contaminated settlements (villages or towns) in Ukraine, Belarus and Russia. The settlements were chosen because thyroid dose reconstruction was considered to have a higher reliability than in other contaminated areas.

Southern Ukraine had relatively small ^{131}I exposures and was used as a control area. Age and sex dependence of thyroid cancer incidence was similar to the incidence in Belarus for which already analytical approximations have been published [6]. To estimate the background risk (number of cases per person-years of observation), these analytical functions were scaled to the thyroid cancer incidence in the period 1991 to 1995 among the birth cohort 1971 to end of May 1986 in southern Ukraine, which was the birth cohort of interest in ref. 6. This scaled function was used to estimate the background risk for the different age groups.

Age specific thyroid doses in the settlements of three contaminated oblasts in the north of Ukraine (Zhytomyr, Kyiv and Chernihiv) were reconstructed on the base of 150 000 measurements of ^{131}I activiies in human thyroids, that were performed with collimated detectors in the period 15 May to 15 June 1986 [7, 8]. Correlations of thyroid doses with caesium deposition, and distance and direction relative to the Chernobyl NPP were used to derive results for settlements with less than twelve measurements. Among the evacuees from the town Pripjat 4969 measurements of ^{131}I activities in thyroids were performed and these measurements were assumed to be representative for the 49 000 inhabitants [9].

In the contaminated areas of Belarus measurements of ^{131}I activities in grass, soil and milk were performed. Based on these measurements a radioecological model for age-specific thyroid doses was developed [10] and applied for the present work to the settlements of seven rayons in the Gomel and Mogilev oblasts. In this area the radioecological model could be validated with measurements of ^{131}I activities in human thyroids. For 91 settlements more than 15 measurements of ^{131}I activities in thyroids were available for the age group 13-17. For 95% of these settlements the results of the radioecological model and the measurements agree within a factor of 4. Because of the availability of ^{131}I activity measurements in human thyroids also the capital Minsk could be included in the study.

The dose reconstruction in six rayons and the capital of Bryansk oblast in the Russian Federation was based on 12 737 measurements of ^{131}I activities in human thyroids [4]. The detectors were uncollimated. For a derivation of the contribution of radionuclide activities outside of the thyroid to the count rate, more than 1000 measurements were performed in a second position: over the thigh. Results of 1000 measurements of total beta activity in milk and interviews of people and local authorities about begin of grazing period, distribution of stable iodine and prohibition of local milk consumption were used to determine the time dependence of the ^{131}I activity in the human thyroid.

The excess absolute risk per unit thyroid dose of a population group i, EARPD$_i$, was calculated according to

$$EARPD_i = (L_i/PY_i - r_i) / D_i, \qquad (1)$$

where L$_i$ is the number of cases, PY$_i$ the person-years of observation, r$_i$ the background risk, and D$_i$ the average thyroid dose in the population group. Poisson regression over all 5821 settlements and straightforward calculations with average values gave consistent results for point estimates of EARPD$_i$. It is stressed that the excess absolute risk calculated here is just the quantity that can be calculated with the lowest uncertainty, e.g. the uncertainty of the background risk has a relatively large influence on the excess relative risk in a situation with large excess risks. The use of the excess absolute risk does not imply that a constant excess absolute risk describes the time dependence better than e.g. a constant excess relative risk. The observation time after the Chernobyl accident is too short to decide about such time dependencies. The rise of the cancer incidence in the period 1989 to 1995 expresses the onset of the effect and should not be compared with models of constant absolute or relative risk.

Conventional Poisson regression was considered to be not appropriate to calculate confidence intervals of risk estimates, because it does not take into account uncertainties of dose estimates. Confidence intervals of EARPD$_i$, were assessed by assuming uncertainty distributions of the four input variables in eq.(1)

100

and using the Monte Carlo method [11]. The program system Crystal Ball[1] was used for the calculations.

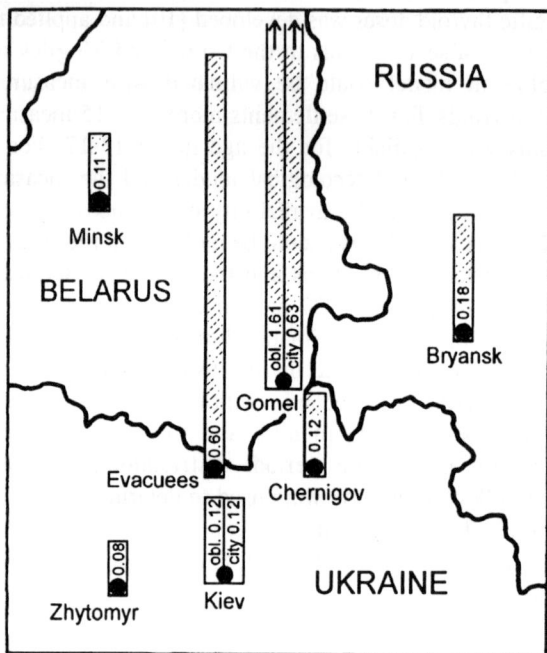

Fig. 1. Cumulative thyroid cancer incidence (number of cases per thousend persons) in the period 1991 to 1995 among the birth cohort 1971 to end of May 1986 in the study area. 'Gomel oblast' indicates the result for seven rayons in Gomel and Mogilev oblast.

Uncertainties of average thyroid doses are mainly used due to systematical errors and representativeness of data: Due to the large number of persons (several hundred thousand) in each of the considered population groups, stochastic fluctuations are negligible. The limits of the 95% confidence interval of average thyroid doses was assumed to be separated by a factor of two from the best estimate. The number of observed cancer cases L_i was assumed to follow a normal distribution with a standard deviation of sqrt(L_i); the number of person·years of observation a normal distribution with a standard deviation of 10%. The variability

---

[1] *Crystal Ball, Forecasting and Risk Analysis for Spreadsheet Users.* DECISIONEERING, Denver, Colorado 80204-9849, USA

of the background risk was derived from the cancer incidence in the period 1986 to 1988: It differed in the northern part of Ukraine by a factor of 1.5, and in Belarus and Bryansk by a factor of two from the incidence in southern Ukraine.

3   Results

The cumulative thyroid cancer incidence in the subarea with average thyroid doses among the birth cohort 1971 to end of May 1986 of more than 0.4 Gy (7 rayons in Gomel and Mogilev oblasts, Gomel city and the evacuees) is considerably larger than in the subarea with average thyroid doses below 0.2 Gy (Zhytomir, Kiev and Chernigov oblasts, 6 rayons in Bryansk oblast + Bryansk city, Kiev city and Minsk city), see Figure 1.

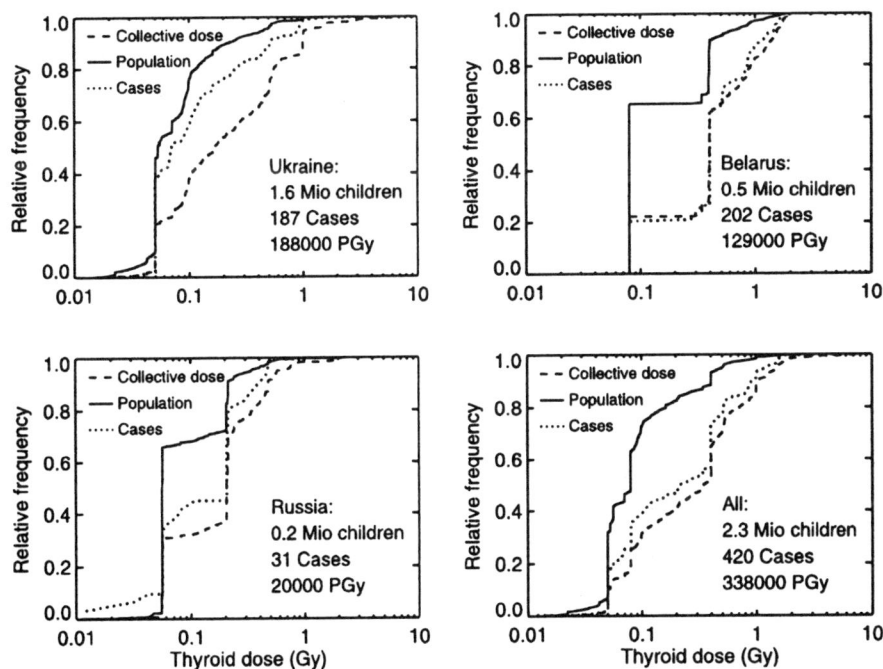

Fig. 2. Cumulative dose distributions of population, collective dose and thyroid cancer cases in the period 1991 to 1995 among the birth cohort 1971 to end of May 1986 in the study area.

Cumulative distributions of population, collective dose and number of thyroid cancer cases as a function of the average thyroid dose in the 5821 settlements are shown in Figure 2. The cities with low average thyroid doses Kiev (0.05 Gy), Minsk (0.08 Gy) and Bryansk (0.06 Gy) contribute significantly to the population of the study area and less to the collective thyroid dose and to the number of thyroid cancer cases. For the study area in Belarus and for the whole study area the cumulative distributions of the collective dose and of the number of thyroid cancer cases are similar, indicating a close relation of these two quantities. In Ukraine and Russia the situation is less obvious. In the study area about 75% of the population has thyroid doses below 0.1 Gy, contributing about 35% to the collective thyroid dose and the number of thyroid cancer cases. 10% of the population has thyroid doses above or equal to 0.4 Gy, also contributing about 35% to the collective thyroid dose and to the number of thyroid cancer cases.

In the study area the excess absolute risk per unit thyroid dose (EARPD) does not depend on age at exposure for the birth cohort 1968 to 1985 (Table 1). The risk for those born in the first five months of 1986 is about a factor of two smaller than in the other age-at-exposure groups, the difference is at the border of being statistically significant. The excess absolute risk of females is about a factor of 2 higher than that of males, again the difference is at the border of being statistically significant.

Table 1. Observed number of thyroid cancer and excess absolute risk per unit thyroid dose (per 10^4 person-year·Gy, median values and 95% confidence intervals) in 5821 settlements in Ukraine, Belarus and Russia.

Birth period	Boys	Girls	Both
1968-1970	10/ 1.1 (-0.2; 3.5)	50/ 6.5 (2.0; 17)	60/ 4.0 (1.2; 10)
1971-1975	17/ 0.9 (0.2; 2.2)	57/ 3.0 (1.1; 6.8)	74/ 2.0 (0.8; 4.4)
1976-1979	29/ 1.8 (0.8; 4.1)	71/ 4.6 (2.0; 11)	100/ 3.3 (1.4; 7.6)
1980-1985	94 /2.2 (1.0; 4.7)	137/ 3.3 (1.5; 6.8)	231/ 2.8 (1.3; 5.8)
Jan-May 1986	3/ 0.5 (-0.1; 1.6)	12/ 2.1 (0.7; 5.0)	15/ 1.3 (0.5; 3.0)

4 Discussion

Although studies of thyroid cancer after external exposures during childhood had a longer time of follow-up than the observation time after the Chernobyl accident and partly the observation started later (atomic bomb survivors), it is interesting to compare the results.

The EARPD for ages at exposure of 0 to 15 years found in this study for ^{131}I exposures after the Chernobyl accident is comparable to the risk observed after external exposures [12, 13].Among the atomic bomb survivors, the EARPD for ages at exposure of 0-9 years was by a factor of 1.6 higher than for ages at exposure of 10-19 years [14]. However, the difference to the finding of the present study (no age-at-exposure effect) is statistically not significant.

Among atomic bomb survivors with age at exposure of 0-9 years the excess relative risk of females was the same as for males. In this paper results on excess relative risks were not presented because of the large uncertainty of the spontaneous risk in the study area (This does not influence very much the EARPD because in the study area the ratio of observed to estimated spontaneous cases was with the exception of the Zhytomir oblast larger than 5). In the background risk used in this study the incidence among the age-at-accident group of 0-9 years was for females by a factor of 2.5 higher than for males. So the findings on the sex dependence of the risk after external exposures (atomic bomb survivors) and of the present study for ^{131}I incorporations are similar.

5 Conclusions

The present study indicates a large potential of studies of thyroid cancer cases among people exposed by the Chernobyl accident to derive information on the risk due to ^{131}I incorporations. It motivates research to evaluate, whether an aggregate study is appropriate under these conditions. Confounding factors like the screening effect need to be better quantified. The sensitivity analysis not described in this paper indicates that uncertainties of dose estimates are the large contributor to the uncertainties of the results. Research needs to be performed to improve estimates of thyroid doses and their uncertainties.

6 Acknowledgements

This study was supported by the INCO-COPERNICUS project IC15CT960306 of the European Commission, and by the project 'Scientists help Chernobyl children' supported by the German Electricity Companies (VDEW).

References

1. Hall P, Mattson A, Boice JD (1996) Thyroid cancer after diagnostic administration of iodine-131. *Radiat Res* **145**: 86-92

2. Hamilton P, Chiacchierini R, Kacmarek R (1989) *A follow-up of persons who had iodine-131 and other diagnostic procedures during childhood and adolescence.* Publication FDA 89-8276. CDRH-Food and Drug Administration, Rockville, MD

3. Kerber RA, Till JE, Simon SL, Lyon JL, Thomas DC, Preston-Martin S, Rallison ML, Lloyd RD Stevens W (1993) A cohort study of thyroid disease in relation to fallout from nuclear weapons testing. *JAMA* **270**: 2076-2082

4. Zvonova IA, Balonov MI (1993) Radioiodine dosimetry and prediction of consequences of thyroid exposure of the Russian population following the Chernobyl accident. In *The Chernobyl Papers. Vol. I. Doses to the Soviet population and the early health effects studies,* Mervin SE, Balonov MI (eds.) pp 71-125. WA Research Enterprises : Richland, WA

5. Jacob P, Goulko G, Heidenreich WF, Likhtarev I, Kairo I, Tronko ND, Bogdanova TI, Kenigsberg J, Buglova E, Drozdovitch V, Golovneva A, Demidchik EP, Balonov M, Zvonova I, Beral V (1998) Thyroid cancer risk to children calculated. *Nature* **392**: 31-32

6. Heidenreich WF, Kenigsberg Y, Jacob P, Buglova E, Goulko G, Paretzke HG, Demidchik EP (1998) Time trends of childhood thyroid cancer in Belarus. Acccepted by *Radiat. Res.*

7. Likhtarev I, Sobolev B, Kairo I, Tabachny L, Jacob P, Pröhl G, Goulko G (1996) Results of large scale thyroid dose reconstruction in Ukraine. *Proc. First International Conference of the European Commission, Belarus, Russian Federation and Ukraine on the Radiological Consequences of the Chernobyl Accident, Minsk.* Report EUR 16544 EN, pp. 1021-1036. European Commission, Luxembourg.

8. Goulko GM, Chepurny NI, Jacob P, Likhtarev IA, Pröhl G, Sobolev BG (1998) Chernobyl thyroid dose assessments and thyroid cancer incidence for the Zhytomyr region (Ukraine). *Radiat. Environ. Biophys.* **36**: 261-273

9. Goulko G, Chumak VV, Chepurny NI, Henrichs K, Jacob P, Kairo IA, Likhtarev IA, Repin VS, Sobolev BG, Voigt G (1996) Estimation of ^{131}I thyroid doses for the evacuees from Pripjat. *Radiat. Environ. Biophys.* **35**: 81-87

10. Drozdovitch VV, Goulko GM, Minenko VF, Paretzke HG, Voigt. G., Kenigsberg YI (1997) Thyroid dose reconstruction for the population of Belarus after the Chernobyl accident. *Radiat Environ Biophys* **36**: 17-23

11. Hoffman FO, Hammonds JS (1994) Propagation of uncertainty in risk assessments: The need to distinguish between uncertainty due to lack of knowledge and uncertainty due to variability. *Risk Analysis* **14**, 707-712

12. Ron E, Lubin JH, Shore RE, Mabuchi K, Modan B, Pottern LM, Schneider AB, Tucker MA, Boice JD (1995) Thyroid cancer after exposures to external radiation: A pooled analysis of seven studies. *Radiat Res* **141**: 259-277

13. Thompson DE, Mabuchi K, Ron E, Soda M, Tokunaga M, Ochikubo S, Sugimoto S, Ikeda T, Terasaki M, Izumi S, Preston DL (1994) Cancer incidence in atomic bomb survivors. Part II: Solid tumors, 1958-1987. *Radiat Res* **137**: S17-S67

THYROID CANCER IN NEW CALEDONIA

SHIRLEY BALLIVET[1], ELIZABETH CHUA[3], GEORGE BAUTOVICH[2], JOHN R TURTLE[3]

[1]Gaston Bourret Hospital, New Caledonia, [2]Royal Prince Alfred Hospital, and [3]Department of Medicine, University of Sydney, Sydney, Australia

INTRODUCTION

New Caledonia is a French overseas territory in the Pacific, located between Australia and Fiji with 196,000 inhabitants (1996 census) of various ethnic groups (Melanesians, Europeans, Polynesians and Asians). As early as 1985, a trend for an increasing rate of thyroid cancer was noted in this population. The average annual incidence rate of thyroid cancer was 5.8/100,000 population in 1985 and 10.8/100,000 in 1992. Female Melanesians have an annual incidence rate of 35/100,000, the highest incidence rate ever reported.[1,2] The overall incidence rate is still increasing, and is reported to be >20/100,000 population in 1996 [unpublished data].

Thyroidectomies are performed in Noumea, the capital of New Caledonia or at Royal Prince Alfred Hospital (RPAH) in Sydney, Australia. After thyroidectomy, most patients are reviewed at RPAH for radioiodine treatment and follow-up. In this study, the outcome of patients with well-differentiated thyroid cancer treated with ^{131}I was evaluated over a 14-year period. Factors associated with prognosis were identified.

PATIENTS & METHODS

All cases of primary thyroid cancer, diagnosed between 1 January 1980 and 31 December 1993, in males or females of any age, and living in New Caledonia at the time of diagnosis, were identified from the Cancer Registry of New Caledonia. After thyroidectomy, the slides were initially reported by a pathologist in Noumea and subsequently sent to Sydney for review. Histologic diagnoses were based on the 1988 World Health Organisation histological classification of thyroid tumours[3]. Pathology slides of the cases diagnosed between 1985 to 1989 were reviewed and reclassified as necessary by two pathologists in Noumea; slides prior to 1985 were no longer available for review. Patients who had ^{131}I treatment in Sydney were identified. A nuclear physician reviewed the [131]I (diagnostic and post-treatment) scans and reported the number and sites of uptake using a standardised form. Medical records from the hospital, letters of attending physicians and when available, patients' records during follow-up in New Caledonia were reviewed.

Initial scans were performed at least 4-6 weeks after thyroidectomy. Preparation for subsequent scans involved withdrawing thyroxine 28 days before the diagnostic scans, substituting tri-iodothyronine for the first 14 days off thyroxine, then withdrawing all thyroid medications for the last 14 days before the scan. Diagnostic scans were performed between 48 and 72 hours after the oral administration of 5 mCi (185 MBq) of [131]I. Medium energy, parallel hole collimation was used, both for whole body scans (Searle LFOV camera) and planar views of the neck and other regions of interest (Searle LFOV and GE 500 cameras). Patients requiring ^{131}I therapy were admitted at RPAH for treatment and scanned again on discharge when the retained activity was less than 15 mCi (600 MBq).

Patients were reviewed and treated with ^{131}I every 3-4 months until they were considered to be disease-free. Therapeutic doses used were 100 mCi (3700 MBq) for ablation of the thyroid remnant, and 200 mCi (7400 MBq) for metastases. The end of the follow-up period was set at 31 December 1994.

The thyrotrophin-stimulating hormone (TSH), thyroglobulin (Tg) levels, and full blood counts done prior to each scan were recorded. Thyroglobulin levels were determined by radioimmunoassay (RIA) from 1980 to October 1989 and by immunoradiometric assay (IRMA) from November 1989 onwards.

Kaplan-Meier product limit method was used to study the survival function and Cox proportional hazards model was used to estimate the relative probability of achieving a disease-free state (occurrence of a negative scan) according to different prognostic factors. Mann-Whitney test was used to estimate the difference between groups with $p<0.05$ considered as significant.

RESULTS

A total of 161 cases of thyroid cancer diagnosed between 1 January 1980 and 31 December 1993 were collected from the Cancer Registry of New Caledonia. Most patients in whom an initial diagnosis of anaplastic carcinoma was made were identified in New Caledonia as having a poor prognosis and were not referred to Sydney. Patients who only had hemi-thyroidectomies, who had previous ^{131}I treatment elsewhere prior to coming to RPAH, or whose records or scans were incomplete were excluded from the study. The remaining 98 patients reviewed in Sydney after total thyroidectomy constituted the study population. There were 86 (88%) females and 12 (12%) males, with a mean age of 46 years. 81% were Melanesians, 10% Europeans, and 9% of mixed background. 76% had papillary carcinoma and 24% had follicular carcinoma.

Initial assessment

Iodine-131 scans:
On the first ^{131}I total body scans done after thyroidectomy, 100% of subjects had radioiodine uptake in the thyroid bed. In addition, metastatic foci were already detectable in 23 patients (24%). Eleven had papillary carcinoma (14% of the papillary carcinoma group) and twelve had follicular carcinoma (52% of the follicular carcinoma group). Metastasis on the first scan was significantly associated with follicular cancer ($p<0.001$).

Thyroglobulin levels
Among the 90 patients whose initial Tg levels were available, 77 were measured at the time of the first scan post-total thyroidectomy. Eleven were measured prior to the second scan, which was within 4 months from the first visit. Initial Tg levels were significantly higher ($p<0.001$) among patients with metastases detected on the first scan than among patients with no detectable metastases. Initial Tg levels were also higher in patients with follicular cancer compared to patients with papillary cancer ($p=0.02$) (Table 1). The mean number of sites of metastases, however, was not significantly different ($p=0.85$) between the 2 groups (papillary=5.18, follicular=5.75). In 90% of cases with metastases on the first scan, the Tg levels were $> 20\mu g/L$.

Table 1. Mean Thyroglobulin Levels at Initial Scan Post-total Thyroidectomy

	With Metastases	No Metastases	With or without Metastases
Papillary	739 ± 1,359	140 ± 395	230 ± 659
Follicular	13,326 ± 18,698	388 ± 1,117	6,857 ± 14,523[†]
Pap & Foll	7,332 ± 14,736*	180 ± 572	

Reference range of Tg: $<20\mu g/L$ in normal population and $<1\mu g/L$ post-total thyroidectomy
*$p<0.01$ compared to patients with no metastases
†$p=0.02$ compared to patients with papillary carcinoma

Follow-up
Follow-up period ranged from 3 to 175 months (14.4 years) with a mean of 46 ± 35 months (3.8 ± 2.9 years).

Attaining a disease-free state:
After ^{131}I treatment, 73.5% were considered to be disease-free, that is, no scan evidence of disease on follow-up. This was achieved after 1 or 2 therapeutic doses

of 100 mCi with a mean cumulative dose of 118.0 ± 34.3 mCi. In the Cox model, initial Tg ≤20μg/L and no metastases on the initial scan were associated with higher probability of attaining a negative scan on follow-up (Table 2).

Table 2. Prognostic Factors For Achieving Disease-free State Using Cox Model

Variables	Relative Probability	p-value	95% CI
Age < 55	1.72	0.091	0.92-3.22
Papillary carcinoma	1.44	0.363	0.66-3.15
No metastases on initial scan	2.27	0.062	0.96-5.36
Initial Tg ≤ 20μg/L	1.87	0.033	1.05-3.32

Thyroglobulin levels

Among patients who had no detectable metastases on initial and follow-up scans, 73.8% had initial Tg levels of ≤20μg/L, and 26.2% had Tg levels >20μg/L. Among the latter group, two patients (Tg levels of 1617 & 305μg/L) had widespread metastases already present at time of operation. Both died within a year after initial treatment. Two other patients (Tg levels of 301 & 76μg/L) had clinical recurrence within three years. The others (Tg ≤65μg/L, except for one with Tg of 174μg/L) had decreasing Tg levels on follow-up.

Eight patients with thyroid bed uptake only on the initial scan had metastases detected on subsequent scans. In all eight cases, the initial Tg levels were >20μg/L (range: 55-3730). Clinical metastasis was already present at initial consult in one patient. In three patients, metastases were detected on subsequent scans within the first 12 months of follow-up. The other four patients presented with lymph node recurrence within 3 years. Distribution of initial Tg levels according to metastatic status based on scan is shown in Table 3.

Table 3: Initial Tg Levels According to Metastatic Status Based on ^{131}I scan

	Tg ≤ 20μg/L n (%)	Tg > 20μg/L n (%)
Metastases on initial scan (n=21)	2 (9.6%)	19 (90.4%)
Metastases on follow-up scans (n=8)	0 (0%)	8 (100%)
No detectable metastases (n=61)	45 (73.8%)	16 (26.2%)

Cases with Metastases
The most common sites of metastases were regional lymph nodes in papillary carcinoma and bone metastases in follicular carcinoma. In 83% of cases, there were more than two sites of radioiodine uptake on the scans. Three patients with extensive metastatic disease decided not to have further radioiodine treatment. The Tg levels on each follow-up for the 23 patients are shown in Figure 1. Overall, Tg levels in papillary carcinoma showed a general decreasing trend compared to follicular carcinoma. Eight out of eleven patients with metastatic papillary cancer were considered to be disease-free after ^{131}I treatment. One of these who had extensive metastases with eight sites of uptake on scan, had Tg levels decreased from 1584 to 14µg/L with subsequent negative scans after receiving a cumulative dose of 1,600 mCi over a period of six years. Among patients with metastatic follicular cancer, three patients (2 with previous quadriplegia and 1 with paraplegia) were able to ambulate again after ^{131}I therapy and further surgical decompression followed by radiotherapy to the metastatic foci. At the end of the study period, one patient was disease-free after two therapeutic doses while five had ongoing ^{131}I treatment. There were six deaths, two of which had refused further treatment.

Complications
The cumulative dose was > 2,000 mCi in three patients, 1,000-2,000 mCi in eleven patients and 500-1,000 mCi in five patients. Pancytopaenia occurred in three patients who had extensive metastatic disease with bone involvement after receiving a mean cumulative dose of 1002 ± 444 mCi. All three were able to have further ^{131}I treatment after recovery of the bone marrow. Three patients reported swelling of the salivary gland or neck. No other complications were noted.

Survival
There were 11 deaths (5 papillary and 6 follicular) during the follow-up period. The overall survival rate was 92% at 2 years and 84% at 5 years. Survival rate for papillary carcinoma was 96% at 2 years and 92% at 5 and 8 years. For follicular carcinoma, survival rate was 90% at 2 years, 66% at 5 years and 50% at 8 years. Because of the small number of deaths, a Cox proportional hazard model could not be performed. Survival curves according to age, histology, Tg level and metastatic status on the initial scan are shown in figure 2. The risk of death was increased in cases with age $\geq$65, follicular carcinoma, metastatic disease on scan and/or initial Tg > 20µg/L.

DISCUSSION
Radioactive iodine has been used for both ablation of surgical remnants and treatment of metastatic disease for many years and many studies have shown that treatment with ^{131}I increases disease-free interval and survival.[4,5] Although used

extensively, controversies still persist regarding ablation doses, treatment intervals, maximum cumulative dose allowable, and safety of giving such high doses.[6]

This is a review of 98 cases of well-differentiated thyroid carcinoma treated at one institution over a period of 14 years. The diagnostic evaluations, mode of treatment and follow-up of patients were relatively homogeneous. Treatment consisted of total thyroidectomy, ^{131}I ablation for residual tissue and/or metastases, and life-long TSH suppression by thyroid hormones. When indicated, patients had tumour embolisation followed by debulking of metastatic foci. Occasionally, radiotherapy may also be administered. Patients received therapeutic doses (100-200 mCi) every 3-4 months until they were considered to be disease-free. 19% of patients had cumulative doses of > 500 mCi given at 3-4 monthly intervals. This form of treatment is far more intensive than that advocated by other institutions.[7,8] However, complications were minimal and response to treatment was excellent.

Uptake of ^{131}I by residual normal thyroid tissue is more efficient than by metastatic tissue.[9] Metastases are therefore frequently not visualised on the initial scan. In this review, metastatic foci were already detectable in 24% of patients on the first scan done after total thyroidectomy, suggesting that the course in this population is quite aggressive. Patients with metastases on presentation had worse outcome in both attaining a disease-free state and long-term survival.

On the other hand, metastatic foci may occasionally fail to take up the radioiodine resulting in a false negative scan.[10] This could explain some of the cases with high initial Tg, but with no detectable metastases on scans. It was not until 1995 when patients with high Tg levels and negative scans were given therapeutic doses of [131]I.

Thyroglobulin has been widely used as a tumour marker for well-differentiated thyroid cancer.[11,12] In this study, 90% of cases with metastases on the first scan had Tg levels >20µg/L. Furthermore, in 8 of the 8 cases that had metastasis detected only on subsequent scans, the initial Tg levels were >20µg/L. These results suggest that a Tg level >20µg/L at initial consult is a good indicator of presence of metastatic disease even when there is no detectable metastases on ^{131}I scan.

Long-term survival for well-differentiated carcinoma is good and exceeds survival rates of most cancers.[13] The results of this study further support this fact, in that patients without metastases had 8-year survival rates of 100% in both papillary and follicular type. In extensive metastatic disease, however, the course could be aggressive resulting in poor outcome. Therefore, in patients with metastatic disease, additional modes of therapy should be considered in order to improve the outcome. For example, patients with significant metastatic tumour masses may benefit from debulking.[14] Because these tumours are extremely vascular, embolisation prior to surgery often decreases blood loss significantly.[15] After reduction of tumour bulk,

[131]I treatment may be more effective. Furthermore, it can improve patient's mobility, giving them a better quality of life.

Well-differentiated thyroid carcinoma is a major health problem in New Caledonia because of its high incidence and aggressive behaviour. However, the present management, in the form of intensive ^{131}I treatment, tumour embolisation, and resection of metastatic foci, suggests that most patients have excellent long-term survival.

ACKNOWLEDGEMENTS
The authors wish to thank Dr Luc Letenneur (Universite Victor Segalen, France) for advice on statistical analysis. The study would not have been possible without the cooperation and dedication of many medical officers who were involved in the management of patients with thyroid disease in New Caledonia.

Figure 1A

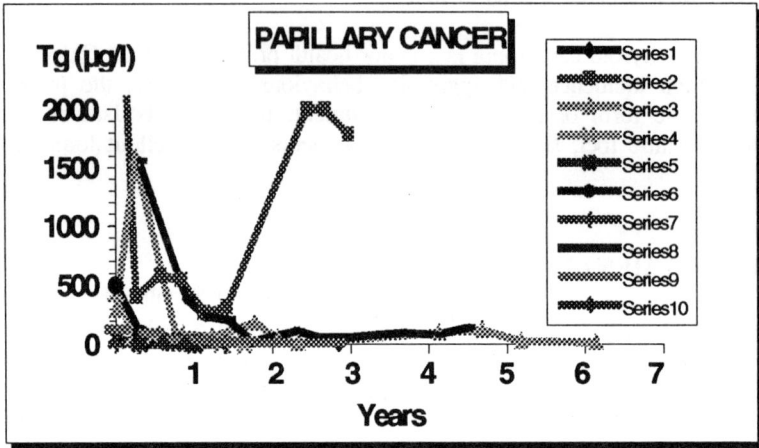

Figure 1B

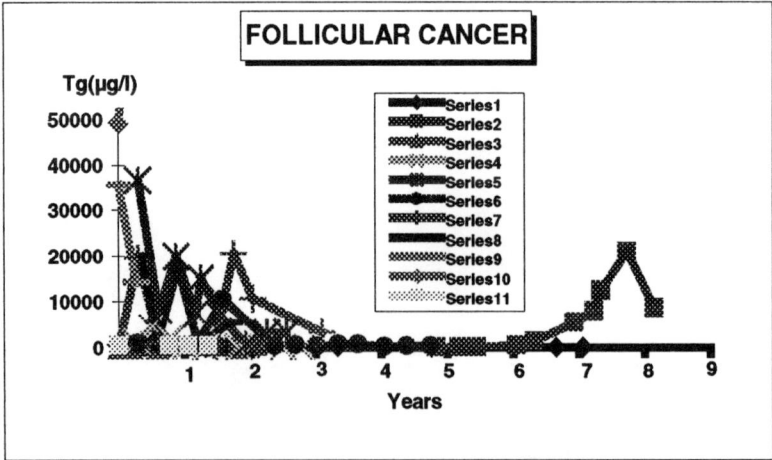

Figure 1
Thyroglobulin levels during folow-up period in patients with metastases at initial scan.
*Note difference in Y axis scale of Papillary cancer compared to follicular cancer.
A. Patients with papillary cancer (n=11)
B. Patients with follicular cancer (n=12)
One patient from the papillary group and one from the follicular group had only one thyroglobulin level available.

Figure2A

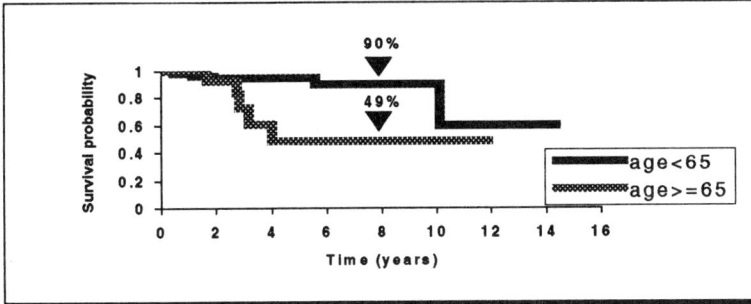

Figure2B

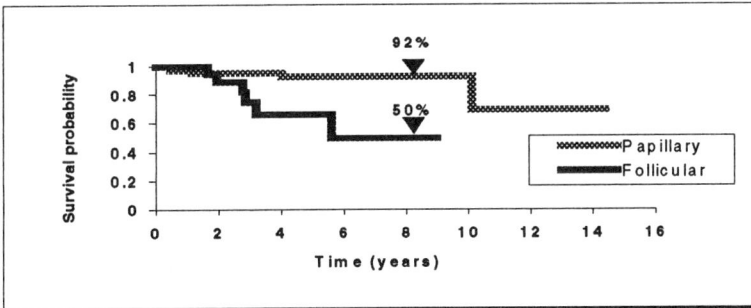

Figure 2C

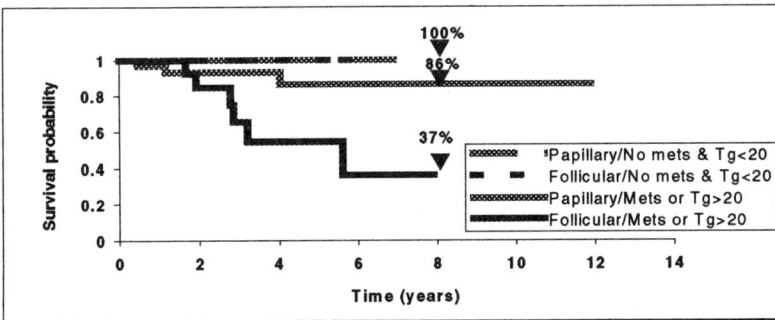

Figure 2
Survival in various subgroups of patients with well-differentiated thyroid carcinoma.
A. According to age, p=0.02 comparing age <65 to age ≥65.
B. According to histology, p<0.01 comparing papillary cancer to follicular cancer.
C. According to metastatic status on initial scans post-total thyroidectomy.

116

REFERENCES

1. Ballivet S, Rachid Salmi L, Dubourdieu D, Bach F. Incidence of thyroid cancer in New Caledonia, South Pacific, during 1985-1992. *Am J Epidemiol* 1995; **141**: 741-746.
2. Blot WJ, Le Marchand L, Boice JD, Henderson BE. Thyroid cancer in the Pacific. *J Natl Cancer Inst* 1997; **89**: 90-91.
3. Hedinger CE. Histological typing of thyroid tumours. In: Hedinger CE, ed. *International Histological Classification of Tumours*, Berlin: Springer-Verlag, 1988: vol 11.
4. Mazzaferri EL, Jhiang SM. Long-term impact of initial surgical and medical therapy on papillary and follicular thyroid cancer. *Am J Med* 1994; **97**: 418-428.
5. Samaan NA, Schultz PN, Hickey RC, et al. Well-differentiated thyroid carcinoma and the results of various modalities of treatment. A retrospective review of 1599 patients. *J Clin Endocrinol Metab* 1992; **75**: 714-720.
6. Dulgeroff AJ, Hershman JM. Medical therapy for differentiated thyroid carcinoma. *Endocr Rev* 1994; **15**: 500-515.
7. Mazzaferri EL. Papillary thyroid carcinoma: factors influencing prognosis and current therapy. *Semin Oncol* 1987; **14**: 315-332.
8. Pacini F, Cetani F, et al. Outcome of 309 patients with metastatic differentiated thyroid carcinoma treated with radioiodine. *World J Surg* 1994; **18**: 600-604.
9. Sweeny DC, Johnston GS. Radioiodine therapy for thyroid cancer. *Endocrinol Metab Clin North Am* 1995; **24**: 803-839.
10. Schlumberger M, Mancusi F, Baudun E, Pacini F. I-131 therapy for elevated thyroglobulin levels. *Thyroid* 1997; **7**: 273-276.
11. Ruiz-Garcia J, Ruiz de Almodovar JM, Olea N, Pedraza V. Thyroglobulin level as a predictive factor of tumoural recurrence in differentiated thyroid cancer. *J Nucl Med* 1991; **32**: 395-398.
12. Spencer CA, Wang CC. Thyroglobulin Measurement: techniques, clinical benefits and pitfalls. *Endocrinol Metab Clin North Am* 1995; **24**: 841-863.
13. Correa P, Chen VW. Endocrine gland cancer. *Cancer [Suppl]* 1995; **75**: 338-352.
14. Niederle B, Roka R, Schemper M, et al. Surgical treatment of distant metastases in differentiated thyroid cancer: indication and results. *Surgery* 1986; **100**: 1088-1096.
15. Wood WJ, Singletary SE, Hickey RC. Current results of treatment for distant metastatic well-differentiated thyroid carcinoma. *Arch Surg* 1989; **124**: 1374-1377.

THYROID CANCER AMONG THE POPULATION OF SEMIPALATINSK REGION EXPOSED TO IONIZING RADIATION DUE TO NUCLEAR WEAPON TESTS. CORRELATIONAL STUDY

Zh. ABYLKASSIMOVA

The Research Institute for Radiation Medicine and Ecology, po.b. 16, Semipalatinsk, 490046, Republic of Kazakstan
E-mail: salex@irl.semsk.su, zhanata@yahoo.com

The population of the Semipalatinsk Region was exposed to acute and chronic irradiation in different doses due to nuclear tests carried out in nuclear tests site from 1949 to 1989. The region territory was divided into five zones of radiation risk according to dose of exposure. The comparison between the thyroid gland cancer incidence in the population of zones of high and low radiation risk was carried out. The correlation epidemiological study was done in order to determine the thyroid gland cancer cumulative incidence, relative risk, attributive risk, attributive risk percent, and confidential interval. The study results have shown that the relative risk of thyroid gland cancer in high-exposed group was significantly higher than in low exposed group.

1. Introduction

Semipalatinsk region is located in the North-East of Kazakhstan, former Soviet Republic and newly independent state. The population of this region is more than 800 thousands people. The nuclear test site (STS) is located in 150 km from Semipalatinsk city, the regional center with population more than 400,000.

A unique radiation situation has existed around the STS. During forty years thirty-eight on-the-ground, 86 atmospheric, and 340 underground (totally – 456) blasts from 1949 through 1989 caused radioactive contamination of vast territories in the Region and exposed hundreds of thousands of people to multiple acute and chronic irradiation in different, mostly low-level doses (1). Up to 1963 the atmospheric and on-the-ground tests were carried out. Later only underground blasts were conducted.

2. Materials and methods

We have prepared the research materials on the retrospective evaluation of the parameters of ground and atmospheric nuclear explosions throughout the testing period. These materials convincingly prove that the exposure doses on the ground (in the "controlled" areas of the Semipalatinsk Region) were measured at the level of 10 to 25 R (roentgen). The external doses calculated from these explosion parameters ranged from 7.0 to 16.0 cGy. Every nuclear explosion at the Semipalatinsk test site contaminated the entire Region with radioactive products and local fallout from radioactive clouds that exposed population of 374 settlements of the Region to multiple acute and chronic irradiation. The doses of exposure were ranging from 0.2 to 502.0 cSv. According to absorbed radiation dose distribution the territory of Region has been divided to four zones of radiation risk: A-zone of extremely radiation risk (100 to 448 cSv); B-zone of maximal radiation risk (35 to 99 cSv); C-zone of increased radiation risk (7 to 34 cSv); D-zone of minimal radiation risk (1,0 to 6,9 cSv) (Figure 1).

Semipalatinsk area

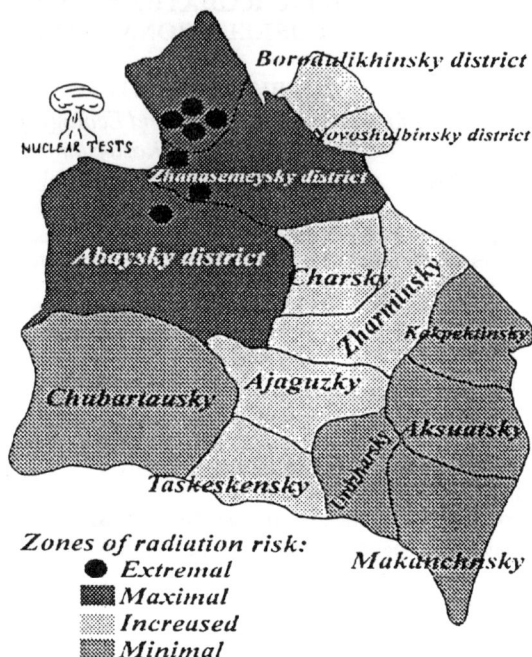

Fig. 1. Zones of elevated radiation in the Semipalatinsk region

To investigate the possible relationship between radioiodine exposure and thyroid cancer we conducted a case review of 100 pathological findings in the patients who underwent the surgery because of nodular goiter during fourteen years period 1980 to 1993. All cases were separated in two groups: residents of A- and B- zones (I group - exposed to high doses) – 72 cases; and residents of D-zone (II group - nonexposed) – 28 cases. The age distribution of thyroid gland cases and the prevalence rate are shown in the Table 1.

Table 1. The thyroid cancer rate per 1,000 of population and age-distribution of cases.

Age	Group I, exposed to high doses			Group II, nonexposed		
	Number of population	Number of cases	Rate per 1,000 pop.	Number of population	Number of cases	Rate per 1,000 pop.
<25 years	40,500	4	0.10	48,000	4	0.08
25-34	11,625	15	1.29*	18,000	7	0.39
35-45	7,500	41	5.47*	15,500	8	0.52
>45 years	15,375	12	0.78	18,500	9	0.49
Total	75,000	72	0.96*	100,000	28	0.28

* - p <0.05

As you can see, the most of thyroid cancer cases for group I were verified at the age of 25 to 44. It means, that the participants of this group were born from 1949 to 1962, during the period of time, when principal dose of exposure was formed. It is well known, that children thyroid gland is many times more sensitive to radiation exposure than adults.

3. Study results
The study results are shown in the table 2.

Table 2. Thyroid cancer study in the Semipalatinsk area.

	Group I	Group II
Prevalence per 100,000	96,0*	28,0*
SIR	1.14*	0.27*
RR - 4.22		CI 0.95% (2.72; 6.8)
AR - 0.87		CI 0.95% (0.60; 1.04)
AR% - 76.3%		

* - p < 0.05

According to number of each zone population the prevalence rate of the thyroid gland cancer was calculated (table 2). In the Group I it was equal 96.0/100,000 population, in the Group II – 28/100,000 population. Age adjusted incidence rate were calculated, using as a standard combine population of both groups. Standardized incidence rate in the Group I was equal 1,14 °/∞ and in the Group II – 0,27°/∞. The relative risk of thyroid cancer among exposed to high doses of radiation was 4,22 times greater than among exposed to low radiation doses (CI 95% 2.72; 6.8). The attributive risk of radiation exposure in high doses was equal 0.87. And attributable risk %, which shows the percent of the risk of thyroid cancer in the Group I that can be attributed to high dose irradiation, was equal 76,3%.

Taking in consideration that radiation induced thyroid cancer is mostly presented by such histological type of cancer like papillary carcinoma we have analyzed all our cases. The distribution of thyroid cancer by pathological type of tumor is presented in the Table 3.

Table 3. The histological type distribution of thyroid gland cancer in observed groups of population exposed to different doses of irradiation.

Histological type of thyroid cancer	Group I Residents of zones A and B	Group II Residents of zone D
Papillary carcinoma	44 (80.5%)	19 (67.9%)
Follicular carcinoma	12 (16.6%)	5 (17.9%)
Others types	16 (2.9%)	4 (14.2%)
Total	72 (100%)	28 (100%)
p	>0.05	>0.05

4. Discussion

We established a clear-cut verifiable dynamics for the growth of the thyroid cancer incidence at every subsequent calendar stage. In thirteen years (1980--1993), the thyroid cancer morbidity rates for the exposed population rose almost fourfold per 100,000 population. Most of the revealed thyroid cancer cases for Group I was verified at the age of 25 to 44. The papillary cancer amounted to 80.5 percent, the follicular cancer to 16.6 percent, and carcinomas' mixed forms to 2.9 percent of these cases. The absence of statistically significant difference between both Groups by pathological type distribution can be explained by following reason. The Semipalatinsk region is endemic area for thyroid gland disorders because of iodine deficiency in soil and water. As is well known the iodine balance problem may lead to developing of the follicular thyroid gland carcinoma (3). So this side of problem needs to be investigated in future additional studies.

A closer look at the list of participants in our research most of whom (Group I) were born from 1949 to 1962, leaves no doubt that, as for the thyroid cancer incidence, people exposed to irradiation in infancy and childhood happened to be most radiological sensitive. Many other researchers (3,4) back up this conclusion. As is shown in the Table 4, our data are correlated with data of other researches.

Table 4. The comparison of the relative and attributive risk of thyroid gland cancer in different groups of population.

Study population	Relative risk (CI)	Attributive risk (CI)
Japanese	-	0.3 (0.16; 0.47)
Russian	2.2	0.2 (0.06; 0.34)
Semipalatinsk region	4.22 (2.72; 6.8)	0.87 (0.60; 1.04)

A higher thyroid cancer incidence for Group I permits us to conclude that the actual primary irradiation doses for this Group were higher. This conclusion also supports the view of many C.I.S. scientists that local radioactive fallout across the Semipalatinsk Region had an uneven drop rate. The "downwind territories" and/or the areas lying closer to the Polygon were in reality contaminated by fusion products more often and on a wider scale. The population participants who made up Group I in fact lived in the most contaminated towns, villages and settlements of these territories. We believe that a thorough epidemiological study involving numerically larger radiation risk groups from among the populace residing in the areas less contaminated by fusion products will provide answers about the emerging pathology and the low-level ionizing radiation.

Such research will enable scientists to calculate relative risks of cancer incidence and cancer mortality rate among the population of the Semipalatinsk Region who were exposed to low level ionizing radiation. It will also allow them to extrapolate the received data on other regions of Kazakhstan that find themselves in similar or identical radiation and hygienic situations.

References

1. Gusev BI, Abylkassimova Zh, Apsalikov KN. The Semipalatinsk nuclear test site: a first assessment of the radiological situation and the test related radiation doses in the surrounding territories. *Radiat Environ Biophys* 1997; **36**: 201-204.
2. International basic safety standards for protection against ionizing radiation and for safety of radiation sources. *Safety series* No 115. IAEA, Vienna, 1996.
3. Tsyb AF. Medical consequences of the Chernobyl Accident. *Med Radiol and Radiat Safety* 1998; **43(1)**: 18-23.
4. Yamashita Sh. Proposal for establishment of skreening of thyroid diseases around Semipalatinsk Nuclear test site. In: Hosi M., Takada R., Kim R., and Nitta Y., ed. *Effects of low level radiation for residents near Semipalatinsk nuclear test site.* Proceed. Of the Second Hirosima Intern.Symp., Hirosima, july 23-25, 1996, 225-234.

FACTORS RELATED TO LATENCY PERIOD IN POST-CHERNOBYL CARCINOGENESIS

A. KOFLER, TH. ABELIN

Department of Social and Preventive Medicine, University of Bern, Finkenhubelweg 11, CH-3012 Bern, Switzerland

I. PRUDYVUS, Y. AVERKIN

Belarus State Research Institute for Oncology and Medical Radiology, Lesnoy, Minsk, Belarus

In connection with post-Chernobyl thyroid cancer, more cases with short latency periods have been observed than ever before. Short latency periods were shown in districts with higher exposure and higher incidence rates, whereas lower age at exposure and higher susceptibility seem to be associated with a prolonged increase of incidence rates and thus a higher mean latency period. These associations should be studied during longer observation periods and with respect to information on completeness and screening activities.

1   INTRODUCTION AND OBJECTIVES

When early in 1992, a first detailed epidemiological analysis of post-Chernobyl thyroid cancer cases was submitted for publication, one of the reasons given for refusal was that latency periods below seven or eight years were too short to be credible. Meanwhile, an updated version of this analysis has been published[1] and the fact of childhood thyroid cancer related to the Chernobyl disaster has been generally accepted[2]. Nevertheless, the questions remain unanswered whether (a) the observation of cases soon after the Chernobyl nuclear accident represents merely the extreme left end of a normal distribution of latency periods, where a very rare phenomenon has become more visible due to the large number of cases involved; or whether (b) a strong exposure, such as occurred following the Chernobyl accident, selectively shortens the latency period; or whether (c) the observed short latency period is explained by the young age at exposure, which may not only lead to a higher thyroid cancer incidence, but also to a shorter latency period. The purpose of this communication is to test these explanations in the light of available data.

2   METHODS

A database of 6090 persons who had a diagnosis of thyroid cancer between 1986 and 1997 was developed on the basis of data from the Belarus Cancer Registry. Double reportings were eliminated and multiple cases with similar but not identical information were examined closely by means of probabilistic data linkage software newly developed by the team of the authors. Where available, place of residence in 1986 rather than at the time of diagnosis was used. 805 persons with thyroid cancer had been under 15 years old in 1986 and represent the present study population. Population data by district (rayon), gender and age were obtained from the 1989 population census. Cohort incidence rates by rayon were computed and presented in graphical form by means of MapStudio, a geographic information system developed by Konstantin Krivoruchko, International Sakharov Institute of Radioecology, Minsk. All cases observed up to age of 26 at diagnosis were included in order to count all cases in the cohorts aged   0-14 in 1986 and observed through 1997.

For the analyses of latency periods, the data from the cities of Gomel and Minsk were excluded, as more intensive medical attention common in large cities might have led to difficulties in interpretation of differences in latency periods. Latency periods were determined as the interval between the time of the accident (end of April, 1986) and the month of diagnosis of thyroid cancer. Distributions of latency periods were then examined for districts with higher or lower incidence rates, and for persons younger or older at the time of the accident.

3   RESULTS

3.1   Incidence rates

Thyroid cancer incidence rates among those aged 0-14 in 1986 reached 3.34 per 10,000 person-years in the most exposed rayon, but half of the cases occurred in districts with rates of 0.56 per 10,000 person-years or less. Figure 1 shows geographically incidence rates by districts, and suggests not only a clear association with distance from the Chernobyl reactor site, but also reflects the wind directions toward northwest observed during the first days following the accident.

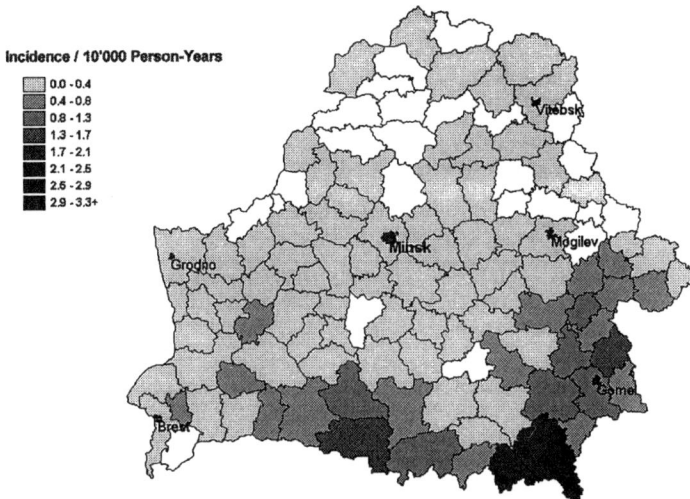

Fig. 1. Thyroid cancer rates per 10'000 person-years of individuals aged 0 - 14 in 1986. Belarus, by district

In Figure 2, average latency periods per district are plotted against average yearly incidence rates of the same district. A very conspicuous correlation cannot be seen, but there seems to be a relative lack of early cases in districts with low incidence. However, this visual impression should be viewed with caution, as the figure does not reflect the size of the districts and the number of cases involved. More detailed analyses are needed to interpret this finding satisfactorily.

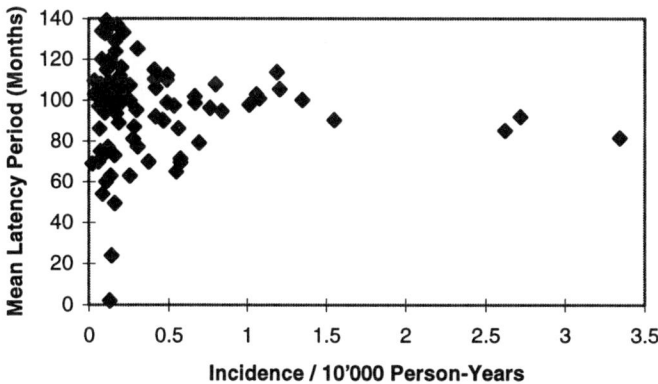

Fig. 2. Plot diagram of districts by mean latency period and thyroid cancer incidence rates, Belarus 1986 - 1997

In Table 1, latency periods (derived from the year of diagnosis) are cross-tabulated against 4 categories of districts with different thyroid cancer incidence rates. There is a significant trend with high incidence districts showing an excess of short latency cases (p for trend = 0.019).

Table 1. Cases of thyroid cancer among persons aged 0 - 14 in 1986 in 4 categories of districts, by incidence rates and latency periods. Category 1 : highest incidence; category 4 : lowest incidence. 1986 - 93 : latency period of 0 - 7 years; 1994 - 97 : latency period of 8 - 11 years

Category	1986 -1993	1994 -1997	Total
1:	73	75	148
2:	57	93	150
3:	62	89	151
4:	48	93	141
All Categories	240	350	590

Figure 3 suggests that indeed up to 1993, cases in high incidence regions were especially numerous compared to those in low incidence areas. More recently numbers and the difference in high incidence areas have diminished, which led to an excess of short latency cases in high incidence areas.

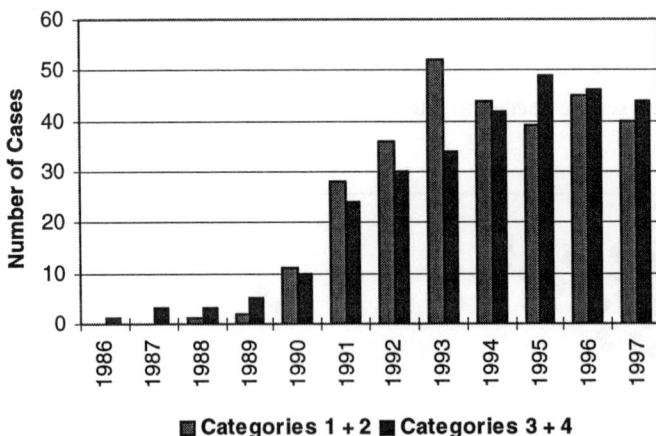

■ Categories 1 + 2 ■ Categories 3 + 4

Fig. 3. Number of yearly cases of thyroid cancer diagnosed 1986 - 97 in Belarus among persons aged 0 - 14 in 1986, by incidence rate in their rayon of residence in 1986

3.2   Age at exposure

Figure 4 shows the trend of the number of diagnosed cases by age at exposure. It indicates that incidence is and remains highest among those exposed at the youngest age. But, as Figure 4 suggests and Table 2 demonstrates more clearly, there are significantly more cases with a short latency period among those aged 5-14 than among those aged 0-4 years at the time of the Chernobyl accident (p=0.0009). This confirms an observation made by Pacini et al[3], who also reported increased latency periods for patients exposed at young age. Longer observation periods are needed to definitely distinguish whether the principal phenomenon is a relative lack of very short latency periods among those exposed at a younger age, or an early decline of cases among those exposed at a higher age.

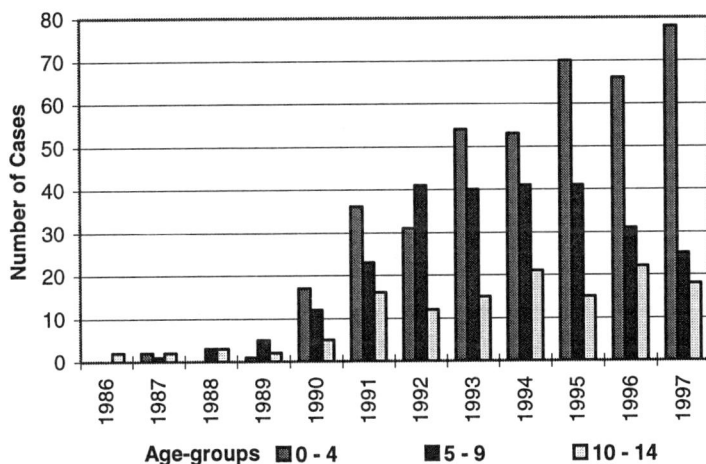

Fig. 4. Number of yearly cases of thyroid cancer diagnosed 1986 - 97 in Belarus among persons aged 0 - 14 at exposure, by age in 1986

Table 2.   Cases of thyroid cancer among persons aged 0 - 14 in 1986 by age in 1986 and latency periods. New cases 1986 - 93 : latency period of 0 - 7 years; 1994 - 97 : latency period of 8 - 11 years.

Age at Exposure	1986 -1993	1994 -1997	Total
0 - 4	106	202	308
5- 9	91	98	189
10 - 14	44	49	93
All Age Groups	241	349	590

3.3 Incidence rates and age at exposure

If for each level of susceptibility a certain threshold level of radiation exposure has to be reached for clinical expression of cancer, we would expect relatively more highly susceptibles in areas with low exposure than in areas with high exposure. This means that cases in low incidence areas would have a higher susceptibility, both of which would be compatible with longer latency periods. However, as Table 3 shows, in areas with low incidence, the proportion of cases aged 0-4 in 1986, was significantly lower and not higher than in areas with high incidence rates (p for trend = 0.004). An easy biological explanation is therefore not possible. On the other hand, here again a longer observation period may allow for distinguishing between basic patterns and temporary observations due to differences in incidence trends.

Table 3. Distribution of cases of thyroid cancer among persons aged 0 - 14 in 1986 by incidence rate and age in 1986

Category	0 - 4 Years	5 - 14 Years	Total
1:	81	67	148
2:	94	56	150
3:	75	76	151
4:	58	83	141
All Categories	308	282	590

As Figure 4 shows, a steep initial increase (which is associated with short observed latency periods) can lead to high incidence rates remaining high over a prolonged period (as is the case for those aged 0-4 in 1986), or reach a lower peak followed by an early decline (as among those 5-9 years old in 1986). The many cases in 1995 to 1997 among those exposed at an age of 0-4 lead to a long average latency period, whereas the decline observed after 1995 among those aged 5-9 at exposure leads to a short average latency period.

4 DISCUSSION AND CONCLUSION

Latency periods as short as four to five years observed in the first cases of post-Chernobyl childhood thyroid cancer had been rarely reported before. Recently, a combined analysis of data from several studies of medical use of radiation and thyroid cancer showed that similar latency periods can be seen, if the total number of cases studied is sufficiently large (4). The present analysis shows that the study of latency periods will pose methodological problems, as long as new cases continue to appear. Although the absolute number of those who were youngest at the time of exposure is highest among the cases with short latency periods, this may simply reflect the fact that this is the age cohort with the largest number of cases, and not a phenomenon relating to latency period specifically. On the other hand, since about 1993, incidence has continued to increase for this youngest cohort but has decreased or remained stable for those older when exposed. If these trends continue, the mean latency period will increase more strongly among those with low age at exposure than among those who were older at the time of the Chernobyl accident, and this could turn out to reflect a special biological feature of persons with high susceptibility.

Present data also suggest that in districts with high incidence rates (and exposure) there were relatively more cases with an early age at exposure. As Figure 3 suggests, this is related to a steep early increase of cases in the high incidence districts, with a peak in 1993, whereas in lower incidence districts, the increase was less steep, and its peak was in about 1995. In other words, high incidence districts seem to have had relatively more short latency period cases. However, further follow-up of these cohorts and detailed knowledge of case characteristics is needed, in order to properly interpret these trends, as they could also be due to such factors as temporary underreporting of cases or to the effect of screening campaigns for selected age groups in particular areas.

Acknowledgements

Thanks are due to the Swiss Federal Office of Public Health for financial support.

130

References

1. Abelin T, Averkin Y, Egger M et al. Thyroid cancer in Belarus post-Chernobyl. Improved detection or increased incidence? *Soz Präventivmed* 1994; **39**: 189-197.
2. Baverstock K. Chernobyl and public health. Editorial. *Brit Med J* 1998; **316**: 952-953.
3. Pacini F, Vorontsova T, Demidchik EP et al. Post-Chernobyl Thyroid Carcinoma in Belarus Children and Adolescents: Comparison with Naturally Occurring Thyroid Carcinoma in Italy and France. *J Clin Endocrinol Metab* 1997; **82**: 3563-9.
4. Ron E, Lubin JH, Shore RE et al. Thyroid Cancer after Exposure to External Radiation: A Pooled Analysis of Seven Studies. *Radiation Research* 1995; **141**: 259-277.

EPIDEMIOLOGY OF THYROID CANCER AMONG CHILDREN HAVING BEEN EXPOSED TO RADIATION IN CONSEQUENCE OF THE CHERNOBYL ACCIDENT

BOMKO E. I.

Scientific Center for Radiation Medicine, Academy of Medical Science of Ukraine
Address: 53, Melnikov St., 252051, Kiev, Ukraine
E-mail: elena@okey.kiev.ua

The present paper is of definite interest as the characterization of pediatric population exposed to direct impact of radiation factor after Chernobyl NPP accident.

The aim of this survey is to form an estimate of cases of the thyroid cancer which was revealed during first 11 years after the Chernobyl disaster among the children 0-14 years old at the time of the accident (Chernobyl accident time, CAT).

The prospective epidemiological investigation for cohort of 40 000 persons born in 1972-1986 was organized. Cohort was divided into two subcohorts: Subcohort 1 consisted of persons evacuated from Prypiat city and residing in city of Kiev. And residents of countryside of Kiev's and Zhytomyr's regions polluted with radionuclides formed the subcohort 2.

Simultaneous exposition to iodine, cesium, etc. was the criterion for sampling. Members of the subcohort 1 were exposed to acute influence of the isotopes mentioned above and were evacuated from Prypiat city in 36 hours after the CAT. Persons of the subcohort 2 were exposed to radioactive iodine for 10 days and further lived in contaminated territories for several years and were being exposed to long-term influence of the radioactive isotopes of cesium, etc.

Parameters per 1 000 children population (by size of children population in 1986) after the Chernobyl accident constituted 1.0 for evacuated persons and 0.42 for the residents, standardized parameters are 1.08 and 0.9 respectively; cumulated parameter per 100 000 person-years – 3.5 and 3.0 respectively.

In subcohort of evacuated persons the average-aged thyroid doses range was 200-280 cGy; mode of integral effective equivalent dose for cesium – 11.5 mSv. In subcohort of the residents the wider range of thyroid irradiation doses was present: from 14.5 to 270.4 cGy; mode of integral effective equivalent dose for cesium – 21.8 mSv.

It was found out that children who were the most close by the Chernobyl nuclear disaster hypocenter and exposed to the short-term irradiation with radioiodine in high doses are now subject to the highest risk of thyroid cancer. The younger kids are under higher risk; females are also under higher risk.

Key words: children population, thyroid cancer, Chernobyl NPP accident.

At present diseases induced by radiation as it is universally recognized are pathologies oncologically or genetically stipulated. The present work is fragment of the research concerning evaluation of low radiation dose effects among pediatric population exposed to direct irradiation in consequence of the Chernobyl accident [1, 2]. But that's rightful to mention the low radiation doses only towards the cesium, strontium and other long-living radionuclides. The main biologically dangerous effector for children was the iodine-131 [3, 4]. Thyroid cancer problem became even more actual after the Chernobyl accident in spite of already carried out wide-scale studies [5].

The present study aim was to make estimation of thyroid cancer cases that occurred during first 11 years after the Chernobyl accident among children 0-14 years old at the time of the accident (Chernobyl accident time, CAT) who was evacuated from Pripyat city or residing in the contaminated territories.

Prospective epidemiological investigation for cohort of 40 000 persons born in 1972-1986 was organized. Persons and cases available for registration were included in the cohort, including those relocated from contaminated territories after 1986. The cohort was divided into two subcohorts. Subcohort 1 consisted of persons evacuated from Prypiat city and residing in city of Kiev. And residents of countryside of Kiev's and Zhytomyr's regions polluted with radionuclides formed the subcohort 2.

Character of the combined irradiation by iodine-131, cesium-137, strontium-90, etc. and distance from accident site were used as the sampling criterion. Members of the subcohort 1 were exposed to acute influence of the isotopes mentioned above. They were very close by the disaster hypocenter and were evacuated from town Prypiat in 36 hours after CAT. Persons of the subcohort 2 were moved away the polluted territories on first decade of May 1986 in order to make them healthier during several months. So they were exposed to radioactive iodine for 10 days. And then they came back and lived there for several years and were exposed to long-term influence of the radioactive isotopes of cesium, strontium, etc.

In studied subcohorts the most wide-spread diseases of non-tumor types were: subcohort 1 – nervous system diseases first of all due to autonomous nervous system-vascular dystonia, subcohort 2 – mental disorders of non-psychiatric character; gastrointestinal tractus non-specific diseases were characteristic for both cohorts.

Thyroid cancer incidence rates per 1 000 pediatric population (by size of children population in 1986) in permanent residence locations after the Chernobyl accident amounted to 1.0 for the evacuated persons and 0.42 for the residents. Cumulative parameter for 11 year for average-year pediatric population per 1 000 evacuated persons amounted to 1.43, residents of contaminated territories – 1.37; for 100 000 person-years – 3.5 and 3.0 respectively. Standardized parameters were 1.08 and 0.9 respectively. World Standard Population was used as calculation standard.

Risk calculation for 100 000 person-years was carried out in age groups of 0-4, 5-9 and 10-14 years old at CAT. In both subcohorts the parameter excess is present among groups 0-4 years old at CAT. The sex-dependent standardization revealed higher insurability of females.

In the subcohort of evacuated persons the calculated average-age thyroid dose range constitutes 200-280 cGy; mode of integral effective equivalent dose for cesium – 11.5 mSv. In the subcohort of residents the wider range of thyroid irradiation doses were evaluated – from 14.5 to 270.4 cGy; mode of integral effective equivalent dose for cesium – 21.8 mSv.

Before the Chernobyl accident no thyroid cancer cases were registered on studied territories, i.e. there were no of them. To reveal the differences between the studied subcohorts the IPE-INFO Program was used. Additional and relative risk indices were obtained for subcohort 1 in comparison with subcohort 2 (95% confidential interval):

```
          Analysis of Single Table
      Odds ratio = 2.35 (0.87<OR<6.12*)
      Cornfield 95% confidence limits for OR
*Cornfield not accurate. Exact limits preferred
      Relative risk = 2.35 (0.96<RR<5.76)
      Taylor Series 95% confidence limits for RR
      Ignore relative risk if case control study

                  Chi - Squares    P - values
Uncorrected          3.69                      0.0546358
Mantel - Haenszel    3.69                      0.0546386
Yates corrected      2.67                      0.1020336
Yates corrected      2.67                      0.1020336
Fisher exact:        1 - tailed P — value      0.0590790
                     1 - tailed P — value      0.0775754
An expected cell value is less than 5.
Fisher exact results recommended.
```

The present study results may be estimated as the preliminary ones. Our study is limited with pediatric age period, because on evaluating thyroid cancer cases among persons having left children age group it is necessary to estimate a number of additional factors. Also the adequate control group is hardly available as identification of iodine component in dose formation for whole territory of Ukraine is going on so is evaluation of uncertainty of the thyroid radioiodin direct measurements. Dose reconstruction models are under changes too. The inversive method application is more appropriate in the field of "Radiation and Thyroid Cancer" problem (i.e. that from cases to inducing factors).

So on the present stage of work we can say that children who were the most close by the Chernobyl disaster hypocenter zone and exposed to the short-term irradiation with radioiodine in high doses are now subject to the highest risk of thyroid cancer. The younger are kids the higher is the risk; females are subject to the highest risk.

References

1. Elena I. Bomko. Morbidity estimation in changeable cohort of children being chronically exposed by low level doses of radiation in consequence Chernobyl accident. *New risk frontiers. 10th Anniversary the Society for Risk Analysis – Europe. Stockholm,* 1997:783-789.
2. Bomko, A.E. Romanenko, A.A. Bomko. Estimation of health effects of long-term chronic exposure of the low level radiation among children exposed in consequence of the disaster at the Chernobyl nuclear power plant. *Low doses of ionizing radiation: biological effects and regulatory control. International Conference held in Seville, Spain,* 1997:326-329.
3. Lester Van Middlesworth, Ph.D., MD. Nuclear Reactor Accidents and the Thyroid. *Thyroid Today, Vol. X, №2,* 1987:1-5.
4. Vasylenko, MD. Hygienic Estimation of Iodine Isotopes. *Hygiene and Sanitary,* 1987, **2:** 64 - 67.
5. Arthur B. Schneider, MD, Ph.D. Thyroid Nodules. Following Childhood Irradiation: A 1989 Update. *Thyroid Today, Vol. XI, №2,* 1989:1-7.

COMPARATIVE ANALYSIS OF THYROID CANCER INCIDENCE RATE IN NEIGHBORING TERRITORIES OF UKRAINE, BELARUS, AND RUSSIA AFTER THE CHERNOBYL ACCIDENT

A. PRYSYAZHNYUK, V. GRISTCHENKO, A. CHEBAN

Research Center for Radiation Medicine, 53, Melnikov st., Kiev, 254050, Ukraine.

Z. FEDORENKO, L. GULAK

Ukraine institute of Oncology and Radiology, 33/43, Lomonosov st., Kiev, 254022, Ukraine.

A. OKEANOV

Belarus institute of Oncology and Medical Radiology, Lesnoye, Minks, 223052, Belarus.

V. STARINSKY, L.REMENNIK

Moscow ontological institute of P.A. Gertsen, 2-nd, Botkinsky bystr., 3, Moscow, 125284, Russia.

Statistical data on ontological service or Ukraine, Belarus, and Russia on the number of new patients with thyroid cancer in 1989-1996 in 12 regions (with 19.1mln population) adjacent to the Chernobyl NPP are generalized. There was performed detailed retrospective (since 1980) and current study to identify all cancers (including thyroid) in the most contaminated area in vicinity of Chernobyl where at the moment of accident had been living 274,000 including 59,200 children under 15 years

Since 1990 in all analyzed territories there were registered increase of thyroid cancer incidence rate, especially in children and adolescents. In the last time period most significant increase was registered in 10-14 and 15-19 age groups. In adult population there were increase of incidence rate in relatively younger groups and latent period was more prolonged

Because of different average per capita and collective population dose burden there were observed different increase of thyroid cancer incidence rate in analyzed territories.

Territorial variation of this pathology was increased and ratio max/min, coefficient of variation there increased as well.

The analysis of correlation between average per capita thyroid dose equivalent and thyroid cancer incidence rate was performed and suggest about statistically relationship between this values

1. Introduction

Most of reports and publications devoted to study of the thyroid cancer incidence rate due to the Chernobyl accident described the only part of problems within restricted areas or separate age groups - children, adolescents, adults (1,2,3, 8,9,10). As a result there is lack of comprehensive picture reflected the problem upon the whole. There are a few publication covered all territories of the three most affected by Chernobyl accident states - the Ukraine, Belarus, Russia (6,7). This studies have to be continued.

The main task of our study is to investigate spatio and temporal models of thyroid cancer incidence rate in neighbouring regions of the Ukraine, Belarus and Russia with substantial thyroid dose burden and to learn relationship between both this values.

2. Materials and methods

To estimate thyroid dose burden after Chernobyl accident available publication have been analyzed (4,5) and some dosimetric data presented on scientific meeting in Obninsk, Russia (11). On this base there were determined average per capita dose equivalent due to iodine-131 in 10 most affected region of Ukraine, Belarus and Russia.

To study spatio-temporal models of thyroid cancer incidence rate in affected territories there were utilized next sources of information:

-statistical data of oncological servicies on the number of thyroid cancer in 1989-1996, the number of population in each administrative unit (six region in Ukraine, two region in Belarus, and four region in Russia), totally numbering 19,13 mln people at the accident period;

-data of local cancer register established in 1987 and covered 150 000 population living in vicinity of Chernobyl (retrospective since 1980 and nowadays study);

- statistical data thyroid cancer in Ukraine in 1977-1979 (A.Ye Prysyazhnyuk study, 1985) and statistical data of thyroid cancer in Belarus in 1981-1985 (A.Ye Okeanov study, 1988)

Ade- specific and age-adjusted incidence rate have been calculated on the basis of available statistical data. There was used direct method of standardization. As a standard was used age distribution of the population former USSR in 1979 at the moment of All-Union census.

There was performed mapping procedure for spatial and temporal analysis of ditterencies of thyroid cancer incidence rate.The data of annual average incidence rate separately for 1989-1992 and 1993-1996 have been transferred on a model of geographyical map of the study regions.Correlation and regression analysis between thyroid cancer incidence rate in 1989-1992 and 1993-1996 and between average per capita thyroid dose equivalent and incidence rate for two periods has been carried out.

3. Analysis of materials

There is observed substantial increase of thyroid cancer incidence rate in most the territories of interest. Analysis of age-specific incidence rate suggests that in 1996 most significant increase was notified in age-groups 10-14 and 15-19 years - 11 and 14 times respectively. In other age-groups there was observed less pronounced increase - in 3-5 times and in oldest age-group - (75 and older) practically the same level as in preaccidental period.

Thyroid cancer incidence rate in preaccidental period in the territories of interest variated in range 1.03-1.36 per 100 000. This figures are very important because its actually reflects spontaneous level of morbidity before radiation factor has been in operation.

In postaccidental period incidence rate increased (table 1). It is very remarkable that in period of 1993-1996 max/min ratio sharply increased from 1,3 to 4,9 time as well as coefficient of variation from 10,2% to 49,2%.

Table 1 - Territorial variation in thyroid cancer incidence rate in neighbouring region of Ukraine, Belarus and Russia 1981-1985, 1989-1992,1993-1996

Years	Incidence rate per100000		Ratio	Coefficient of varieties
	maximum	minimum	max/min	(%)
1981-1985	1.36	1.03*	1.3	10.2
1989-1992	4.62	1.03	3.5	37.8
1993-1996	9.36	1.91	4.9	49.5

*Ukraine in 1977-1979

We evaluate new figure of collective and average per capita thyroid dose equivalent in region of Ukraine, Belarus, Russia based on (4,5,11).

New estimation of average per capita thyroid doze equivalent in Ukraine are in 1,4 times, in Belarus in 1,8 in Russia in 2,35 times higher then in (5). There is impressed the high value of average per capita dose equivalent in vicinity of

Chernobyl which is differe by an order of magnitude from rest of territories. Because of this value require different model for description dose-reponce then rest of figures presented in table we omitted data of this area for calculation.

The was performed mapping analysis of thyroid cancer incidence rate of the surveyed area in 1989-1992,1993-1996. This maps show close coincide of region with low, intermediate and high level thyroid incidence rate.

Correlation and regression analysis suggest about very close relation between figures of incidence rate in 1989-1992 and 1993-1996 .Value of correlation coefficientis, r= 0.772, p<0.01 suggest about statistically strong relationship between both values. Only Orel region is far much higher from 95% confidential interval. Because of that we have omitted date of Orel region from next calculation.

Correlation and regression analysis between average per capita thyroid dose equivalent and thyroid cancer incidence rate in 1993-1996 suggest about existence of close relationship between this values (r=0.678, p<0.05). Presented data could be good background for evaluation of dose- effect risk coefficient.

4. Discussion

That is notable that in preaccidental period the value of incidence rate was very low and its variation very small. After Chernobyl accident there was observed remarkable increase of thyroid cancer incidence rate in most studied territories of Ukraine, Belarus and Russia. There is statistically signiticant dependence between average per capita thyroid dose equivalent and level of morbidity (excluding Orel region). Analysed data suggest that epidemiologycal and dosimetric studies should be directed for improvement of dosimetric data and evaluation of thyroid cancer incidence rate. On this base could be possible to study dose-effect relation and determine coefficient of risk.

References

1. Abelin T., Averkin J.I., Okeanov A.E. and Bleuer J.P. Thyroid Cancer in Belarus: the epidemiological situation. The Radiological consequences of the Chernobyl accident. Proceedings of the first international conference. Minsk, Belarus, 18 to 22 March 1996. Editors A.Karaoglou, G.Desmet, G.N.Kelly and H.G.Mezel. EUR 16544 EN. ECSC-EC-EAEC. Brussels Luxembourg. 1996: 727-730.

2. Bogdanova T., Bragarnik M., Tronko N.D. et al. The pathalogy of thyroid cancer in Ukraine post Cernobyl. The radiological concequences of the Cernobyl accident. Proceedings of the first international conference. Minsk, Belarus, 18 to 22 March 1996. Editors A.Karaoglou, G.Desmet, G.N.Kelly and H.G.Mezel. EUR 16544 EN. ECSC-EC-EAEC. Brussels Luxembourg. 1996: 785-790.

3. Demidchik E.P., Drobyshevskaya I.M., Cherstvoy E.D. et al. Thyroid cancer in children in Belarus. The radiological concequences of the Cernobyl accident. Proceedings of the first international conference. Minsk, Belarus, 18 to 22 March 1996. Editors A.Karaoglou, G.Desmet, G.N.Kelly and H.G.Mezel. EUR 16544 EN. ECSC-EC-EAEC. Brussels Luxembourg. 1996: 785-790.

4. Health concequences of the Cernobyl accident. Results of the IPHECA pilot projects and related national programmes Scientific Report WHO, Geneva, 1996: 248-253.

5. Ilyin L.A., Balonov M.I. Buldakov L.A. et al. Radiocontamination patterns and possible health concequences of the accident at the Cernobyl nuclear power station. J. Radiol. Prot. 1990:10(1):3-29.

6. Prisjazhniuk A.Ye. Spatio-temporal models for incidence of malignant neoplasms in the area subjected to radioactive contamination after the Cernobyl accident. The Cernobyl papers. Vol 1. Doses to the soviet population and early health effected studies. Editors: Steven E.Mervin, Michail J.Balonov. Research Enterprises. Richland, Washington, 1993: 399-423.

7. Prisjazhniuk Anatoly, Fedorenko Zoya, Okeanov Alexey et al. Epidemiology of cancer in population living in contaminated territories of Ukraine, Belarus, Russia after the Cernobyl accident. The radiological concequences of the Cernobyl accident. Proceedings of the first international conference. Minsk, Belarus, 18 to 22 March 1996. Editors A.Karaoglou, G.Desmet, G.N.Kelly and H.G.Mezel. EUR 16544 EN. ECSC-EC-EAEC. Brussels Luxembourg. 1996: 909-921.

8. Sobolev B., Likhtarev I., Kairo I. et al. Radiation risk assessment of the thyroid cancer in Ukrainian children exposed due to Chernobyl. The radiological concequences of the Cernobyl accident. Proceedings of the first international conference. Minsk, Belarus, 18 to 22 March 1996. Editors

140

A.Karaoglou, G.Desmet, G.N.Kelly and H.G.Mezel. EUR 16544 EN. ECSC-EC-EAEC. Brussels Luxembourg. 1996: 741-748.

9. Tsyb A.F., Parshkov E.M., Shakhtarin V.V. et al. Thyroid cancer in children and adolescents of Bryansk and Kaluga regions. The radiological concequences of the Cernobyl accident. Proceedings of the first international conference. Minsk, Belarus, 18 to 22 March 1996. Editors A.Karaoglou, G.Desmet, G.N.Kelly and H.G.Mezel. EUR 16544 EN. ECSC-EC-EAEC. Brussels Luxembourg. 1996: 691-698.

10. Tronko N., Bogdanova T., Komissarenko I. et al. Thyroid cancer in children and adolescents in Ukrainian after Chernobul accident (1986-1995). The radiological concequences of the Cernobyl accident. Proceedings of the first international conference. Minsk, Belarus, 18 to 22 March 1996. Editors A.Karaoglou, G.Desmet, G.N.Kelly and H.G.Mezel. EUR 16544 EN. ECSC-EC-EAEC. Brussels Luxembourg. 1996: 683-690.

11. Workshop on health effects of low dose radiation and/or low dose rate-exposure. Obninsk, Russian Federation, 16-18 September 1997. Personal communiation.

THYROID CANCER IN THE ALTAI REGION POPULATION EXPOSED TO FALLOUT FROM THE NUCLEAR TESTS AT THE SEMIPALATINSK TEST SITE

Ya. N. SHOIKHET AND A. F. LAZAREV
Altai State Medical University, 40 Lenin Ave, 656049, Barnaul, Russia

E. V. ZAITSEV, V. I. KISELEV AND I. B. KOLYADO
Institute of Regional Medico-Ecological Problems, P.O.Box 4663, Barnaul 656043, Russia
E-mail: zev@biomed.altai.su

Altai Region (Russian Federation) borders in the south-west on the Semipalatinsk Test Site where atmospheric nuclear tests were conducted from 1949 through 1962.

Essential distinctions in thyroid cancer incidence in Altai Region comparing to the national rate have been registered. Thyroid cancer incidence rate in Altai Region has been stated to exeed the average one for Russian Federation, particularly among women, and to be high for young persons. Particularities of occurrence of some histological cancers in different areas of Altai Region with different exposure rate during 39 years have been detected.

Epidemiological studies of the prevalence of thyroid diseases in subjects exposed as children have been carried out. A high rate of nodules and thyroid cancer have been stated.

1 INTRODUCTION

Altai Region is an administrative unit of the Russian Federation located in the south of Western Siberia and bordering in the south-west on the Semipalatinsk Test Site (STS). Atmospheric nuclear tests were conducted at the STS from 1949 through 1962. Weather conditions in this region resulted in most fission products being transported towards Altai Region with the greatest contribution from the August 29, 1949 nuclear test[1]. As a result of the fallout from this test, effective doses in certain settlements in the south-west of Altai Region exceeded 1 Sv. Radioactive iodine isotopes were one of the major components of test products and made a considerable contribution to the thyroid dose[1].

2 ANALYSIS OF THYROID CANCER INCIDENCE IN THE RUSSIAN FEDERATION AND ALTAI REGION

Analysis of standardised incidence rates in Altai Region and the Russian Federation[2] in 1989-1994 showed a higher incidence rate of thyroid cancer in Altai Region (Table 1), being even more noticeable in women.

Table 1. Thyroid cancer incidence in the Russian Federation and Altai Region population in 1989-1994 (per 100,000 residents).

Area	Standardised incidence rates by calendar year					
	1989	1990	1991	1992	1993	1994
Russia	2.1	2.0	2.0	2.7	2.4	2.6
Altai Region	3.2	2.9	3.0	3.3	2.8	3.5
p	<0.001	<0.001	<0.001	<0.001	<0.001	<0.001

In the structure of cancer diseases thyroid cancer has a higher portion in Altai Region than in the Russian Federation. Among different age groups, in contrast to the Russian Federation where the highest contribution was made by the age group ≥60 (34,5%), in Altai Region the highest contribution was made by the age group <40 (34,9%).

3 RETROSPECTIVE ANALYSIS OF THYROID CANCER INCIDENCE

Upon analysis of data of the registry on 969 histologically verified thyroid cancers, it has been determined that with the time passing from 1949-1962 (when atmospheric nuclear tests were conducted) the share of the group affected under 20 years of age declines and the one of the age group 60 and more years of age grows.

The histologic structure of thyroid cancers has also undergone characteristic changes (Table 2).

Among rayons of Altai Region the highest incidence rate has been registered in Rubtsovski rayon which is adjacent to the STS. In 1994 the thyroid cancer incidence rate exceeded in 1.9 and 2.4 times the average rate in Altai Region and the Russian Federation respectively. This trend was even more noticeable in women.

Table 2. Morphological structure of thyroid malignant neoplasms in Altai Region in 1956-1994.

Years	Follicular cancers (1)		Papillary cancers (2)		P_{1-2}	Lowly differentiated cancers (3)		P_{1-3}	P_{2-3}
	n	%	n	%		n	%		
56-70	3	5.2	31	53.4	<0.001	24	41.4	<0.001	>0.05
71-80	14	10.5	88	66.6	<0.001	31	23.3	<0.001	<0.001
81-90	198	39.4	267	53.2	<0.01	37	7.4	<0.001	<0.001
91-94	119	43.1	145	52.5	<0.05	12	4.3	<0.001	<0.001
Total	334	34.5	531	54.8	<0.001	104	10.7	<0.001	<0.001

4 THYROID EXAMINATION STUDY

In 1996-1997, i.e. 47-48 years after the first nuclear test, the epidemiological study of prevalence of thyroid diseases was carried out in Altai Region.

The main objective of the study was to determine by uniform and sensitive thyroid screening the occurrence of nodular disease and thyroid cancer in population groups exposed as children to radioactive fallout from the STS nuclear tests.

1171 individuals 0-14 years of age on August 29, 1949 were studied. The subjects were selected from the IRMEP register. Thyroid dose from the 1949 test ranged among exposed from 0.3 to 77 Gy. Thyroid examinations included palpation by endocrinologists and ultrasound examinations. Fine needle aspiration biopsy was recommended for subjects with nodules of any size, when thyroiditis was suspected and when the thyroid had diffused enlargements. Blood specimen were taken for thyroid function tests and thyroid antibody measurements.

In the course of screening nodules were found in 273 subjects (23.3%). Among them, 53 individuals had palpable lesions. More than one nodule were detected in 84 subjects. The smallest nodule detected was 2 mm, and the largest was 74 mm (mean, 12 mm)

FNA biopsy was performed in 309 subjects (26.4%). Results of cytological assays are given in Table 3. When malignant tumours were suspected, subjects were sent for surgery and followed by public health care system. By now 11 histopathological specimens have been studied with diagnoses being confirmed for all 11 cases.

Collection and study of histopathological specimens is going on. Afterwards an analytical study of dose response relationship will be performed.

Table 3. Cytopathological diagnoses after FNA biopsies (n=309).

Diagnosis	N	%
Benign neoplasm	203	65,7
Papillary carcinoma	22	7,1
Follicular neoplasm	11	3,6
Possible neoplasm	8	2,6
Other diagnosis	19	6,1
Inadequate sample	59	19,1

References

1. Djachenko VI, Gabbasov MN, Kiselev VI, Lagutin AA, Loborev VM, Markovtsev AS, Shoikhet YN, Sudakov VV, Volobuyev VM, Zelenov VI. Estimation of the Altai Region Population Exposure Resulting from the Nuclear Tests at the Semipalatinsk Test Site. In: Shapiro CS, Kiselev VI, Zaitsev EV, eds. *Nuclear Tests: Long-Term Consequences in the Semipalatinsk/Altai region*, NATO ASI series, Partnership sub-series 2. Environment; vol. 36. Berlin Heidelberg: Springer-Verlag, 1998: 107-132.
2. Dvoirin VV, Aksel EM, Trapeznikov NN. *Statistcs on malignant tumors in Russia and some other countries of the CIS in 1994* (in Russian). Moscow: Russian Academy of Medical Sciences, 1995; **1-2.**

THYROID CARCINOMA POST CHERNOBYL IN THE RUSSIAN FEDERATION: A PATHOLOGICAL STUDY

A.Yu.ABROSIMOV, E.F.LUSHNIKOV, A.F.TSYB

Medical Radiological Research Centre RAMS, Koroliov street 4, Kaluga oblast, Russia

E-mail: mrrc@obninsk.ru

G.A.THOMAS, E.D.WILLIAMS

TCRG, University of Cambridge, Strangeways Research Laboratory, Wort's Causeway, Cambridge CB1 4RN, UK

E-mail: gat1000@cam.ac.uk

We have reviewed the pathology of a total of 50 selected cases of thyroid carcinoma diagnosed in the Russian Federation between 1993 and 1997, 47 of these coming from the exposed oblasts of Kaluga, Bryansk, Oriol and Tula, including 28 children under the age of 15 at the time of operation. We have excluded an initial group of cases where some of the material from the peripheral hospitals was inadequate for diagnosis. 24 of the 28 childhood thyroid cancers were papillary in type, 1 was follicular and 3 could not be classified due to too little tumour present in material obtained from peripheral hospitals for classification. 18 of the 22 cases over the age of 15 at operation were papillary carcinomas, 2 were follicular, 1 medullary and 1 showed a tumour with the morphology associated with familial polyposis coli. One of the papillary carcinomas from the older group showed the features of a microcarcinoma. 24 childhood papillary carcinoma could be subclassified: 13 of these were of solid follicular type (54%) and 7 of classical type (29%) and 4 of other types (17%). These figures are intermediate between the distribution of subtypes seen in England and Wales and the distribution seen in Belarus and Ukraine. A peak of incidence at the age of 11-12 is also seen in Belarus and Ukraine, and is compatible with a cohort effect resulting from the increased sensitivity of very young children to the carcinogenic effect of exposure to fallout from the Chernobyl accident.

1 INTRODUCTION

Thyroid carcinoma is relatively rare disease, forming about 1% of all malignant tumours in human. But a significant increase of frequency of thyroid carcinoma has been reported in children from the several regions of Belarus and Ukraine near Chernobyl[1,2]. The same trend occurs in Bryansk, Kaluga, Oriol and Tula oblasts of the Russian Federation contaminated with radionuclides after the Chernobyl accident. The most considerable increase occurs in younger age groups of the population.

The objective of this work is a study of the pathology of childhood thyroid carcinoma in the exposed oblasts of the Russian Federation after the Chernobyl.

2 MATERIAL AND METHODS

Histological sections of a total of 50 selected cases of thyroid carcinoma diagnosed in the Russian Federation between 1993 and 1997 have been examined by pathologists from Obninsk and Cambridge centres. 47 of these cases coming from the exposed oblasts of Bryansk, Kaluga, Oriol and Tula. A number of cases from Bryansk oblast where the original diagnosis could not be confirmed has been excluded. There are 28 children under the age of 15 at the time of operation and 22 adolescents over the age of 15 but under 20 at the operation. 42 cases were diagnosed at the Medical Radiological Research Centre RAMS (Obninsk), 8 other cases were primarily diagnosed at peripheral hospitals in Bryansk, Kaluga, Oriol and Tula. Histological material (paraffin blocks and formalin fixed tissue) from these cases was obtained from the hospitals concerned. Paraffin blocks from each case were cut in Cambridge, sections were stained with haematoxylin and eosin.

All cases of thyroid carcinoma were classified in accordance with the criteria of the WHO International Histological Typing of Thyroid Tumours (1988)[5].

Immunocytochemistry (ICC) and in situ hybridisation (ISH) techniques were carried out also in the Cambridge centre. The indirect immunoperoxidase technique has been applied on serial paraffin sections by using primary polyclinal rabbit antihuman antibodies for calcitonin and thyroglobulin (DAKO). Dilutions of primary antibodies were 1::2,000 for calcitonin and 1:8,000 for thyroglobulin. Secondary swine antirabbit antibodies conjugated with horseradish peroxidase (DAKO) were used after dilution to a concentration of 1:100. ISH was used to localize m-RNA for calcitonin and thyroglobulin in thyroid cells. Appropriate positive and negative controls were also used.

3 RESULTS AND DISCUSSION

The 50 cases included 30 females and 20 males. The mean age for females was 14.3 and for males 13.2. There were 28 children (13 females and 15 males) under the age of 15 at the time of operation and 22 case (17 females and 5 males) over the age of 15 byt under 20 at operation. The average age of patients under 15 at operation was 11.3, and the sex ratio 0.9:1 (f:m), whereas the average age of those over 15 was 17.1, and the sex ratio was 3.4:1 (f:m). The age distribution of thyroid carcinoma diagnosed in children under the age of 15 at operation is shown in the figure 1.

The age distribution of the cases shows a slightly bell shaped curve, although, in part due to the small number of cases observed in Russia, this is not as marked as that observed in Belarus and Ukraine[6].

In common with thyroid carcinoma in age matched series from Belarus and Ukraine, the majority of the cases are of the papillary type. Papillary carcinomas are subclassified on the dominant histological phenotype into solid follicular, classic papillary, follicular variant, papillary microcarcinoma and diffuse sclerosing variant. Where the tumour is clearly of the papillary type but either primary tumour is not present in the section examined or there is too little tumour present for subclassification to be carried out the tumour is assigned "PTC not otherwise specified". Medullary carcinoma and follicular carcinomas are classified separately.

All cases of papillary and follicular carcinoma were positive for thyroglobulin ICC and ISH, except for occasional cases with individual C cells. Tumour cells of one medullary carcinoma were positive for calcitonin and negative for thyroglobulin.

number of cases

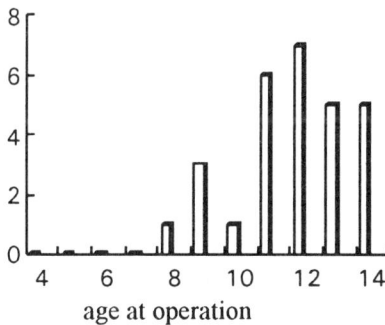

age at operation

Fig. 1. Age distribution of cases of thyroid carcinoma diagnosed in children from the Russian Federation (1993-1997) under the age of 15 at operation.

24 of 28 childhood thyroid cancers in children under 15 at the time of operation were papillary in type, 1 was follicular and 3 could not be classified due to too little tumour present in material obtained from peripheral hospitals for classification. 24 papillary carcinomas could be subclassified: 13 of these were of solid follicular type (54%) and 7 of classical type (29%) and 4 of other types (17%). These figures are intermediate between the distribution of subtypes seen in England and Wales and the distribution seen in Belarus and Ukraine. The age distribution of these cases is different from that seen in England and Wales[4] with a peak incidence at the age of 11-12 rather than a smooth increase with age. This peak is also seen in Belarus and the Ukraine, and is compatible with a cohort effect resulting from the increased sensitivity

of very young children to the carcinogenic effect of exposure to fallout from the Chernobyl accident.

18 of the 22 cases over the age of 15 at operation were papillary carcinomas, 2 follicular, 1 medullary and 1 showed a tumour with the morphology associated with familial polyposis coli[3]. 18 papillary carcinomas could be subclassified: 3 of these were solid follicular type (17%), 8 of classical type (44%), 1 showed the features of a microcarcinoma (6%), and 6 of other types (33%).

We carried out an analysis of thyroid carcinoma subtypes in individual Russian oblasts in patients under 15 and between 15 and 20 at operation. The 28 cases of thyroid carcinoma in children under 15 included 21 patients from Bryansk oblast, 1 from Kaluga, 1 from Oriol and 5 from Tula. A solid follicular variant of papillary carcinoma was present in 13 cases (46%), non solid follicular variant in 11 cases (40%), other types of thyroid carcinoma in 4 cases (14%). The 22 cases of thyroid carcinoma in patients over 15 and under 20 at operation included 6 cases from Bryansk oblast, 3 from Kaluga 4 from Oriol, 6 from Tula and 3 from other oblasts. A solid follicular variant of papillary carcinoma was present in 3 cases (14%), non solid follicular variant in 16 cases (72%), other types of thyroid carcinoma in 3 cases (14%).

The major difference between the two age groups is the much lower proportion of papillary carcinomas of the solid follicular variant in the older age group. The high relative frequency of the solid follicular type of papillary carcinoma in children from the exposed areas of Belarus and the Ukraine suggests that this type may be specifically associated with radiation. However, there appears only to be a low proportion of the solid follicular variant in the older age groups in Belarus and Ukraine, which perhaps suggest that a larger proportion of the cases in the older Russian age group are also not related to radiation exposure, but represent the natural incidence of thyroid carcinoma in this region. However, the bell shaped age distribution curve of the younger age group and the type of histology suggests that a significant proportion of cases in the younger group may be related to radioiodine in fallout from Chernobyl. Although the numbers are small, there is a suggestion that more of the type of tumour seen in the exposed population in the Ukraine and Belarus are found in Bryansk than the other oblasts.

References

1. Baverstock K, Egloff B, Pinchera A, Ruchti C, Williams D. Thyroid cancer after Chernobyl. *Nature* 1992; **359:** 21-22.
2. Bogdanova T, Bragarnik M, Tronko ND, Harach HR, Thomas GA, Williams ED. Childhood thyroid cancer after Chernobyl. *J Endocrinol* 1995; **144:** 25.
3. Harach HR, Williams GT, Williams ED. Familial adenomatous polyposis associated thyroid carcinoma: a distinct type of follicular cell neoplasm. *Histopathology* 1994; **25:** 549-561.
4. Harach HR, Williams ED. Childhood thyroid cancer in England and Wales. *Br J Cancer* 1995; **72:** 777-783.
5. Hedinger Ch, Williams ED, Sobin LH. Histological typing of thyroid tumours. In: *International Histological Classification of Tumours,* 2nd edn. WHO, Springer: Berlin, 1988.
6. Williams ED. Effects on the thyroid in population exposed to radiation as a result of the Chernobyl accident. In: *One Decade after Chernobyl. Summing up the consequences of the accident,* IAEA, Vienna, 1996.

MORPHOLOGICAL FEATURES AND ANALYSIS OF RADIATION RISK OF DEVELOPMENT OF POST-CHERNOBYL THYROID CARCINOMA IN CHILDREN AND ADOLESCENTS OF UKRAINE

T. BOGDANOVA, V. KOZYRITSKY AND M. TRONKO

Institute of Endocrinology and Metabolism of the Academy of Medical Sciences of Ukraine, Vyshgorodska Str. 69, Kyiv 254114, Ukraine
E-mail: tb@viaduk.net

I. LIKHTAREV, I. KAIRO, M. CHEPURNOY AND V. SHPAK

Research Centre of Radiation Medicine of the Academy of Medical Sciences of Ukraine, Melnikov Str. 52, Kyiv 252050, Ukraine
E-mail: vil@rpi.kiev.ua

Morphological analysis was performed in 296 cases of thyroid carcinoma which were removed for the period 1986 to 1997 in children aged 4 to 14 years (241 cases) and adolescents aged 15 to 18 years (55 cases). Most of carcinomas - 225 in children (93.4%) and 50 in adolescents (90/9%) - were verified as papillary carcinomas. Among papillary carcinomas tumors of solid-follicular structure (79.8% in children and 69.6% in adolescents) prevailed. Such carcinomas, as compared with tumors of typical papillary structure, were characterized by more pronounced signs of extrathyroid and intrathyroid spreading, vascular invasion, metastatic spreading in regional lymph nodes. An analysis of thyroid exposure doses showed a marked increase in the incidence of tumors of the above solid-follicular structure as well as an increase of relative risk of their development with increase of the exposure dose, what points out the radiation genesis of the carcinomas under study.

Numerous investigations showed a significant increase in thyroid carcinoma incidence in children of Ukraine after the Chernobyl accident.[1-3] It has also been established that a large majority of thyroid malignant tumors in children were papillary carcinomas, among which tumors of solid-follicular structure prevailed. Incidence of this solid-follicular variant of papillary carcinoma in children of Ukraine was significantly higher as compared with children of Great-Britain, whose tumors were considered as a control group. Moreover, tumors with the above structure in children of Great-Britain were noted mainly in the younger age group (under 10 years), while in children of Ukraine they were also observed in the elder age group (10 to 14 years).[4,5]

The aim of this work was a comparative analysis of morphological structure of papillary carcinomas in children of Ukraine aged 4 to 14 years and adolescents aged 15 to 18 years, as well as a study of the incidence and relative risk of development of solid-follicular variant of papillary carcinoma in children depending on thyroid exposure dose.

Morphological analysis was performed in 296 cases of thyroid carcinomas removed for the period 1986 to 1997 in children aged 4 to 14 years (241 cases) and adolescents aged 15 to 18 years (55 cases). The data presented evidence that, with rare exception, post-Chernobyl thyroid carcinomas both in children and adolescents of Ukraine are represented by papillary forms (Table 1).

Table 1. Main types of the thyroid carcinoma in children and adolescents in Ukraine after Chernobyl.

Type of carcinoma	Children		Adolescents		Total	
	N	%	N	%	N	%
Papillary	225	93.4	50	90.9	275	92.9
Folliculary	8	3.3	3	5.5	11	3.7
Medullary	7	2.8	–	–	7	2.4
Oxyphilic cell poorly differention	1	0.5	–	–	1	0.3
Anaplastic	–		2	3.6	2	0.7

Only in 5 cases (children) and in one case (adolescent) tumors measuring less than 1 cm (0.7 - 0.8 cm on the average) were revealed, which were verified as papillary microcarcinomas (2.2% among papillary carcinomas).

Papillary carcinomas were subdivided into the following histological subtypes: typical papillary variant, solid-follicular variant, and diffuse-sclerotic variant. Typical papillary variant was revealed in 10.7% of cases in children and in 26.0% of cases in adolescents; solid-follicular variant in 79.8% of cases in children and in 69.6% of cases in adolescents; diffuse-sclerotic variant in 7.5% of cases in children and in 2.2% of cases in adolescents.

A detailed histological analysis, taking into account the possibility of estimating the features of malignant growth, infiltrative, invasive properties of tumors, has been performed in 178 cases of papillary carcinoma (148 in children and 30 in adolescents).

In case of typical variant of papillary carcinoma in adolescents, no signs of tumoral spreading out of the thyroid capsule or blood invasion were revealed. In children signs of extrathyroid spreading were noted in 41.6% of cases, and there were no signs of blood invasion either. Signs of lymphatic invasion in children were revealed in 41.7% of cases, and in adolescents they were 1.3 times more rare - in 33,3% of cases.

Papillary carcinomas of solid-follicular structure, as compared with typical papillary variant, both in children and adolescents showed more often signs of intraglandular and extrathyroid tumoral spreading, lymphatic and blood invasion. However, probably, because of the non equivalence of the groups compared at the expense of a small number of cases of typical papillary carcinoma, only differences revealed in the presence of extrathyroid tumoral spreading and lymphatic invasion had a trustworthy character. It should be noted that in children the above signs manifested themselves more distinctly than in adolescents.

In this variant of papillary carcinoma we may note the constant presence of solid loci in zones of infiltrative tumoral growth. Clusters of tumoral cells in vessels also have, as a rule, the aspect of solid formations. On the basis of this observation, it is not excluded that aggressive behaviour of the tumor in case of a mixed histological structure would probably depend on tumor's solid component.

Metastases of papillary carcinoma in regional lymph nodes were registered in children in 65.5% of cases, and in adolescents 1.6 time more rarely (40.3% of cases). Most often metastases were revealed in children in case of solid-follicular variant of papillary carcinoma: in 71.9% of cases (in case of typical papillary variant they were revealed only in 50.0% of cases observed).

Metastases of papillary carcinoma in lymph nodes had a typical papillary structure or more often a mixed one, with presence of papillary and follicular areas. In case of solid-follicular variant in 54.0% of cases tumor's metastases contained vast solid areas, which sometimes completely replaced lymph node tissue.

Taking into account that the possible cause of development of papillary carcinomas of solid-follicular structure in children of Ukraine was radiation exposure as a result of the Chernobyl accident, we have analysed the relationship between the incidence of development of tumors with the above structure and the thyroid exposure dose received.

In order to establish a probable relationship between thyroid irradiation and development of solid-follicular variant of papillary carcinoma, we have analysed 168 morphologically studied cases of papillary carcinomas in children aged under 15 years, who were operated from 1990 to 1995, i.e. at the period of a trustworthy increase of thyroid cancer incidence in Ukraine.

As a characteristic of thyroid exposure rate, we have used the estimate of the average I-131 exposure dose in inhabitants (of the corresponding age) of the settlement where the patient-children or patient-adolescent was residing at the moment of the accident. Dose estimate was performed as a result of a thyrodosimetric passportization of settlements of Ukraine.[6]

The study performed has revealed a progressive increase in the incidence of solid-follicular variant of papillary carcinoma with increase of thyroid dose. So, this variant of tumor in children from non contaminated regions (thyroid doses were less than 0.05 Gy) was revealed in 51.1% of cases observed. In children with a thyroid dose 0.05 to 0.2 Gy this variant was noted 1.4 time more frequently, in 69.6% of cases; in children with a dose 0.2 to 1 Gy - 1.65 time more frequently, in 84,4% of cases; and, finally, in children with a dose 1 Gy and higher this variant was revealed in 87.5% of cases or 1.7 time more frequently as compared with the dose zone < 0.05 Gy.

Estimate of the relative risks has also shown that the increase in children's thyroid dose within the range of the above dose zones was accompanied with an increase in relative risk (odds ratio) of development of thyroid papillary carcinoma with described structure (Table 2)

Table 2. Radiation doses to histological subtype of the papillary thyroid carcinoma relationship.

Histological subtype	% of cases in the dose zones (in Cy)			
	<0.05	0.05–	0.2–	1.0–
Solid-follicular variant of PTC	51.1	69.6	84.4	87.5
odds ratio for every dose zone		2.19	5.18	6.68

Therefore, we may conclude that thyroid carcinomas removed in children and adolescents after the Chernobyl accident were represented in a large majority of cases by papillary forms, mainly with solid-follicular structure. Solid-follicular variants of tumors manifested high invasive properties, showing signs of intraglandular and extrathyroid spreading, lymphatic and blood invasion. In children these indices were more pronounced, pointing out a more aggressive biological behavior of tumor, what was confirmed by the incidence of metastases revealed in lymph nodes.

Our analysis has confirmed the correctness of distinguishing the solid-follicular variant of papillary carcinoma in children as a special subtype of papillary carcinoma connected with previous exposure as a result of the Chernobyl accident. Moreover, it has been established an increase in relative risk of development of tumors with this morphological structure with increase of thyroid exposure dose, what evidences radiation genesis of these tumors and suggests a direct relationship between thyroid exposure dose in children and subsequent effect in the form of an increase in the incidence of carcinoma of the structure described. However, to have final conclusions in this way, we need to carry out long-term investigations with a comparative analysis in different age groups.

References

1. Likhtarev IA, Sobolev BG, Kairo IA, Tronko ND, Bogdanova TI, Oleinic VA, Epshtein EV, Beral V. Thyroid cancer in the Ukraine. *Nature* 1995; **375**: 365.
2. Tronko N, Bogdanova T, Bolshova E, Komissarenko I, Oleynik V, Tereschenko V, Epstein E, Chebotarev V. Thyroid cancer in children and adolescents in Ukraine after the Chernobyl accident. In: *The radiological consequences of the Chernobyl accident,* Brussels-Luxemburg: ECSC-EC-EAEC, 1996: 683-690.
3. Jacob P, Goulko G, Heidenreich WF, Likhtarev I, Kairo I, Tronko ND, Bogdanova TI, Kenigsberg J, Buglova E, Drozdovitch V, Golovneva A, Demidchik EP, Beral V. Thyroid cancer risk to children calculated. *Nature* 1998; **392:** 31-32.
4. *Molecular, cellular, biological characterization of childhood thyroid cancer,* Williams ED and Tronko ND, ed. Brussels-Luxemburg: ECSC-EC-EAEC, 1996: 105 p.
5. Tronko M, Bogdanova T. *Thyroid cancer in children of Ukraine (Consequences of the Chernobyl accident).* Kyiv: Chornobylinterniform, 1997: 200 p (in russian).
6. Likhtarev IA, Sobolev BG, Kairo IA, Tabachny L, Jacob P, Prohl G. Gulko G. Results of large scale thyroid dose reconstruction in Ukraine. In: *The radiological consequences of the Chernobyl accident,* Brussels-Luxemburg: ECSC-EC-EAEC, 1996: 1021-1034.

THE MOLECULAR BIOLOGY OF RADIATION CARCINOGENESIS

M.J. ATKINSON

GSF-Institut für Pathologie, Postfach 1129, D85758 Oberschleissheim, Germany

E-mail atkinson@gsf.de

The molecular biological principles governing the carcinogenic process are now well understood. A panoply of genes has been identified whose mutation is causally linked to the malignant transformation of cells. The malignant phenotype is the result of the gene mutations causing dysregulation of the cell cycle. This may be due to either upregulation of stimulatory gene action (proto-oncogenes) or loss of cell cycle repressive gene function (tumor suppressor genes). A number of novel tumor genes, with more diverse roles in the carcinogenic process, have also been implicated in the carcinogenic process. These include cell adhesion, DNA repair, and cell death (apoptosis) genes. The important contribution of these genes to radiation carcinogenesis is only beginning to be recognized. In the last few years yet another group of genes, the tumor susceptibility genes, have been identified. Multiple allelic forms of these genes are distributed throughout the population, and groups of them act in concert to modify the susceptibility of an individual to carcinogenesis.

Mutation of specific subsets of tumor genes is usually associated with a distinct tumor entity. These same genes are also affected in radiation-induced malignancies, although the question of radiation-specific mutational events remains open. Consequently caution is urged in attributing specific gene mutations to ionizing radiation. Moreover the role of susceptibility genes in determining sensitivity to radiation carcinogenesis should be considered.

GENETIC BASIS OF CANCER

Although epigenetic mechanisms may contribute to the carcinogenic process, the primary causal mechanisms have their origins in acquired or inherited genetic alterations. Evidence supporting the genetic basis of cancer can be found in the transmission of the malignant phenotype from a tumorous cell to its progeny. This may also occur through the germ line, where a mutated gene is passed from parent to offspring. Inheritance of the mutated gene can increase the risk of cancer developing in affected individuals, manifesting itself as one of the familial cancer syndromes. That the genome itself is responsible is documented by the ability of so-called naked DNA to confer the malignant phenotype upon a hitherto normal cell. This transforming DNA may be introduced by experimental manipulation (gene transfer) or by a biological agent (retrovirus) (see review by Cooper).[1]

TUMOR GENES

Investigations into the nature of the transforming DNA have revealed the existence of two closely related sets of genes with oncogenic properties. The viral oncogenes (*v-onc*) are a family of genes that appear to have been derived from cellular homologues by a process of viral capture and mutation. These genes are potent transforming agents that usually exhibit cell and tissue selectivity in their oncogenic action. The cellular homologues of the viral oncogenes (*c-onc*) are not, as a rule, independently capable of cell transformation in a non-mutated form. Their biological function as positive regulators of the rate of cell proliferation is under normal circumstances tightly controlled. However, in tumors, cellular and viral oncogenes are present in an activated form, enabling them to overcome regulatory processes and to act in an autonomous manner.

Studies of several familial cancer syndromes have established the existence of an additional set of cancer genes, with actions quite distinct to those of the oncogenes. Initially identified in familial retinoblastoma through the pioneering work of Knudson, the tumor suppressor genes represent a class of molecule acting normally to slow the rate of cell proliferation. [2] Although functionally antagonistic to the oncogenes the suppressor genes act upon quite distinct cellular processes. The mode of gene mutation occurring in suppressor genes is also quite distinct to that seen in oncogenes. As defined by the two-hit model of suppressor gene inactivation, the oncogenic potential of suppressor genes is only revealed when both copies of the gene are subjected to inactivating mutation. Usually this is achieved by the mutation of one allele at a tumor suppressor locus accompanied by the deletion of the remaining allele. Thus, in individuals inheriting two genetically distinguishable alleles at a given suppressor gene locus (heterozygosity), the deletion of one allele will give the appearance of homozygosity at the locus in tumor cells (loss of heterozygosity). Consequently loss of heterozygosity is considered an indicator of the presence of a tumor suppressor gene.

ONCOGENES ARE ACTIVATED, SUPPRESSORS INACTIVATED

Conventional wisdom has always asserted that the activation of oncogenes is the result of gene mutation. An example of this is the well described series of point mutations of the *ras* family of oncogenes. However, a number of oncogenes are activated other genetic mechanisms that lead to overexpression of a non-mutant protein. These include gene amplification that retains endogenous regulatory elements driving transcription (e.g. *c-myc* and *mdm2*), gene translocation that places the oncogene under an inappropriate transcriptional control (*c-myc* and *bcl2*). Translocation events may also fuse parts of two genes together, resulting in the production of chimeric proteins. These may be constitutively active proteins due to lack of normal regulatory domains or the inclusion of an inappropriate activation domain.

Suppressor gene mutation usually, but not exclusively, involves the generation of either a null (inactive) allele or of an inactive protein. Under normal circumstances expression from the remaining allele would compensate and would be no oncogenic consequence. However, loss of the remaining wild type allele can unmask the presence of the mutation, and will lead to a complete loss of function. This allelic loss may occur via a number of different chromosomal events including loss of chromosomal material spanning the suppressor gene locus or duplication of the mutated gene. However, non-mutational events leading ton suppressor gene inactivation are also observed. In a recent example the p73 suppressor gene located on chromosome 1p was found to require only the mutation of one allele. The remaining allele was found to have been inactivated in somatic cells by paternal imprinting. [3]

In addition to mutational inactivation, the loss of suppressor gene function may be induced by complexing of the suppressor gene product by proteins encoded by oncogenic viruses.[4] A number of such proteins have been identified, including SV40 virus large T antigen, papilloma virus protein E6, and adenovirus protein E1b, all of which bind and inactivate p53. The Sv40 large T antigen and the papilloma E7 protein are able to form complexes with the retinoblastoma protein. One can assume that these viral agents influence the carcinogenic process in infected individuals, and that they may even contribute to the process of radiation carcinogenesis.

THE CELL CYCLE IS NOT THE SOLE TARGET OF TUMOR GENE ACTION

The great majority of the tumor genes described to date act directly upon cell cycle regulatory pathways, or are themselves components of the regulatory process. However, a growing number of tumor genes have biological activities that are not immediately connected to cell cycle progression. These include genes involved in such diverse processes as cell-cell adhesion (E-cadherin),[5] DNA damage repair (Atm), [6] DNA mismatch repair genes, [7] and cell death by apoptosis (Bcl2). [8] Mutation of these genes (or over-production in the case of bcl2) directly contributes to carcinogenesis without direct involvement of cell cycle control.

In addition to these non-classical tumor genes an additional subset of genes contributes, albeit indirectly, to the tumorigenic process. A number of these genes (estimated to be over 200) interact to determine the background level of tumor susceptibility of an individual. It is these genes that are responsible for the well-characterized variation in tumor susceptibility between different inbred mouse strains.[9] It is precisely this variability that is permitting the isolation and identification of these genes.

TRANSLOCATION EVENTS ARE SEEN IN SOLID TUMORS

Activation of tumor genes by chromosomal translocation is commonly encountered in hematological malignancies such as lymphoma and leukemia. One possible explanation for the high frequency of translocation events in these tissues is the presence of somatic gene rearrangement activity necessary for generating T-cell receptors and immunoglobulin diversity. This has prompted the erroneous belief that such recombination events are exclusive to these tissues.

Translocation events are seen in a restricted set of solid tissue malignancies. These include the Pax/Forkhead translocation in Rhabdomyosarcoma,[10] the EWS/FLI1 translocation in Ewings sarcoma,[11] the Cyclin D1/PTH translocation in Parathyroid tumors[12] and of course the RET/PTC translocations in Thyroid cancer (discussed elsewhere in this volume). Two features mark the tissues affected by these translocations. Firstly, the cells are capable of only limited self-renewal due to the absence of a stem cell population, and secondly, the cells are transcriptionally highly active, leading to overproduction of the chimeric gene product.

MUTATIONS ARE TUMOR SPECIFIC AND NOT RADIATION SPECIFIC

Many experimental studies have demonstrated that ionizing radiation induces a highly reproducible set of mutations in DNA. These studies have show that high LET radiation primarily generates large deletions and translocations, whilst low LET causes predominantly small deletions and point mutations.[13, 14] However, caution must be exercised in interpreting these observations as the majority of these studies have used artificial experimental systems. In almost all of the studies a DNA target conferring a selectable phenotype e.g. *lac-z*, *Hpr*, or *Aprt*, was chosen for studying the effects of the irradiation. The post-irradiation selection of mutated DNA may artificially skew the spectrum of mutations observed in these systems. There is no evidence that the changes observed in these targets would be the same as those seen in more physiological targets such as the tumor genes discussed above.

Considerable effort has been put into identifying radiation-specific gene mutations in cancerous tissues arising after irradiation. A number of these studies have succeeded in identifying frequent gene mutations in these tumors. However a closer comparison with the mutations seen in non-radiation induced tumors suggests that the evidence for a direct radiation fingerprint is at the best circumstantial.

A series of studies of the *ras* oncogene have identified frequent point mutations in radiation-induced rat lung neoplasia. High LET (^{239}Pu) irradiation was associated with a 48% mutation rate in the *Ki-ras* gene,[15] whilst low LET (X-ray) induced tumors exhibited a less than 3% mutation rate in the same gene.[16] The discrepancy in mutation rate is not due to radiation, as in both studies the mutation rate was indistinguishable from that seen in non-radiation induced lung neoplasias. The difference in mutation rate seen in the two experiments is presumably due to differences in tumor progression, which can influence the frequency of *Ki-ras* mutations.[17]

In man, mutations of *Ki-ras2* have been described in 2 of 5 (40%) liver angiosarcomas associated with thorotrast exposure. In spontaneous examples of this rare tumor a comparable *Ki-ras2* mutation rate was seen (5 of 19)(26%).[18] Again the similarity in mutations frequency between radiation-induced and „spontaneous" tumors suggests no specific radiation effect. The same is true of the leukemia arising after exposure to atomic bomb irradiation. Here *N-ras* and *K-ras* mutations were seen in 8/25 (32%) of the leukemia from exposed subjects, whilst a rate of 13/47 (28%) was observed in leukemia from a non-exposed population.[19]

In the case of the tumor suppressor gene p53 a series of studies have failed to provide evidence of a radiation-specific effect. An initial study of lung tumors is radon-exposed subjects found a high incidence of 16/53 (31%) for one specific p53 mutation affecting codon 249.[20] Despite great effort this potential radiation fingerprint was not seen in similar, but not identical populations exposed to inhaled alpha-emitting irradiation.[21, 22] In all of these studies the rate of p53 mutation is equivalent to that reported in lung tumors arising in a non-exposed non-smoking collective.[23]

Mutations in p53 have been described in cases of radiation-induced tumors arising after radiation therapy. A case report of a radiation-field glioblastoma revealed a 3 base deletion within p53,[24] whilst 21/24 post-irradiation sarcomas contained p53 mutations. In neither of these two studies is there any evidence that the mutation frequency and mutation spectrum differ from tumors arising by „spontaneous" means.

Our own study of mouse osteosarcoma induced by the bone seeking alpha-particle emitting radionuclide [227]Thorium revealed that p53 gene deletions were present in 4/18 (22%) tumors and that point mutations were present in only 1/18 (6%) cases. This led us to believe that the deletion events were directly attributable to the high LET energy irradiation. Indeed, a survey of nine non-radiation induced murine osteosarcomas yielded no deletions and only 1 point mutation. However, these tumors were induced by v-fos oncogene containing FBR murine sarcoma virus,[25] and the low rate of p53 involvement suggests the v-fos transformation mechanism is independent of p53. The high rate of p53 deletion events in radiation-induced osteosarcomas may in fact be a general feature of non-viral osteosarcoma. In man a study of p53 in spontaneous osteosarcoma revealed deletion events in 8/76 (24%) cases whilst point mutations were less frequent, occurring in 12/76 (16%) tumors.[26] Indeed, in a small-scale study of mouse osteosarcoma induced by γ-irradiation Ootsuyama found evidence of an excess of p53 gene deletion events.[27] The alternative explanation, that the high rate of p53 deletions in spontaneous human osteosarcoma is due to unrecognized irradiation events, would require that a quarter of these tumors were radiation-induced.

Two instances where possible radiation-induced genetic effects may be identifiable are acute myeloid leukemia (AML) of the mouse and papillary thyroid cancer in man. In both of these cases there is not yet sufficient evidence to exclude a molecular fingerprint of radiation.

In radiation-induced AML there is a nearly ubiquitous interstitial deletion affecting chromosome 2. This event is independent of the radiation quality, with both X-rays, γ-rays and neutron-induced AMLs exhibiting chromosome 2 losses.[28] The deletion of chromosome 2 sequences are seen in individual bone marrow cells isolated as early as 24 hours post-irradiation, indicating a direct causality.[29] However, as AML is an extremely rare tumor type, there is little information on chromosome 2 status in non-radiation induced tumors. Consequently the formal possibility exists that chromosome 2 losses are an essential part of the leukemiogenesis process, and are not indicative of radiation damage.

In papillary thyroid cancer a series of chromosomal translocations serve to generate a constitutively active RET protein kinase. In radiation-induced tumors of this type there is some preliminary evidence suggesting that one specific *Ret* translocation is more frequent (see elsewhere in this volume). Before this mutation can be accepted as a specific radiation-induced event it is essential to exclude the possibility that the mutation may be specific to all papillary thyroid cancers arising in very young subjects in these population groups.

In conclusion, the causal relationship between ionizing radiation and specific tumor gene mutations in malignant tissue has not yet been established. In the cases reviewed above both the mutation type and frequency seen in radiation-induced malignancies was comparable to that seen in the appropriate control tumors. In cases where doubt remains the lack of appropriate control samples precludes a firm conclusion.

GENETIC BACKGROUND CONTRIBUTES TO RADIATION-INDUCED CANCER

The genetic background of an individual can influence susceptibility to carcinogenesis. Germ line mutations in tumor suppressor genes such as retinoblastoma or p53 results in an increased prevalence of both spontaneous and induced tumors. A range of these inherited germ line mutations has been shown to increase sensitivity to the carcinogenic effects of ionizing radiation. These include the *Apc* gene mutation which makes *min* mice hypersensitive to radiation induced colorectal cancer [30] and the DNA protein kinase mutation in SCID mice which increases sensitivity to X-ray induced thymic lymphoma.[31] Loss of p53 gene function in p53 null (knockout) mice increases their sensitivity to radiation-induced cancer in several tissues.[32, 33]

In addition the inheritance pattern of normal allelic variants at multiple loci can also govern sensitivity to carcinogens. This is illustrated by the different inbred mouse strain sensitivities to radiation-induced AML and osteosarcoma.[29, 34]

CONCLUSIONS

Analysis of the genetic mechanisms of radiation carcinogenesis shows us that some caution must be exercised in the interpretation of the genetic events responsible for radiation-induced (thyroid) cancer.

Firstly, the nature of the gene mutations (single bases, small deletions, large deletions, and translocations) must bear some mechanistic relationship with the causal irradiation.

Secondly, the tumor genes involved (in papillary thyroid cancer these include p53, ras, G_S, and Ret) are all implicated in sporadic malignancy. Demonstration of their selective involvement in radiation-induced tumors requires a careful analysis of biologically equivalent tumors from a non-irradiated matched population.

Thirdly, given the importance of genetic background, the prevalence of tumor-disposing genotypes (potential founder gene effects) must be considered. This is particularly true of small isolated populations with a limited gene pool.

Acknowledgements

The work of my group mentioned in this paper was funded by a grant from the European Commission Radiation Protection Program (F14PCT950008b).

References

1. Cooper G, Lane M. Cellular transforming genes and oncogenesis. *Biochim Biophys Acta* 1984, **738**: 9-20

2. Knudson AG. Antioncogenes and human cancer. *Proc Natl Acad Sci (USA)* 1993, **90**: 10914-10921

3. Dickman S. First p53 relative may be a new tumor suppressor. *Science* 1997, **277**: 1605-1606

4. Weinberg R. The cat and mouse games that genes, viruses, and cells play. *Cell* 1997, **88**: 573-575

5. Guilford P, *et al.* E-cadherin germline mutations in familial gastric cancer. *Nature* 1998, **392**: 402-405

6. Gilad S, *et al.* Genotype-phenotype relationships in ataxia-telangiectasia and variants. *Am J Hum Genet* 1998, **62**: 551-561

7. Peltomaki P. DNA mismatch repair gene mutations in human cancer. *Environ Health Perspect* 1997, **105 Suppl 4**: 775-780

8. Crossen P. Genes and chromosomes in chronic B-cell leukemia. *Cancer Genet Cytogenet* 1997, **94**: 44-51

9. Nagase H, Bryson S, Fee F, Balmain A. Multigenic control of skin tumor development in mice. *Ciba Found Symp* 1996, **197**: 156-168

10. Davis R, Bennicelli J, Macina R, Nycum L, Biegel J, Barr F. Structural characterization of the FKHR gene and its rearrangement in alveolar rhabdomyosarcoma. *Hum Mol Genet* 1995, **4**: 2355-2362

11. May W, *et al.* Ewing sarcoma 11;22 translocation produces a chimeric transcription factor that requires the DNA-binding domain encoded by FLI1 for transformation. *Proc Natl Acad Sci (U S A)* 1993, **90**: 5752-5756

12. Arnold A, Kim H, Gaz R, Eddy R, Fukushima Y, Byers M, Shows T, Kronenberg H. Molecular cloning and chromosomal mapping of DNA

rearranged with the parathyroid hormone gene in a parathyroid adenoma. *J Clin Invest* 1989, **83:** 2034-2040

13. Thacker J. The nature of mutants induced by ionising radiation in cultured hamster cells. III. Molecular characterization of HPRT-deficient mutants induced by gamma-rays or alpha-particles showing that the majority have deletions of all or part of the hprt gene. *Int J Radiat Biol* 1986, **50:** 1-30

14. Grosovsky AJ, de Boer JG, de Jong PJ, Drobetsky EA, Glickman BW. Base substitutions, frameshifts, and small deletions constitute ionizing radiation-induced point mutations in mammalian cells. *Proc Natl Acad Sci (U S A)* 1988, **85:** 185-188

15. Stegelmeier BL, Gillett NA, Rebar AH, Kelly G. The molecular progression of plutonium-239 induced rat ling carcinogenesis: K-ras expression anmd activation. *Mol Carcinog* 1991, **4:** 43-51

16. Belinsky SA, Middelton SK, Picksley SM, Hahn FF, Nikula KJ.Analysis of the K-ras and p53 pathways in X-ray induced lung tumors of the rat. *Radiation Res* 1996, **145:** 449-456

17. Cazorla M, *et al.* Ki-ras gene mutations and absence of p53 gene mutations in spontaneous and urethane-induced early lung lesions in CBA/J mice. *Mol Carcinog* 1998, **21:** 251-260

18. Przgodzki RM, *et al.* Sporadic and thorotrast-induced angiosarcomas of the liver manifest frequent and multiple point muttations in K-ras2. *Lab Invest* 1997, **76:** 153-159

19. Tanaka K, Takechi M, Kamada, N. Mutation of ras oncogene in atomic bomb radiation-exposed leukemia. *J Rad Res (Tokyo)* 1991, **32:** 378-388

20. Taylor JA, Watson MA, Devereux TR. p53 mutation hotspots in radon-associated lung cancer. *Lancet* 1994, **343:** 86-87

21. Vähäkangas KH, Samet JM, Metcalf RA, Welsh JA, Bennett WP, Lane DP, Harris CC. Mutations of p53 and ras genes in rdaon-associated lung cancers from uranium miners. *Lancet* 1992, **339:** 576-580

22. Hollenstein M, *et al.* p53 gene mutation analysis in tumors of patients exposed to alpha-partilces. *Carcinogenesis* 1997, **18:** 511-516

23. Takagi Y, *et al.* p53 mutations in non-small-cell lung cancers occurring in individuals without a past history of active smoking. *Br J Cancer* 1998, **77:** 1568-1572

24. Tada M, Sawamura Y, Abe H, Iggo R. Homozygous p53 gene mutation in a radiation-induced glioblastoma 10 years after treatment for an intracranial germ cell tumor. *Neurosurgery* 1997, **40:** 393-396

25. Rüther U, Garber C, Komitowski D, Müller R, Wagner EF. Deregulated c-fos expression interferes with normal bone development in transgenic mice. *Nature* 1987, **325**: 412-416

26. Toguchida J, *et al.* Mutation spectrum of the p53 gene in bone and soft tissue sarcomas. *Cancer Research* 1992, **52**: 6194-6199

27. Ootsuyama A, Makino H, Nagao M, Ochiai A, Yamauchi Y, Tanooka H. Frequent p53 mutation in mouse tumors induced by repeated b-irradiation. *Mol Carcinogenesis* 1994, **11**: 236-242

28. Bouffler SD, Meijne EIM, Huiskamp R, Cox R. Chromosomal abnormalities in neutron-induced acute myeloid leukemias in CBA/H mice. *Radiation Res* 1996, **146**: 349-352

29. Bouffler SD, Breckon G, Cox R. Chromosomal mechanisms in murine radiation acute myeloid leukemogenesis. *Carcinogenesis* 1996, **17**: 655-659

30. Ellender M, Cox R. *personal communication*

31. Liebermann M, Hansteen GA, Waller EK, Weissman IL, Sen-Majumdar A. Unexpected effects of the severe combined immunodeficiency mutation on murine lymphomagenesis. *J Exp Med* 1992, **176**: 399-405

32. Kemp CJ, Wheldon T, Balmain A. p53-deficient mice are extremely susceptible to radiation-induced tumorigenesis. 1994, **8**: 66-69

33. Lee JM, Abrahamson JLA, Kandel R, Donehower LA, Bernstein A. Susceptibility to radiation-carcinogenesis and accumulation of chromosomal breakage in p53 deficient mice. 1994, **9**: 3731-3736

34. Luz A, *et al.* Bone tumor induction after incorporation of short-lived radionuclides. *Radiat Environ Biophys* 1991, **30**: 225-227

EXPERIMENTAL THYROID CARCINOGENESIS IN RODENTS: ROLE OF RADIATION AND XENOBIOTIC CHEMICALS

CC CAPEN

Department of Veterinary Biosciences, The Ohio State University, Columbus

RA DELELLIS

Department of Pathology, New York Hospital, Cornell Medical Center, New York

ED WILLIAMS

Thyroid Carcinogenesis Research Group, Strangeways Research Laboratories, Cambridge

The results of a re-evaluation of thyroid histopathology are summarized in this report from an important (previously reported) large study in female Long-Evans rats (3000 animals randomly assigned to ten treatment groups) exposed at six weeks of age to varying doses of either ^{131}I or localized X-rays to the thyroid or localized X-rays to the pituitary with and without the thyroid. There was close agreement in the diagnosis of follicular cell carcinoma between the two independent evaluations of thyroids; in eight of ten treatment groups the diagnosis was either identical or differed by one. The concordance was not as good for adenomas, most likely due to the category of focal hyperplasia of follicular cells utilized in the current review. However, the results of the re-evaluation support the overall conclusion of this study that the proportion of animals developing thyroid carcinoma was similar for internal ^{131}I irradiation and localized external X-rays within the dose ranges utilized. In addition, major mechanisms are discussed by which nongenotoxic xenobiotic chemicals disrupt thyroid hormone economy and increase the development of thyroid follicular cell tumors in chronic studies in laboratory rodents.

1 THYROID CARCINOGENESIS AND RADIATION: EXTERNAL (LOCALIZED) X-RAYS COMPARED TO INTERNAL ^{131}I IRRADIATION

Epidemiologic studies in humans and early animal studies have suggested that the risk of developing thyroid cancer following exposure to external (localized) X-rays is greater than exposure to internal ^{131}I irradiation.[3,6] However, results of a large animal study supported by the US Food and Drug Administration (FDA) in female Long-Evans rats (3,000 animals divided into ten equal treatment groups administered a single dose of irradiation at six weeks of age [^{131}I doses of 0, 80, 330, and 850 rads; X-ray doses localized to thyroid of 0, 94, 410, and 1060 rads; X-ray localized to pituitary 410 rads and pituitary plus thyroid 410 rads] and all surviving animals killed after two years) revealed that the proportion of animals with thyroid carcinomas was similar for ^{131}I and X irradiation within the dose range of 0-1000 rads.[4] A National Cancer Institute (NCI) advisory committee suggested a review of the thyroid microscopic slides upon which the conclusions were based because: 1) the effectiveness ratio between X-rays and ^{131}I was not consistent with that previously reported in the literature from earlier animal and human studies where X-rays were reported to be a factor of approximately 10 times more effective than ^{131}I; 2) the high reported incidence of thyroid medullary (C-cell) tumors; and 3) the medical and societal significance of the conclusions from this study.

The authors of the present report, at the request of the NCI and with the cooperation of the FDA Center for Devices and Radiological Health, conducted a detailed review of the thyroid microslides in a blind manner without knowledge of treatment groups from this large animal study and compared the thyroid findings with those in the original published report. A total of 2,818 microslides of thyroid glands representing approximately 10,000 levels of thyroid tissue from 2,727 experimental rats were available for review from Lee *et al.*[4] The microslides were evaluated at the same time by the three pathologists and a consensus histopathologic diagnosis was tabulated for the thyroid lesions for subsequent analysis. In addition, the following data was tabulated for each rat: size of thyroid lesion, architecture, invasion, histologic pattern, cytology, lesion frequency, and lesion multiples, quality of histologic preparation, parathyroid presence and nodularity, and conclusion for the thyroid follicular cell and C-cell lesions. The key to the radiation exposure given each animal was not available until the end of the microscopic review of the thyroid microslides. The microslides were reviewed using a Zeiss microscope fitted with a Sony Trinitron color television camera, a DXC1850 camera control unit, and a Panasonic CT1010M color video monitor that provided excellent image reproduction with little difference in resolution between viewing the sections through the microscope or on the monitor screen. The numbers of levels of thyroid tissue were recorded for each rat and the histologic quality was assessed for each slide evaluated. The mean levels of thyroid available for evaluation ranged from 2.86 ± 0.38 to 4.50 ± 2.3 with no apparent variation between treatment groups.

There was a significant dose-dependent increase in follicular cell carcinomas in rats administered ^{131}I or exposed to external X irradiation (Fig. 1). In rats given the high dose (HD) of ^{131}I, 7.3% (19/260) developed follicular cell carcinoma compared to 0.4% (1/276) in controls. By comparison, 8.9% (22/247) of rats administered the HD of X-ray developed follicular cell carcinoma compared to 0.4% (1/265) in control rats. A small number of anaplastic carcinomas were observed in the HD irradiation groups for both [131]I (2 rats) and X-rays (3 rats). If these rats were included, the respective figures increased to 8.1% (21/260) for the HD ^{131}I group and 10.1% (25/247) for the HD X-ray group.

There also was a significant dose-dependent increase in follicular cell adenomas in rats administered ^{131}I or exposed to external X-irradiation (Fig. 1). Of the rats receiving the HD ^{131}I, 8.5% (22/260) developed adenomas compared to 1.1% (3/276) in controls. External X-rays resulted in an 18.6% (46/247) incidence of adenomas in rats administered the HD compared to 2.6% (7/265) in controls.

When the total thyroid follicular cell tumor incidence (adenoma and carcinoma) was evaluated, there was a significant increase to 16.6% (43/260) in the HD ^{131}I group compared to 1.4% (4/276) in controls and a 28.7% (71/247) incidence in the HD X-ray group compared to 3.0% (8/265) in controls.

Focal hyperplastic lesions of follicular cells were recorded in addition to evaluating thyroid tumors following exposure to ^{131}I and external X-rays. There was a dose-related increase in focal hyperplastic lesions of follicular cells in rats following administration of external X-rays but not in rats given ^{131}I (Fig. 1). Rats receiving the HD of X-rays had a 9.7% (24/247) incidence of focal hyperplasia compared to 1.9% (5/265) in controls. By comparison following administration of the HD ^{131}I, 1.9% (5/260) of rats developed focal follicular cell hyperplasia compared to 2.5% (7/276) in controls.

The cytology and size of follicular cell lesions was evaluated independent of conclusion. There was a significant dose-dependent increase in less well-differentiated follicular cell lesions in both the ^{131}I and X-ray treated groups (Fig. 2). Larger (> 5mm) follicular cell lesions developed more frequently in the HD group with both ^{131}I and external irradiation (Fig. 3).

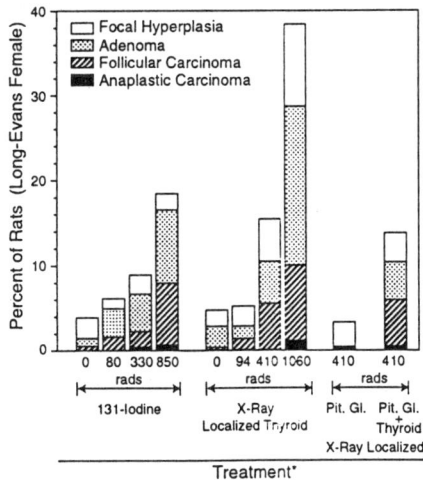

Fig. 1. Thyroid Follicular Cell Lesions vs Radiation Exposure

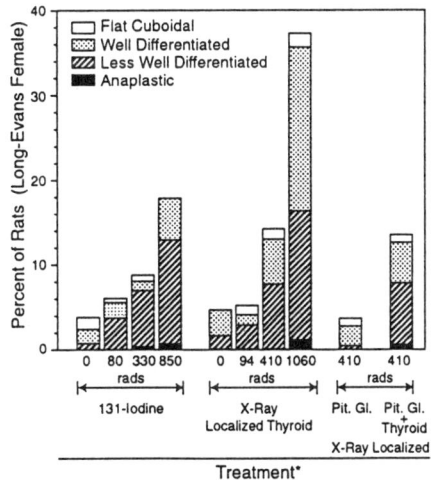

Fig. 2. Thyroid Follicular Cell Cytology vs Radiation Exposure

There was a slight increase in C-cell carcinomas in the mid (MD) and HD groups for ^{131}I (3.4%; 9/267) and 3.5% (9/260 rats), respectively, compared to control (0.7%; 2/276) rats (Fig. 4). C-cell carcinomas were increased (4.9%; 13/263) in the MD X-ray group compared to controls (0.8%; 2/265) but the incidence in the HD group decreased and was similar (0.8%) to that in controls. The incidence of C-cell adenomas was high in both groups (^{131}I--21.4%; X-rays--

15.9%) and did not appear to be increased by administration of either [131]I (HD 21.5%) or external X-rays (HD 15%). Focal C-cell hyperplasia also was a frequent finding both in the control rats ([131]I--10.5%, X-rays--11.3%) and in those receiving a HD of [131]I (11.0%), but there was a significant decrease in the incidence in the HD X irradiation (3.6%) group (Fig. 4).

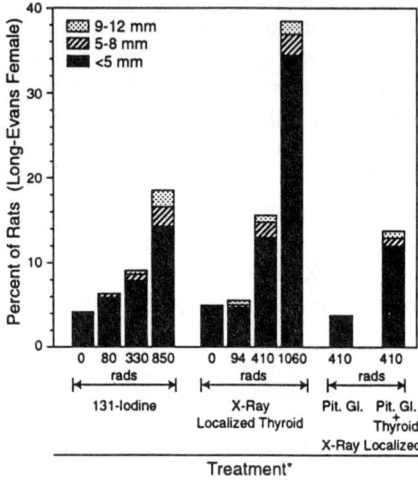

Fig. 3. Thyroid Follicular Cell Lesion Size vs Radiation Exposure

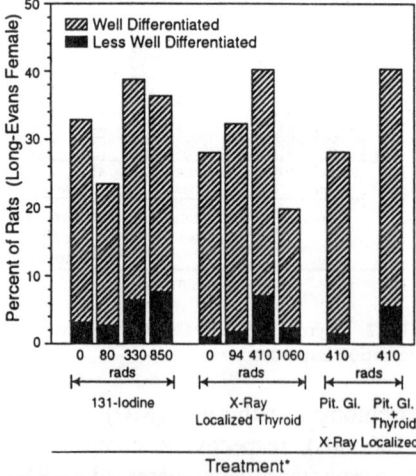

Fig. 4. Thyroid C-Cell Lesions vs Radiation Exposure

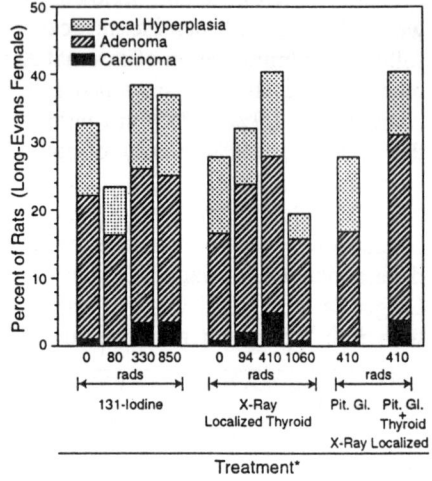

Fig. 5. Thyroid C-Cell Cytology vs Radiation Exposure

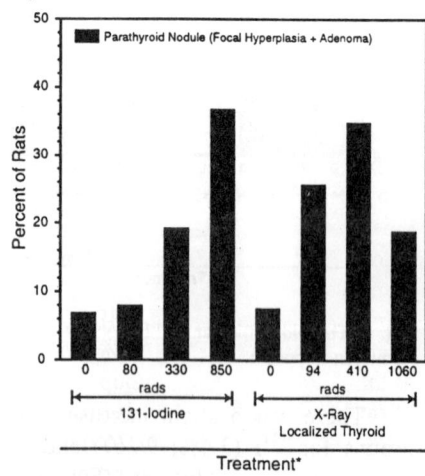

Fig. 6. Parathyroid Nodular Proliferative Lesions vs Radiation Exposure

C-cell lesions were predominantly composed of well differentiated C-cells in all groups (Fig. 5); however, there was a trend for the lesions to be composed of less well differentiated C-cells following MD (6.0%) and HD (7.3%) of ^{131}I irradiation. The sections from all animals were evaluated for the presence and nodularity of parathyroid tissue. No attempt was made to separate parathyroid adenoma from focal hyperplasia. Parathyroid tissue was present in approximately 80% of all rats, although it was identified less frequently in the HD irradiation groups. There was a significant dose-dependent increase for parathyroid nodules (focal hyperplasia plus adenomas) from 6.8% in controls to 36.7% in the HD ^{131}I treated rats (Fig. 6). In X irradiated rats the parathyroid nodules increased from a control value of 7.5% to 25.6% (LD) and 34.8% (MD) but decreased to 18.8% for the HD group.

Summary: Comparison of the Thyroid Pathology in the Original Evaluation (Lee, et.al.[4]) and the Re-evaluation Conducted for NCI.

There was close agreement in the diagnosis of follicular cell carcinoma between the two independent histopathologic evaluations of thyroids from this important experiment, in that for 8 of 10 treatment groups the number of carcinomas diagnosed was either identical or differed by one (Fig. 7). The total number of follicular carcinomas diagnosed in the whole experiment (93) was identical in both evaluations. The concordance was not as good for follicular cell adenomas, most likely due to the separate category of focal follicular cell hyperplasia in the current NCI review. Similarly, comparisons of the incidence of C-cell proliferative lesions was difficult since the NCI review classified these into focal hyperplasia, adenoma, and carcinoma; while the original evaluation published data only for medullary (C-cell) tumors without further analysis. However, the overall trend for changes in C-cell lesions was similar for both evaluations. No comparison was possible for parathyroid lesions, since they were not reported in the original study.
Although the numbers of follicular cell lesions detected was similar between the two evaluations, the number of animals used in the data analysis differed because in the current (NCI) review rats were excluded when the sections were severely autolysed or where the thyroid tissue was uninterpretable for other reasons. The combination of these changes plus the slightly higher number of follicular cell carcinomas recorded in the HD X-ray group increased the percentage of carcinomas from 7.9% (21/267) to 10.1% (25/247). By comparison, follicular cell carcinomas in the HD ^{131}I irridation group were identical in the two evaluations and the number of rats used for data analysis differed only slightly, resulting in a small change from 7.6% (21/276) to 8.1% (21/260).
It also is important to point out that follicular cell adenomas were present in larger numbers in the HD X-ray group than in the corresponding HD ^{131}I group in both the original report and current review data. It has been suggested in the

literature that follicular cell carcinomas in the rat may arise from preexisting follicular adenomas.[5]

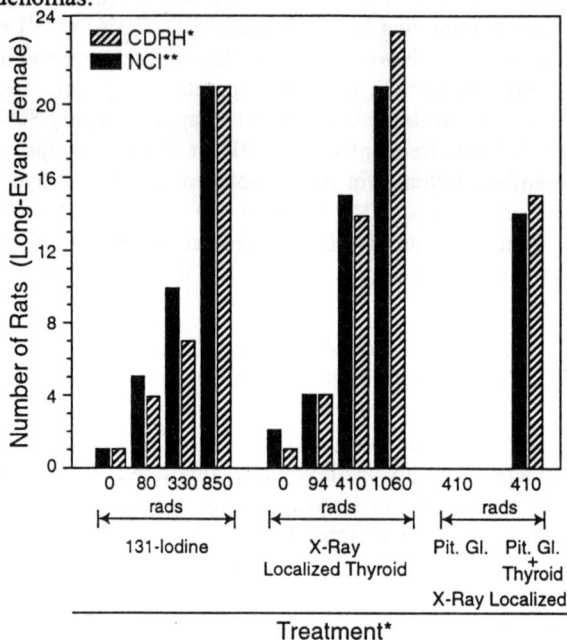

Fig. 7. Comparison of Rats with Thyroid Follicular Cell Carcinoma in Two Independent Pathological Evaluations. *CDRH = Center for Devices and Radiological Health; **National Cancer Institute

2 THYROID CARCINOGENESIS AND XENOBIOTIC CHEMICALS

Xenobiotic chemicals in large doses may disrupt thyroid function in rodents either by a direct effect on the thyroid influencing synthesis or secretion of thyroxine (T4) and triiodothyronine (T3) or by adversely influencing the peripheral metabolism of thyroid hormones.[2] Review of the US Physicians Desk Reference (1994) reveals a number of marketed drugs that result in a thyroid tumorigenic response when tested at high concentrations in rodents, particularly in rats. A broad spectrum of product classes is represented including antibiotics, calcium-channel blockers, antidepressants, and hypolipidemic agents amongst others. Amiodarone (an antiarrhythmic drug) and iodinated glycerol (an expectant) are highly iodinated molecules that disrupt thyroid hormone economy by mechanisms similar to the food color, FD&C Red No. 3.

The major mechanisms by which non-genotoxic xenobiotic chemicals disrupt the hypothalamic-pituitary-thyroid axis can be summarized (Fig. 8) as follows: First, a direct thyroid effect by blocking either the uptake of iodine, inhibiting the important thyroperoxidase enzyme that disrupts iodine binding and the coupling reaction or the proteolysis of colloid and the release of active thyroid hormones, all of which result in low blood levels of T4 and T3. Second, inhibition of 5'-deiodinase in peripheral tissues (such as liver and kidney) that normally converts T4 (the major secretory product of the thyroid) to T3 (the principal thyroid hormone that interacts with receptors in target cells). When the 5'-diodinase is inhibited by highly iodinated compounds such as Amiodarone and FD&C Red No. 3, T4 is converted preferentially to reverse T3 (rT3) which is biologically inactive and does not exert negative feedback on the pituitary and hypothalamus. Third, induction of hepatic microsomal enzymes such as T4-UDP glucuronyl transferase, which increases the conjugation of thyroid hormones with glucuronic acid and excretion of conjugated T4 and T3 in the bile, again resulting in lower blood levels of thyroid hormones. A number of xenobiotics have been reported to act by this mechanism including CNS-acting drugs, calcium-channel blockers, steroids, retinoids, chlorinated hydrocarbons, and polyhalogenated biphenyls.[2]

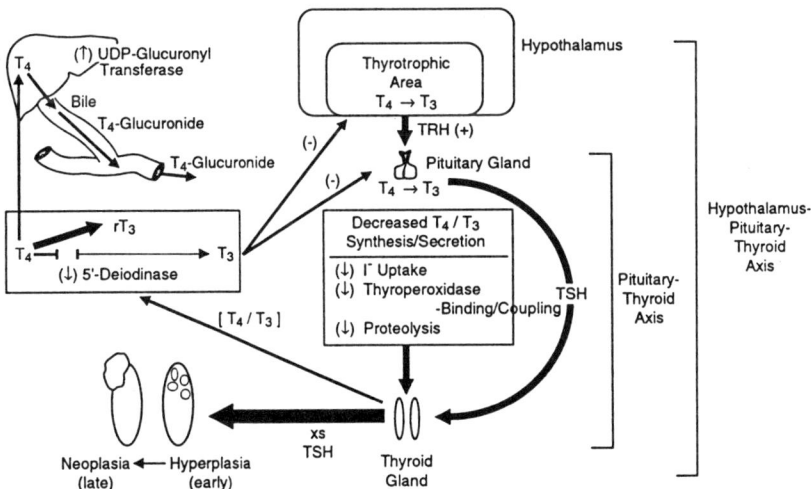

Fig. 8. Disruption of Hypothalamic, Pituitary, Thyroid Triad by Xenobiotic Chemicals

With each of these seeming different mechanisms, the hypothalamus-pituitary axis senses the lower circulating thyroid hormone levels and increases the production of thyroid stimulating hormone (TSH). The rodent thyroid is very sensitive to TSH and follicular cells respond by undergoing hypertrophy and hyperplasia initially and, if sustained, by the development of thyroid tumors (usually adenomas occasionally carcinomas). The human thyroid responds in a different manner to chronic increased blood levels of TSH by frequently undergoing hyperplasia (resulting in "goiter" or clinical enlargement of the thyroid as a common response to iodine deficiency) but rarely develops thyroid tumors as a response to long-term stimulation by TSH.

The proliferative lesions that develop from rodent thyroid follicular cells in response to a chronic increase in TSH represent a morphologic continuum from hyperplasia, to benign tumors (adenomas), and occasionally to malignant tumors (carcinomas). It is difficult with the techniques currently available to accurately determine when a focal proliferative lesion becomes autonomous and continues to proliferate in the absence of the inciting stimulus. Reversibility studies with compounds that produce a high incidence of focal proliferative lesions early, such as methimazole, have been helpful and suggest that many of the small focal lesions classified as adenomas in the thyroid and other endocrine tissues of rodents are reversible when the hormonal imbalances return to normal.[8]

A number of chemicals disrupt thyroid function in rodents by inhibiting the important thyroperoxidase. These include thiourea, propylthiouracil, sulfonamides, methimazole, aminotriazole, and acetoacetamide, amongst others. Chemicals that inhibit thyroperoxidase result in: decreased iodination of tyrosine due to a failure of oxidation of iodide ion to iodine (I_2) and the inhibition of the coupling of iodotyrosines to form active iodothyronines such as T4 and T3. A contemporary example of a chemical acting as a thyroperoxidase inhibitor is sulfamethazine. This is a widely used antibacterial compound in food-producing animals with a current permissible tissue residue level of 100 ppb. Carcinogenicity studies completed at the National Center for Toxicologic Research reported a significant increase in thyroid tumors in male Fischer 344 rats administered the HD (2,400 ppm) of sulfamethazine. The incidence of thyroid tumors was increased in both male and female $B_6 C_3 F_1$ mice after two years in the HD (4,800 ppm) group but not in the lower dose groups.[7]

References

1. Capen CC. Toxic responses of the endocrine system. In: Klaassen CD, ed. *Cassarett and Doull's Toxicology: The Basic Science of Poisons*, 5th ed. New York: McGraw Hill, 1995: 617-640.
2. Capen CC. Mechanistic data and risk assessment of selected toxic endpoints of the thyroid gland. *Toxicol Pathol* 1997; **25**: 39-48.
3. Doniach I. Effects including carcinogenesis of ^{131}I and X ray on the thyroid of experimental animals: A review. *Health Phys* 1963; **9**: 1357-1362.
4. Lee W, Chiacchierini RP, Shleien B, Telles NC. Thyroid tumors following ^{131}I or localized X irradiation to the thyroid and pituitary glands in rats. *Radiat Res* 1982; **92**: 307-319.
5. Lindsay S, Sheline GE, Potter GD, Chaikoff IL. Induction of neoplasms in the thyroid gland of the Rat by X-Irradiation of the Gland. *Cancer Res* 1961; **21**: 9-16.
6. Maxon HR, Thomas SR, Saenger EL, Buncher CR, Kereiakes JC. Ionizing radiation and the induction of clinically significant disease in the human thyroid gland. *Am J Med* 1977; **63**: 967-978.
7. McClain RM. The use of mechanistic data in cancer risk assessment: case example-Sulfanamides. In: *Low Dose Extrapolation of Cancer Risk: Issues and Perspectives*. Washington, DC: International Life Sciences Institute Series (ILSI), 1995: 163-173.
8. Todd GC. Induction and reversibility of thyroid proliferative changes in rats given an antithyroid compound. *Vet Pathol* 1986; **23**: 110-117.

BIOLOGICAL MECHANISMS UNDERLYING RADIATION INDUCTION OF THYROID CARCINOMA

ED WILLIAMS
Thyroid Carcinogenesis Group, University of Cambridge,
Strangeways Research Laboratory, Wort's Causeway,
Cambridge, UK, CB4 8RN
email: edw1001@cam.ac.uk

A brief review of radiation carcinogenesis highlights three points, the age related change in sensitivity to the carcinogenic effect of radiation on the thyroid, the apparent lack of carcinogenic risk following radioiodine therapy of Graves Disease, and the relevance of thyroid growth to carcinogenesis. The thyroid is a stable tissue, it completes most of its growth during development and is unlike either permanent tissues such as neurones which lose the ability to divide in adult life or renewing tissues such as the colon where growth and differentiation continue throughout life. The growth potential of the thyroid is limited, and because of the sequential acquisition of somatic mutations during the carcinogenic process, growth after the initial mutagen exposure is essential for carcinogenesis. The importance of post mutagen growth was demonstrated experimentally and estimation of the rate of growth of the human thyroid follicular cells shows that the availability of post mutagen growth could explain much of the age related change in sensitivity to radiation carcinogenesis in the human thyroid and the lack of carcinogenic risk following radioiodine therapy for Graves disease.

1   INTRODUCTION

There is no doubt that radiation to the thyroid can lead to the development of cancers derived from the follicular cell from studies both in animals and in man. Exposure of animals to external radiation from X-rays[1] or radiation from radioactive isotopes of iodine[2] has led to both benign and malignant tumours of the thyroid.   Carcinogenesis is more effective if exposure is followed by an elevation in TSH, and a very effective model for thyroid carcinogenesis in rodents is administration of iodine 131 followed by prolonged goitrogen treatment[3].   The relative effectiveness of radiation from iodine 131 and from X-rays in causing thyroid cancer is of considerable importance, early studies suggested that iodine 131 was only about a tenth as effective as X-rays[4] but a very large study in rats reached the conclusion that their relative effectiveness was close to equality[5]. While an increased TSH following radiation exposure has been shown to increase tumour frequency in animals, abolishing TSH secretion either by hypophysectomy or by high dose thyroxine treatment immediately after the animals have been exposed to radiation abolishes all tumour formation[6,7].

The carcinogenicity to the thyroid in rodents of exposure to both external and internal radiation has long been accepted; in man the carcinogenic potential of internal radiation has been questioned, while that of external radiation has been accepted. Early studies showing the link in man came from what has been called the "thymus obsession"; the use of X-rays to the thymus to treat a variety of respiratory and other ailments in children, and also from the use of X-rays to treat a range of conditions in the head and neck, again in children[8-10]. High dose X-ray therapy to the neck in adults has been associated with the later development of anaplastic carcinoma[11]. In contrast studies have failed to show any carcinogenic risk to the human thyroid from the use of iodine 131 in the treatment of Graves Disease[12] although the incidence of thyroid carcinoma increased in the population of the Marshall Islands after exposure to fallout from atomic testing, and has increased in children exposed to fallout from the Chernobyl accident[13,14].

For both X-rays and radioactive iodine there is evidence that children are more susceptible to the carcinogenic effect to the thyroid than adults. This has been shown for X-rays in a pooled analysis of several studies[15] and in a large study of the consequences of the atomic bomb in Japan[16]. Radioactive iodine is considered to be the component of fallout causing the increased incidence of thyroid carcinoma in those exposed in the Marshall Islands and in the areas around Chernobyl, in both instances children showed a much greater relative increase in thyroid carcinoma than did adults[13,14], (fig 1).

Figure 1: Effect of age on susceptibility to internal radiation. Data from Chernobyl studies. The expected data are based on figures from England and Wales.

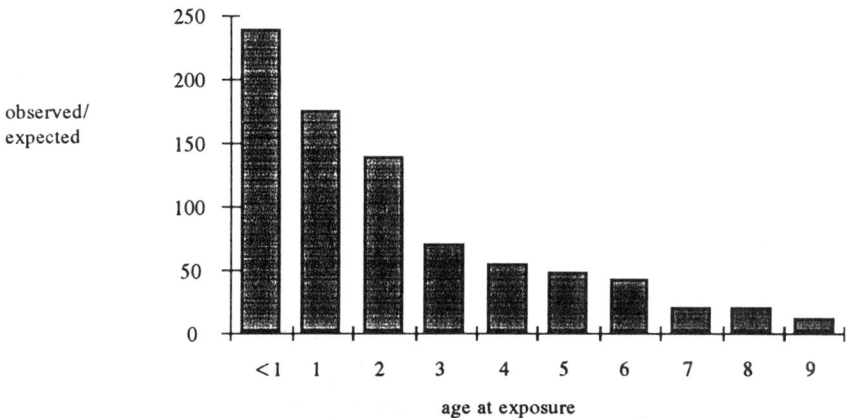

This report is not concerned with the molecular mechanisms that link radiation exposure to thyroid carcinogenesis, but with some of the cell biological features of the thyroid that are relevant to that link. The introduction has highlighted a number of specific points that need consideration, including the age related changes in sensitivity to the carcinogenic effect of radiation, the apparent lack of carcinogenic risk following radioiodine therapy of Graves Disease and the importance of thyroid growth in thyroid carcinogenesis.

In considering the biological mechanisms underlying thyroid carcinogenesis, it is first necessary to put the thyroid into context with other tissues. Mammalian tissues generally can be divided into permanent, stable and labile. Permanent tissues are those which are made up of cells which have finished all growth by birth or soon afterwards, the cells remain fully differentiated throughout life but accumulate mutations, and if they die are not replaced. Neurons are good examples of permanent cells. Stable tissues are made up of cells which complete most of their growth before the individual reaches maturity, but retain a capacity for growth on demand. That capacity may be limited, as has been shown for fibroblasts, in the so called "Hayflick limit", the thyroid is a good example of a

180

stable tissue. Labile tissues are made up of cells which continually replicate the cycle of growth, differentiation and cell loss, with stem cells giving rise to daughter cells which are normally equally divided between cells that give rise to the next generation of stem cells and cells that continue to divide, the latter giving rise to cells that eventually all differentiate, lose the capacity for growth and die. The colon is a typical stem cell tissue. The relationship between growth and differentiation and the three types of tissue is shown diagrammatically in **Figure 2** below.

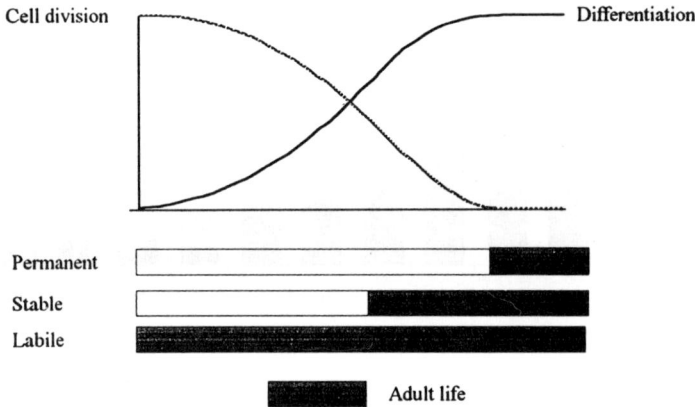

The thyroid is a stable cell tissue, it grows rapidly in fetal and early life but by adult life cell divisions are rare. It retains the capacity to grow when exposed to a high level of TSH, but in response to prolonged TSH stimulation the weight of the gland in rodents reaches a plateau, with the late development of tumours (fig 3).

Analysis of the variables involved shows that a high TSH level is quickly reached, and maintained, but the mitotic response rapidly returns to pretreatment levels, even though the functional response to TSH remains high[17]. Further studies showed that there was no additional growth if the stimulus was withdrawn and reinstated[18]. It seems likely that the same principles, shown experimentally in rodents apply also to man, indeed it is obviously necessary that there should be a limit to the growth response, otherwise the thyroid gland would grow to a huge size in the face of continued stimulation. In Graves Disease, where the thyroid is stimulated by an antibody to the TSH receptor, mimicking the effect of TSH but not subject to feed-back control, the gland usually grows to two or four times its normal size. The symptoms relating to overproduction of thyroid hormone are cured by removal of three quarters of the gland, the remnant in most cases is not able to regenerate to replace the lost tissue. In man and in rodents, the thyroid grows during development, the growth of the gland drops to very low levels in adult life, with the weight reaching a plateau, stimulation leads to further growth, reaching a second plateau which represents the "Hayflick limit" for the thyroid.

Figure 3: Diagram of response of thyroid gland to prolonged growth stimulation, first growing rapidly then reaching a plateau, then giving rise to tumours.

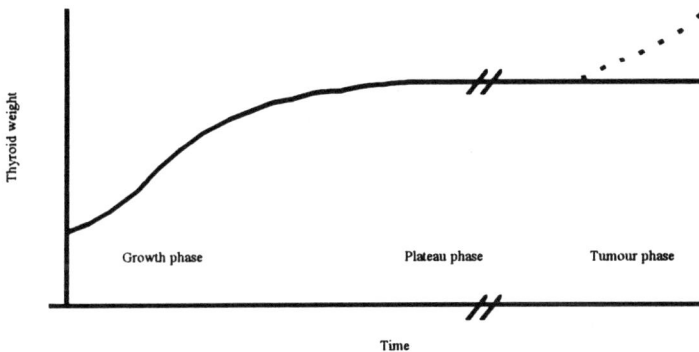

The significance of these observations to carcinogenesis relate to the concept that carcinogenesis depends on somatic mutation and clonal selection. The development of malignancy theoretically needs at least 4 somatic mutations - loss of activity of both copies of a tumour suppressor gene, gain of activity of an oncogene and gain of activity of a gene causing invasion and metastasis[19]. In practice it may well be that many more genes are involved, indeed 6 or 7 have been implicated in the genesis of carcinoma of the colon[20], and somatic mutations in genes involved in DNA repair may well be important. Gain of function mutations can occur through specific chromosomal rearrangements or through point mutations, the latter usually necessarily affect specific codons, while loss of function mutations can occur through a wide range of deletions or rearrangements, or a wide range of point mutations. Radiation or any other mutagen can affect any part of the genome, although some regions show a greater likelihood of mutation, the so called "hot spots". Because of the large number of genes whose function is relevant to cell survival, a dose of mutagen high enough to give a significant chance of causing all the appropriate somatic mutations needed for malignancy in one cell would almost certainly lead to cell death because of the high frequency of other mutations. The mutations needed for carcinogenesis are therefore acquired selectively and sequentially. The evidence from the thyroid showing that increased post mutagen growth increases neoplasia, while abolition of post mutagen growth abolishes neoplasia suggests either that the initial mutations which lead eventually to malignancy do not confer independent growth of a sufficient amount to initiate the clonal selection sequence or that the mutagen exposure causes genomic instability in subsequent cell divisions, or both. Post mutagen growth is therefore critical to the development of malignancy - in permanent cells there is no post mutagen exposure and no malignancy, in labile cells there is continuous post mutagen exposure growth, while in stable cells post mutagen exposure growth is facultative and correlates with the development of malignancy. To test the role of post mutagen growth we have performed an experiment, the results of which will be described in detail elsewhere[21]. Half of a group of 60 male Wistar rats were given 3 months goitrogen treatment, so that they had reached their thyroid growth plateau. After exposure to external radiation (0, 1 or 5 Gy) all animals were then given 9 months goitrogen treatment before the thyroids were removed, step sectioned and the number of tumours counted. The experimental design is shown graphically (fig 4A) and the results are shown in fig 4B.

Figure 4A: Effect of post mutagen growth on thyroid carcinogenesis: experimental design.

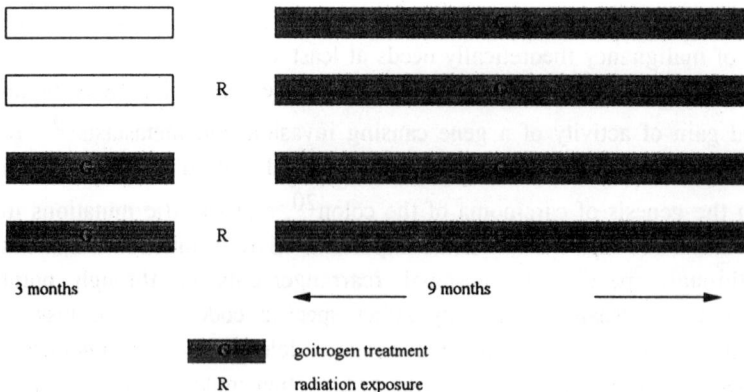

| 3 months | 9 months |

goitrogen treatment

R   radiation exposure

Figure 4B: Effect of post mutagen growth on thyroid carcinogenesis: results

■ Growth stimulus after radiation

☐ Growth stimulus before and after radiation

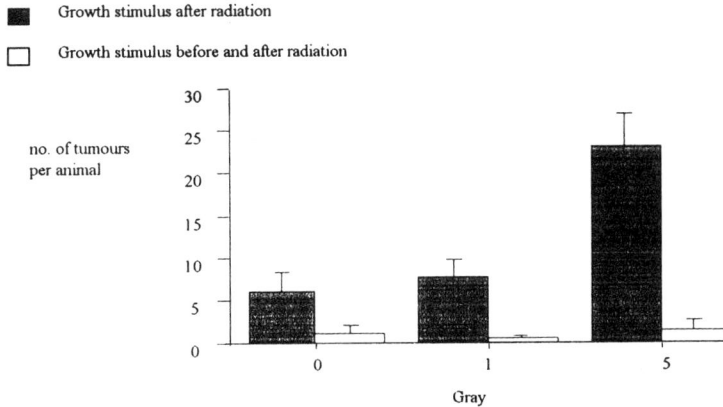

The animals which received no goitrogen before radiation, so that the goitrogen given after exposure induced post mutagen growth showed very many more tumours than did the animals in which growth took place before rather than after mutagen exposure. These differences are significant for the groups given 1 Gy and 5 Gy. The differences in the groups which did not receive radiation are not significant, but might be influenced by an age related difference in DNA repair processes, so that errors occurring during growth at a young age are better repaired than errors occurring during growth at a later age. These findings confirm the importance of post mutagen exposure growth in the genesis of thyroid carcinoma and show that it is the growth induced by TSH that is important, not simply the presence of an elevated TSH.

There are therefore theoretical reasons why post mutagen exposure growth is important in carcinogenesis, and practical evidence confirming the theory. In considering how this applies to radiation carcinogenesis and particularly to age related sensitivity it is important to estimate how much growth occurs in the human thyroid. At birth the weight of the gland is approximately 1.5 g. The size of the adult gland depends on the dietary iodide intake, in the United States and much of Northern Europe the weight of the adult gland is of the order of 16 - 20 g. However during growth the relative volume of follicular cells and colloid changes, with the colloid space rising from approximately 30% at birth to about 60% in young adult life and the follicular cell volume falling from about 50% at birth to

20% in adulthood [22]. These UK figures are compatible with a follicular cell mass rising from about 0.75 g at birth to about 3 to 4 g in maturity (fig 5).

Figure 5: Human thyroid weight during development

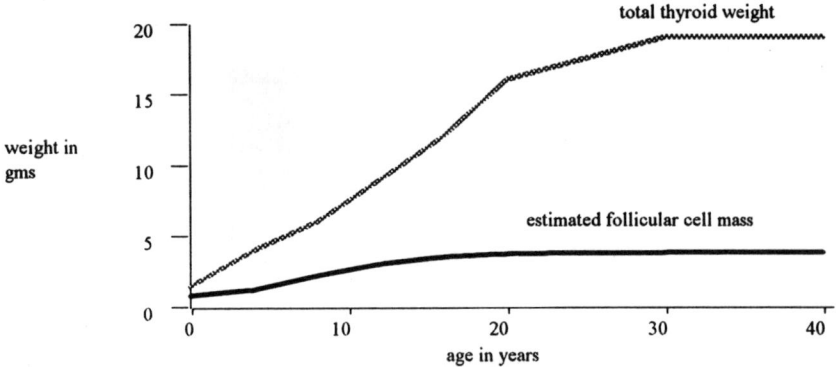

While changes in average follicular cell volume would affect the calculations, these figures suggest that the observed growth can be accounted for by two or three generations of growth occurring in each follicular cell present at birth. If in the thyroid all cells at birth have two generations of growth remaining, it can be shown that the number of these cells will drop rapidly during the first few years of life, and the number with one generation remaining will initially rise, later falling (from about 5 years of age in one model) while the number of cells which have ceased to divide continues to rise (fig 6). A mutation occurring during cell division in a cell with two generations of growth left will be able to acquire a further mutation in only one subsequent cell cycle. While there are more cells undergoing the second cell division a mutation at this time will not be followed by a second opportunity for a cell division related event. Similar arguments apply for the induction of genomic instability (whether due to mutations in DNA repair genes or other mechanisms); as the number of cells passing through the second postnatal division increases, so the chance of future mutations arising from genomic instability decreases. If the mutations required to generate significant independent growth include tumour suppressor gene loss, non-disjunction is a potentially important mechanism, but only in the mitosis subsequent to the one in which the original mutation occurred. In addition to all these points the mitotic rate of follicular cells declines with age, whether expressed per 1000 cells or per gland, so that the effectiveness of mutagens that are partly or wholly cell cycle dependent will also decline with age.

Figure 6: Model of number of cells with 0, 1, or 2 generations of growth remaining (based on 2 cell generations between birth and maturity and the estimayted follicular cell number in man.

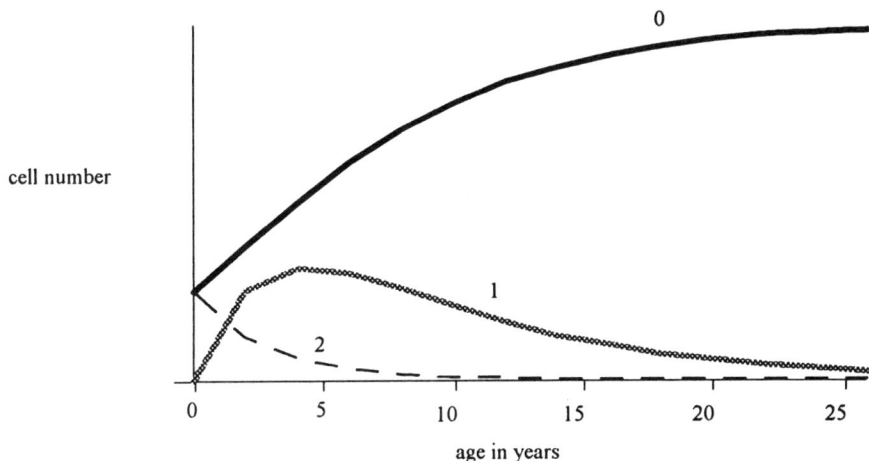

Whatever the mechanisms operating, it is clear from experimental observations that post mutagen exposure growth is important in thyroid carcinogenesis, and that it is likely to be a major factor in explaining the age related change in sensitivity to exposure of the thyroid to both external and internal radiation, with, for internal radiation, the added factor of the age related change in radioiodine uptake, largely related to increased milk consumption of very young children. In man it is also likely to be relevant to situations in which growth follows mutagen exposure in adults; tumours have been recorded in patients who had received radiation to the neck, for example, for breast cancer therapy, and later developed Graves Disease[23]. External radiotherapy to the neck in adult life has also been associated with later development of undifferentiated carcinoma, here it is possible that a pre-existing tumour was radiated and growth continued in the tumour after radiation.

An understanding of cell biology of the thyroid follicular cell, as part of a stable tissue with a limited growth capacity combined with a recognition of the importance of post mutagen exposure growth is necessary to understand some of the unusual features of thyroid carcinogenesis. It provides an explanation for the marked age related sensitivity for carcinogenesis after radiation exposure, with young children having a high mitotic rate and a high remaining growth potential, while adults have a low mitotic rate and a low residual growth potential. It explains the lack of carcinogenicity when radiation is used to treat adults with Graves disease - as growth potential is probably very low, while allowing the possibility of progression in glands that already contain a tumour. The restricted growth potential, which has been "used up" by the growth at the start of Graves Disease, is also relevant to the high incidence of late hypothyroidism not only after radiation therapy where cell sterilisation plays a role, but also after surgery.

187

References

1. Lindsay S, Sheline GE, Potter GD, Chaikoff IL. Induction of neoplasms in the thyroid gland of the rat by x irradiation of the gland. Cancer Research 1961, 21, 9-16
2. Doniach I. Experimental induction of tumours of the thyroid by irradiation. Brit Med. Ball 1958, 14, 181-183
3. Doniach I. The effect of radioactive iodine alone and in combination with methylthiourakil upon tumour production in rats thyroid gland. Brit J Cancer 1953, 7, 181 - 202
4. Doniach I. Comparison of the carcinogenic effect of x irradiation with radioactive iodine in rats thyroid. Brit J Cancer 1956, 11, 67 - 76
5. Wah Lee, Chiacchierini RP, Shleien B and Telles NC. Thyroid Tumours following ^{131}I or Localized X irradiation to the Thyroid and Pituitary Glands in Rats. Radiation Research 1982, 92, 307 - 319
6. Nadler NJ, Mandavia M, Goldberg M. The effect of hypophysectomy on the experimental production of thyroid neoplasms. Cancer Res. 1970, 30, 1909 - 1911
7. Jemec B. Studies of the goitrogenic and tumorigenic effect of two goitrogens in combination with hypophysectomy or thyroid hormone treatment. Cancer 1980,45, 2138 - 2148
8. Duffy BJ, Fitzgerald PJ. Thyroid cancer in childhood and adolescence; a report on 28 cases. J Clin Endocrinol Metab 1950, 10, 1296 - 1308
9. Hanford JM, Quimby EH, Frantz UK. Cancer arising many years after irradiation therapy. Incidence after irradation for benign lesions in the neck. JAMA 1962, 181, 404 - 410
10. DeGroot L, Paloyan E. Thyroid Carcinoma and Radiation. A Chicago Endemic. JAMA 1973, 225, 487 - 491
11. Getaz EP, Shimaoka K. Anaplastic carcinoma of the thyroid in a population irradiated for Hodgkin's Disease. J Surg. Oncol, 1979, 12, 181 - 189
12. Holm LE, Dahlqvist I, Israelsoon A, Lundell G. Malignant thyroid tumours after iodine 131 therapy - a retrospective cohort study. N. Engl. J. Med 1980, 303, 188 - 191
13. Dobyns BM, Hyrmer BA. The surgical management of benign and malignant thyroid neoplasms in Marshall Islanders exposed to hydrogen bomb fallout. World J Surg 1992, 16, 126 - 140
14. Williams ED. Effects on the thyroid in populations exposed to radiation as a result of the Chernobyl accident; in, One decade after Chernobyl, summing up the consequences of the accident. International Atomic Energy Agency, Vienna 1996
15. Ron E, Lubin JH, Shore RE, Mabuchi K, Modan B, Pottern LM, Schneider AB, Tucker MA and Boice JB. Thyroid Cancer after Exposure to External Radiation: A Pooled Analysis of Seven Studies. Radiation Research 141, 259 - 277, (1995)
16. Ezaki H, Takeichi N and Yoshimoto Y. Thyroid Cancer: Epidemiological Study of Thyroid Cancer in A-Bomb Survivors from Extended Life Span Study Cohort in Hiroshima. J. Radiat .Res. Supplement, 193 - 200 (1991)
17. Wynford-Thomas D, Stringer BMJ, Williams ED. Dissociation of growth and function in the rat thyroid during prolonged goitrogen administration. Acta Endocrinol (Copenh) 1982: 101; 210 - 216

18 .Wynford Thomas D, Stringer BMJ, Williams ED. Desensitisation of rat thyroid to the growth-stimulating action of TSH during prolonged goitrogen administration. Acta Endocrinologica 1982, 101: 562 - 569

19. GA Thomas, D Williams and ED Williams. Reversibility of the malignant phenotype in monoclonal tumours in the mouse. Br. J. Cancer 1991, 63: 213 - 216

20. Fearon ER. Molecular genetic studies of the adenoma-carcinoma sequence. Adv.Int. Med 1994, 39, 123 - 147

21. Thomas GA, Horler K and Williams ED. Post mutagen exposure growth and thyroid neoplasia. In preparation

22. Roberts PF. Variation in the morphometry of the normal human thyroid in growth and ageing. J Pathol 1974, 112, 161 - 168

23. Doniach I, Eadie DGA, Hopestone HF. The development of multiple adenomata in primary hyperthyroidism in previously irradiated thyroid glands. Brit. J. Surg, 1966, 53, 681 - 685

THYROID CANCER IN ATOMIC BOMB SURVIVORS

SHIGENOBU NAGATAKI

Radiation Effects Research Foundation
5-2 Hijiyama Park, Minami-ku, Hiroshima 732-0815, Japan
E-mail: nagataki@rerf.or.jp

The Life Span Study (LSS) cohort includes a large number of atomic bomb survivors, both males and females, who were exposed at a wide range of ages to ionizing radiation and who been followed up for five decades. Data from this cohort study afford a unique opportunity to study patterns of cancer risk as they relate to age, time and sex. The latest published LSS incidence data show a strong linear dose response for thyroid cancer. An estimated excess relative risk (ERR) per Sv of 1.15 for thyroid cancer is one of the highest found for solid cancers. The thyroid cancer risk is strongly dependent on age at exposure, much more strongly so than for many other solid cancers, with the ERR decreasing significantly with increasing age at exposure. There is no evidence of significant variation in the ERR with time since exposure, attained age or sex.

1. INTRODUCTION AND BACKGROUND

A large number of epidemiological studies have demonstrated that exposure to ionizing radiation, especially during childhood, is capable of causing thyroid cancer. There is, however, much uncertainty about the magnitude of thyroid cancer risk associated with radiation exposure given during adult life, and the temporal patterns of the risk, which are affected by age and sex, have not been well characterized. The Life Span Study cohort includes a large number of atomic bomb survivors of both sexes who were exposed to a range of radiation doses at a wide range of ages. The cohort has been followed up for over 50 years. Data from this cohort study afford a unique opportunity to examine the temporal patterns and provide the keys for synthesizing information from different populations exposed at different ages.

Thyroid cancer was one of the solid cancers found to be increased among the survivors of the atomic bombings of 1945 in Hiroshima and Nagasaki. Over the last 50 years, a number of thyroid cancer studies have been conducted in the LSS cohort and the Adult Health Study (AHS) clinical sub-cohort of atomic bomb survivors. As one of the earliest, organized efforts to ascertain thyroid cancer cases in a systematic manner, the prevalence of thyroid cancer was studied in the Adult Health Study sample – a clinical sub-cohort of the LSS – during 1958-1959 (1), which demonstrated an increased frequency of this cancer in proximally exposed subjects. Subsequent AHS prevalence studies provide further supporting evidence of the increased thyroid cancer risk (2-4). An extensive study undertaken of autopsy materials during 1957-1967 also demonstrated the frequency of thyroid carcinoma, largely "latent"(as defined by being <1.5 cm in diameter) to increase with an increasing radiation dose (5).

2. A-BOMB INCIDENCE DATA

While these prevalence, or cross-sectional, data provide some useful information, incidence data obtained longitudinally are essential in determining the temporal patterns of cancer risk. Such incidence data for the LSS have recently become available through linkage to the population-based tumor registries in Hiroshima and Nagasaki. The Hiroshima and Nagasaki tumor registries, started in 1957/58, are among the oldest and considered among the best registries in Japan, characterized by high histological verification and low death-certificates only rates (6).

The latest published LSS cancer incidence data obtained for the period of 1958-1987 included a total of 8,613 first primary solid cancers among the 79,972 LSS subjects who were alive as of 1958 and for whom DS86 dose estimates are available (7). Of these, 225 were thyroid cancer cases. Diagnoses were confirmed histologically for 93% of the thyroid cancer cases.

The analysis revealed a strong linear dose response for thyroid cancer, with an estimated excess relative risk (ERR) per Sv of 1.15, one of the highest for solid cancers. However, the most important feature of the thyroid cancer ERR is that it is highly dependent on age at exposure with the ERR being highest among those exposed as children and decreasing with increasing age at exposure (Table 1).

Table 1: Fitted ERR at 1 Sv for Thyroid Cancer by Sex and Age at Exposure

	Age at exposure				
Sex	0-9	10-19	20-39	40+	All ages
Male	9.39	2.60	-0.23	-0.23	1.08
	(7)	(7)	(10)	(12)	(36)
Female	9.47	3.12	0.42	-0.23	1.17
	(26)	(44)	(65)	(54)	(189)
Both	9.46	3.02	0.34	-0.23	1.15
	(33)	(51)	(75)	(66)	(225)

(Number of cases in parentheses)

This trend is well described by a log-linear decrease in the ERR with age at exposure as shown in Figure 1 (8). The rate with which the thyroid cancer ERR decreases with age at exposure (about 73% decrease for each 10 year increase in age at exposure) is about twice as fast as than for other solid cancers. However, there is no evidence that the ERR depends on sex. The ERR also does not vary significantly with either time since exposure or attained age.

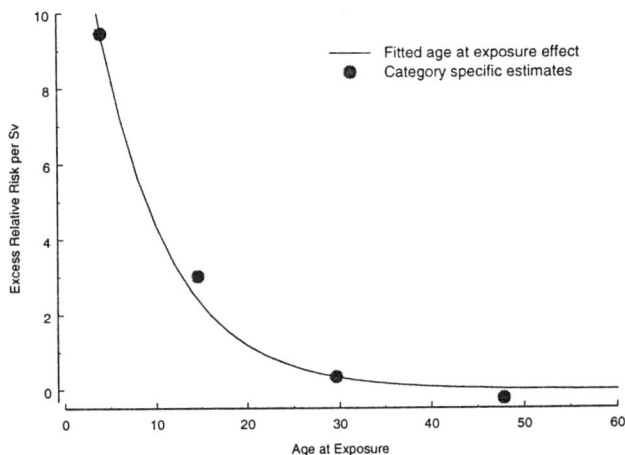

Fig. 1: Age-at exposure dependence of thyroid cancer incidence excess relative risk in the atomic bomb survivors 1958 – 1990 (From Preston DL, 1998)

3. FUTURE

Currently, an in-depth LSS incidence study of thyroid tumors is nearing completion (9); this study involves a panel of pathologists who have reviewed all cases for diagnostic confirmation and morphological characterization. Preliminary data show the predominance of papillary carcinomas in this population and support the previously reported age- and temporal pattern of radiation-induced thyroid cancer risk. A second independent review recently conducted by a panel of international pathologists of cases selected from the above series has found that the solid follicular papillary carcinomas, a type which dominates the post-Chernobyl childhood cases, are rarely seen in the mostly adult-onset LSS cases.

More than 50 years after exposure to the atomic bombings, about half of the survivors in the LSS are alive. Furthermore, the majority (about 90%) of those survivors who were exposed to the bombs during infancy and childhood are currently alive and now entering into ages in which natural (background) cancer rates are increased. In view of the very strong tendency for the thyroid cancer ERR to increase with decreasing age at exposure, the future course of the thyroid cancer ERR among the young survivors is of special importance in assessing the thyroid cancer risk associated with radiation exposure. It is, therefore, of utmost importance that we continue to follow the atomic bomb survivor cohort with respect to cancer incidence in general and thyroid cancer in particular.

Acknowledgement

The author grateful acknowledge the helpful assistance of Dr. Kiyohiko Mabuchi in the preparation of this manuscript.

References

1. Hollingsworth DR, Hamilton HB, Tamagaki H, Beebe GW. Thyroid disease: A study in Hiroshima, Japan. Medicine 1963; **42**: 47-71.
2. Socolow EL, Hashizume A, Neriishi S, Niitani R. Thyroid carcinoma in man after exposure to ionizing radiation. New Engl J Med 1963; **268**: 406-410.
3. Wood JW, Tamagaki H, Neriishi S, Sato T, Sheldon WF, Archer PG, Hamilton HB, Johnson KG. Thyroid carcinoma in atomic bomb survivors, Hiroshima and Nagasaki. Am J Epidemiol 1969: **89**: 4-14.
4. Parker LN, Belsky JL, Yamamoto T, Kawamoto S, Keehn RJ. Thyroid carcinoma after exposure to atomic radiation: A continuing survey of a fixed population, Hiroshima and Nagasaki, 1958-71. Ann Intern Med 1974; **80**: 600-604.
5. Sampson RJ, Key CR, Buncher CR, Iijima S. Thyroid carcinoma in Hiroshima and Nagasaki. I. Prevalence of thyroid carcinoma at autopsy. J Am Med Assoc 1969; **209**: 65-70.
6. Mabuchi K, Soda M, Ron E, Tokunaga M, Ochikubo S, Sugimoto S, Ikeda T, Terasaki M, Preston DL, Thompson DE. Cancer incidence in atomic bomb survivors. Part I. Use of the tumor registries in Hiroshima and Nagasaki for incidence studies. Radiat Res 1994; **137**: s1-s16.
7. Thompson DE, Mabuchi K, Ron E, Soda M, Tokunaga M, Ochikubo S, Sugimoto S, Ikeda T, Terasaki M, Izumi S, Preston DL. Cancer incidence in atomic bomb survivors. Part II. Solid tumors, 1958-1987. Radiat Res 1994; **137**: s17-s67.
8. Preston DL. Radiation risk estimates for thyroid cancer in atomic bomb survivors and their application to Chernobyl data. Report prepared for the Japan Radiation Research Association, Tokyo, Japan, 1998.
9. Hayashi Y, Tsuda N, Akiba S, Fujita S, Tokunaga M, Tokuoka S, Shimaoka K, Ron E, Land CE, Mabuchi K. Studies of thyroid tumor incidence among the RERF Life Span Study cohort, 1950-1987, RERF Research Protocol 6-91, 1991.

CAN THE CHERNOBYL ACCIDENT PROVIDE ANSWERS REGARDING THE RELATIVE RISK OF ^{131}I- VS. SLNS

A.B. BRILL
Vanderbilt University, Nashville, TN 37232, USA.
E-mail: brillab@ctrvax.vanderbilt.edu
M. STABIN
Oak Ridge Associated Universities, Oak Ridge, TN, 37831,USA
E-mail: stabinm@orau.gov
A. BOUVILLE
Radiation Effects Branch, National Cancer Institute, Bethesda, MD,20892 USA
E-mail: ab76o@nih.gov
L. ANSPAUGH
Radiobiology Division, University of Utah, Salt Lake City, UT, 84112 USA
E-mail: LAnspaugh@aol.com
V.T. KHROUCH, Y.I. GAVRILIN, AND S.M. SHINKAREV
Institute of Biophysics, Moscow, Russia
E-mail: msavkin@rcibph.dol.ru

Thyroid and breast doses were calculated based on deposited activity of ^{131}I in Gomel City and Hoiniki Raion. Estimates of integrated deposition of SLNs in these regions were used to generate dose estimates from ingestion and inhalation. The dose from SLNs is less than 10% of the dose from ^{131}I and all estimates have wide uncertainties. It seems unlikely that we will learn the relative risk of SLNs from this experience

1   INTRODUCTION

Prior to the Chernobyl accident the only population in which there was a clear increase in thyroid cancer following ^{131}I was in the Marshall Islanders, and only 15% of their thyroid dose was estimated to come from ^{131}I. Epidemiological studies, however, included few young children, and the low statistical power of these studies could account for their failure to detect an effect. In this paper we calculate dose to the breast in lactating women, to their thyroids, and to the thyroids of newborn infants from the consumption of breast and cows' milk for persons residing in regions with different ^{131}I- and SLN fallout patterns.

2   ABSORBED DOSE CALCULATIONS

Environmental dosimetry models are used to calculate relevant radionuclide intake levels, and absorbed dose using ICRP Dose Conversion Factors (DCFs). Dose from the ingestion of ^{131}I and other radionuclides in contaminated milk is calculated according to the following equation:

$$D = \mu \times F \times DD \times \alpha \times MPD \times f_m \times L \times DCF \times \frac{1}{\lambda}, \qquad (1)$$

for which the parameters are defined as follows:

μ = Correction coefficient (Varies from ~0.1-1 in different settlements)
F = Ratio of integrated deposition of the radionuclide to that of ^{131}I,
DD= Deposition density of ^{131}I, MBq m^{-2};
α = Mass-interception fraction for fallout retained on vegetation, m^2 kg^{-1};
MPD = Mass (dry) per day of pasture consumed by a cow, kg day^{-1};
f_m = Fraction of cow's intake that is secreted in milk, day L^{-1};
L = Consumption rate of milk, L day^{-1};
DCF = Dose-conversion factor for the organ of interest, Gy kBq^{-1}; and
λ = Effective rate of loss of radionuclide from vegetation, day^{-1}.

Values of F were estimated for Gomel City to be 0.2 for ^{133}I and ^{132}Te; for Hoiniki raion (excluding the 30 km zone) the value is 0.5. The values of μ and DD are estimated to be 0.22 and 0.26 and 2.3 MBq m^{-2} and 11.5 MBq m^{-2} for Gomel and Hoiniki, respectively. Values for the other parameters are given elsewhere.[1-3]

For the dose to the infant's thyroid from drinking mothers' milk a modified form of eqn (1) is:

$$D = \mu \times F \times DD \times \alpha \times MPD \times f_m \times L \times f_{mm} \times L_i \times DCF_i \times \frac{1}{\lambda}, \qquad (2)$$

where the additional parameters are:

f_{mm} = Fraction of mother's intake that is secreted in milk, day L^{-1},
L_i = Consumption rate of milk by infant, L day^{-1}.

The dose from inhalation is

$$D = F \times DD \times \frac{1}{v_g} \times BR \times DCF, \qquad (3)$$

where:
v_g = Deposition velocity of iodine and tellurium on the ground, m day^{-1}; and

$BR=$ Breathing rate, m^3 day^{-1}.

The dose to the infant from drinking milk contaminated by the mother's inhalation of activity is

$$D = F \times DD \times \frac{1}{v_g} \times BR \times f_{mm} \times L_i \times DCF_i . \qquad (4)$$

Based on the above equations and assumptions, the doses estimated for the different target tissues in Gomel City and Hoiniki residents are given in Table 1

The above eqns (1-4) are multiplicative chains with each parameter having the form of a geometric mean. As the distribution of each parameter is assumed to be lognormal, i.e., the logarithms of each value are distributed normally, the product of the chain could also be calculated by summing the logarithms of each value and exponentiating the sum. More importantly, this assumption provides for a convenient analytical method of propagating uncertainties. Thus, the logarithms of the geometric standard deviations (GSDs) have the behavior of a standard deviation of a normal distribution, and the usual rules of error propagation can be used. Thus, for a multiplicative chain of i independent variables, the variance of the logarithm of the product is equal to:

$$(\ln GSD_p)^2 = \sum_i (\ln GSD_i)^2 , \qquad (5)$$

and the GSD of the product is

$$GSD_p = \exp\left[\sqrt{\ln(GSD_p)^2} \right] . \qquad (6)$$

In a rigorous sense geometric means should not be summed, but the geometric means should be converted to arithmetic means and variances before summing and error propagation. However, in situations where one single term dominates the sum and the distribution, only a small error is introduced by summing geometric means and by assuming that the GSD of the sum is equal to the GSD of the dominant term.

3   CONCLUSIONS

The infant drinking cows' milk receives a higher thyroid dose from ^{131}I than does a nursing infant. The mother passes most of the radioiodine from the cow's milk she drinks into her urine, thus diminishing the amount passed to her child. The thyroid dose in Hoiniki is about 6 fold higher than in Gomel City, and the contribution from SLNs is about 2 times higher. The fractional contribution of SLNs is much smaller than was reported for the Marshall Island exposures, and it seems unlikely that the increased incidence in Chernobyl-exposed children can be attributed to SLNs.

Table 1
Total Dose (Gy) and Fraction from SLNs

Organ/ Source		Gomel City				Hoiniki Raion			
		Dose (Gy)		Fraction due to SLNs		Dose (Gy)		Fraction due to SLNs	
Mother's Thyroid		Geo Mean	GSD	Geo Mean	GSD	Geo Mean	GSD	Geo Mean	GSD
	Inhalation	0.0022	4.2	0.071	3	0.014	4.2	0.26	3
	Ingestion	0.078	3.5	0.0036	3	0.46	3.5	0.009	3
	Total	0.08	3.5	0.0054	3	0.48	3.5	0.013	3
Thyroid- Nursing Infant									
	Inhalation	0.0024	4.2	0.095	3	0.016	4.2	0.21	3
	Ingestion	0.017	4.3	0.0053	3	0.1	4.3	0.013	3
	Mother's inhalation	0.0015	5	0.08	3	0.0097	5	0.18	3
	Total	0.021	4.3	0.021	3	0.13	4.3	0.051	3
Mother's Breasts									
	Inhalation	1.3 E-06	4.5	0.22	3	1.0 E-05	4.5	0.41	3
	Ingestion	4.5 E-05	3.7	0.022	3	2.7 E-04	3.7	0.052	3
	Total	4.6 E-05	3.7	0.027	3	2.8 E-04	3.7	0.066	3
Thyroid-Cow milk-drinking Infant									
	Inhalation	0.0024	4.2	0.095	3	0.016	4.2	0.21	3
	Ingestion	.0.24	3.5	0.0053	3	1.5	3.5	0.013	3
	Total	0.25	3.5	0.0062	3	1.5	3.5	0.015	3

References

1. Gavrilin YI, Khrouch VT. Shinkarev SM, Drozdovitch V, Minenko V, Shemyakina E, Bouville A, Anspaugh L. Estimation of thyroid doses received by the population of Belarus as a result of the Chernobyl accident. The radiological consequences of the Chernobyl accident. Proceedings of the first international conference, Minsk, Belarus, 18 to 22 March 1986 (Editors: A. Karaoglou, G. Desmet, G. N. Kelly and H. G. Menzel). European Commission report EUR*16544 EN*. Luxembourg; 1996:1011-1020.
2. Gavrilin YI, Khrouch VT, Shinkarev SM, Krysenko NA, Skryabin AM, Bouville A, Anspaugh L Chernobyl accident: Reconstruction of thyroid dose for inhabitants of the Republic of Belarus. Health Phys.; submitted.
3. Anspaugh L, Bouville A, Stabin M, Brill AB, Khrouch VT, Gavrilin YI, Shinkarev SM. Radioactive iodine dose to the breast and thyroid in lactating women and nursing infants from the Chernobyl accident. Health Phys, in preparation.

RELATIVE BIOLOGICAL EFFECTIVENESS OF EXTERNAL RADIATION VS. I-131: REVIEW OF ANIMAL DATA

H. D. ROYAL, M.D.

Mallinckrodt Institute of Radiology, 510 S. Kingshighway Blvd.
St. Louis, Missouri 63110, USA
E-mail: royal@mirlink.wustl.edu

The increase in thyroid cancers among children exposed to radioiodine due to the Chernobyl accident has renewed interest in carcinogenic potential of radioiodine exposure. The purpose of the paper is to review existing animal data to determine if this data gives a reliable estimate of the RBE of radioiodine when compared to external radiation. This review is limited to papers where 1) the same investigators exposed groups of animals to I-131 and other groups of animals to external radiation and 2) the endpoint of interest was thyroid cancers. I-131 is the radioiodine of greatest interest due to its use in medicine and it importance in environmental contamination due to nuclear weapons production and testing as well as due to nuclear accidents.

Early animal studies were focused on determining the potential carcinogenic effects of therapeutic doses of I-131. These early studies generally indicated that the RBE of I-131 was 2-20 times less effective than external radiation in causing thyroid cancer. In addition to the high doses used, these early studies had many flaws that limit their scientific value. One more recent study that used younger animals and lower doses suggest that I-131 is as effective as external radiation in causing thyroid cancer. No relevant papers have been published since 1982.

1. INTRODUCTION

1.1 Problems with Human Data

The increase in thyroid cancers among children exposed to radioiodine due to the Chernobyl accident has renewed interest in carcinogenic potential of radioiodine exposure. Prior to the Chernobyl accident, there was no human data that could be used to estimate the carcinogenic risk coefficient for radioactive iodines. Follow-up studies of patients who had diagnostic studies or treatment revealed no measurable excess in thyroid cancer that could be attributed to I-131[1-4]. However, these studies included few children and studies of external radiation have shown that children are much more sensitive to the carcinogenic effects of radiation than are adults[5].

Although the increased risk for thyroid cancer in children exposed as a result of the Chernobyl accident is now widely accepted, calculating the risk coefficient for the carcinogenic effect of radioiodine in humans continues to be problematic. In order to calculate a risk coefficient, the dose and the effect need to be measured with reasonable certainty. Individual doses are better than group doses. There is much more certainty in individual thyroid doses due to medical exposures involving external radiation there is in individual thyroid doses due to accidental exposure to radioiodine. For external radiation due to medical procedures, the exposure occurs in a controlled setting and the dose is absorbed over a very brief period of time. Individual thyroid doses can be calculated with reasonable accuracy using simple assumptions about the exposure rate and duration, energy of the radiation and geometry of the thyroid gland and the surrounding tissues. The dosimetry for accidental radioiodine exposure is much more complex and therefore inherently uncertain. Major factors to be considered include 1) source of food, particularly milk; 2) quantity of food ingested; 3) fraction of ingested iodine incorporated into the thyroid gland; 4) size of the thyroid gland and 5) biological halflive of iodine in the thyroid gland.

Estimating the effect of thyroid exposure, whether due to external radiation or radioiodines, is also more difficult for thyroid cancer than with other types of cancer for two major reasons. First, thyroid cancer is an uncommon cancer which fortunately is fatal in only 5-10% of people in whom it occurs. Large numbers of people must be studied in order to have a stable measure of the mortality rate. If incidence rates are used, they are prone to error since clinically inapparent thyroid disease is common. The numbers of thyroid cancers detected can increase severalfold simply due to increased surveillance [5].

1.2 Advantages and Limitations of Animal Studies

Because of the difficulties in determining the risk coefficient for thyroid cancer due to radioiodine in humans, estimates of the relative biological effectiveness of radioiodines have been based on animal studies. There are two principal advantages of animal studies. First, the radiation exposure can be given in a controlled setting so that the radiation dose to the thyroid is known with more certainty than is possible when humans are exposed unintentionally. Second, the radiation dose can be varied while potentially confounding factors are kept constant. Despite these two advantages, animal studies introduce other important difficulties. There are major differences in radiation sensitivity between species therefore it is unclear whether a risk coefficient measured in animals is relevant to humans. In addition, the search for microscopic thyroid cancer in animals is much more exhaustive than the search is in humans. Typically in animal studies, all animals are autopsied and the number of thyroid cancers is determined by careful histologic examination of the thyroid. Under normal circumstances in humans, the only thyroid cancers that are discovered are those that become clinically apparent, usually as a palpable neck mass.

1.3 Purpose of this Review

This review is limited to animal studies in which investigators 1) systematically exposed groups of animals to I-131 and other groups of animals to external radiation and 2) had thyroid cancer as the radiation effect of interest. By requiring the same investigators to present their results for both types of exposure, control over confounding variables is enhanced and problems due to varying definitions of thyroid cancer are minimized. This review is limited to I-131 because the effects of I-131 exposure have been studied more extensively than any other radioiodine. Interest in the carcinogenic effects of I-131 is great because of the use of I-131 in medicine and because large quantities of I-131 have been released into the environment by the atmospheric testing of nuclear weapons (20 billion curies) and by rare accidents such as Chernobyl (40 - 50 million curies)[6]. The purpose of this review is to revisit the animal data cited in NCRP Report No. 80[7] and to update the report with any animal data that was subsequently published. Some discussion of the scientific validity of these studies will also be presented

2. Review of Animal Studies

2.1 General Concepts

Conceptually measuring the relative biological effectiveness (RBE) in an animal model seems simple. For most solid tumors, the dose-effect relationship is envisioned to be a simple linear regression. This simple relationship is often appropriate because the data used to determine the dose-effect relationship is sparse and does not support more sophisticated model fitting. In reality, many factors affect the RBE including factors related to the radiation (dose, dose rate, energy, uniformity of deposition), the animal model used (species, genetics, sex, age, hormonal status) and the endpoint that is measured (thyroid ablation, goitrogenesis, carcinogenesis). Recognition that all these factors may affect the RBE means that many experiments would need to be done in order to determine the effects of each of the potentially important variables. Unfortunately, valid studies require the use of large numbers of animals and are therefore be expensive to perform. It is also an oversimplification to think that the RBE of I-131 will be accurately represented by a single number since the effectiveness of I-131 in causing the endpoint of interest may vary significantly based on the factors listed above.

2.2 Early Animal Studies

The early animal studies (Studies 1-4 in table 1) reviewed in NCRP Report No. 80[7] to estimate the thyroid carcinogenic effects of I-131 compared to external radiation were exploratory rather than scientifically definitive. These early studies were motivated by concerns that the medical use of I-131 for the treatment of a benign condition (hyperthyroidism) might eventually result in the treatment-induced thyroid cancers. Given this concern about the possible effects of I-131 treatment, relatively large amounts of I-131 (25-30 μCi in rats; 3 μCi in mice) were injected intraperitoneally resulting in thyroid doses in the range of 2,000 - 24,000 cGy. In addition, older rats of both sexes were used. Experience in human with external radiation has subsequently indicated the important effect of age on risk[5]. In some experiments, goitrogens were used to enhance the carcinogenic effect.

Table 1. Animal studies

Study Number	Author	Animal Model	X-ray Dose (cGy)	I-131 Dose (cGy)	Estimated RBE
1	Doniach (1957)[8]	160 Lister male and female rats Average age - 3 months Surviving - 116	1100	2000-24000	1/2 - 1/20
2	Lindsey et al. (1957)[9] Lindsey et al. (1961)[10]	I-131 550 male and female Long-Evans rats Age: 6-12 weeks Surviving - 354 Xray 450 male Long-Evans rats Age: 8-12 weeks Surviving - 107	1000	~5,000	1/5
3	Walinder (1972)[11]	700 male CBA mice Age: 110-130 days of age	475-1430	5400-16,000	1/4-1/11
4	Walinder (1972)[12]	815 male, 696 female CBA mice Age: 18th day of gestation	180	1900-7,300	????
5	Lee et al (1982)[13]	3,000 female Long-Evans rats Age: 6 weeks Surviving - 2762	94-1060	80-850	1/1 for Ca 1/2 for adenomas

In addition, these early experiments suffered from use of relatively small numbers of animals in each their experimental groups. In these early studies, only animals that survived the planned period of observation had their thyroids examined histologically. For most of these studies, the death rate was very high, approaching

80% in x-ray portion of study 2. No assurances were given in these early studies, that the person performing the histologic examination was blinded to the animal's exposure history.

2.3 Study of Lee et al.

In contrast to the early studies, the study by Lee et al[13] is better designed and is therefore scientifically more defensible. Prior to performing their study, a dosimetric study was performed to accurately measure the thyroid dose from both I-131 and x-rays[14]. The authors used a new dosimetric model for I-131 and they indicated that earlier studies had probably overestimated the dose that was received by the thyroid from I-131 by 60-70%. Such an error would have resulted in the underestimation of the RBE for I-131.

The Lee study used younger (6 week old) rats of the same type (Long-Evans) as Lindsey[9]. Use of younger rats may have an important effect on the results of the study given what we now know about the increased sensitivity of children to external radiation. The thyroid doses used in this study were lower than those used in the earlier studies and were in a range than is more relevant for environmental and diagnostic exposures. Much larger numbers of rats were used in each experimental group (10 groups of 300 animals each). In addition, histologic examination of the thyroid was performed in a much higher proportion of the animals. The histologic examination was performed without knowledge of the exposure history of the animal. In recognition of the potential value of the data produced by the experiment, an independent blinded review of the thyroid sections was performed and confirmed the findings of the original authors. The results of the independent review was reported in another paper presented at this symposium.

This study concluded that the RBE for thyroid cancer was similar for external radiation and for I-131, that the risk was proportional to the square root of the dose, and that the risk was independent of dose rate (Fig. 1). The dose response curves obtained for adenomas were different that the dose response curves for thyroid cancer. I-131 appeared to be approximately half as effective in causing adenomas as was external radiation (Fig. 2). This study also demonstrated that in this experimental model pituitary radiation had no effect on the occurrence of thyroid cancers. A group of animals given pituitary irradiation were included in this study because of the first reports of the Israeli tinea capitus study had been published[15, 16] and concern had been raised that the combination of thyroid and pituitary irradiation had a synergistic effect on thyroid carcinogenesis.

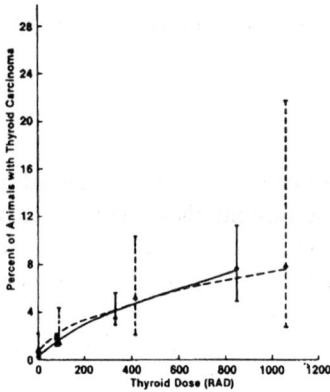

Fig. 1 . Dose-response curve for thyroid carcinoma

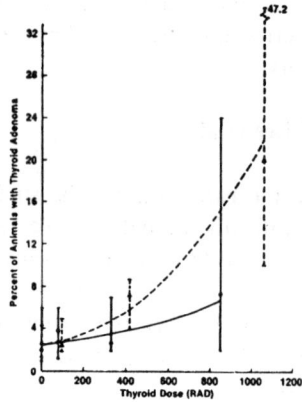

Fig. 2. Dose-response curve for thyroid adenomas

3. CONCLUSIONS

Since the Lee study that was published in 1982, there has been no new animal data published in the English literature. In the last decade, dose reconstructions for U.S. and former Soviet nuclear production facility and for atmospheric testing have indicated that large populations have been exposed to potentially significant doses of I-131. These dose reconstructions as well as the experience following the Chernobyl accident highlight the need to better determine the risk from environmental releases of I-131. Given the paucity of useful existing animal data, consideration should be given to funding several high quality animal studies to better determine the RBE for I-131 and other radioiodines. The relevance of data obtained from animal experiments will be questioned, however, data obtained from animals studies may improve our understanding of the carcinogenic effects of I-131 especially when that animal data can be interpreted in the context of human data. Human data should be forthcoming not only from Chernobyl but also from population exposed from nuclear weapons production facilities and from atmospheric testing of nuclear weapons.

References

1. Hall, P & Holm, LE. Cancer in iodine-131 exposed patients. *J Endocrinol Invest* 1995; **18**, 147-9.
2. Hall, P & Holm, LE. Late consequences of radioiodine for diagnosis and therapy in Sweden. *Thyroid* 1997; **7**, 205-8.
3. Hall, P, Mattsson, A & Boice, JD, Jr. Thyroid cancer after diagnostic administration of iodine-131. *Radiat Res* 1996; **145**, 86-92.
4. Hall, P, Furst, CJ, Mattsson, A, et al. Thyroid nodularity after diagnostic administration of iodine-131. *Radiat Res* 1996; **146**, 673-82.
5. Ron, E, Lubin, JH, Shore, RE, et al. Thyroid cancer after exposure to external radiation: a pooled analysis of seven studies. *Radiat Res* 1995; **141**, 259-77.
6. Becker, DV, Robbins, J, Beebe, GW, Bouville, AC & Wachholz, BW. Childhood thyroid cancer following the Chernobyl accident: a status report. *Endocrinol Metab Clin North Am* 1996; **25**, 197-211.
7. *NCRP Report No. 80: Induction of thyroid cancer by ionizing radiation* . Bethesda, MD: National Council on Radiation Protection and Measurement, 1985: 1-93.
8. Doniach, I. Comparison of the Carcinogenic Effect of X-Irradiation With Radioactive Iodine on the Rat's Thyroid. *Brit. J. Cancer* 1957; **11**, 67-76.
9. Lindsay, S, Potter, GD & Chaikoff, IL. Thyroid Neoplasms in the Rat: A Comparison of Naturally Occurring and I-131-Induced Tumors. *Cancer Research* 1957; , 183-189.
10. Lindsay, S, Sheline, GE, Potter, GD & Chaikoff, IL. Induction of Neoplasms in the Thyroid Gland of the Rat by X-Irradiation of the Gland. *Cancer Research* 1961; **21**, 9-17.
11. Walinder, G. Late Effects of Irradiation of the Thyroid Gland in Mice - I. Irradiation of adult mice. *Acta Radiologica Therapy Physics Biology* 1972; **11**, 433-451.
12. Walinder, G & Sjoden, A. Late Effects of Irradiation of the Thyroid Gland in Mice - II. Irradiation of mouse foetuses. *Acta Radiologica Therapy Physics Biology* 1972`; **11**.
13. Lee, W, Chiacchierini, RP, Shleien, B & Telles, NC. Thyroid tumors following 131I or localized X irradiation to the thyroid and pituitary glands in rats. *Radiat Res* 1982; **92**, 307-19.
14. Lee, W, Shleien, B, Telles, NC & Chiacchierini, RP. An Accurate Method of I-131 Dosimetry in the Rat Thyroid. *Radiat Res* 1979; **79**, 55-62.
15. Modan, B, Ron, E & Werner, A. Thyroid cancer following scalp irradiation. *Radiology* 1977; **123**, 741-4.
16. Ron, E & Modan, B. Benign and malignant thyroid neoplasms after childhood irradiation for tinea capitis. *J Natl Cancer Inst* 1980; **65**, 7-11.

FUNCTIONAL AND HISTOMORPHOLOGICAL CHANGES OF THYROCYTES UNDER DIFFERENT IODINE INTAKE AND EXTERNAL IONIZING RADIATION IN RATS

C. HOANG-VU, C. BOLTZE, C. SEKULLA AND H. DRALLE

Klinik für Allgemeinchirurgie, MLU Halle, Magdeburger Str. 18, 06097 Halle
Germany
E-mail: hoang-vu@medizin.uni-halle.de

R. GERLACH AND J. DUNST

Klinik für Strahlentherapie, MLU Halle, Voßstr. 1, 06112 Halle
Germany

H. J. HOLZHAUSEN

Institut für Pathologie, MLU Halle, Magdeburger Str.14, 06097 Halle
Germany

G. BRABANT

Abt. Klinische Endokrinologie , MHH, 30625 Hannover
Germany

To test the influence of external ionizing radiation and the protective role of iodine supplementation we investigated the changes in functional and histological parameters of the thyroid in rats following X-ray radiation under high, normal and low dietary iodine (LID). Iodine rich diet stimulated increased TSH plasma level twofold as compared to controls. Plasma T3 and T4 level were not significantly changed in both groups, whereas T3 decreased about 80% and T4 about 30% in the LID-group. TSH levels increased after 10 weeks in all LID-animals. TSH secretion fluctuated significantly between 5 and/or 8 weeks. This observation was only found in LID-animals but not in iodine supplemented litter mates. Irradiation led to increased T4 with a constant T3 initially, followed by a slight reduction of both thyroid hormones. Histological evaluations revealed clear hyperplasia of thyroid follicles and it was only detected by LID. Irradiation with 4 Gy and LID mostly destroyed follicle structures of the thyroid, whereas these changes were not detected in the iodine supplemented animals. The data provide evidence that iodine has a protective effect in the initial phase of external ionizing radiation.

Introduction

Epidemiological studies in euthyroid patients with diffuse euthyroid goitre revealed an increase rather than a decrease in TSH serum levels with unchanged thyroid hormone levels [1,2]. In healthy volunteers experimentally induced decrease in iodine supply lowered but did not stimulate TSH secretion [3]. These data suggest an increased sensitivity to TSH in iodine deficiency, which may contribute to goitre formation, as Tg synthesis and secretion were stimulated leading to enlarged colloid diameter, thereafter increased follicle sizes [1]. Increased follicle size is an indicator for endemic iodine dependent goitre [4]. Exposure of cells to ionizing radiation can result in genetic mutations, chromosomal aberrations, oncogenic transformations, and cell death. Epidemiological studies proved the primary data on cancer risk in human after exposure to ionizing radiation. After the Chernobyl accident the frequency of thyroid cancer in children from Belarus is increasing by a factor of 20 since 1990. To systematically test the potential influence of external ionizing radiation and a protective role of iodine supplementation we investigated the changes of functional and histological thyroid parameters due to external radiation in rats under iodine deficiency as well as under high iodine diet.

Material and methods

Adult male Sprague-Dawley rats (Han:SPRD, 30 d old) were maintained under pathogen-free conditions in individual cages in a temperature- (24±1°C, 50-70% relative humidity) and light-controlled (Illuminated from 6.00-18.00h) room. Litter mates were separated in 3 groups and maintained in 3 different chambers. They were fed with a standard diet of 7µg Iodine (I^-) /100g BW/d or iodine deficient diet of <420ng I^- /100g BW/d (LID) and standard diet with supplemented iodine (KI - substitution in the drinking water 72 µg I^- /100g BW/d). Destilled water was available ad lib. A single external irradiation of the animals took place at the age of 40 days with a dose of either 1,0 or 4,0 Gy. Weekly blood samples were taken for the measurement of the thyroid hormones and TSH. After 15 weeks the animals were killed and the thyroid glands were removed for histological and morphological studies. Plasma TSH was measured using a TSH radioimmunoassay kit kindly provided by the NIDDK, USA. The lower limit of sensitivity was 360 pg/ml. T_3 and T_4 were measured with commercial kits for use in human serum (EIA, Boehringer Mannheim, Germany).

Results

The TSH levels were constant during the experimental period in the controls. Iodine rich diet significantly stimulated TSH plasma levels twofold ($p<0.01$). The plasma concentrations of T_3 and T_4 were not significantly changed in iodine rich and control groups. In the group with iodine deficiency T_3 clearly decreased about 80% ($p<0.001$) and T_4 about 30% ($p<0.05$). Parallel to the decrease of thyroid hormones TSH levels increased after approx. 10 weeks under iodine deficiency in all animals. Mean T_3 and T_4 plasma levels were not altered, whereas TSH levels were moderately increased by radiation in animals with standard diet (Fig 1). In LID animals external radiation had no additional effect on the secretion of thyroid hormones and TSH. However, iodine supplementation led to an increase of TSH plasma concentration compared to the controls. External radiation caused a decrease of TSH plasma levels (Fig 1).

Fig 1: T_3, T_4 and TSH plasma concentrations (x ± SEM, n=8) 15 weeks after a single dose of external radiation either with 1 Gy (B) or with 4 Gy (C) compared with controls (no radiation, A). Diagonal hatch bar: controls, standard diet (7μg I/100g BW/d); solid bar: low iodine diet (>420 ng I/100g BW/d); crosshatch bar: iodine supplementation (79 μg I/100g BW/d)

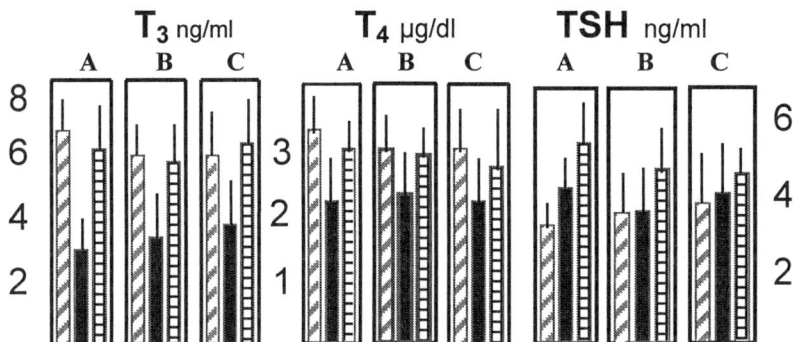

Fig 2: Representative light micrographs of thyroid glands 15 weeks after radiation (x40). Standard: Standard diet; I-: Low iodine diet; I+: Iodine supplementation (see Fig 1). Control: No radiation, 4 Gy: Single external ionizing radiation with 4 Gy.

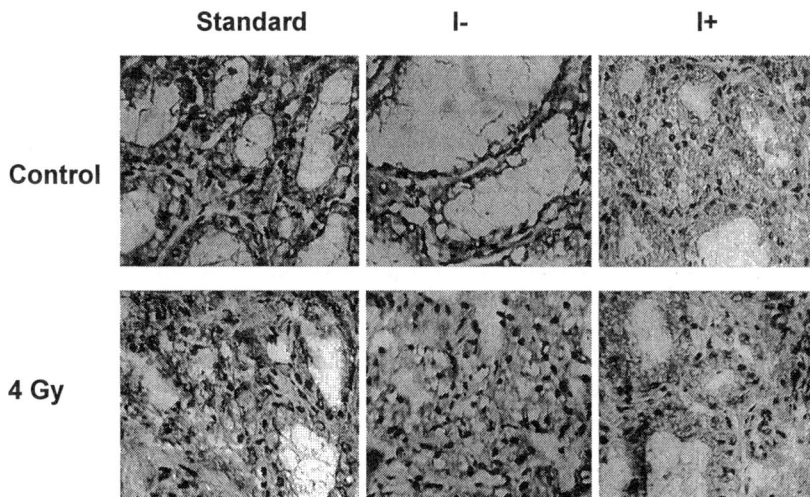

Compared to the controls LID led to a significant decrease of the follicle number (62 vs. 81 follicles/mm²) and a significant increase of colloid diameter (205 vs. 132

μm). Iodine supplementation for 15 weeks induced a marginal increase in the number of follicles (82 vs. 81 follicles/mm^2), and decrease in the colloid diameter from 132 μm to 97 μm (Fig 2). Clear hyperplasia of thyroid follicles and was only detected in the animals under iodine deficiency.

Irradiation with 1 Gy and an additional iodine deficiency did not alter the structure of thyroid cells. However, an external ionizing radiation with 4 Gy and iodine deficiency for 15 weeks clearly induced destroyed follicles of the thyroid (Fig 2), whereas these changes were not detected in the iodine supplemented animals.

Discussion

Iodine deficiency in laboratory animal experiments is accompanied with an increase in plasma TSH levels, which induced an increase in thyroid weight (data not showed). However, increased thyroid weight means not only an increase in cell number (hyperplasia), but may also mean hypertrophy of cell and follicles. This hypertrophy is not related to growth but is consequence of an increase of specific functions of the thyroid, such as increased Tg production[3]. An additional stimulus, such as external ionizing radiation, led to clear histomorphological changes of the thyroid, whereas these changes could not be found in the iodine supplemented animals indicating a protective effect of iodine in this time. The preliminary data provide evidence that the presented animal model is useful to systematically test the effects of external ionizing radiation on thyroid morphology and function.

Acknowledgements
The excellent technical assistance of Mrs. H. Renftel-Heine is gratefully acknowledged. The study was supported in part by Deutsche Krebshilfe.

References
1. Fenzi F, C Ceccarelli, E Macchia, Monzani F, Bartalena L, Giani C, Ceccarelli P, Lippi F, Baschieri L, Pinchera A. Reciprocal changes of serum thyroglobulin and TSH in residents of a moderate endemic goitre area. *Clin Endocrinol 23: 115-122, 1985.*

2. Gutekunst R, Smolarek H, Hasenpusch U, Stubbe P, Friedrich HJ, Wood WG, Scriba PC. Goitre epidemiology: thyroid volume, iodine excretion, thyroglobulin and thyrotropin in Germany and Sweden. *Acta Endocrinol (Copenh.) 112: 494-501, 1986.*

3. Brabant G, Bergmann P, Kirsch CM, Köhrle J, Hesch RD, von zur Mühlen A. Early adaptation of thyrotropin and thyroglobulin secretion to experimentally decreased iodine supply in man. *Metabolism 41: 1093-1096, 1992.*

4. Bray GA. Increased sensitivity of the thyroid in iodine-depleted rats to the goitrogenic effects of thyrotropin. *J Clin Invest 47: 1640-1647, 1968.*

CHARACTERIZATION OF LYMPHOID INFILTRATION IN POST-CHERNOBYL CHILDHOOD THYROID CARCINOMA IN UKRAINE

T. BOGDANOVA, L. ZURNADZHY AND M. TRONKO

Institute of Endocrinology and Metabolism of the Academy of Medical Sciences of Ukraine,
Vyshgorodska Str.,69, Kyiv 254114, Ukraine
E-mail: tb@viaduk.net

G.A. THOMAS AND E.D. WILLIAMS

Thyroid Carcinogenesis Group, Strangeways Research Laboratory,
Wort's Causeway, Cambridge CB1 4RN, UK
E-mail: gerry.thomas@srl.cam.ac.uk

In 127 cases of thyroid tumours in children of Ukraine, frequency, severity and type of lymphoid infiltration (LI) have been studied. LI was classified as tumour (T), peritumour (PT) and background (BG). There were 81 papillary carcinomas (PTC), 6 follicular carcinomas (FC), and 40 follicular adenomas (FA). FA and FC were analysed together as follicular tumours (FT). CD45 showed more LI in PTC than in FT (T - 26% versus 7% ; PT - 84% versus 37%; BG - 47% versus 39%). There was no significant difference in LI in PTC and FT in children from more and less exposed areas. PTC studies with antibodies to B cells (CD79A), T cells (CD4; CD8), macrophages (CD68) and dendritic cells (S100) showed that T cells were more often revealed in T, while B cells were dominant in PT and BG. Macrophages (MF) and dendritic cells (DC) mainly infiltrated T. A positive reaction for CD45, CD68 and S100 was associated with regional metastases in 73%, 88%, 87% of cases, and distant metastases in 17%, 14% and 15% of cases. Thus, LI was more often associated with PTC than with FT. Presence in T MF and DC did not prevent from development of regional or distant metastases.

The relationship between development of thyroid carcinoma, in particular of papillary carcinoma, and lymphoid infiltration was studied in numerous investigations, but for the present this point remains unclear. Lymphoid infiltration in papillary carcinoma is considered as a positive prognostic factor;[1,2] in other works chronic thyroiditis is associated with a high risk of development of papillary carcinoma,[3] with an increase of intraglandular tumour spreading.[4] The capacity of lymphoid cells for producing growth factors which stimulate tumoral growth has been also shown.[5] Moreover, all the above investigations were performed on carcinomas of adult patients, without analysis of a possible previous effect of radiation. Only one work points out that lymphoid infiltration in post-Chernobyl papillary thyroid carcinomas in children of Belarus was revealed 2.3 times more frequently than in carcinomas of children of Italy who have not been exposed to radiation factors.[6]

The aim of this work was to study the frequency, localization, severity and type of lymphoid infiltration in post-Chernobyl thyroid tumours in children of Ukraine. We have studied 127 thyroid tumours which were removed in children aged 9 to 14 years in 1995-1997. 90 tumours were removed in children from most exposed areas of fallout from Chernobyl (Kyiv oblast, including city of Kyiv, Chernihiv, Zhytomir, Cherkasy and Rivne oblasts), and 37 tumours were removed in children from other less exposed regions of Ukraine. 81 tumours were verified as papillary carcinoma, 6 as follicular carcinoma, and 40 as follicular adenoma. Subsequently, because of the uniformity of the changes observed, follicular carcinomas and adenomas were gathered in one group of "follicular tumours". The mean age of children with papillary carcinoma made 12.1 years, and with follicular tumour 12.7; the sex ratio (F:M) was 2.1:1 and 4.1:1, respectively, for PTC and FT.

Lymphoid infiltration was subdivided into tumour (T), peritumour (PT) and background thyroid (BG). Lymphoid infiltration was estimated by immunohisto-chemistry with antibodies to the pan lymphocytic marker CD45 (Table 1).

Table 1. Overall details.

	PTC	FT
No of cases	81	46
Mean age	12.1	12.7
Sex ratio (F:M)	54:27=2.0:1	37:9=4.1:1
Dominant lymph. infiltr. (CD45): Tumour	2 (2.5%)	2 (4.3%)
Peritumour	60 (74.1%)	12 (26.1%)
Background	15 (18.5%)	19 (41.3%)
Nunber with lymphoid infiltration	77 (95.1%)	33 (71.7%)

In papillary carcinoma lymphoid infiltration is observed more often than in follicular tumours. Moreover, lymphoid infiltrates in papillary carcinoma are predominantly peritumour, while in follicular tumours the lymphoid's foci are more often dispersed in extratumoral tissue.

A comparative analysis of frequency and dominant localization of lymphoid infiltration depending on the exposure rate of the area where the child with thyroid tumour was residing, showed no significant differences in the above indices.

The severity of the lymphoid infiltration was determined according the intensity of immunohistochemical reaction with antibodies to CD45 from + to ++++, where + reflects a weak-spread reaction, and ++++ reflects a wide-spread diffuse reaction equivalent to that observed in Hashimoto's thyroiditis. Differences between papillary carcinomas and follicular tumors were observed both after the presence of lymphoid infiltration in tumour, peritumour or background thyroid, whether dominant or not, and after the intensity of reaction to CD45. A comparison between papillary carcinomas and follicular tumours showed that immunopositivity for CD45 (of any degree of intensity) was revealed in tumour in 26% of papillary carcinomas and in 7% of follicular tumours ($p<0.01$); in peritumour in 84% of papillary carcinomas and in 37% of follicular tumours ($p<0.001$), and in background thyroid in 47% of papillary carcinomas and in 39% of follicular tumours ($p>0.05$). A highly intensive reaction (grades +++, ++++) was also observed more often in papillary carcinoma than in cases of follicular tumours. In peritumour such reaction was oberved in 19/81 (23%) of papillary carcinomas and only in 4/46 (8)% of follicular tumours, $p<0.05$, and in background thyroid in 18% of papillary carcinomas and 4% of follicular tumours (Table 2).

Table 2. No of cases with different severity of lymphoid infiltration (CD45): whether dominant or not.

	PTC			FT		
	T	PT	B	T	PT	B
++++	–	3	8	–	–	2
+++	1	16	7	1	3	–
++	5	23	3	2	5	5
+	15	26	20	–	9	11
Number of cases	81	81	81	46	46	46

The dominant peritumour localization of lymphoid infiltration noted in papillary carcinoma does not depend on the child's age, but the frequency of severe diffuse thyroiditis in extrathyroid tumoral tissue (grades +++, ++++) is somewhat higher in children aged 12 to 14 years (19.7%) as compared to younger children aged 9 to 11 years (16.0%, p>0.05).

The type of lymphoid infiltrate, both peritumour and background, is uniform. They often contain germinal centres and are represented by B cells (CD79A), T helper and T suppressor cells (CD4, CD8) with dominant B cells. In contrast to this, in tumour lymphocytes are, as a rule, represented by T cells, namely, CD8 cells.

Macrophages were revealed in 42 of 47 (89%), and dendritic cells in 39 of 47 (83%) of the papillary carcinomas. Practically in all cases, both macrophages and dendritic cells mainly infiltrated the tumour; in peritumour area and background thyroid isolated immunopositive cells were revealed in 28% of cases.

Localization of macrophages or dendritic cells differs depending on the histological structure of the carcinoma. So, macrophages in papillary areas are revealed mainly in interpapillary space and rarely in the papilla stroma. In follicular areas they are dominant inside the follicles, and in solid areas in the stroma surrounding the clusters of tumoral cells. Dendritic cells are mainly localized in solid areas, namely, in the stroma separating the solid foci or in the foci of squamous metaplasia. In papillary areas they are not numerous and concentrated in the papilla stroma.

When dividing the papillary carcinomas into the three main subtypes (classical papillary, solid-follicular and diffuse-sclerosing), most of tumours with positivity for CD45, CD68 and S100 belong to solid-follicular variant of PTC: 55 of 81 (68%) for CD45, 30 of 47 (64%) for CD68, and 27 of 47 (57%) for S100 cells.

Lymphoid infiltration in the papillary carcinomas studied, as well as tumour infiltration by macrophages or dendritic cells did not exclude development of regional and distant metastases. A positive reaction for CD45, CD68 and S100 was associated with the presence of regional metastases in 73%, 88% and 87% of cases, respectively. A positive reaction for CD45, CD68 and S100 and the presence of distant metastases in lungs were associated in 17% for CD45, in 14% for CD68, and in 15% for S100. In all series metastases were dominant in case of solid-follicular variant of papillary carcinoma.

The data obtained diverge with those presented in the work of Fiumara et al.[1] who revealed a negative correlation between development of distant metastases and the presence of lymphoid infiltration or dendritic cells. Probably, one may explain this by the fact that the authors studied carcinomas in adult patients among which, as known, tumours with classical papillary structure were dominant. and not solid-follicular variant, which is the most frequent in our series. It is evident that further studies are necessary in this way.

Thus, these investigations allowed to establish that lymphoid infiltration is more often associated with papillary carcinoma than with follicular tumour, with dominant localization around the tumour, and not diffusely in the background. This points out that diffuse thyroiditis was not the cause of development of papillary carcinomas in children of Ukraine. Also, there were no significant differences in the frequency and localization of lymphoid infiltration depending on more or less exposed to fallout from Chernobyl, and depending on the child's sex and age.

Studies of the type of lymphoid infiltrates showed that among lymphocytes infiltrating the tumour, T lymphocytes (CD8 cells) are revealed more frequently, while in peritumour areas and extratumoral tissue B lymphocytes are dominant. Macrophages and dendritic cells mainly infiltrated the tumour, and, moreover, the positive reaction for CD45, CD68 and S100 was associated with the presence of regional and distant metastases, what does not allow to consider the lymphoid infiltration as a favourable prognostic factor. Furtherly, in order to elucidate the contribution of lymphoid infiltration to the tumoral growth, one plans to study in the cases presented the different growth factors and oncogenes.

References

1. Fiumara A, Belfiore A, Russo G, Salomone E, Santonocito GM, Ippolito O, Vignery R. In situ evidence of neoplastic cell phagocytosis by macrophages in papillary thyroid cancer. *J Clin Endocrinol Metab* 1997; **82:** 1615-1620.
2. Rashima K, Yokoyama S, Noguchi S, Murakami N, Yamashita H, Watanabe S, Uchio S, Toda M, Sasaki A, Daa T. Chronic thyroiditis as a favorable prognostic factor in papillary thyroid carcinoma. Thyroid 1998; **8:** 197-202.
3. Wirtschafter A, Schmidt R, Rosen D, Kundu N, Santoro M, Fusco A, Multhaupt H. Expression of the RET/PTC fusion gene as a marker for papillary carcinoma in Hashimoto's thyroiditis. *Laryngoscope* 1997; **107:** 95-100.
4. Asanuma K, Sugenoya A, Kasura Y, Itoh N, Kobayashi S. The relatioship between multiple intrathyroidal involvement in papillary thyroid carcinoma and chronic non-specific thyroiditis. *Cancer Lett* 1998; **122:** 177-180.
5. Takahashi MN, Thomas GA, Williams ED. Evidence for mutial interdependence of epithelium and stromal lymphoid cells in a subset of papillary carcinomas. *Brit J Cancer* 1995; **72:** 813-817.
6. Pacini F, Vorontsova T, Demidchik E, Molinaro E, Agate L, Romei C, Shavrova E, Cherstvoy E, et al. Post-Chernobyl thyroid carcinoma in Belarus children and adolescents: comparison with naturally occuring thyroid carcinoma in Italy and France. *J Clin Endocrinol Metab* 1997; **82:** 3563-3569.

THE RET GENE IS INVOLVED IN DIFFERENT TUMORAL DISEASES

M. SANTORO, G. SALVATORE, G. CHIAPPETTA, A. FUSCO AND G. VECCHIO

Centro di Endocrinologia ed Oncologia Sperimentale del CNR/Dipartimento di Biologia e Patologia Cellulare e Molecolare, Universita' di Napoli "Federico II", via S. Pansini 5, 80131 .and Istituto Nazionale dei Tumori di Napoli, Fondazione Senatore Pascale, via M. Semmola, Napoli- Italy.

E-mail: vecchio@unina.it.

G.A. THOMAS AND E.D. WILLIAMS

Thyroid Carcinogenesis Group, University of Cambridge, Strangeways Research Laboratory, Cambridge, UK

E-mail: gat1000@cam.ac.uk

The RET gene encodes a tyrosine kinase receptor for neurotrophic molecules. RET is a valuable example of how different mutations of a single gene may cause different diseases. Inactivating mutations of RET are associated with Hirschsprung's disease. On the other side, different point mutations activate RET in familial multiple endocrine neoplasia syndromes. Finally, gene rearrangements activate the oncogenic potential of RET in human thyroid papillary carcinomas; these rearrangements are particularly frequent in Chernobyl-associated thyroid papillary carcinomas. The detailed knowledge of the specific RET mutations provides relevant tools for the clinical management of these human tumor diseases.

1. RET function

RET encodes a tyrosine kinase (TK) receptor for growth factors of the glial cell line derived neurotrophic factor (GDNF) family. GDNF family comprises TGF-β-related molecules, including GDNF and neurturin (NTN), which have trophic influences on a variety of neuronal populations. They mediate their action through multicomponent receptor systems composed by a ligand-binding glycosyl-phosphatidylinositol (GPI)-linked protein (designated GFRα) and the RET kinase. Two GPI-linked proteins have been isolated: GFRα1 and GFRα2. GDNF and NTN activate RET by interacting with either GFRα1 or GFRα2; GDNF is the preferred ligand for GFRα1 while NTN binds preferentially GFRα2.[1-6] Recently, a novel GDNF-related neurotrophic factor, designated persephin (PSP), and a novel GFRα-like receptor, GFRα3, have been isolated, but it is still unclear whether they are able to stimulate RET.[7-8] RET *null* mice show severe defects in the innervation of the hindgut and branching of the ureteric bud.[9] GDNF *null* mice showed a similar phenotype.[10-12] Accordingly, RET mutations have been described in patients affected by Hirschsprung's disease. These mutations cause a "loss-of-function" of RET mediated by different molecular mechanisms.[13-15]

2. RET activation in MEN2 syndromes

Point mutations of RET are responsible for the inheritance of familial medullary thyroid carcinoma (FMTC), multiple endocrine neoplasia type 2A (MEN2A) and type 2B (MEN2B).[13] These diseases are characterized by medullary thyroid carcinomas (MTC), pheochromocytomas, parathyroid adenomas and mucosal neuromas. In most of the cases mutations associated to MEN2A and FMTC cause the substitutions of extracellular cysteines with other residues. These mutations activate RET transforming potential.[16] Indeed, RET-MEN2A products, as a consequence of the loss of a cysteine residue, are constitutively dimerized through disulfide bridges, and, consequently, their transforming and neuronal differentiating potential is constitutively activated. More than 80% of MEN2A cases involve cysteine 634, while in about 50% of FMTC cases, cysteine 618 or 620 are affected.[13] The FMTC mutations have been found to be able to activate RET, but at a lower extent than the MEN2A mutation. This offers a plausible basis of the diversity of the disease phenotype between the two syndromes.[17-18] In contrast, in the great majority of cases, the MEN2B mutation determines the substitution of methionine 918, of the TK domain of RET, with a threonine residue. This mutation activates RET without causing a constitutive dimerization; a change in the substrate specificity seems to be the molecular basis of the RET-MEN2B transforming potential.[16]

3. RET oncogenic activation in human thyroid papillary carcinomas

Specific rearrangements of RET have been found in human thyroid carcinomas of the papillary subtype. These rearrangements lead to the fusion of the RET TK domain to the 5'-terminal regions of heterologous genes, generating chimeric oncogenes designated RET/PTC. RET fusion partners are the H4, RI, RFG(ELE1), and RFG5 genes in the case of RET/PTC1, 2, 3 and 5, respectively.[19-22] In the case of RET/PTC4, the fusion between RFG and RET genes includes also the transmembrane encoding domain of RET.[23] By substituting the RET transcriptional promoter with those of the fusion partners, these rearrangements drive the expression of RET in the thyroid gland; moreover, the fusion partners contain coiled-coil domains which cause a constitutive dimerization and kinase activation of the rearranged RET products. RET/PTC oncogenes are present in about 40% of human papillary carcinomas and are absent in other tumoral subtypes.[24] A dramatic increase in the incidence of papillary carcinomas has been reported in Belarus and Ukraine following the Chernobyl nuclear accident in 1986.[25-26] RET/PTC rearrangements, mainly the RET/PTC3 type, have been reported to occur with a high frequency in these Chernobyl-associated papillary carcinomas.[27-31] It is conceivable that ionizing radiations promote the occurrence of these RET alterations. In the framework of the European Community Project FI4C-CT96-0003, we have examined RET/PTC activation in papillary carcinomas occurred in Ukraine after the Chernobyl accident. The tissue samples were collected by Prof. Cherstvoy (Institute of Pathology of Minsk) and Prof. Tronko (Institute of Endocrinology and Metabolism of Kiev) and analysed by RT-PCR. Through this analysis, we have confirmed that RET/PTC oncogenes are frequently involved in Chernobyl-associated thyroid tumors and that, in particular, the RET/PTC3 isoform is typical of the solid-follicular subtype. Indeed, 17 out of 28 papillary carcinomas examined showed RET rearrangements. Five cases were RET/PTC1- and 12 were RET/PTC3-positive. Eighteen of these tumors were of the solid subtype. Nine of the solid tumors were RET/PTC3-positive, while only one was RET/PTC1-positive.

4. Conclusions

Understanding the specificity of RET mutations associated with the different tumor diseases has a fundamental clinical relevance. Genetic screening for RET mutations is a powerful diagnostic tool for the unambigous diagnosis of MEN2 gene carriers, which allows presymptomatic thyroidectomy at an early stage of the disease process.[32] The identification of RET/PTC rearrangement may be of help in the differential diagnosis of thyroid tumoral diseases, in particular for the differentiation between highly aggressive anaplastic thyroid tumors (which are negative for this rearrangement) and papillary carcinomas. Finally, the identification of RET activation as a rate-limiting step in the development of these human tumoral disease supports the attractive possibility of novel therapeutic strategies which will target RET oncogenic derivatives.

Acknowledgements

This work was supported by the E.C. grant FI4C-CT96-0003.

References

1. Jing S, Wen D, Yu Y, Holst PL, Luo Y, Fang M, Tamir R, Antonio L, Hu Z, Cupples R, Louis JC, Hu S, Altrock BW, Fox GM. GDNF-induced activation of the Ret protein tyrosine kinase is mediated by GDNFR-alpha, a novel receptor for GDNF. *Cell* 1996; **85:** 1113-1124.

2. Treanor JJS, Goodman L, de Sauvage F, Stone DM, Poulsen KT, Beck CD, Gray C, Armanini MP, Pollock RA, Hefti F, Phillips HS, Goddard A, Moore MW, Buj-Bello A, Davies AM, Asai N, Takahashi M, Vandlen R, Henderson CE, Rosenthal A. Characterization of a multicomponent receptor for GDNF. *Nature* 1996; **382:** 80-83.

3. Trupp M, Arenas E, Fainzilber M, Nilsson AS, Sleber BA, Grigoriu M, Kilkenny C, Salazar-Grueso E, Pachnis V, Arumae U, Sariola H, Saarma M, Ibanez CF. Functional receptor for GDNF encoded by the c-Ret proto-oncogene. *Nature* 1996; **381:** 785-789.

4. Durbec P, Marcos-Gutierrez CV, Kilkenny C, Grigoriu M, Wartiowaara K, Suvanto P, Smith D, Ponder B, Costantini F, Saarma M, Sariola H, Pachnis V. GDNF signalling through the Ret receptor tyrosine kinase. *Nature* 1996; **381:** 789-793.

5. Klein RD, Sherman D, Ho WH, Stone D, Bennett GL, Moffat B, Vandlen R, Simmons L, Gu Q, Hongo JA, Devaux B, Poulsen K, Armanini M, Nozaki C, Asai N, Goddard A, Phillips H, Henderson CE, Takahashi M, Rosenthal A. A GPI-linked protein that interacts with Ret to form a candidate neurturin receptor. *Nature* 1997; **387:** 717-721.

6. Buj-Bello A, Adu J, Pinon LG, Horton A, Thompson J, Rosenthal A, Chinchetru M, Buchman VL, Davies AM. Neurturin responsiveness requires a GPI-linked receptor and the Ret receptor tyrosine kinase. *Nature* 1997; **387:** 721-724.

7. Milbrandt J, de Sauvage FJ, Fahrner TJ, Baloh RH, Leitner ML, Tansey MG, Lampe PA, Heuckeroth RO, Kotzbauer PT, Simburger KS, Golden JP, Davies JA, Vejsada R, Kato AC, Hynes M, Sherman D, Nishimura M, Wang LC, Vandlen R, Moffat B, Klein RD, Poulsen K, Gray C, Garces A, Johnson EM Jr. Persephin, a novel neurotrophic factor related to GDNF and neurturin. *Neuron* 1998; **20:** 245-253.

8. Jing S, Yu Y, Fang M, Hu Z, Holst PL, Boone T, Delaney J, Schultz H, Zhou R, Fox GM. GFRalpha-2 and GFRalpha-3 are two new receptors for ligands of the GDNF family. *J Biol Chem* 1997; **272:** 33111-33117.

9. Schuchardt A, D'Agati V, Larsson-Blomberg L, Costantini F, Pachnis V. Defects in the kidney and enteric nervous system of mice lacking the tyrosine kinase receptor Ret. *Nature* 1994; **367**: 380-383.

10. Sanchez M, Silos-Santiago I, Frisen J, He B, Lira SA, Barbacid M. Renal agenesis and the absence of enteric neurons in mice lacking GDNF. *Nature* 1996; **382**: 70-73.

11. Pichel JG, Shen L, Sheng HZ, Granholm AC, Drago J, Grinberg A, Lee EJ, Huang SP, Saarma M, Hoffer BJ, Sariola H, Westphal H. Defects in enteric innervation and kidney development in mice lacking GDNF. *Nature* 1996; **382**: 73-76.

12. Moore MW, Klein RD, Farinas I, Sauer H, Armanini M, Phillips H, Reichardt LF, Ryan AM, Carver-Moore K, Rosenthal A. Renal and neuronal abnormalities in mice lacking GDNF. *Nature* 1996; **382**: 76-79.

13. Pasini B, Ceccherini I, Romeo G. RET mutations in human disease. *Trends Genet* 1996; **12**: 138-144.

14. Pasini B, Borrello MG, Greco A, Bongarzone I, Luo Y, Mondellini P, Alberti L, Miranda C, Arighi E, Bocciardi R, Seri M, Barone V, Radice MT, Romeo G, Pierotti M. Loss of function effect of RET mutations causing Hirschsprung disease. *Nature Genet* 1995; **10**: 35-40.

15. Carlomagno F, De Vita G, Berlingieri MT, de Franciscis V, Melillo RM, Colantuoni V, Kraus MH, Di Fiore PP, Fusco A, Santoro M. Molecular heterogeneity of RET loss of function in Hirschsprung's disease. *EMBO J* 1996; **15**: 2717-2725.

16. Santoro M, Carlomagno F, Romano A, Bottaro DP, Dathan NA, Grieco M, Fusco A, Vecchio G, Matoskova B, Kraus MH, Di Fiore PP. Germ-line mutations of MEN2A and MEN2B activate RET as a dominant transforming gene by different molecular mechanisms. *Science* 1995; **267**: 381-383.

17. Carlomagno F, Salvatore G, Cirafici AM, De Vita G, Melillo RM, de Franciscis V, Billaud M, Fusco A, Santoro M. The different RET-activating capability of mutations of cysteine 620 or cysteine 634 correlates with the multiple endocrine neoplasia type 2 disease phenotype. *Cancer Res* 1997; **57**: 391-395.

18. Chappuis-Flament S, Pasini A, De Vita G, Fusco A, Lyonnet S, Lenoir G, Santoro M, Billaud M. MEN2 mutations affecting specific extracytoplasmic cysteines exert a dual effect on the RET receptor. *Oncogene* 1998, *in press.*

19. Grieco M, Santoro M, Berlingieri MT, Melillo RM, Donghi R, Bongarzone I, Pierotti MA, Della Porta G, Fusco A, Vecchio G. PTC is a novel rearranged

form of the ret proto-oncogene and is frequently detected in vivo in human thyroid papillary carcinomas. *Cell* 1990; **60:** 557-563.

20. Bongarzone I, Monzini N, Borrello MG, Carcano C, Ferraresi G, Arighi E, Mondellini P, Della Porta G, Pierotti MA. Molecular characterization of a thyroid tumor-specific transforming sequence formed by the fusion of ret tyrosine kinase and the regulatory subunit RI alpha of cyclic AMP-dependent protein kinase A. *Mol Cell Biol* 1993; **13:** 358-366.

21. Santoro M, Dathan NA, Berlingieri MT, Bongarzone I, Paulin C, Grieco M, Pierotti MA, Vecchio G, Fusco A. Molecular characterization of RET/PTC3: a novel rearranged version of the RET proto-oncogene in a human thyroid papillary carcinoma. *Oncogene* 1994; **9:** 509-516.

22. Klugbauer S, Demidchik EP, Lengfelder E, Rabes HM. Detection of a novel type of RET rearrangement (PTC5) in thyroid carcinomas after Chernobyl and analysis of the involved RET-fused gene RFG5. *Cancer Res* 1998; **58:** 198-203.

23. Fugazzola L, Pierotti MA, Vigano E, Pacini F, Vorontsova TV, Bongarzone I. Molecular and biochemical analysis of RET/PTC4, a novel oncogenic rearrangement between RET and ELE1 genes, in a post-Chernobyl papillary thyroid cancer. *Oncogene* 1996; **13:** 1093-1097.

24. Tallini G, Santoro M, Helie M, Carlomagno F, Salvatore G, Chiappetta G, Carcangiu ML, Fusco A. RET/PTC oncogene activation defines a subset of papillary thyroid carcinomas lacking evidence of progression to poorly differentiated or undifferentiated tumor phenotypes. *Clin Cancer Res* 1998; **4:** 287-294.

25. Baverstock K, Egloff B, Pinchera A, Ruchti C, Williams D. Thyroid cancer after Chernobyl. *Nature* 1992; **359:** 21-22.

26. Williams D. Epidemiology. Chernobyl, eight years on. *Nature* 1994; 371: 556.

27. Fugazzola L, Pilotti S, Pinchera A, Vorontsova TV, Mondellini P, Bongarzone I, Greco A, Astakhova L, Butti MG, Demidchik EP, Pacini F, Pierotti MA. Oncogenic rearrangements of the RET proto-oncogene in papillary thyroid carcinomas from children exposed to the Chernobyl nuclear accident. *Cancer Res* 1995; **55:** 5617-5620.

28. Klugbauer S, Lengfelder E, Demidchik EP, Rabes HM. High prevalence of RET rearrangement in thyroid tumors of children from Belarus after the Chernobyl reactor accident. *Oncogene* 1995; **11:** 2459-2467.

29. Klugbauer S, Lengfelder E, Demidchik EP, Rabes HM. A new form of RET rearrangement in thyroid carcinomas of children after the Chernobyl reactor accident. *Oncogene* 1996; **13:** 1099-1102.

30. Nikiforov YE, Rowland JM, Bove KE, Monforte-Munoz H, Fagin JA. Distinct pattern of ret oncogene rearrangements in morphological variants of radiation-induced and sporadic thyroid papillary carcinomas in children. *Cancer Res* 1997; **57:** 1690-1694.

31. Klugbauer S, Demidchik EP, Lengfelder E, Rabes HM. Molecular analysis of new subtypes of ELE/RET rearrangements, their reciprocal transcripts and breakpoints in papillary thyroid carcinomas of children after Chernobyl. *Oncogene* 1998; **16:** 671-675.

32. Wells SA Jr, Chi DD, Toshima K, Dehner LP, Coffin CM, Dowton SB, Ivanovich JL, DeBenedetti MK, Dilley WG, Moley JF, Norton JA, Donis-keller H. Predictive DNA testing and prophylactic thyroidectomy in patients at risk for multiple endocrine neoplasia type 2A. *Ann Surg* 1994; **220:** 237-247.

MOLECULAR BASIS OF TUMOUR INITIATION AND PROGRESSION IN THE THYROID FOLLICULAR CELL: IN VITRO MODELS

DAVID WYNFORD-THOMAS

Cancer Research Campaign Laboratories, Department of Pathology, University of Wales College of Medicine, Heath Park, Cardiff CF4 4XN, U.K.

Tel: (44)-1222-742700
Fax: (44)-1222-744276
Email: KingTD@Cardiff.ac.uk

ABSTRACT

Tumours of the thyroid follicular cell are proving to be one of the most informative models for "dissecting" the molecular genetics of multi-stage human tumorigenesis. Early thyroid tumour development is closely correlated with activating mutations of five alternative proto-oncogenes - ras, ret, trk, gsp and the TSH receptor - associated with different tumour phenotypes, providing an excellent example of genotype/phenotype correlation. For two of these genes - ras and ret - there is also direct experimental evidence from gene transfer studies that they are sufficient to initiate tumorigenesis, one of very few situations where such proof of causality has been obtained for a human tumour. Similar data has recently been obtained for the TSH-receptor. Much less is known of the molecular basis of malignant transformation in thyroid, although loss of the tumour suppressor gene p16 [INK4a] appears to be a promising candidate. The rare, further progression to undifferentiated (anaplastic) cancer provides a particularly clear-cut illustration of the role of the tumour suppressor gene p53 in human cancer. Furthermore, in vitro data suggest the intriguing possibility that the anaplastic phenotype results from a combination of p53 mutation together with a spontaneous switch in differentiation programme, i.e. co-operation between a genetic and an epigenetic event. There is now a real hope that the entire sequence of multi-step progression in follicular cell neoplasia will soon be reconstructed in vitro by gene transfer beginning with nomal human thyrocytes.

1. INTRODUCTION

Tumours arising from the thyroid follicular cell represent a particularly attractive model for molecular analysis. Multiple stages can be clearly defined and furthermore readily obtained from surgery, thus allowing the possibility of correlating successive genetic abnormalities with the progression of the tumour phenotype, resembling in this respect the "classic" model of multi-step carcinogenesis - colorectal tumours [18.] Unlike the latter, however, thyroid offers the additional advantage of not only displaying multiple stages but also multiple "routes" of tumour development (Fig. 1), arising from the same cell, the strikingly different clinico-pathological behaviour of papillary versus follicular tumours providing a unique opportunity to correlate genotype with phenotype. Finally, from the experimental standpoint the ability to obtain and culture normal human follicular cells has made it possible to reconstruct the earliest stages of tumour development by in vitro gene transfer, in a way which has not been possible for most other human tumour types.

Figure 1.   Multi-step, multi-route thyroid tumorigenesis

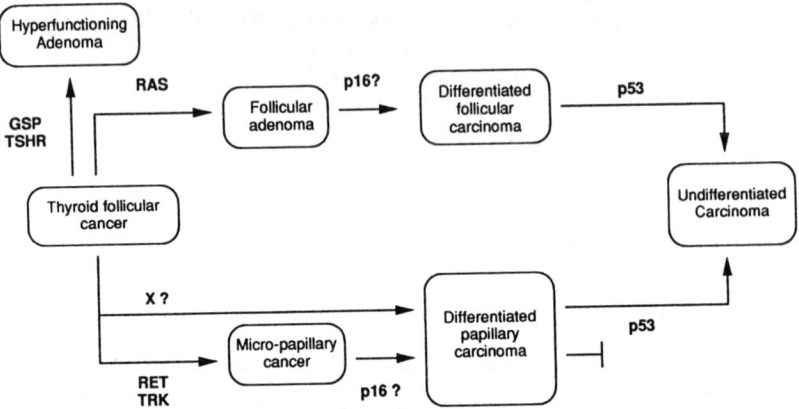

A summary of the main genes known or suspected of playing a role in the development of thyroid tumours, indicating their likely stage of involvement. Others remain to be identified, particularly at the benign/malignant interface. As indicated by the alternative pathways to papillary cancer, recent data[47] also suggest the need to identify new initiating gene(s) in a sub-group of these tumours with greater potential for progression.

2.   TUMOUR INITIATION

Normal adult thyroid follicular cells exhibit a very low rate of proliferation and a correspondingly low death rate [27.] In principle, therefore, a tumour can arise following any somatic mutation which results in a sustained increase in proliferation rate. This could result from activation of stimulatory signal pathways within the cell whose components are coded for by oncogenes, or conversely from loss of inhibitory signals through inactivation of the products of tumour suppressor genes (TSGs) [48,57,63.] Since, however, inactivation of TSGs usually requires both alleles to be affected, whereas activation of oncogenes requires only one "hit", it is not surprising that in practice thyroid tumours appear to arise predominantly through oncogene activation.

In theory, one might expect a wide range of possible oncogenic mutations since there are potentially at least four mitogenic intracellular signalling pathways active in the follicular cell [57], each with multiple components. In practice, however, only a very restricted sub-set of these appears to be capable of generating sustained proliferation.

2.1 Activation of Ras Oncogenes

Although not specific to thyroid, the mitogenic pathway which appears to be most frequently activated in follicular tumours is that which contains the products of the ras oncogene family (H-, K- and N-ras)[6]. These genes code for small G proteins which transduce signals from a wide variety of growth factor receptors, particularly those of the tyrosine kinase superfamily [35]. Although many such receptors operate in normal follicular cells (notably the EGF receptor), it is not yet clear to what extent ras proteins are important as physiological growth signal transducers in these cells (studies on the WRT rat thyrocyte line have suggested that they may form one arm of a bifurcating TSH signal pathway [1]). What is now clear though is the importance of mutated forms of ras for thyroid tumorigenesis.

A series of observational studies of clinical material has established the high incidence of point mutation of all three ras genes in follicular tumours of all stages, from the earliest adenomas available for study[37], through differentiated to anaplastic cancer[28], strongly suggesting an early and essential role in this tumour pathway (Fig. 2). (The situation in papillary cancers is more controversial [44,58]).

Figure 2.   Multi-step tumorigenesis in the thyroid follicular cell

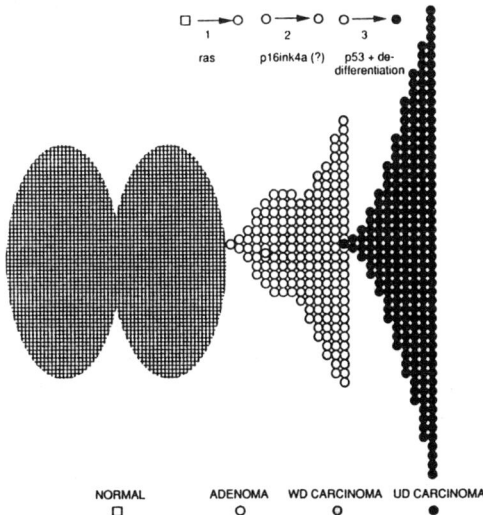

This simplified schematic illustrates our current view of clonal selection in the development of "follicular" (as opposed to "papillary") tumours. Note that although the roles of ras and p53 mutation in steps [1] and [3] respectively are well established, much of the evidence for loss of p16 is still limited to in vitro studies. Note also the suggestion here that the essential genetic event [2] driving the adenoma -> carcinoma transition may need to occur in a very early "window" of tumour development, which may explain the usual absence of obvious co-existing adenoma and carcinoma.
Key: WD = well-differentiated; UD= undifferentiated (anaplastic) carcinoma

Such observational data cannot, however, prove that ras mutation is sufficient by itself to initiate tumour development in the absence of co-operating mutations. In vitro gene transfer experiments [4,29] on the other hand have provided compelling evidence for such a causal role.

Introduction of mutant ras into normal adult follicular cells in monolayer culture results in a dramatic stimulation of proliferation (much greater than any known combination of growth factors) which is sustained for up to 20 - 25 population doublings, and can even give rise in an artificial tissue culture matrix to three-dimensional clones containing structures highly reminiscent of some types of human follicular adenoma[4]. Furthermore, in contrast to data obtained from rodent cell line models[19], expression of mutant ras in these follicular cells does not entail extinction of differentiated functions[29], consistent again with the phenotype of early adenoma. Transgenic data[42] are broadly in agreement.

Clearly then, constitutive activation of ras generates a signal which is not subject to the early desensitisation seen with external growth factor stimulation, either because it turns on a qualitatively different set of pathways, because it is downstream of the point of action of such desensitising controls, or because the magnitude of the signal is simply too high to be downregulated effectively. Candidate downstream effectors for mutant ras in thyroid currently include the raf -> MAP Kinase Kinase -> MAP Kinase pathway[35] and, more indirectly, autocrine stimulation via secretion of IGF-1[10]. It may also increase response to paracrine stimulation (in vivo) through upregulation of expression of the receptor for stromally-derived hepatocyte growth factor (encoded by the met gene)[22].

2.2 Activation of Ret and Trk Oncogenes

An intriguing feature of tumours of the thyroid follicular cell is the existence of two distinct sub-types of differentiated cancer termed, rather confusingly, "papillary" and "follicular", which display widely different clinico-pathological behaviour[52,53]. Amongst other differences, papillary cancers metastasise predominantly via lymphatics both within and outside the gland, in sharp contrast to their follicular counterparts where haematogenous dissemination is the rule.

These phenotypic differences appear to be strikingly associated with a major genotypic difference, namely the occurence in papillary, but not follicular tumours, of an unusual oncogenic abnormality, activation of the ret (or trk) oncogenes[46,47]. These encode growth factor receptors[13,26] which curiously, are normally expressed not on follicular cells but on cells of neuro-ectodermal origin such as the C-cell component of the thyroid[15]. Activation is by gene rearrangement which results in the inappropriate expression of a constitutively activated receptor. Why the follicular cells should be so exquisitely sensitive to this signal is a mystery. A plausible explanation, however, is that it reflects a degree of shared differentiation between follicular and C-cells, which may relate to the long-postulated common embryological origin of a sub-set of these cells[31].

As with ras and follicular tumours, so too with ret and papillary tumours, activation has been found in the earliest lesions available - so-called "occult" or micro-carcinomas[51], hence pointing to an initiating role.

Complementing this observational evidence, we have shown in gene transfer experiments[4] that introduction of an activated ret gene into normal follicular cells results in outgrowth of proliferating colonies of thyrocytes, which interestingly show major phenotypic differences from those induced by ras, consisting of a more migratory pattern of growth and the formation of characteristic papilliform structures. Such data strongly suggests that the "choice" of initiating oncogene (e.g. ret vs ras) determines the resulting tumour phenotype.

2.3 Activating Mutations of the TSH Receptor and GαS

The most predictable (but as it turns out not the most frequent) site of activating mutation is the tissue-specific signal pathway which normally mediates the physiological growth response to thyroid stimulating hormone (TSH).

The TSH receptor appears to be particularly prone to activating point mutations, in at least 20 different amino acids[40]. Predictably, the phenotype usually associated with this molecular abnormality is that of autonomously functioning thyroid adenoma ("hot" nodule)[39] since activation of the receptor will stimulate thyroid function as well as growth. Occasional examples in "cold" lesions (both benign or malignant)[43] are probably explained by the presence of additional abnormalities resulting in loss of differentiation.

An equivalent phenotype may also result from activating mutation of the GαS protein[33,38] which normally transduces the signal from TSH receptor to adenylate cyclase. The range of possible activating mutations in this protein is more restricted (to just 2 amino acids), which may account for the relative rarity of GαS compared to TSHR mutations in thyroid tumours[33,38,44]. Furthermore, in vitro gene transfer experiments[23] show that, unlike the activated TSH receptor[32] activated gsp is unable alone to stimulate sustained proliferation of normal human follicular cells, suggesting that it acts in concert with other genetic abnormalities.

3 TUMOUR PROGRESSION

3.1 Differentiated Cancer

It is now generally accepted that clinically significant cancers do not arise from a single genetic abnormality, but require multiple, successive mutations generating waves of clonal expansion, which eventually result in a clone with sufficient autonomous proliferative capacity to produce an invasive/metastatic lesion (Fig. 2). Epidemiological and pathological observations have long suggested that well-differentiated, minimally-invasive follicular carcinomas represent a genetic progression from follicular adenoma[53], although the absence of adjacent benign and malignant components has made this harder to prove than in the adenoma/carcinoma sequence in colon. One reason for this may be that (as indicated in Fig.2) the progression event in follicular adenoma must occur in an early "window" of its development[61], and that by the time such a lesion has reached clinically-detectable dimensions, its cellular proliferation rate has dropped to such an extent that it is effectively no longer liable to further mutation ie. most adenomas are essentially "burnt out" lesions. Similarly, although there is no definitive proof, it is highly likely that clinically-evident papillary cancers arise by a rare progression event occurring early in the development of what would otherwise remain as a micro-carcinoma.

In the case of follicular tumours the major phenotypic differences between the adenoma and well-differentiated, minimally-invasive carcinoma relates to the ability of the latter to invade blood vessels and surrounding tissue, pointing to an abnormality of the genes regulating invasion eg those coding for metalloproteinases. Although changes in expression have been observed in such genes, however, no primary mutations have as yet been reported. Instead, it would appear that tumour progression is determined rather by genes which control proliferative lifespan ie the number of times a cell can divide before it undergoes spontaneous growth arrest (so-called replicative "senescence"). Both activated ras and ret for example induce only a self-limiting period of proliferation, clones spontaneously ceasing growth after around 25 population doublings (enough to give between 10^7 and 10^8 cells)[4]. This programmed growth arrest can be brought about by a number of intracellular cell-cycle inhibitor pathways, coded for by products of tumour suppressor genes, which appear to represent an important "brake" against tumour expansion.

3.1.1   Loss of the tumour-suppressor gene, p16^{INK4a}

In the thyroid, as in many other cancers, a major player in this growth-limiting control system is the TSG p16^{INK4a} which encodes an inhibitor of a key component of the cell cycle machinery, the cyclin kinases CDK4 and 6[20]. In cell lines derived from both follicular and papillary thyroid cancers a very high frequency of p16 inactivating mutations has been observed, ranging from large-scale deletion of the locus through point mutation to promoter methylation[24,25].

There is increasing evidence that this is not merely a cell culture artefact but that similar lesions occur also in the primary tumours[14]. Analysis of these is complicated by dilution with admixed non-neoplastic DNA which limits the ability to convincingly detect deletions or point mutations. Our laboratory has attempted to circumvent this by analysing the epithelial component of tumours isolated in primary culture and, so far, p16 abnormality has been observed in 30% of a small series of well-differentiated follicular and papillary cancers.

The relevance of such abnormalities is supported by in vitro gene transfer experiments which show that experimental inactivation of the signal pathway normally regulated by p16 (the cyclin D1/CDK4/pRb pathway) e.g. by expression of the human papillomavirus gene HPV E7, can greatly extend the proliferative lifespan of thyroid cells growing under the influence of an activated ret oncogene and furthermore, conveys on them the ability to grow in a three-dimensional culture matrix (Ivan & Wynford-Thomas - unpublished).

3.1.2 Other tumour suppressor genes

The search for other candidate TSG abnormalities in differentiatied thyroid cancer has been rather disappointing. A particularly strong candidate was the APC gene, given its synergistic role with ras in colon cancer[18] and the association of thyroid cancer with inherited APC mutation in Gardner's syndrome[41]. Despite this, however, several groups have failed to observe somatic mutation in sporadic thyroid cancers[8,9,64].

More hopeful has been a recently identified TSG responsible for Cowden disease, another inherited cancer syndrome which features thyroid tumours. This gene, PTEN (or MMAC1)[30], located on chromosome 10q23 encodes a dual-specificity phosphatase[36] which may be involved in turning off mitogenic kinase signalling cascades. Loss of heterozygosity (LOH) at the PTEN locus was recently demonstrated in a significant proportion of follicular adenomas with, interestingly, the highest frequency in atypical adenomas[34]. Surprisingly, however, given the occurrence of thyroid carcinomas in Cowden disease, no LOH was detectable in the 10 follicular carcinomas analysed, suggesting that it is not responsible for tumour progression[34]. Clearly, further work will be needed to clarify the role of this gene.

3.1.3 Telomerase

It is now becoming clear that a major biological clock responsible for turning off cell proliferation after a pre-determined number of cell divisions is based on the progressive shortening of the specialised ends of chromosomes - telomeres - which occurs with every successive round of chromosome replication[56]. To overcome this mortality barrier, most cancer cells activate an enzyme, telomerase, which prevents telomere erosion by synthesising more telomeric sequences. Indeed, the expression of telomerase is such a characteristic feature that it has been suggested as a diagnostic maker of malignancy.

Several groups, including our own, have analysed telomerase status in thyroid but unfortunately the results are as yet incomplete and contradictory[21,50]. It is clear that telomerase is expressed in probably the majority of papillary, and at least some, follicular cancers but there is dispute over the all-important question of whether it is expressed in benign adenomas, and no data yet on papillary micro-carcinomas.

3.2 Undifferentiated Cancer

While the evidence for direct progression from adenoma to carcinoma and from micro-papillary to clinical papillary cancer remains circumstantial, there is less dispute over the origin of undifferentiated (anaplastic) cancer from a pre-existing differentiated component (which may be either follicular or papillary)[7]. Molecular genetic analysis has also revealed a very clear cut association between this progression event and the occurrence of mutation in the p53 tumour suppressor gene[11,12,16]. p53 mutation is of course the commonest genetic abnormality in human cancers overall and the specific association with undifferentiated as opposed to differentiated thyroid cancer illustrates very well the role of this genetic abnormality in progression of cancer rather than in malignant transformation per se.

Why p53 mutation is required for this step is still not clear but again most probably relates to the role of p53 in the limitation of proliferative lifespan[59,62]. The situation is more complex than with p16, however, since we have shown that by itself experimental abrogation of p53 function in thyroid cells - whether normal or derived from differentiated cancers - has little or no phenotypic effect[54] and (in contrast to some other published experimental models[2,17]) does not directly cause loss of differentiation[55].

Work from our laboratory suggests that the conversion to anaplastic cancer requires not only p53 muation but also a spontaneous switch in differentiation programme from an epithelial to a pseudo-mesenchymal phenotype[5]. Since both of these events have to occur independently in the same cell this readily accounts for the (fortunate) rarity of progression to anaplastic cancer.

4   UNRESOLVED QUESTIONS

The simplest scenario based on the above data is that thyroid tumours are initiated by activation of a dominant oncogene, eg ras or ret, the nature of which determines the subsequent "route" of tumour development.   Further progression is then dependent on the sequential loss of tumour suppressor genes allowing escape from successive senescence barriers.

There are, however, several unresolved problems which complicate this scheme. For example, it now appears that the frequency of ret mutation is much lower in undifferentiated cancers than would be expected given the proportion which arise from papillary precursors[47]. This suggests that papillary cancers initiated by ret may lack the potential for progression and leaves open the nature of the initiating oncogenic event for those papillary cancers from which undifferentiated tumours can arise.

A more subtle problem concerns the role of p53. Recent data strongly suggests that it acts as a downstream effector of telomere erosion in mediating cell senescence[60]. If, as now seems likely, most well-differentiated cancers have already activated telomerase, with as a result stable telomeres, it is difficult to understand why their subsequent growth should ever activate a p53 dependent growth arrest mechanism. Perhaps, again, undifferentiated cancers will be found to arise from a restricted sub-set of differentiated precursors, in this case characterised by absence of telomerase.

References

1. Al-alawi N, Rose DW, Buckmaster C, Ahn N, Rapp U, Meinkoth J. and Feramisco JR. Thyrotropin-induced mitogenesis is ras dependent but appears to bypass the Raf-dependent cytoplasmic kinase cascade. Mol Cell Biol. 1995;15 (3): 1162-1168.

2. Battista S, Martelli ML, Fedele M, et al. A mutated p53 gene alters thyroid cell differentiation. Oncogene 1995; 11:2029-2037.

3. Bond J, Dawson T, Lemoine N, Wynford-Thomas D. Effect of serum growth factors and phorbol ester on growth and survival of human thyroid epithelial cells expressing mutant ras. Mol Carcinogen 1992; 129-135.

4. Bond JA, Wyllie FS, Rowson J, Radulescu A, Wynford-Thomas D. In vitro reconstruction of tumour initiation in a human epithelium. Oncogene 1994; 9: 281-290.

5. Bond JA. Ness GO, Rowson J, Ivan M, White D, Wynford-Thomas D. Spontaneous de-differentiation correlates with extended lifespan in transformed thyroid epithelial cells: An epigenetic mechanism of tumour progression? Int J Cancer 1996; 67: 563-572.

6. Bos JL. Ras oncogenes in human cancer: a review. Cancer Res 1989; 49: 4682-4689.

7. Carcangiu ML, Steeper T, Zampi G and Rosai J. Anaplastic thyroid carcinoma. Am. J . Clin Path 1985; 83: 135-158.

8. Colletta G, Sciacchitano S, Palmirotta R, et al. Analysis of adenomatous polyposis coli gene in thyroid tumours. Br J Cancer 1994; 70: 1085-1088.

9. Curtis L, Wyllie AH, Shaw JJ, et al. Evidence against involvement of APC mutation in papillary thyroid carcinoma. Eur J Cancer 1994; 30A: 984-987.

10. Dawson TP, Radulescu A, Wynford-Thomas D. Expression of mutant p21ras induces insulin-like growth factor 1 secretion in thyroid epithelial cells. Cancer Res 1995;55: 915-920.

11. Dobashi Y, Sugimura H, Sakamoto A, et al. Stepwise participation of p53 gene mutation during de-differentiation of human thyroid carcinomas. Diag Mol Path 1994; 3: 9-14.

12. Donghi R, Longoni A, Pilotti S, Michieli P, Della Porta G and Pierotti MA. Gene p53 mutations are restricted to poorly differentiated and undifferentiated carcinomas of the thyroid gland. J Clin Invest 1993; 91: 1753-1760.

13. Durbec P, Marcos-Gutierrez CV, Kilkenny C, et al. GDNF signalling through the Ret receptor tyrosine kinase. Nature 1996; 381: 789-793.

14. Elisei R, Shiohara M, Koeffler HP, Fagin JA. Inactivating mutations of p15INK4b and p16INK4a are common in human thyroid carcinoma cell lines, but rare in primary thyroid tumours. J Endocrinol Invest 1996; 19 (S6) p.70.

15. Fabien N, Paulin C, Santoro M, Berger N, Grieco M, Dubois PM and Fusco A. The RET proto-oncogene is expressed in normal human parafollicular thyroid cells. Int J Oncology 1994; 623-626.

16. Fagin JA, Matsuo K, Karmakar A, Lin Chen D, Tang S-H and Koeffler HP. High prevalence of mutations of the p53 gene in poorly differentiated human thyroid carcinomas. J Clin Invest 1993; 91: 179-184.

17. Fagin JA, Tang S-H, Zeki K, Di Lauro R, Fusco A and Gonsky R. Re-expression of thyroid peroxidase in a derivative of an un-differentiated thyroid carcinoma cell line by introduction of wild-type p53. Cancer Res 1996; 56: 765-771.

18. Fearon ER. Molecular Genetics of Colorectal Cancer. *Ann. New York Acad Sci.* 1995; 768: 101-110.

19. Fusco A, Berlingieri MT, Difiore PP, Portella G, Grieco M, Vecchio G. One- and two-step transformations of rat thyroid epithelial cells by retroviral oncogenes. Mol Cell Biol 1987;7:3365-3370.

20. Hall M and Peters G. Genetic alterations of cyclins, cyclin-dependent kinases, and Cdk inhibitors in human cancer. Adv in Cancer Res 1996; 68: 67-108.

21. Haugen BR, Nawaz S, Markham N et al. Telomerase activity in benign and malignant thyroid tumours. Thyroid 1997; 7:337-342.

22. Ivan M, Bond JA, Prat M, Comoglio PM and Wynford-Thomas D. Activated ras and ret oncogenes induce over-expression of c-met (hepatocyte growth factor receptor) in human thyroid epithelial cells. Oncogene 1997, 14: 2417-2423.

23. Ivan M, Ludgate M, Gire V, et al. An amphotropic retroviral vector expressing a mutant gsp oncogene: Effects on human thyroid cells in vitro. J Clin Endocrinol & Metab 1997; 82: 2702-2709.

24. Ivan M, Wynford-Thomas D and Jones CJ. Abnormalities of the p16INK4a gene in thyroid cancer cell lines. Euro J Cancer 1996; 32A: 2369-2370.

25. Jones CJ, Shaw JJ, Wyllie FS, Gaillard N, Schlumberger M, Wynford-Thomas D. High frequency deletion of the tumour suppressor gene p16INK4a (MTS1) in human thyroid cancer cell lines. Mol Cell Endocrinol 1996; 116: 115-119.

26. Kaplan DR, Hempstead BL, Martin-Zanca D, Chao MV, Parada LF. The trk proto-oncogene product: A signal transducing receptor for nerve growth factor. Science 1991; 252: 554-558.

27. Leblond CP. Classification of cell populations on the basis of their proliferative behaviour. Nat Cancer Inst Monograph 1964; 14: 119-150.

236

28. Lemoine NR, Mayall ES, Wyllie FS, Williams ED, Goyns M, Stringer B, Wynford-Thomas D. High frequency of ras oncogene activation in all stages of human thyroid tumorigenesis. Oncogene 1989;4: 159-164.

29. Lemoine NR, Staddon S, Bond J, Wyllie FS, Shaw JJ, Wynford-Thomas D. Partial transformation of human thyroid epithelial cells by mutant Ha-ras oncogene. Oncogene 1990; 5: 1833-1837.

30. Liaw D, Marsh DJ, Li J et al. Germline mutations of the PTEN gene in Cowden disease, an inherited breast and thyroid cancer syndrome. Nature Genetics 1997; 16: 64-67.

31. Ljungberg O. Histogenesis of thyroid carcinoma. Med. Hypotheses; 1984; 14: 253-257.

32. Ludgate M, Gire V, Crisp M, Ajjan R, Weetman A, Ivan, M & Wynford-Thomas D. Contrasting effects of activating mutations of GαS and the thyrotropin receptor on proliferation and differentiation of thyroid follicular cells. Submitted.

33. Lyons J, Landis CA, Harsh G, et al. Two G protein oncogenes in human endocrine tumours. Science 1990; 249:655-659.

34. Marsh DJ, Zheng Z, Zedenius J et al. Differential loss of heterozygosity in the region of the Cowden locus within 10q22-23 in follicular thyroid adenomas and carcinomas. Cancer Res, 1996; 57:500-503.

35. Marshall CJ. Ras effectors. Curr Op Cell Biol 1996; 8:197-204.

36. Myers MP, Stolarov JP, Eng C et al. P-TEN, the tumour suppressor from human chromosome 10q23, is a dual-specificity phosphatase. Proc Natl Acad Sci, USA 1997; 94: 9052-9057.

37. Namba H, Rubin SA, Fagin JA. Point mutations of ras oncogenes are an early event in thyroid tumorigenesis. Mol Endocrinol 1990; 4: 1474-1479.

38. O'Sullivan C, Barton CM, Staddon SL, Brown CL, Lemoine NR. Activating point mutations of the gsp oncogene in human thyroid adenomas. Mol Carcinogen 1991; 4: 345-349.

39. Parma J, Duprez L, Van Sande J, et al. Somatic mutations in the thyrotropin receptor gene cause hyperfunctioning thyroid adenomas. Nature 1993; 365: 649-651.

40. Paschke R and Ludgate M. The molecular biology of the TSH receptor in thyroid diseases. N Eng J Med 1997; 337: 1675-1681.

41. Plail R, Bussey H, Glazer G, Thompson J. Adenomatous polyposis: an association with carcinoma of the thyroid. Br J Surg 1987; 74: 377-380.

42. Rochefort P, Caillou B, Michiels F-M, Ledent C, Talbot M, Schlumberger M, Lavelle F, Monier R AND Feunteun J. Thyroid pathologies in transgenic mice

expressing a human activated Ras gene driven by a thyroglobulin promoter. Oncogene 1996;12: 111-118.

43. Russo D, Aturi F, Schlumberger M, et al. Activating mutations of the TSH receptor in differentiated thyroid carcinomas. Oncogene 1995; 11: 1907-1911.

44. Said S, Schlumberger M, Suarez H. Oncogenes and anti-oncogenes in human epithelial thyroid tumours. J Endocrinol Invest 1994; 17: 371-379.

45. Santoro M, Carlomagno F, Hay ID, et al. Ret oncogene activation in human thyroid neoplasms is restricted to the papillary cancer sub-type. J Clin Invest 1992; 89: 1517-1522.

46. Santoro M, Sabino N, Ishizaka Y et coll. Involvement of RET oncogene in human tumours: specificity of RET activation to thyroid tumours. Br.J Cancer 1993; 68: 460-464.

47. Santoro M, Tallini G, Carlomagno F et al. Activation of the ret proto-oncogene in human thyroid tumours. J Endocrinol Invest 1996; 19 (S6): p4.

48. Sherr CJ and Roberts JM. Inhibitors of mammalian G1 cyclin-dependent kinases. Genes & Dev. 1995; 9: 1149-1163.

49. Suarez HG, Du Villard JA, Severino M et al. Presence of mutations of all three ras genes in human thyroid tumours. Oncogene 1990; 5: 565-570.

50. Umbricht CB, Saji M, Westra WH et al. Telomerase activity: A marker to distinguish follicular thyroid adenoma. Cancer Research 1997; 57: 2144-2147.

51. Viglietto G, Chiappetta G, Martinez-Tello FJ, et al. RET/PTC oncogene activation is an early event in thyroid carcinogenesis. Oncogene 1995; 11: 1207-1210.

52. WHO Histological Typing of Thyroid Tumours. Chr. Hedinger, Williams ED AND Sobin LH (ed.) 2nd ed. 1988: Berlin, Springer-Verlag.

53. Williams DW, Williams ED. The pathology of follicular thyroid epithelial tumours. In: Wynford-Thomas D, Williams ED, (ed.). Thyroid Tumours: Molecular Basis of Pathogenesis. Edinburgh, Churchill Livingstone, 1989: pp 57-65.

54. Wyllie F, Haughton M, Blaydes J, Schlumberger M, Wynford-Thomas D. Evasion of p53-mediated growth control occurs by three alternative mechanism in transformed thyroid epithelial cells. Oncogene 1995; 10: 49-59.

55. Wyllie FS, Haughton MF, Rowson JM & Wynford-Thomas D. Human thyroid cancer cells as a source of iso-genetic, iso-phenotypic cell lines with or without functional p53. Submitted Br J Cancer.

56. Wynford-Thomas D AND Kipling D. Telomeres, Cancer and the knock-out mouse. Nature 1997; 389: 551-552.

57. Wynford-Thomas D. Molecular genetics of thyroid cancer. Trends in Endocrinol and Metabol 1993;4:224-232.

58. Wynford-Thomas D. Molecular genetics of thyroid cancer. Curr. Op. Endocrinol & Diab. 1995; 2: 429-436.

59. Wynford-Thomas D. p53: guardian of cellular senescence. J Path 1996; 180:118-121.

60. Wynford-Thomas D. Proliferative lifespan checkpoints: Cell-type specificity and influence on tumour biology. Eur. J Cancer 1997; 33: 716-726.

61. Wynford-Thomas D. Thyroid Cancer. *In:* N Lemoine, J Neoptolemos & T Cooke (ed). Cancer: A molecular Approach. Oxford, Blackwell Scientific Publications, 1994: pp 192-222.

62. Wynford-Thomas D. Mutation de la p53 dans les cancers humains: existent-elle pour faire sauter l'obstacle de la senescence cellulaire? Medecine/Sciences 1994; 10: 912-913.

63. Wynford-Thomas D. Origine et progression des tumeurs épithéliales: vers les mécanismes cellulaires et moléculaires. Médecine/Sciences 1993; 9: 66-75

64. Zeki K, Spabalg D, Sharifi N, Gonsky R, Fagin J. Mutations of the adenomatous polyposis coli gene in sporadic thyroid neoplasms. J Clin Endocrinol Metab 1994; 79: 1317-1321.

TRANSGENIC MODELS OF THYROID TUMORIGENESIS: RELATION TO CHERNOBYL CANCERS

COPPÉE, F., LEDENT, C., CLEMENT, S., DESSARS, B., GOFFART, J.C., PARMA, J., PARMENTIER, M., SCHURMANS, S. AND DUMONT, J.E.

Institute of Interdisciplinary Research, (IRIBHN) University of Brussels, School of Medicine, Campus Erasme, B - 1070 Brussels, Belgium.

Studies in vitro have allowed some extent clarification of the signal transduction cascades which lead to mitogenesis of thyroid cells: carried out on primary cultures they only allow us to follow cells during a few cell cycles. Cell lines allow more prolonged studies but they are only distantly related to their in vivo counterparts. Genetic studies on human thyroid cancers have demonstrated the involvement of some oncogenes. However by the time they can be studied tumors are already far in their evolution. To bridge the gap between in vitro work and human tumors, transgenic models allow the study of the consequences, over an animal life time, of a single well defined oncogenic event. The existing thyroid models are
- constitutive activation of the TSH cAMP cascade (adenosine A2 receptor, mutated TSHR, Gs α, or cholera toxin)
- constitutive activation of both the cAMP and the PIP2 phospholipase C cascade (mutated α1 β adrenergic receptor)
- constitutive activation of a growth factor cascade (mutated RET, viral RAS)
- inactivation of p53 tumor suppressor (E6 from HPV16)
- inactivation of Rb tumor suppressor (E7 from HPV16)
- combinations of the above (E7-A$_2$R, E6-E7, SV40LT)

The relation of these models to human thyroid tumors and in particular to irradiation induced thyroid cancers is discussed.

1 INTRODUCTION

The use of animal experimental models for the development of diagnostic and therapeutic tools applicable to human patients is of obvious importance. On the fundamental point of view transgenic and knockout models allow to study under in vivo conditions and over a long timespan the precise role of genes and proteins which are considered as important on the basis of in vitro work on cell lines or primary cultures lasting a few weeks at the most. On the other hand, in vivo models involve complex systems and interorgan relations which may make it very difficult to interpret results. General expression or suppression of an active gene in many cell types further complicates the problem. Inserting or « knocking out » an active gene in one cell type of course reduces this complexity.

In the case of the thyroid, the isolation and characterization of the thyroglobulin promoter first gave us the means to selectively target expression of an exogenous gene to the thyrocyte (Christophe et al., 1989). By using this promoter upstream of a reporter gene, chloramphenicol acetyltransferase, to generate transgenic mice, C. Ledent showed that indeed this promoter is organ specific (Ledent et al, 1990). Interestingly this promoter which confers cyclic AMP responsiveness to thyroglobulin gene expression also confers TSH and cyclic AMP responsiveness to the transgene. This promoter has then been used by several laboratories to generate transgenic mice expressing various putative protooncogenes, oncogenes, or even herpes virus thymidine kinase in thyrocytes (Tallini et al, 1997). They will be called Tg-X mice (Tg for the promoter, X for the gene downstream). In this short review we shall describe the models of thyroid tumorigenesis and their relation to the thyroid tumours (Suarez, 1998) especially those encountered in patients irradiated after the Chernobyl accident.

2 CONTROL OF THYROID CELL PROLIFERATION

In vitro work on thyroid cells in primary cultures or thyroid cell lines has allowed delineation of major pathways involved in the control of thyroid cell proliferation and differentiation. On the basis of this work it was possible to predict the phenotypes of mice in which these pathways are altered by selective gene or protein activation or expression.

As in other cell types, the thyrocytes can be induced to proliferate in response to various growth factors : epidermal growth factor (EGF), hepatic growth factor (HGF), fibroblast growth factor (FGF), insulin like growth factor (IGF1), etc.. The panel of growth factors active in a given model depends on the species, and the model (eg the cell line) and even on the history of the cell line. For example FRTL5 cells replicated many times (« old ») respond to EGF while the original FRTL5 cells (« young ») did not (Golstein unpublished).

Classical growth factors act by stimulating their protein tyrosine kinase receptors and their downstream cascades involving phosphorylations of proteins on tyrosines, resulting in the activation of protooncogene ras, of PI_3 kinase, etc... In dog and human thyroid cells some of these growth factors (EGF, HGF) induce proliferation and a loss of expression of specific differentiation genes (thyroglobulin, thyroperoxidase, sodium iodide symporter, TTF1, etc). Others such as insulin or IGF1, do not induce mitogenesis but are necessary for the mitogenic effect of other factors ; they increase to some extent the expression of some differentiation genes (Dumont et al. 1992). Phorbol esters, which are long acting analogs of diacylglycerol, activate protein kinase C and through a protein serine phosphorylation cascade induce proliferation and loss of differentation expression in these cells. TSH, through the cyclic AMP cascade enhances both proliferation and differentiation in the same cells at the same time (V. Pohl et al. 1990, Dumont et al. 1992, Uyttersprot et al. 1997). All the mitogenic pathways finally converge on the phosphorylation and inactivation of the antioncogenic proteins of the Rb family (Rb, p107, p130) (Coulonval et al 1997). If these data can be extrapolated to

241

long term in vivo situations it is easy to predict the in vivo consequences of overactivation or repression of a gene or protein of these cascades (table 1).

1   TABLE 1

2   PREDICTED CONSEQUENCES OF MUTATION OF THYROID SIGNAL TRANSDUCTION GENES AND PROTEINS

Consequences of mutation on			Example: effect On cascade		
FUNCTION	DIFFERENTIATION	PROLIFERATION	BIOCHEMISTRY	CELL population	LESION PHENOTYPE
↗	++	↗	↗cA cascade	↗	HYPERFUNCTIONING ADENOMA AUTONOMY
↗	++	-	↗cA cascade and lack of IGF or loss of proliferation potential	-	0
↘	↘↘	↗	↗GF cascade	↗	COLD ADENOMA CARCINOMA
↘	-	↘	↘cA cascade	↘	DISAPPEARANCE OF MUTATED CELL
-	-	↘	↘GF cascade	↘	DISAPPEARANCE OF MUTATED CELL

3   THYROID TRANSGENIC MODELS (TABLE 2)

3.1. Tg-TSHR*

The TSH receptor is the first intermediate in the TSH cAMP cascade. Mutations confering constitutive activation to this receptor have been shown to be responsible for 80% of human thyroid autonomous adenomas and congenital hyperthyroidism (neomutation or hereditary). Expression of constitutively activated TSHR* in the thyroid has already been obtained in several labs. Preliminary communications suggest a mild or no phenotype (small growth, mild hyperthyroidism) (Di Lauro, personal communication).

Table 2 – Thyrocyte transgenic and knockout models
Overexpression and/or activation of genes of SD proteins (dominant)

Constructs	Biochemical effects	Phenotype
Tg-TSHR*	$\vee$ cAMP	?
Tg-Gsα*	$\vee$ cAMP	autonomous thyroid adenomas
Tg-cholera toxin	$\vee$ cAMP	autonomous thyroid
Tg-Adenosine A2	$\vee$ cAMP	autonomous toxic goitrous thyroid adenomas
Tg-α$_1$BAR*	$\vee$ cAMP, PLC, Ca^{++}, DAG	autonomous thyroid
Tg-IGF-1	Y kinases	?
Tg-IGF-1R	Y kinases	?
Tg-RET* Tg-PTC1	Y kinases	hypothyroidism multiple papillary carcinoma
Tg-HaRas*	$\vee$ Ras MAPK cascade	some adenomas ($\vee$ with goitrogens)
Tg-HPV16 E6	p53 sequestrations	little change
Tg-HPV16 E7	Rb sequestration	simple goiter
Tg-HPV16 E7+A$_2$R	$\vee$ cAMP $\neg$ Rb	Follicular carcinoma ?
Tg-SV40LT	p53 and Rb sequestration	anaplastic carcinoma

3.2. Tg-A$_2$R

The adenosine A$_2$ receptor is positively coupled to adenylate cyclase As it desensitizes poorly and as most cells release adenosine as a by product of their metabolism, this receptor behaves, in systems in which there is no potent deactivating mechanism, as a constitutive stimulant of adenylate cyclase and the cyclic AMP cascade. As could be predicted from the biochemistry, Tg A$_2$R mice develop a homogeneous goiter with a great enhancement of the cell proliferation rate and hyperthyroidism. In fact they behave as autonomous adenomas involving the whole gland. In time nodules develop and in old animals some become invasive. These mice represent good models of autonomous adenomas and congenital hyperthyroidism, in which the cAMP cascade is activated by mutations of the TSH receptor, or Gsα, and even of Graves disease in which the cAMP cascade is stimulated by thyroid stimulating immunoglobulins which activate the TSH receptor (Ledent et al. 1992).

3.3. Tg-Gsα*

Gsα is the GTP binding protein activating adenylate cyclase. Point mutations conferring constitutive activity have been described. When expressed in mice thyroids such mutated Gsα exhibited a rather mild phenotype (Tg-Gsα*): thyroid hyperplasia with papillary foci but no gross enlargement; adenomas appear after 8 months; T4 and T3 levels were slightly elevated. Serum hormone levels were markedly elevated in mice with adenomas (Michiels et al 1994, Feunteun et al 1997).

3.4. Tg-CholTox

Cholera toxin specifically activates Gsα the G protein controlling adenylate cyclase. Tg-Chol Tox mice develop a mild phenotype of thyroid hyperplasia and hyperthyroidism. Although papillary infoldings in follicles were observed no adenoma developed even under methimazole treatment (Zeiger et al 1997). Tg-Gsα* and Tg-Chol Tox also represent models of autonomous adenomas and congenital hyperthyroidism with a mild phenotype.

3.5. Tg-α₁ B AR*

The α_1 B hamster adrenergic receptor is normally coupled to the phospholipase C cascade. Its mutated form (Arg 288 Lys, Lys 230 His, Ala 293 Leu) is a constitutive activator of both the phospholipase C and the cAMP cascade.

The Tg α_1 B AR* transgenics are characterized by goiter and hyperthyroidism as the TgA2R mice. However the phenotype varies quantitatively from one line to another in relation with the level of expression. Cell proliferation , as well as iodide uptake are enhanced. The follicles become pseudostratified with numerous papillary infoldings. A major characteristic is the appearance of many necrotic cells and debris. With age, nodules appear which progressively invade the capsula and generate metastases. Both of these latter characteristics are attributed to the stimulation of the phospholipase C cascade which, in the thyroid, activates H_2O_2 generation leading to cell degeneracy, mutations and the transformation of thyroid cells. Indeed the PIP2 cascade has not been shown to be mitogenic in thyroid but rather activates the H2O2 generating system, thus also oxygen radicals formation and iodide oxidation. Thus, in this case, the combination of the activation of two non oncogenic cascades leads to oncogenesis (Ledent et al 1997).

3.6. Tg-E7

The HPV16-E7 gene codes for a protein which sequesters the cell cycle regulatory proteins of the Rb family (Rb, p107, p130). It may interfere with other proteins. Rb inhibits the entry of the cells in DNA synthesis and has a differentiating effect. Tg-E7 mice develop a euthyroid goiter with intense thyrocyte proliferation. Although the thyroid function is normal on the whole, the efficiency of the thyroid to synthesize and secrete thyroid hormones, as expressed by the ratio of the each variable to the weight of tissue, and therefore to the cell mass, is decreased. However iodide uptake or relative TSHR, TPO or Tg expressions are not decreased. This suggests only a partial degree of dedifferentiation of the cell. After 4 months, foci of proliferating thyrocytes appear which presumably are at the origin of later appearing nodules, leading to capsular invasion and in rare cases differentiated lung metastases (Ledent et al 1995). These mice might therefore be models of euthyroid sporadic goiter.

3.7. Tg-Ki Ras* Tg-HaRas*

Ki and Ha Ras activate the Ras cascades. Mutated and activated Ki Ras expressed downstream a thyroglobulin promoter induces only mild abnormalities and some adenomas. Treatment with goitrigens of these animals induces adenomas in most of them and even follicular carcinomas in some (Santelli et al 1993).
Expression of activated Ha Ras gave more severe phenotypes, with tumors resembling human papillary carcinomas. However these tumours did not metastasize (Rochefort et al 1996).

3.8. Tg-PTC1 = Tg - Ret*

Ret is a tyrosine kinase receptor for GDNF normally not expressed in thyrocytes. In a fraction of human thyroid papillary cancers, due to a series of chromosome rearrangements, truncated. Ret is expressed as a chimeric protein with, as N terminal, a fragment of a protein normally expressed in the thyroid. The chimeric coding sequence is under the control of the promoter of this gene and thus expressed in the thyrocyte. Tg-PTC1 transgenic mice develop hypothyroidism and multiple Ret expressing typical papillary carcinomas (Jhiang et al 1996, Sagartz et al 1997).

3.9. Tg SV40LT

The SV40 large T antigen, besides other effects, binds and sequestrates two major antioncogenes : p53 and Rb. It therefore acts on the last steps of the mitogenic cascade. Tg SV40LT mice models exhibit an early hyperplasia and goiter, and hypothyroidism. The animals die rapidly from hypothyroidism and tracheal compression. Hyperplasia with loss of follicular structure is homogenous but becomes heterogenous, with numerous nodules, in older animals. Some criteria of differentiation (such as the pertechnetate uptake/weight of tissues) are still satisfied but iodide oxidation and thus thyroid hormone synthesis as well as thyroid hormone secretion are severely reduced. This tumour resembles human thyroid anaplastic carcinomas (Ledent et al 1991).

3.10. Tg-A2R* - E7

TgA2R-E7 models expressing both A2R on E7.in their thyroid develop early a phenotype which combines the consequences of each oncogene : they develop a huge goiter with intense cell proliferation and severe hyperthyroidism. However they also develop nodules, hypervascularity and rapidly capsular and vascular invasion, and finally pulmonary metastases. Even the metastatic cells retain a degree of differentiation as they take up radioiodide (Coppée et al 1996). The categorization of these tumors in human terms is not evident : the follicular appearance, as well as the hematogenic dispersion suggest a follicular carcinoma, but the aspect of the nucleus is compatible with a human papillary carcinoma. A rather similar although less dramatic and slower developing phenotype can be obtained by treating E7 mice with methimazole, i.e. by a treatment that decreases thyroid hormones, increases TSH blood levels and thus leads (as the A2R) to chronic stimulation of the cAMP cascade.

4 ROLE OF THE THYROGLUBLIN PROMOTER IN THE EXPRESSION OF A PHENOTYPE

The control of an oncogene by the thyroglobulin promoter has consequences which are not trivial. Indeed the transcription of the thyroglobulin promoter is not only thyrocyte specific but also cAMP dependent. This, in transgenes of genes involved in the cAMP cascade, will lead to a positive feedback : the expressed protein such as A2R will enhance cAMP accumulation and thus the expression of A2R. On the other hand, for an oncogene of the growth factor cascade such as Ret the expression of the oncogene could cause a repression of the transcription of thyroid specific and cAMP dependent genes and therefore of the oncogene itself. In this case the oncogene exerts a negative feedback on its own expression. A similar result is obtained with SV40 large T which dedifferentiates the cell and should therefore repress its Tg promoter dependent expression.

5 THE PROBLEM OF THE VARIABILITY OF PHENOTYPE FOR ONCOGE ACTIVATING THE SAME CASCADE

The severity of the phenotypes of cAMP hypergenerating thyroids with regard to hyperthyroidism, goiter and development of adenomas are in the order : Tg-A2R > Tg Chol Tox >Tg-Gs* > = Tg TSHR*.

In fact this severity may reflect the degree of activation of the cascade, as when investigated before eventual adenoma generation, the same order of severity is observed for hyperthyroidism. This degree itself partially reflects the level of expression of the protooncogene as was shown in Tg-α1 B AR* models. Indeed in the case of Tg-Gsα* models the mRNA expression of mutated Gs was lower than the natural expression of Gs (Michiels et al 1994). The phenotype of Tg-α1 B AR* mice is quite variable in its intensity and in its timing of appearance from one transgenic mice line to another (Ledent et al 1997). This variability was correlated to the level of expression of the transgene. A similar variety of expression was observed previously for the chloramphenicol acetyltransferase gene under the control of the thyroid promoter (Ledent et al 1990). This is believed to depend on the site of integration of the transgene in the genome. There is always a possibility that A2R could have other effects than activating adenylate cyclase, such a stimulating phospholipase C. However such a dual stimulation in Tg α1β* AR mice does not lead to higher growth or function but rather to necrosis of thyrocytes.

In regulating the level of the transgene protein expression the long term chronic adaptation of the cell to this transgene should also be taken into account. The regulation at transcription will be similar for all transgenes, as they bear on the same thyroglobulin promoter. However for protein synthesis at translation , protein processing and protein disposal the controls and feedbacks could vary from one transgene protein to another. To relate expression to severity of phenotype it would therefore be better to measure protein level and activity.

6 STEPWISE TUMORIGENESIS

The genesis of cancer is generally ascribed to the sequential activation of protooncogenes and inactivation of antioncogenes. A given series of mutagenic events, not necessarily in the same order, leading to a defined form of tumor. This concept is exemplified in the case of A2R -E7 models in which the combination of two partial oncogenes, each one causing by itself a goiter but not an invasive tumor, leads to tumorigenesis, invasiveness and metastasis.

The occasional tumors appearing in hyperplastic thyroids of the other models presumably derive from previous foci of multiplying cells, generating adenomas and then carcinomas. A similar but general and faster evolution is seen in Tg SV40 models. The discrete appearance of foci suggests an additional mutation of a cell and clonal propagation. The long delay of appearance and spatial segregation of the adenomas and their multiplicity are compatible with this hypothesis. In some cases the necessary additional steps may be the exogenous stimulation provided by chronic TSH stimulation resulting from the administration of goitrigens. In that regard the thyroid transgenic models represent good examples of sequential tumor developments. They raise the question of the nature of these secondary genetic events leading to tumorigenesis.

7 THYROID TRANSGENIC MODELS AND « CHERNOBYL » TUMOURS

The clinical, morphological and genetic aspects of thyroid tumours developed after the Chernobyl accident are reviewed elsewhere in these proceedings. These tumors are papillary cancers. We have not been able to demonstrate a TSH receptor mutation in any of the tumors we have investigated. In fact the major and only mutagenic event observed in these tumors are chromosome rearrangements leading to heterotypic expression of an activated Ret receptor in the tumours. The best transgenic model for such tumours are the Tg-PTC1 transgenes.

Acknowledgments

The authors would like to thank for their support
- The Fonds de la Recherche Scientifique Médicale and Télévie, the Fonds Cancérologique de la CGER, the Association contre le Cancer and Association Sportive contre le Cancer and the Radioprotection program of the Commission of European Communities (CT 960304).

References

1. Christophe D, Gérard C, Juvenal G, Bacolla A, Teugels E, Ledent C, Christophe-Hobertus C, Dumont JE, Vassart G. Identification of a cAMP-responsive region in thyroglobulin gene promoter. *Mol Cell Endocrinol.* 1989;64:5-18.
2. Coppée F, Gérard AC, Denef JF, Ledent C, Vassart G, Dumont JE, Parmentier M. Early occurrence of metastatic differentiated thyroid carcinomas in transgenic mice expressing the A2a adenosine receptor gene and the human papillomavirus type 16 E7 oncogene. *Oncogene.* 1996;13:1471-1482.
3. Dumont JE, Lamy F, Roger PP, Maenhaut C. Physiological and pathological regulation of thyroid cell proliferation and differentiation by thyrotropin and other factors. *Physiological Rev.* 1992;72:667-697.
4. Feunteun J, Michiels F, Rochefort P, Caillou B, Talbot M, Fournes B, Mercken L, Schlumberger M, Monier R. Targeted oncogenesis in the thyroid of transgenic mice. *Horm Res.* 1997;47:137-139.
5. Jhiang SM, Sagartz J, Tong Q, Parker-Thornburg J, Capen CC, Cho JY, Xing S, Ledent C. Targeted expression of the ret/PTC1 oncogene papillary thyroid carcinomas. *Endocrinology.* 1996;137:377-378.
6. Ledent C, Denef JF, Cottecchia S, Lefkowitz R, Dumont JE, Vassart G, Parmentier M. Costimulation of adenylyl cyclase and phospholipase C by a mutant alpha1B-adrenergic receptor transgene promotes malignant transformation of thyroid follicular cells. *Endocrinology.* 1997;138:369-378.Abstract.
7. Ledent C, Dumont JE, Vassart G, Parmentier M. Thyroid adenocarcinomas secondary to tissue-specific expression of Simian virus-40 large T-antigen in transgenic mice. *Endocrinology.* 1991;129:1391-1401.
8. Ledent C, Dumont JE, Vassart G, Parmentier M. Thyroid expression of an A2 adenosine receptor transgene induces thyroid hyperplasia and hyperthyroidism. *EMBO J.* 1992;11:537-542.
9. Ledent C, Marcotte A, Dumont JE, Vassart G, Parmentier M. Differentiated carcinomas develop as a consequence of the thyroid specific expression of a thyroglobulin-human papillomavirus type 16 E7 transgene. *Oncogene.* 1995;10:1789-1797.
10. Ledent C, Parmentier M, Vassart G. Tissue-specific expression and methylation of a thyroglobulin-chloramphenicol acetyltransferase fusion gene in transgenic mice. *Proc Natl Acad Sci USA.* 1990;87:6176-6180.
11. Ledent C, Parmentier M, Vassart G. Tissue-specific expression and methylation of a thyroglobulin-chloramphenicol acetyltransferase fusion gene in transgenic mice. *Proc Natl Acad Sci U S A.* 1990;87:6176-6180.

12. Michiels FM, Caillou B, Talbot M, Dessarps-Freichey F, Maunoury MT, Schlumberger M, Mercken L, Monier R, Feunteun J. Oncogeneic potential of guanine nucleotide stimulatory factor alpha subunit in thyroid glands of transgenic mice. *Proc Natl Acad Sci USA*. 1994;**91**:10488-10492.

13. Pohl V, Roger PP, Christophe D, Pattyn G, Vassart G, Dumont JE. Differentiation expression during proliferative activity induced through different pathways: in situ hybridization study of thyroglobulin gene expression in thyroid epithelial cells. *J Cell Biol*. 1990;**111**:663-672.

14. Rochefort P, Caillou B, Michiels FM, Ledent C, Talbot M, Schlumberger M, Lavelle F, Monier R, Feunteun J. Thyroid pathologies in transgenic mice expressing a human activated Ras gene driven by a thyroglobulin promoter. *Oncogene*. 1996;**12**:111-118.

15. Sagartz JE, Jhiang SM, Tong Q, Capen CC. Thyroid stimulating hormone promotes growth of thyroid carcinomas in transgenic mice with targeted expression of ret/PTC1 oncogene. *Lab Invest*. 1997;**76**:307-318.

16. Santelli G, de Franciscis V, Portella G, Chiappetta G, D'Alessio A, Califano D, Rosati R, Mineo A, Monaco C, Manzo G, Pozzi L, Vecchio G. Production of transgenic mice expressing the Ki-ras oncogene under the control of a thyroglobulin promoter. *Cancer Res*. 1993;**53**:5523-5527.

17. Suarez HG. Genetic alterations in human epithelial thyroid tumours. *Clinical Endocrinology*. 1998;**48**:531-546.

18. Tallini G, Costa J. Unraveling the pathogenesis of thyroid tumors using transgenic mice. *Lab Invest*. 1997;**76**:301-305.

19. Uyttersprot N, Allgeier A, Baptist M, Christophe D, Coppée F, Coulonval K, Deleu S, Depoortere F, Dremier S, Lamy F, Ledent C, Maenhaut C, Miot F, Panneels V, Parma J, Parmentier M, Pirson I, Pohl V, Roger PP, Savonet V, Taton M, Tonacchera M, Van Sande J, Wilkin F, Vassart G, Dumont JE. The cAMP in thyroid. From the TSH receptor to mitogenesis and tumorigenesis. *Advances in Second Messenger and Phosphorylation Research* 1997;**31**:125-140.

20. Zeiger MA, Saji M, Gusev Y, Westra WH, Takiyama Y, Dooley WC, Kohn LD, Levine MA. Thyroid-specific expression of cholera toxin A1 subunit causes thyroid hyperplasia and hyperthyroidism in transgenic mice. *Endocrinology*. 1997;**138**:3133-3140.

MOLECULAR ANALYSIS OF THYROID CARCINOMAS IN CHILDREN AFTER CHERNOBYL: ABSENCE OF RAS, P53, AND GSα MUTATIONS, BUT HIGH PREVALENCE OF SPECIFIC TYPES OF RET REARRANGEMENT

[1]H.M. RABES, [1]V.WALDMANN, [1]B. SUCHY, [2]E. LENGFELDER, [3] E.P. DEMIDCHIK, [1]E. ZEINDL-EBERHART AND [1]S. KLUGBAUER

[1]*Institute of Pathology, Ludwig-Maximilians-University of Munich, Thalkirchner Str. 36, D 80337 Munich, Germany,* [2]*Institute of Radiation Biology, University of Munich,* [3]*Medical High School of Minsk, Belarus*

Papillary thyroid carcinomas (PTC) in children exposed to radioactive fallout after the Chernobyl reactor accident provide information on molecular mechanisms of radiation-induced thyroid carcinogenesis. In contrast to sporadic adult tumors, mutations were neither observed in H-, K- and N-RAS nor p53 or Gsα. A high prevalence of RET rearrangement was found. Among the analyzed 59 childhood PTC which developed till 10 years after Chernobyl, evidence for RET rearrangement was obtained in 61%. The PTC1 type of rearrangement (H4/RET) is less frequent as compared to ELE1/RET (PTC3) which is present in about two thirds of the RET rearrangement-positive tumors. Among PTC3 tumors, several truncated subtypes of ELE1/-RET rearrangements were also detected. Rare cases revealed fusion of an unkown gene (RFG5) with RET (PTC5). All types of rearrangement contain coiled-coil regions with dimerization potential. Dimerization and translocation into the cytoplasm appear to evoke a ligand-independent constitutive activation of RET, its autophosphorylation and interaction with unphysiological substrates. Breakpoint studies revealed small homologous nucleotide sequences in both participating genes suggesting DNA double strand break repair by illegitimate recombination via end-joining.

INTRODUCTION

Recent results in molecular epidemiology support the concept that distinct types of tumors exhibit a specific pattern of molecular alterations that may reflect the exposure to a particular class of carcinogenic factors.[1] Investigations of this kind focused mainly on p53 missense mutations. Type and site of DNA adduct formation of specific carcinogenic chemicals determines the pattern of p53 mutations. For ionizing radiation, the situation is less clear. A p53 mutation hot spot with a G-T transversion at codon 249 has been claimed for radon-associated lung cancer, but has not been confirmed by others.

Thyroid cancer is a most valuable source of information on radiation-induced tumors. Therapeutic irradiation of head, neck or upper thorax increased the risk of thyroid carcinogenesis, in particular during childhood, as evident from epidemiological studies. An increase of thyroid tumors was also observed in individuals exposed to radioactive contamination from nuclear weapons. After the Chernobyl reactor accident, a large population was exposed to radioactive fallout. Radioactive iodine represented the largest fraction of rapidly released radionuclides and led transiently to high thyroid doses. An increased incidence of thyroid carcinomas was observed in children living at the time of the reactor accident in most heavily contaminated regions of Belarus. Tumors were classified as papillary thyroid carcinomas with follicular and solid variants, most with lymph node metastasis at the time of diagnosis.

This unprecedented paradigm of rapid development of a specific tumor type in a cohort of children who were simultaneously exposed for a short time interval to high thyroid doses, provides a unique opportunity to study molecular mechanisms of radiation-induced thyroid carcinogenesis and to elucidate relations between type of exposure and ensuing molecular alteration in tumors. A detailed report on our studies and a complete list of references is given in [2,3].

RESULTS

RAS, GSα and P53

Missense mutations of codon 12, 13 or 61 of H-, K- or N-RAS genes which are critical for constitutive activation of the RAS-dependent intracellular signal transduction pathway, have been reported for thyroid carcinomas of adults. However, these mutations do not play a role in childhood PTC after Chernobyl. In agreement with results of another group we did not find a significant number of RAS mutations in a large series of post-Chernobyl PTC.

A similar lack of missense mutations was observed for another protein participating in signal transduction, Gsα, which mediates stimulation of adenylate cyclase. Oncogenic activation ensues from mutation at codon 201 or 227 of the Gsα gene. In a series of 20 post-Chernobyl PTC in children we did not detect any missense mutations in these codons.

P53 mutations have been found in a large number of various human tumor types, including poorly differentiated thyroid carcinomas of adults. In contrast, in our series of childhood PTC after Chernobyl, P53 mutations were missing. This agrees with published data of just one missense mutation (codon 160) among 33 post-Chernobyl tumors in children.

These results suggest that RAS, GSα and P53 mutations as found in adult thyroid tumors are obviously less relevant for induction or progression of radiation-induced thyroid carcinomas of children after Chernobyl.

RET

RET activation is due to fusion of the carboxyterminal part of the gene, the tyrosine kinase (TK) domain, with 5'regulatory parts of the H4 gene (PTC1), the RIα gene (PTC2) and the ELE1 gene (PTC3). In adult PTC RET rearrangement is found in about 16% with geographical variation. H4/RET (PTC1) is the most frequently observed form in PTC of adults; RIα/RET and ELE1/RET occur in rare cases only.

In our study RET rearrangement was investigated in 59 PTC of children, 21 males and 38 females, between 7 months and 18 years of age at the time of the reactor accident. They underwent thyroidectomy between 1993 and 1996. RT-PCR, identification PCR, direct sequencing and 5'RACE were combined in the analysis. In more than 60% a RET rearrangement was found. The ELE1/RET type was most predominant. About two thirds of the RET rearrangement-positive PTC showed this PTC3 type. In contrast, RIα/RET (PTC2) has not been found at all. H4/RET (PTC1) was observed in significantly fewer cases than PTC3 (Table 1).

Table 1. RET rearrangements in PTC of children from Belarus thyroidectomized during the first decade after the Chernobyl reactor accident (n=59).[3]

Type of rearrangement	n	percent of total number	percent of RET rearrangement-positive cases
No RET rearrangement	23	39.0 %	-
RET rearrangement (all types)	36	61.0 %	100 %
RET/PTC1 (H4/RET)	8	13.6 %	22.2 %
RET/PTC2 (RIα/RET)	0	0	0
RET/PTC3 (ELE1/RET) (incl. subtypes)	23	39.0 %	63.9 %
RET/PTC5 (RFG5/RET)	1	1.7 %	2.7 %
RET/PTCx (unidentified)	4	6.8 %	11.1 %

It is unique to radiation-induced PTC that among the ELE1/RET rearrangements several tumors with a truncated ELE1 part in the fused gene were observed. In 3 tumors the complete ELE1 exon 5 was missing, in one case a truncation by 18 bp of this exon was detected. In all cases of analyzed rearrangement so far, however, the same basic structure of the fused gene is evident: The 5' regulatory regions contain coiled-coil oligomerization domains while the 3'part of the fusion product preserves the RET TK domain, irrespective of the actual length of the fused parts of the participating genes. This holds true also for a recently identified novel form of RET rearrangement (PTC5) which is characterized by fusion of a gene of unknown function (designated RET-fused gene 5, RFG5) and the RET TK domain.

In addition to the fusion transcripts with the regulatory part of H4 or ELE1 at the 5'end, reciprocal RET/H4 or RET/ELE1 transcripts were detected. It is not yet known if the RET-activated carboxyterminal part of H4 or ELE1 has a biological impact on tumor development, because the function of these genes has not yet been unravelled. The presence of reciprocal transcripts argues for rearrangement by a balanced chromosomal inversion at 10q11.2, where both genes are located.

A balanced inversion at this point in ELE1/RET rearrangements was further investigated by breakpoint analyses in genomic DNA of PTC3 tumors. Breakpoints are spread in the ELE1 gene in intron 4 and 5; in RET, they are clustered in intron 11. The germline sequences of RET and ELE1 show at the breakpoints short patches of homologous nucleotides with only minor deletions or additions at the ligated ends. This suggests rapid repair of double strand breaks by recombination preferentially by end-joining processes.

CONCLUSION

The high prevalence of RET rearrangement in post-Chernobyl PTC of children with a predominance of ELE1/RET rearrangements suggests that this molecular alteration is a direct consequence of thyrocyte uptake of high doses of radioactive iodine causing DNA double strand breaks, followed by repair by illegitimate recombination via end-joining processes in the proliferating thyrocyte compartment of the juvenile thyroid gland. In terms of molecular epidemiology, ELE1/RET rearrangements may reflect a dose-dependent effect of a specific class of carcinogenic factors, i. e. radioactive iodine, connected with rapidly developing PTC.

References

1. Harris CC. p53: at the crossroads of molecular carcinogensis and risk assessment. *Science* 1993; **262**: 1980-1981.
2. Klugbauer S, Lengfelder E, Demidchik EP, Rabes HM. High prevalence of RET rearrangement in thyroid tumors of children from Belarus after the Chernobyl reactor accident. *Oncogene* 1995; **11**: 2459-2467.
3. Rabes HM, Klugbauer S. Molecular genetics of childhood papillary thyroid carcinomas after irradiation: High prevalence of RET rearrangement. *Rec Res Cancer Res* 1998; **154**: 249-265.

ASSOCIATION BETWEEN MORPHOLOGICAL SUBTYPE OF POST CHERNOBYL PAPILLARY CARCINOMA AND REARRANGEMENT OF THE RET ONCOGENE

GA THOMAS, H BUNNELL, ED WILLIAMS

Thyroid Carcinogenesis Group, University of Cambridge, Strangeways Research Laboratory, Wort's Causeway, Cambridge, UK, CB1 4RN

E-mail: gat1000@cam.ac.uk

M SANTORO, GC VECCHIO

Department of Cellular and Molecular Biology, University of Naples, Italy

E-mail: masantor@cds.unina.it

TI BOGDANOVA, L VOSCOBOINIK, ND TRONKO

Institute of Endocrinology and Metabolism, Kiev, Ukraine

E-mail: tb@viaduk.net

V POZCHARSKAYA, ED CHERSTVOY

Institute of Pathology, Minsk State Medical Institute, Minsk, Belarus

The large increase in papillary thyroid carcinoma in children following the Chernobyl nuclear accident has enabled us to perform a detailed study of the frequency of activation of the ret oncogene, an oncogene specifically associated with papillary carcinomas of the thyroid, and its relationshp with morphological subtype. Three separate morphological subtypes of papillary carcinoma can be identified; the solid follicular subtype of papillary carcinoma is more frequently found in patients from areas more heavily exposed to radioactive fallout than in a similar age matched population no exposed to fallout from Chernobyl. We have successfully used the reverse transcriptase polymerase chain reaction to study the frequency of the two common rearrangements of the ret oncogene (PTC1 and PTC3) in 116 cases of papillary carcinoma in patients who were under 20 at the time of operation and resident in Ukraine and Belarus. Of these 89 were morphologically classified as solid follicular papillary carcinomas (PTC SF) and 27 as diffuse sclerosing variants (PTC DSV: 11 cases) or classic papillary carcinomas (PTC CP: 16 cases). A ret rearrangement was identified in 28% of PTC SFs, and 37.5% and 60% of PTC CPs. However, when the specific type of ret rearrangement (PTC1 or 3) was correlated with the morphological subtype of papillary carcinoma, PTC1 showed a strong correlation (p<0.001) with the DSV and CP subtype (12 of 26 tumours were positive for PTC1 and none with PTC3) and PTC3 with the SF subtype (17 positive for PTC3 and 8 positive for PTC1).

1. INTRODUCTION

There has been a large increase in thyroid carcinoma in children exposed to fallout from the Chernobyl nuclear accident[1-4]. This increase has been almost exclusively restricted to a specific type of carcinoma derived from the thyroid follicular cell, papillary carcinoma[5]. We have identified three subtypes of papillary carcinoma in children, characterised by their dominant morphological pattern[6]. The classical papillary carcinoma, which is also commonly observed in adults, is composed mainly of of large, crowded, cuboidal epithelial cells with pale staining cytoplasm and a high nuclear cytoplasmic ratio which are arranged in branching papillary structures supported by a fibroblastic core. Psammoma bodies (concentric calcified bodies) and typical nuclear features are also frequently present. A second subtype composed of a combination of solid and follicular areas with less prominent nuclear features of papillary carcinoma, except for the presence of nuclear inclusions, was also identified. This subtype, the solid follicular subtype, is probably different from the follicular variant of papillary carcinoma observed in adults, not only because of the nuclear features but also the lack of even minor papillary infoldings in the follicular areas. The third type is the diffuse sclerosing variant which is uncommon but well described in children and in adults. Here the tumour widely infiltrates the gland and is closely associated with lymphocytic cells and a fibrotic response. In children under the age of 10 years who have not been exposed to fallout from the Chernobyl accident the solid follicular subtype is relatively frequent[6]. This subtype is the most common morphological subtype of papillary carcinoma in children following the Chernobyl accident, and is still the most prevalent type in recent years, despite the fact that the majority of cases are now more than 10 years old at operation[7]. The morphology of any tumour is a reflection of the molecular biological changes which are involved in its genesis. It is therefore of interest to correlate morphological with molecular biological analyses.

Papillary carcinomas are uniquely associated with rearrangements of the ret oncogene[8]. The ret gene is a tyrosine kinase receptor for glial derived neurotophic factor[9], and is not normally expressed in the thyroid follicular cell. The ret tyrosine kinase is activated normally by binding to its ligand which produces dimerization of the receptor. Rearrangement of the 3' end of the ret gene to a second gene which contains coiled-coiled domains permits constitutive activation of the ret tyrosine kinase. Seven different rearrangements of the ret gene have so far been reported, involving four different genes[8, 10, 11, 12, 13, 14]. However, the two most common rearrangements involve an intrachromosomal rearrangement to either the H4 gene (PTC1)[8] or to the ele 1 gene (PTC3)[11]. In each case, with the exception of PTC4, the breakpoint occurs within intron 11. This gives rise to a mRNA transcript the 5' end of which is coded for by exon 12 and subsequent exons of the ret gene, but the 3' end is encoded by exons derived from the gene to which the rearranged ret is fused.

In this study we use the reverse transcriptase polymerase chain reaction (RT-PCR) to document the frequency of PTC1 and PTC3 rearrangements in cases of papillary thyroid carcinoma from Ukraine and Belarus, and have correlated the type of rearrangement present with the morphology of the tumour.

2.   MATERIAL STUDIED

We have examined a total of 136 cases of papillary carcinoma from patients from Ukraine and Belarus aged under 20 at operation. All patients were operated at either the Institute of Endocrinology and Metabolism in Kiev, Ukraine or in Minsk, Belarus. Paraffin sections from representative blocks of material from each case were reviewed by pathologists from the University of Cambridge, UK and either the Institute of Endocrinology, Kiev or the Institute of Pathology in Minsk. The tumours were classified on their dominant pattern of morphology. Frozen material was available for RNA extraction in 58 cases, paraffin material only was available from 76 cases.

RNA was extracted from the available tissue according to standard protocols. One microgramme of RNA was reverse transcribed and then subjected to 35 cycles of PCR with a thermal cycler (Perkin-Elmer-Cetus). The product of the reaction was analysed on a 2% agarose gel and hybridised with a probe complimentary to the tyrosine kinase domain of ret. A common antisense and different forward oligonucleotide primers, specific for the H4 and ele 1 genes were used for PCR, Details of the RT-PCR reaction are the same as those previously reported[15]. Negative controls included PCR without previous RT, PCR in the absense of primers, and RT-PCR carried out to the same protocol on normal thyroid tissue. The quality of the RNA samples was assayed by amplifying the human hypoxanthine phosphoribosyltransferase (HPRT) mRNA. The HPRT primers used corresponded to nucleotides 316-340 and nucleotides and 661-685[16].

3.   RESULTS

There was insuficient material for histological subclassification in 1 case, two others were excluded as they represented the only cases of their particular subtype. Seventeen cases were also excluded as they did not yield amplifiable RNA. Of the 116 cases remaining, 89 were classified as PTC SF, 16 as PTC CP and 11 as PTC DSV. Ret rearrangement (either PTC1 or 3) was demonstrated in 25 of the 89

PTC SFs (28%), 6 of 16 PTC CPs (37.5%) and 7 of 11 PTC DSVs (64%). When the specific type of ret rearrangement was correlated with morphology (table 1) a strong association (c^2: p<0.001) of PTC3 with the solid follicular subtype and PTC1 with non solid follicular papillary carcinomas (PTC CP and DSV) was observed. One PTC DSV showed both PTC1 and PTC3 rearrangements.

Table 1. PTC1 and PTC3 rearrangement in post Chernobyl PTCs

	PTC1	PTC3
PTC SF	8/89 (9%)	17/89 (19%)
PTC non SF	12/26 (46%)	0/26

4. DISCUSSION

Rearrangement of the ret oncogene is known to be uniquely associated with thyroid papillary carcinoma. The frequency of ret rearrangment varies between different studies, irrespective of whether the study population has a history of radiation exposure, However, there have been few studies which have involved large numbers of tumours. We studied only 2 of the seven rearrangements of the ret gene so far documented. In a separate study in which we investigated the frequency of expression of the ret oncogene by RT-PCR for the extracellular region and tyrosine kinase region of the gene and compared this with separate identification of PTC1 and PTC3 in 59 cases. In all cases we were unable to demonstrate expression of the extracellular domain of the gene, suggesting that the reciprocal translocation was not transcribed, contradicting findings from some previous studies[13,14] and were able to demonstrate ret tyrosine kinase expression in a total of 32 cases. In only 5 tumours in which we demonstrated positivity for ret tyrosine kinase expression were we unable to demonstrate either PTC1 or PTC3 rearrangement. This study was carried out blind in two different centres using aliquots of the same RNA samples.These results suggest that the majority of post Chernobyl childhood thyroid carcinomas which carry a ret rearrangement show the previously described intrachromosomal rearrangements characterised as PTC1& 3.

We have demonstrated in this study that the type of ret rearrangement is associated with specific morphological subtypes of papillary carcinoma. This association has been previously suggested in a smaller study [17], where the authors found that PTC3 was more frequently found in papillary carcinomas with a solid morphology. However, several important questions arise from these findings. It is interesting that the activation of the ret gene by rearrangement appears to be restricted not only to tumours of one particular cell type (the thyroid follicular cell), but also to one particular subtype of tumour (papillary) derived from that cell type, particularly as it is generally accepted that the follicular cell does not normally express the gene concerned. However, it is obvious that the follicular cell must contain the downstream machinery neccesary for expression of the growth stimulatory properties of the ret tyrosine kinase. It is of particular interest thet ret mutation, not rearrangement is involved in tumourigenesis of the other epithelial component of the thyroid, the C cell. The genes to which the 3' end of the ret gene is translocated in these tumours may play a role also in defining the morphology of the tumour produced, as the same component (exon 12 onwards) is translocated in both PTC1 and 3. Support for this is found in studies of transgenic mice. Thyroid tumours induced in mice are usually of the follicular type, but mice transgenic for thyroid targetted expression of the PTC1 rearrangement show the typical classical papillary carcinoma morphology we have documented here, including the nuclear changes which are characteristic for papillary carcinoma (grooved nuclei and intranuclear cytoplasmic inclusions)[18].

Finally it is interesting that exposure to radioiodine in fallout appears to be linked to an increase in a particular morphological subtype of papillary carcinoma, which is associated with a particular rearrangement of the ret gene. Paediatric tumours of other tissues have also recently been linked to specific rearrangements e.g. myxoid liposarcoma[19], alveolar rhabdomyosarcoma[20], Ewing's sarcoma and peripheral neuroepithelioma[21], suggesting that specific rearrangements play a major role in the development of the histological phenotype of the tumour generated. It is likely therefore that further investigation of these phenomena will provide insights into the mechanism by which radiation from isotopes of iodine causes double strand DNA breaks and the physiological mechanisms which lead to tumourigenesis of the follicular cell in the young child.

Acknowledgments

This work was supported by EC contract numbers FI4C CT96 003 and IC15 CT96 0304

References

1: Baverstock K, Egloff B, Pinchera A, Ruchti C, Williams D Thyroid cancer after Chernobyl. *Nature* 1992 **359**: 21-22

2: Kazakov VS, Demidchik EP, Astakhova LN Thyroid cancer after Chernobyl. *Nature* 1992 **359**: 21

3: Likhtarev IA, Sobolev BG, Kairo IA et al., Thyroid cancer in the Ukraine. *Nature* 1995 **375**: 365

4: Jacob P, Goulko, Heidenreich WF et al., Thyroid cancer risk to children calculated. *Nature* 1998 **392**: 32

5: Williams ED, E Cherstvoy, B Egloff, et al., Interaction of pathology and molecular characteristics of thyroid cancers. In: The Radiological Consequences of the Chernobyl accident. A Karaoglou, G Desmet, GN Kelly and HG Menzel (eds). 1996 EUR 16544 EN pp699-714

6: Harach HR and Williams ED Childhood thyroid cancer in England and Wales. *British J Cancer* 1995 **72**: 777-783

7: Bogdanova TI, Tronko ND, Bragarnik M, Thomas GA, Williams ED Pathology of post Chernobyl thyroid cancer in Ukraine 1990-1997. 1998 submitted

8: Santoro M, Carlomango F, Hay ID et al., Ret oncogene activation in human thyroid neoplasms is restricted to the papillary cancer subtype. *J Clin Invest* 1992 **89**: 1517-1522

9: Treanor JJS, Goodman L, deSauvage F et al., Characterization of a multicomponent receptor for GDNF. *Nature* 1996 **382**: 80-83

10: Bongarzone I, Monzini N, Borrello MG et al., Molecular characterization of a thyroid tumor-specific transforming sequence formed by the fusion of ret tyrosine kinase and the regulatory subunit of Riα of cyclic AMP-dependent protein kinase A. *Mol Cell Biol* 1993 **13**: 358-366

11: Santoro M, Dathan NA, Berlingieri MT et al., Molecular characterisation of ret/PTC3: a novel rearranged version of the ret proto-oncogene in a human papillary carcinoma. *Oncogene* 1994 **9**: 509-516

12: Fugazzola L, Pierotti M, Vigano E, Pacini F, Vorontsova T, Bongarzone I Molecular and biochemical analysis of RET/PTC4, a novel oncogenic rearrangement between RET and ELE1 genes, in a post Chernobyl papillary carcinoma. *Oncogene* 1996 **13**: 1093-1097

13: Klugbauer S, Demidchik EP, Lengfelder E, Rabes HM Molecular analysis of new subtypes of ELE/RET rearrangements, their reciprocal transcripts and breakpoints in papillary thyroid carcinomas of children after Chernobyl. *Oncogene* 1998 **16**: 671-675

14: Klugbauer S, Demidchik EP, Lengfelder E, Rabes HM Dtection of a novel type of RET rearrangement (PTC5) in thyroid carcinomas after Chernobyl and analysis of the involved RET-fused gene RFG5. *Cancer Res* 1998 **58**: 198-203

15: Viglietto G , Chiappetta G, Martinez-Tello FJ et al., RET/PTC oncogene activation is an early event in thyroid carcinogenesis. *Oncogene* 1995 **11**: 1207-1210

16: Kim SH et al., The organization of the human HPRT gene. *Nucl Acid Res* 1986 **14**: 3103-3118

17: Nikiforov YE, Rowland JM, Bove KE, Monforte-Munoz H, Fagin JA Distinct pattern of ret oncogene rearrangements in morphological variants of radiation-induced and sporadic thyroid papillary carcinomas in children. *Cancer Res* 1997 **57**:1690-1694

18: Jihang SM, Sagartz JE, Tong Q et al., Targetted expression of the ret/PTC1 oncogene induces papillary thyroid carcinomas. *Endorinology* 1996 **137**: 375-378

19: Crozat, A., Aman, P., Mandhal, N., & Ron, D. Fusion of CHOP to a novel RNA binding protein in human myxoid liposarcoma. *Nature*, 1993 **363**: 640-644.

20: Galili, N., Davis, R.J., Fredricks, W.J., et al., Fusion of a head fork domain gene to PAX3 in the solid tumour alveolar rhabdomyosarcoma. *Nat-Genet.*, 1993 **3**: 230-235.

21: Zucman, J., Delattre, O., Desmaze, et al., Cloning and characterisation of the Ewing's sarcoma and peripheral neuroepithelioma t(11:22) translocation breakpoints. *Genes Chrom-Cancer* 1993 **4**: 271 -277.

MOLECULAR GENETIC ANALYSIS OF *RET* REARRANGEMENTS IN PAPILLARY THYROID CARCINOMAS FROM BELARUSSIAN CHILDREN AND ADULTS

J. SMIDA, H. ZITZELSBERGER AND L. LENGFELDER

Institute of Radiation Biology, Ludwig-Maximilians-University, Schillersraße 42,
D-80336 Munich, Germany

K. SALASSIDIS, L. HIEBER AND M. BAUCHINGER

GSF-National Research Center for Environment and Health, Institute of Radiobiology,
D-85758 Neuherberg, Germany
E-mail: Bauchinger@gsf.de

Rearrangements of the *ret* oncogene were investigated in papillary thyroid carcinomas (PTC) from 51 Belarussian children with a mean age of 3 years at the time of the Chernobyl radiation accident. For comparison 32 PTC from adults, 16 PTC from exposed Belarussian and 16 PTC from German patients without radiation history, were included in the study.

Ret rearrangements were detected and specified by RT-PCR and direct sequencing using specific primers for *ret*/PTC1, 2 and 3. Only *ret*/PTC1 and no *ret*/PTC3 was found in the adult patients, with a frequency of 69% for the Belarussian cases but only with a frequency of 19% in the German patients. In contrast, 13 *ret*/PTC3 (25.5%) and 12 *ret*/PTC1 (23.5%) rearrangements were present in PTC from Belarussian children. Allover, our study reveals a similar frequency of *ret*/PTC3 and *ret*/PTC1 which is in contrast to previous studies with lower numbers of cases and exhibiting a high predominance of *ret*/PTC3. A similar ratio (2.5:1) as in the previous investigations (diagnosed 1991-94) was obtained for a subgroup of cases included in our study that were diagnosed in 1993-94.

The present data suggest that *ret*/PTC3 may be typical for radiation-associated childhood PTC with short latency period, whereas *ret*/PTC1 may be a marker for later occurring PTC of radiation-exposed adults and children.

1   Introduction

An increasing incidence of childhood papillary thyroid carcinoma (PTC) among Belarussian children was reported for the first time in 1992 [1]. This development suggests a link between the exposure to radioactive isotopes due to incorporation of ^{131}I in childhood thyroids. As early as 4 years after the Chernobyl accident the first childhood thyroid carcinomas were diagnosed in Belarus. This short latency periods is in contrast to the 18±8 years observed in other radiation-associated thyroid papillary carcinomas [2]. The Belarussian childhood thyroid tumours exhibit a more aggressive behaviour than PTCs without radiation history.

In thyroid carcinomas, different types of *ret* rearrangements were identified, two types *ret*/PTC1 and *ret*/PTC3 have been found to be the predominant alterations in post-Chernobyl PTCs [3,4,5]. The activated forms of the *ret* proto-oncogene result from specific chromosomal rearrangements fusing the tyrosine kinase domain (TK) of c-*ret* with the 5′ domain of other genes.

In the present study, 51 childhood PTC from Belarus were randomly selected from the tumour tissue bank established at the GSF-Institute of Radiobiology and analysed for *ret* rearrangements. The main part of the investigated tumours were diagnosed between 1995 and 1996, i.e. nine to ten years after the Chernobyl accident. The time of surgery was before the age of 16 in all cases. In addition to the childhood tumours, 16 PTC from adult patients from Munich without radiation history and 16 PTC from adult Belarussian patients living in the contaminated area were analysed.

2 Material and Methods

Fresh samples of tumour tissue - obtained from Prof. E.P. Demidchik, Thyroid Tumour Centre Minsk and the Martha-Maria Hospital, Munich - were snap-frozen in liquid nitrogen.

PolyA⁺mRNA was extracted from the homogenised tumour material using a Micro-FastTrack Kit (Invitrogen). The random primed reverse transcription was performed using a cDNA Cycle Kit (Invitrogen, NL). RT-PCR was carried out with 2.5 U Taq DNA polymerase (Gibco BRL) using 100 pmol of each sense and antisense primer in reaction buffer (KCl system, provided by Gibco BRL), containing 1.5 mM $MgCl_2$ and 2mM of each dNTP. To screen for *ret* mRNA expression two fragments corresponding to the tyrosin kinase (TK) and extracellular (EC) domains of the c-*ret* gene were amplified using two intron-spanning primer pairs. Samples demonstrating preferential or exclusive amplification of the TK domain were amplified for detection of *ret* rearrangements with specific primer pairs PTC1, PTC2 and PTC3. Direct sequencing of the amplified DNA fragments was carried out by the dideoxy-nucleotide method, using the same primers as for PCR amplification.

3 Results

Twenty-five (49%) out of 51 childhood PTC exhibited a known rearrangement of the TK domain of the *ret* gene. Among these tumours, 13 *ret*/PTC3 (25.5%) and 12 *ret*/PTC1 (23.5%) but no *ret*/PTC2 rearrangements were found. In addition to these characterised *ret*-rearrangements, in seven cases (14%) the comparison between amplification of the TK and EC domain gave evidence for an obviously enhanced TK-product. This might be indicative for further *ret*-gene alterations, which, however, could not be characterised within this study. Would these be considered to be *ret* rearrangements, the total percentage of all *ret* alterations would increase to 65%.

Thirteen of 16 tissue samples (81%) from Belarussian adults showed an increased amplification of the TK domain of the *ret* gene. Rearrangements of *ret*/PTC1 could be identified in 11 cases (69%), while in two cases (12%) only an increased TK-amplification signal was found.

In contrast to the high prevalence of *ret* rearrangements in the Belarussian adults, in the sixteen PTC without radiation history from Munich adults only three *ret*/PTC1 rearrangements (19%) could be identified. Our results from adult patients show that the overall frequency of *ret* rearrangements is significantly different (χ^2=8.13, P<0.05) between radiation-associated (69%) and thyroid papillary carcinomas from adults without radiation history (19%). In Belarussian radiation-exposed children, the total rearrangement frequency is somewhat less (49%) than in adult patients living in the same contaminated area. In contrast to the adults, in childhood tumours besides *ret*/PTC1 (23.5%) also *ret*/PTC3 (25.5%) occurred leading to a PTC1/PTC3 ratio of about unity.

4 Discussion

Rearrangements of the tyrosine kinase c-*ret* are obviously playing a role in tumourigenesis of the thyroid gland [6]. In post-Chernobyl childhood thyroid tumours it has been demonstrated that activating *ret* rearrangements predominantly *ret*/PTC3 (31 in a total of 56 cases) are highly prevalent [3, 4, 5].

In the present study we investigated 51 cases of childhood, 16 adult PTC from Belarus and 16 PTC from German non-exposed adults. The marked prevalence of *ret* rearrangements (11 out of 16, i.e. 69%) in PTC from Belarussian adults is the most striking difference to the frequency of *ret* rearrangements observed in 'spontaneous' papillary carcinomas without radiation history (3 out of 16, i.e. 19%). Spontaneous thyroid tumours from different geographical areas showed also lower frequencies of *ret* rearrangements, ranging from 3 to 35% [7], however, because these data have been obtained from various tumour types they are not directly comparable with our results. Using nested RT-PCR, Williams et al. [8] found a total of 53% *ret* activation in archived tumour material from the UK. In adult patients with external radiotherapy 16 out of 19 PTC (84%) *ret*/PTC1 were found [2] which is in line with our own data on Belarussian adults (69%). These results suggest a strong correlation between radiation exposure and activating *ret*/PTC1 in adults and children.

Our findings from 51 childhood PTC (49% overall *ret* rearrangements) correspond to other studies [3, 4, 5, 9]. However, our results show a ratio of about unity for *ret*/PTC3 and *ret*/PTC1 frequency which contrasts to the ratio of about 3:1 observed in these studies. This difference may reflect an influence of different latency periods of PTC. Nikiforov et al. [5] studied PTC that occurred as early as 1991-92, Klugbauer et al. [4] investigated tumours from 1993-94. In the present study, 40 tumours (78%) were diagnosed 1995-97 and 11 (22%) 1993-94, reflecting a mean latency period of 9 years. In the 11 earlier diagnosed tumours five *ret*/PTC3 and two *ret*/PTC1 (ratio 2.5:1) were identified. In contrast, in the 40 later diagnosed tumours 8 carried *ret*/PTC3 and 10 *ret*/PTC1 (ratio 0.8:1). Compared with the 38 tumours of shortest latency period [5], harbouring 22 *ret*/PTC3 and 6 *ret*/PTC1 (ratio 3.7:1) our findings of totally 13 *ret*/PTC3 and 12 *ret*/PTC1 in 51 tumours (ratio 1.1:1), is significantly different (χ^2=4.16, P=0.04).

We conclude, that our data confirm the crucial role of the *ret* proto-oncogene in the development of radiation-associated thyroid papillary carcinomas. Only *ret*/PTC1 and *ret*/PTC3 but no *ret*/PTC2 were found. The frequency of both types of *ret* rearrangements is obviously different between tumours from Belarussian children and adults. This is the first comparative analysis of *ret* rearrangements in thyroid PTC of children and adults exposed to radioiodine after the Chernobyl accident. In contrast to previous studies of childhood thyroid carcinomas, *ret*/PTC3 was not found to be the predominant form of *ret* rearrangement. Taking all the data into account, we suggest that *ret*/PTC3 rearrangements are indicative for PTC with a short latency period.

Acknowledgements

Work supported by the EC Nuclear Fission Safety Programme F14PCT95 0008d.

References

1. Baverstock, K., Egloff, B., Pinchera, A., Ruchti, C. and Williams, D., Thyroid cancer after Chernobyl. *Nature*, **359**, (1992) pp. 21-22.
2. Bounacer, A., Wicker, R., Caillou, B., Cailleux, A.F., Sarasin, A., Schlumberger, M. and Suarez, H.G., High prevalence of activating ret proto-oncogene rearrangements, in thyroid tumors from patients who had received external radiation. *Oncogene*, **15**, (1997) pp. 1263-1273.
3. Fugazzola, L., Pilotti, S., Pinchera, A., Vorontsova, T.V., Mondellini, P., Bongarzone, I., Greco, A., Astakhova, L., Butti, M.G., Demidchik, E.P., Pacini, F. and Pierotti, M.A., Oncogenic rearrangements of the RET proto-oncogene in papillary thyroid carcinomas from children exposed to the Chernobyl nuclear accident. *Cancer Res.*, **55**, (1995) pp. 5617-5620.
4. Klugbauer, S., Lengfelder, E., Demidchik, E.P. and Rabes, H.M., High prevalence of RET rearrangement in thyroid tumors of children from Belarus after the Chernobyl reactor accident. *Oncogene*, **11**, (1995) pp. 2459-2467.

5. Nikiforov, Y.E., Rowland, J.M., Bove, K.E., Monforte-Munoz, H. and Fagin, J.A., Distinct pattern of ret oncogene rearrangements in morphological variants of radiation-induced and sporadic thyroid papillary carcinomas in children. *Cancer Res.*, **57,** (1997) pp. 1690-1694.

6. Grieco, M., Santoro, M., Berlingieri, M.T., Melillo, R.M., Donghi, R., Bongarzone, I., Pierotti, M.A., Della Porta, G., Fusco, A. and Vecchio, G., PTC is a novel rearranged form of the ret proto-oncogene and is frequently detected in vivo in human thyroid papillary carcinomas. *Cell*, **60,** (1990) pp. 557-563.

7. Sugg, S.L., Zheng, L., Rosen, I.B., Freeman, J.L., Ezzat, S. and Asa, S.L., ret/Ptc-1, -2, and -3 oncogene rearrangements in human thyroid carcinomas: implications for metastatic potential? *J. Clin. Endocrinol. Metab.*, **81,** (1996) pp. 3360-3365.

8. Williams, G.H., Rooney, S., Thomas, G.A., Cummins, G. and Williams, E.D., RET activation in adult and childhood papillary thyroid carcinoma using a reverse transcriptase-polymerase chain reaction approach on archival-nested material. *Br. J. Cancer*, **74,** (1996) pp. 585-589.

9. Ito, T., Seyama, T., Iwamoto, K.S., Mizuno, T., Tronko, N.D., Komissarenko, I.V., Cherstovoy, E.D., Satow, Y., Takeichi, N., Dohi, K. and et al., Activated RET oncogene in thyroid cancers of children from areas contaminated by Chernobyl accident. *Lancet*, **344,** (1994) p. 259.

ACTIVATION RATE OF RAS AND RET/PTC IN NODULAR THYROID DISEASE DEVELOPING IN THE MARSHALL ISLANDS

RM TUTTLE[1], T TAKAHASHI[2], K FUJIMORI[2], KR TROTT[3], J ANDERSON[1], YY DJUH[1], SL SIMON[4].

[1]Walter Reed Army Medical Center, Washington DC, [2]Tohoku University, Sendai Japan; [3]St Bartholomew's Medical College, United Kingdom; [4]National Academy of Sciences, Washington DC

MAJ RM Tuttle, MD. Assistant Chief, Department of Clinical Investigation, Walter Reed Army Medical Center, 6825 16th Street NW, Washington DC 20307-5001.

In the years following the 1954 Castle-Bravo nuclear weapons testing accident in the Marshall Islands, a dramatic increase in the incidence of nodular thyroid disease has been documented in exposed individuals. While the precise mechanism of radiation induced tumorigenesis is not completely understood, several investigators have proposed a role for both ras and ret/PTC mutations in radiation-induced thyroid tumors. Our objective was to determine the prevalence of ras and ret/PTC mutations in nodular thyroid disease currently developing in the Marshall Islands. Thyroidectomy was performed for clinically indicated reasons in 10 Marshallese subjects in 1994. PCR amplification of each ras oncogene was followed by oligospecific hybridizations to screen for point mutations. RT-PCR was used to detect ret/ptc mutations. Ras mutations were detected in 2/6 (33%) papillary thyroid cancers, 1/3 (33%) follicular thyroid cancers, and 0/10 normal thyroid tissues. Two of the three ras mutations were detected in subjects born after the atomic weapons testing program was completed in the Marshall Islands. No ret/ptc mutations were detected in any of the samples. While activation of ras was detected in a significant number of malignant thyroid tissue samples, the specific pattern of ras activation does not appear to differ significantly from other studies of non-irradiated thyroid neoplasia. Furthermore, activation of the ret/ptc oncogenes does not appear to be a common event in nodular thyroid disease currently developing in the Marshall Islands.

Between 1946 and 1958 the United States detonated over 60 nuclear weapons in a group of coral atolls in the equatorial waters of the Pacific Ocean now known as The Republic of the Marshall Islands[6]. A group of 82 Marshallese people living on Rongelap were not evacuated prior to the March 1st, 1954 nuclear test known as Operation Castle-Bravo[2,6]. The radiation released from this 15 megaton nuclear explosion has resulted in dramatic increases in both benign and malignant thyroid disease in the Marshallese living on the nearby atolls of Rongelap and Utrik at the time of the blast[2].

While the Marshallese have long believed that many of the more distant atolls also received significant radiation exposure as a result of the atomic weapons testing program, support for this hypothesis did not come until 1987 when Hamilton et al demonstrated a higher than expected rate of thyroid nodule formation in the distant southern atolls that varied as a function of distance from the nuclear testing sites[1]. The Marshall Islands government sponsored a Nationwide Radiological Survey to assess the extent of radioactive contamination which eventually came to include an examination of the prevalence of thyroid disease throughout the country[7]. Thyroid samples obtained for standard clinical indications as part of this nationwide survey were preserved for molecular analysis and are the basis of this current report.

With new advances in molecular biology, it is possible to examine precise changes in DNA and messenger RNA sequences associated with malignant transformation. Some investigators have noted a higher than expected prevalence of both ras and ret/ptc mutations in radiation induced thyroid disease[4]. If these oncogenes prove to be biological markers of radiation induced thyroid cancer, it would be of great interest to know whether the nodular thyroid disease currently developing in the Marshall Islands is associated with these specific mutations.

MATERIALS AND METHOD

Thyroidectomy was performed on 10 subjects with thyroid nodules suspicious for malignancy on Majuro in 1994. After obtaining appropriate informed consent, samples of the thyroid nodule and adjacent normal thyroid tissue were surgically removed and immediately frozen.

Nucleic acids were extracted from fresh frozen tissue using standard organic extraction techniques. Nested primer sets specific for regions surrounding codons 12-13 and 61 were designed for each ras gene (Ha, Ki, and N). PCR amplification was done using Perkin-Elmer kits with Amplitaq Gold (Perkin-Elmer) and followed with oligospecific hybridization using radiolabelled oligospecific probes[5]. Several of the PCR products were sequenced using the ABI Prism DyeDeoxy Terminator Cycle Sequencing kit on the 373 DNA sequencer (Perkin-Elmer).

cDNA synthesis and RT-PCR amplification were performed as described by Klugbauer[3] using cDNA clones provided by Dr. Sissy Jhiang (Ohio State University, Columbus Ohio) as positive controls. Investigators performing the molecular studies were blinded to the clinical data.

RESULTS

Samples of thyroid nodules and normal thyroid tissue were available from 10 subjects (mean age 41 + 4 years; range 29-72 years; 7 female). Of the 5 subjects alive in 1954, four lived on Kwajalein atoll and one lived on Majuro atoll. Neither of these atolls is in close proximity to the Bravo test site.

Final histological diagnoses included 1 adenomatous goiter (patient alive in 1954), 3 follicular cancers (1 alive in 1954), and 6 papillary cancers (3 alive in 1954).

Mutations in the ras proto-oncogene was detected in three of the thyroid nodules (See table 1). No ras mutations were detected in the corresponding normal tissue specimens. Ras mutations were detected in 2 of 6 papillary cancers (33%), and 1 of 3 follicular cancers (33%). Two of the ras mutations were detected in subjects born after 1964.

Reverse transcriptase analysis of total RNA demonstrated normal beta-2-microglobulin mRNA in each sample. Specific ret/ptc mutations were readily detected in the cDNA clones for each of the ret/ptc mutations and in other clinical thyroid specimens previously detected to be ret/ptc positive in our laboratory. No ret/ptc mutations were detectable in the thyroid nodules or the adjacent normal thyroid specimens of these subjects.

Table 1. Correlation of ras mutations with histological diagnosis and potential exposure to radiation fallout.

Sample #	Histologic Diagnosis	Alive during nuclear testing	Specific ras mutation
1	Follicular Cancer	Yes	N-ras, codon 61 GLN to ARG
2	Papillary Cancer -	No (Born in 1964)	K-ras, codon 61 GLN to VAL
3	Papillary Cancer	No (Born in 1965)	N-ras, codon 61 GLN to ARG

DISCUSSION

Mutations in the ras proto-oncogene were detected in 33% of a small number of papillary and follicular thyroid cancers that were recently diagnosed and treated in the Marshall Islands. While this rate of ras activation is higher than generally reported in larger studies, the specific types of ras mutations are consistent with those reported in both radiation associated and sporadic thyroid malignancies.

Since the five subjects alive during the time of the nuclear testing were residing on atolls quite distant from the nuclear test sites, it is unlikely that they received significant doses of radioactive iodine from the fallout.

The absence of ret/ptc mutations in these samples may suggest that radioactive iodines were not the major etiologic agent in the development of these thyroid nodules. Analysis of ret/ptc activation in the thyroid samples obtained from the Rongelap and Utrick exposed populations as part of the Brookhaven National Laboratory medical follow up program would provide an additional interesting comparison group.

In summary, ras activation but not ret/ptc activation appears to be a common event in thyroid nodules currently developing in the Marshall Islands. The precise dose of thyroid irradiation to these Marshallese subjects remains uncertain making it difficult to compare these results with those of other nuclear accidents or external beam irradiation.

The opinions and assertions contained herein are the private views of the authors and are not to be construed as official or as reflecting the views of the Department of the Army or the Department of Defense.

REFERENCES

1. Hamilton TE, van Belle G, Logerfo JP. Thyroid neoplasia in Marshall Islanders exposed to nuclear fallout. *JAMA* 1987; **258**: 629-636.
2. Howard JE, Vaswani A, Heotis P. Thyroid disease among the Rongelap and Utirik population – An update. *Health Physics* 1997; **73(1)**: 190-198.
3. Klugbauer, S, et al. High prevalence of RET rearrangement in thyroid tumors of children from Belarus after the Chernobyl reactor accident. *Oncogene* 1995; **11(12)**: 2459-67.
4. Nikiforov, YE, Fagin J. Radiation-induced thyroid cancer in children after the Chernobyl accident. *Thyroid Today* 1998. **XXI(2)**:1-11.
5. Nikiforov, YE, et al. Prevalence of mutations of ras and p53 in benign and malignant thyroid tumors from children exposed to radiation after the Chernobyl nuclear accident. *Oncogene* 1996. **13(4)**: 687-93.
6. Simon SL. A brief history of people and events related to atomic weapons testing in the Marshall Islands. *Health Physics* 1997; **73(1)**: 5-20.
7. Takahashi T, Trott KR, Fujimori K, Simon SL, Ohtomo H, Nakashima N, Takaya K, Kimura N, Satomi S, Schoemaker MJ. *Health Physics* 1997; **73(1)**: 199-213.

CYTOGENETIC ANALYSIS, GENE EXPRESSION AND TUMOURIGENICITY STUDIES OF RADIATION-INDUCED HUMAN THYROID CARCINOMAS

A.C. RICHES, C.M. PEDDIE, P.E. BRYANT AND C.V. BRISCOE
School of Biomedical Sciences, University of St. Andrews, Scotland

H. ZITZELSBERGER, E. LENGFELDER, L. LEHMANN, L. HIEBER. M. BAUCHINGER
Radiobiological Institute, University of Munich and Institute of Radiobiology, GSF, Neuherberg, Germany

E.P. DEMIDCHEK
Center for Thyroid Tumours, Minsk, Belarus

A. SALO, E. ROMPPANEN, M. PERÄLÄ, K. SERVOMAA, T. RYTÖMAA AND R. MUSTONEN
STUK, Helsinki and North Savo Environment Centre, Kuopio, Finland

Radiation-induced human thyroid carcinogenesis has been studied using primary cell cultures from childhood thyroid tumours from Belarus and human thyroid tumour cell lines. These lines were generated from primary tumours appearing in athymic nude mice following irradiation of a human thyroid epithelial cell line (HTori-3) *in vitro* with gamma or alpha particle irradiation.

The cytogenetic characteristics of the primary cell lines were investigated using G-banding, comparative genomic hybridisation (CGH) and spectral karyotyping (SKY). Clonal structural aberrations could be detected as well as non-clonal aberrations involving chromosome 10q and 2p. One of the Belarussian cases revealed a hypertriploid karyotype with marker chromosomes t(7;9;15), t(1;4). t(2;10;17), t(9;13) and chromosomal losses on 1q and 13q and chromosomal gains on 2p and 9q.

The growth properties of the primary cell lines from the childhood carcinomas were investigated. While there was heterogeneity of growth *in vitro*, these cell lines failed to produce tumours in athymic nude mice. However an anaplastic thyroid tumour grew well and two clones derived from what was originally thought to be a case of thyroiditis also produced progressively growing tumours.

Differential display reverse transcription polymerase chain reaction (DDRT-PCR) has been used to compare changes in gene expression between the experimentally-induced human thyroid tumour cell lines and the non-tumourigenic parent cell line. So far 7 gamma- and 3 alpha- induced cell lines have been studied revealing both up-regulation and down-regulation of genes.

These radiation-induced human thyroid tumours are providing a useful model to investigate changes associated with radiation-induced carcinogenesis in the human thyroid.

1. INTRODUCTION

Thyroid carcinoma incidence is increased significantly following exposure of the thyroid to ionizing radiations. After the Chernobyl nuclear power plant accident in April 1986, a markedly increased incidence of thyroid carcinomas was observed in children [1, 2]. Stable chromosomal translocations have been previously investigated in these radiation-induced papillary thyroid carcinomas (PTC's)[3].

2. MATERIALS AND METHODS

Thyroid samples were analysed from 56 Belarus patients (51 PTC's, 3 benign, 2 thyroiditis). Tissue culture and chromosome analysis were performed on these samples [3, 4]. Karyotyping was undertaken after G-banding. Spectral karyotyping (SKY) was performed with 24 painting probes specific for each chromosome and comparative genomic hybridisation (CGH) as previously described [4]. The tumourigenicity of some of these cell lines was tested in athymic nude mice.

Human thyroid tumour cell lines generated from a human thyroid epithelial cell line irradiated *in vitro* [5, 6] were used to examine changes in gene expression using differential display reverse transcription-polymerase chain reaction (DDRT-PCR).

3. RESULTS AND DISCUSSION

Analysis of the G-banded chromosomes revealed examples of clonal structural aberrations in 13 of the 56 cases (23%) (Table 1). Two cases (S9, S48) exhibited very complex structurally rearranged chromosomes which could not be satisfactorily analysed by G-banding. One of these cell lines (S48) was further analysed by SKY revealing a number of translocations [t(7;9;15), t(1;4), t(2;10;17), t(9;13), t(1;6), t(1;6;11), t(2;7;22), t(2;17) and t(6;11)]. CGH revealed chromosomal gains on chromosome 1q21, 2p11.1-pter, 2q11.2-q13, 3q26.2-q26.3, 6p21.3pter, 9q13-q33, 17q11.1-qter and losses on 1q42, 13q21.2-q21.3, 15q11.1-q14.

Of 5 cell lines tested for tumourigenicity only one grew repeatedly. This line was derived from a 14 year old female exhibiting thyroiditis. This presumably suggests that the thyroiditis was associated with a carcinoma and the two cell lines (S48K6 and S48K18) produced from this sample contained tumour cells. In general PTC's did not form tumours. One line from an anaplastic carcinoma grew well (S77).

The initial screening using DDRT-PCR of 6 radiation-induced thyroid tumour cell lines compared to the unirradiated parent cell line (HTori-3) revealed 121 differentially displayed bands. One gene was turned off in 3 different tumour lines (Table 2) and a further 2 genes were up-regulated and 3 genes down-regulated.

Table 1. Clonal chromosome aberrations in childhood thyroid tumours from Belarus.

Case	Pathological diagnosis	Number of metaphases total	abnormal	Aberrant Karyotype
S47	PTC	10	10	10 x 46, XX, t(5;7)(q23;p15)
S95	PTC	12	6	2 x 46, XY, t(1;9)(q42;q34)
S96	PTC	10	10	10 x 46, XX, t(10;22)(q11;q11)
S125	PTC	23	11	2 x 46, XY, t(1;2)(p22;q34)
				2 x 46, XY, t(14;15)(p11;p11)
S166	PTC	15	5	2 x 46, XX,del(16)(q13;qter)
S175	PTC	12	11	10 x 46,XX,t(1;5)(q32;31),
				t(10;16)(q22;q23)
S179	PTC	17	17	17 x 46, XX, t(2;13)(q21;q32)
S206	PTC	43[1]	3[1]	3 x 46, XX, t(1;2)(q42;p25)
		22[1]	4[1]	4 x 46, XX, t(2;9)(p12;q12)
S224	PTC	100[1]	5[1]	5 x 46, XX, t(1;2)(q22;q33)
S253	PTC	100[1]	12[1]	12 x 46, XX, t(10;15)(q11;q22)
S284	PTC	100[1]	45[1]	45 x 46, XX, t(1;10)(p13;q11)
S48	thyroiditis	6	6	6 x near-triploid with several identical marker chromosomes
S71	goitre	10	10	10 x 46, XX, t(1;10)(p32;q26)

[1] translocations confirmed by FISH-painting for chromosomes 1, 6 and 10

Table 2. Differentially expressed genes in radiation-induced thyroid cancer cell lines.

Cell Line	Size (bp)	Gene	EMBL No.	% Homo.
HTG8	230	mRNA7, NADH dehydrog. 4 (-)	MIHSCG	98.4
	230	cytochrome C oxidase II subunit (-)	MTHSCOXII	98.9
	230	EST from fetal brain (-)	HS129G10B	97.4
	100	EST from ovary tumour & C3 gene	HS1273870	98.3
HTG9	100	EST from ovary tumour & C3 gene	HS1273870	98.3
HTG13	100	EST from ovary tumour & C3 gene	HS1273870	98.3
	335	EST from cDNA clone (+)	HS1241544	99.2
	335	EST from mouse (+)	MM1176353	100.0

(-) down-regulated gene ; (+) up-regulated gene

Multiple structural chromosome aberrations as well as complex rearrangements were frequently detected in these putatively radiation-induced thyroid tumours compared to those seen in "spontaneous" thyroid tumours. Novel breakpoints were detected which might serve as a starting point for characterisation and positional cloning of genes involved in radiation-induced tumourigenesis.

While a human thyroid epithelial cell line when irradiated *in vitro* produced undifferentiated tumours, in general PTC's did not produce tumours apart from one interesting example that was initially diagnosed as Hasimoto's thyroiditis.

These human thyroid carcinomas and cell lines provide a unique resource to investigate the molecular mechanisms involved in radiation-induced carcinogenesis.

Acknowledgements

Work supported by the EC Nuclear Fission Safety Programme F14PCT95 0008d.

References

1. Baverstock E, Egloff B, Pinchera A, Rucheti C, Williams D. Thyroid cancer after Chernobyl. *Nature* 1992; **359**; 21-22.
2. Kazakov S, Demidchik EP, Astakhova LN. Thyroid cancer after Chernobyl. *Nature* 1992; **359**; 20-21.
3. Lehmann L, Zitzelsberger H, Kellerer AM, Braselmann H, Kulka U, Georgiadou-Schumacher V, Negele T, Spelsberg F, Demidchik E, Lengfelder E, Bauchinger M. Chromosome translocations in thyroid tissues from Belarussian children exposed to radioiodine from the Chernobyl accident measured by FISH-painting. *Int.J.Rad.Biol.* 1996; **70**; 513-516.
4. Lehmann L, Greulich KM, Zitzelsberger H, Negele T, Spelsberg F, Bauchinger M. Weier HUG. Cytogenetic and molecular genetic characterization of chromosome 2 rearrangement in a case of human papillary thyroid carcinoma with radiation history. *Cancer Genet. Cytogenet.* 1997; **96**; 30-36.
5. Riches AC, Herceg Z, Bryant PE, Wynford-Thomas D. Radiation-induced transformation of SV40-immortalised human thyroid epithelial cells by single and fractionated exposure to γ-irradiation *in vitro*. *Int.J.Rad.Biol.* 1994; **66**; 757-765.
6. Riches AC, Herceg Z, Bryant PE, Stevens DL, Goodhead DT. Radiation-induced transformation of SV40-immortalised human thyroid epithelial cells by single exposure to plutonium α-particles *in vitro*. *Int.J.Rad.Biol.* 1997; **72**; 515-521.

IODINE DEFICIENCY AND THYROID CANCER MORBIDITY FOLLOWING THE ACCIDENT AT THE CHERNOBYL POWER PLANT

V.V.SHAKHTARIN, A.F.TSYB, V.F.STEPANENKO, E.F.LUSHNIKOV, V.P.SNYKOV, M.YU.ORLOV, S.F.TROFIMOVA

Medical Radiological Research Center of the Russian Academy of Medical Sciences, Obninsk

Findings of the study show that the development of thyroid cancer in populations exposed to radiation from the Chernobyl accident at the children's and juvenile age depends on both radiation dose and level of iodine deficiency in the residence area within existing thyroid doses. At radiation dose of 1 Gy, ERR of thyroid cancer in populations living under conditions of a severe iodine deficiency is almost by two times higher than in those living in the area without iodine deficiency. The programs of prophylaxe of iodine deficiency in arease suffered following the Chernobyl accident may be a real contribution to the reduction of manifestations of radiation induced effects on the thyroid gland.

According to available information, the areas of Belarus, Russia, Ukraine which were contaminated following the Chernobyl accident belong to the zone of iodine endemia [3]. The influence of radiation and iodine deficiency on the development of thyroid cancer, the role of independent etiologic factors is widely discussed in the literature [1,2,4,6,7,9]. Nevertheless, the question about their combined influence on the development of thyroid cancer remains open. In this work, the results of investigation of thyroid cancer morbidity in population (children and adolescents only) with irradiated thyroid gland AND in areas with different levels of iodine deficiency are presented.

The investigation was carried out in the area of Bryansk region including three districts with Cs-137 contamination level up to 40 Ci/km^2, three districts - up to 5 Ci/km^2 and four districts - less than 1 Ci/km^2. In these districts, there are 119.785 people, birth years 1968-1986, who received different thyroid doses as a result of the Chernobyl accident at the children's and juvenile age. Collective absorbed thyroid dose (internal iodine-131 irradiation) was estimated according to a semiempiric model [8]. For the investigated population this the value of this dose is 29452 persons *Gy.

The status of iodine endemia in the area was evaluated according to the recommendations of ICCIDD basing on renal iodine excretion determined by cerium-arsenide method. As criterion of iodine deficiency grade indices of iodine in urine recommended by WHO/UNICEF (1992) were used. In total 3083 people living in 75 settlements of mentioned districts were examined. The main examined group was in the age of children and teenagers (2590 people) - from 4 to 18 years. There were 1283 boys and 1307 girls. We examined 493 adults, 18 - 55 years as well. 162 of them were males and 331 were females. On the basis of our investigation, a chart of providing of the population with iodine in the mentioned region divided into areas with iodine content in urine from > 10,0 mg/dl; 10-7,5 µg/dl; 7,5-5,0 mg/dl and < 5,0 mg/dl. Discrepancies in indices of iodine content between separated areas are significant in all cases (p < 0,001 in all cases). The analysis of iodine deficiency grade and thyroid doses suggests a complex relationship of these indices. Various combinations of thyroid dose and iodine deficiency in the populations are observed.

By 1.07.1998 36 thyroid cancers were detected in investigated population. In 32 cases, international commission verification of morphological diagnosis was performed. In 3 cases, morphological diagnosis was confirmed in the Federal Oncological Center of Russia and in one case, the diagnos was established at the Minsk Research Institute. During medical monitoring, it was found that in April - August 1986, 2 of 36 patients with thyroid cancer were outside the surveyd area. Therefore, only 34 patients were included into the program of the analysis.

Table 1.

Number of observed and expected thyroid cancer within 12 years after the Chernobyl accident in persons, birth years 1968-1986, living in the area with different iodine deficiency and their collective organ dose at the expense of I-131

Renal iodine excretion in the area of residence µg/dl	Number of persons, birth	Collective thyroid dose, persons*Gy	Observed number of cancer		Expected number of cancer	
			abs.	For 100000	abs.	For 100000
< 5,0	8325	2043	3	36,0	0,43	5,21
>5,0 - 7,5	60442	21889	24	38,1	3,15	5,21
>7,5 - 10,0	18178	3617	4	22,0	0,95	5,21
>10,0	32840	1903	3	9,1	1,71	5,21
Total:	119785	29452	34	28,4	6,24	5,21

Table 1 presents the characteristic of 34 hyroid cancers according to sex and morphological form. In females, thyroid cancer occurred by 1,5 times more often than in males. In more yhan 90% of cases, papillary thyroid cancer was diagnosed.

Table 2.

Characteristic of thyroid cancers diagnosed within 12 years after the Chernobyl accident according to sex and histological forms in persons birth years 1968-1986, living in inspected areas

Sex	Histological form	Number of cases	Total
Males	Papillary	12	
	Follicular	1	14
	Carcinoma	1	
Females	Papillary	19	
	Follicular	--	20
	Carcinoma	1	
Total			34

Table 2 gives numbers of people, birth years 1968-1986, living in the areas divided according to iodine deficiency grade, their collective radiation dose as well as observed and expected number of thyroid cancers. For calculation of the expected number of diseases the following information was used: age and sex indices of the morbidity from 0-29 years in Russia in 1991, 1993, 1994 , number of the population according to the data of the State census of the population in the year 1989 in each settlement in the surveyed area and age distribution of the population of Bryansk region according to the data of the State statistics. As index of thyroid cancer morbidity, we used the index of excess relative risk (ERR) which was calculated according to the recommendations of UNSCEAR (1994).

The available date allow to analyse the ERR of thyroid cancer morbidity for different values of collective and mean radiation doses and to determine the change of excess relative risk normed according to a mean adiation dose (ERR/Dm) in different iodine in the area of residence.

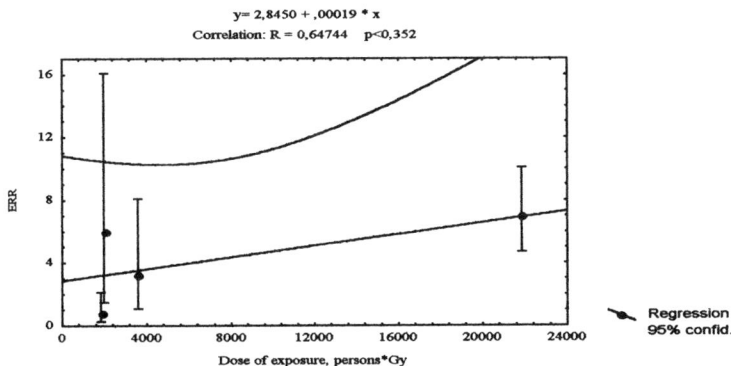

$$y = 2,8450 + ,00019 * x$$
Correlation: R = 0,64744   p<0,352

Fig. 1. Excess relative risk (ERR) of thyroid cancer in different collective organ doses at the expense of I-131

Fig. 1 shows the dependence of ERR on collective thyroid dose. The obtained results suggest the absence of significant dependence of the ERR of thyroid cancer in the given radiation dose range.

y= -0,3979 + 21,379 * X
Correlation: R = 0,95911 p<0,041

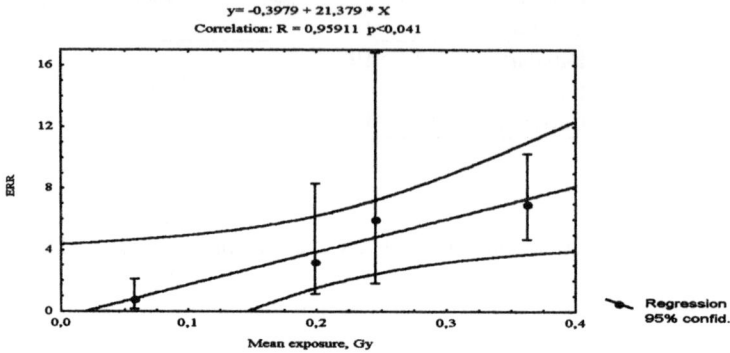

Fig. 2. Excess relative risk (ERR) of thyroid cancer in different mean organ doses at the expense of I-131

Fig. 2 shows the dependence of ERR on mean thyroid dose (Dm) in a range from 0 to 0,4 Gy. The statistical proceding indicates that the dependence of ERR on mean dose can be expressed as follows (as errors two standard deviation are given):

$$ERR = (-0,4 \pm 1,1) + (21,4 \pm 4,5)*Dm \qquad (1)$$

Significance levels for coefficients of the formula (1) are 0,75 and 0,04, i.e. the significance of the Determination of a free member in the formula is small, and the slope (risk coefficient) is determined with a sufficient significance and accuracy of about 20%. This coefficient measures 1/Gy.

y = 27,071 - 1,164 * x
Correlation: r = -0,9595 p<0,04

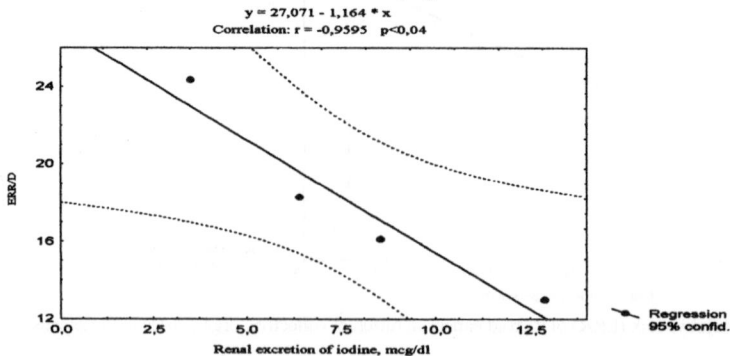

Fig. 3. Relationship of ERR to the level of iodine deficiency, ERR is normalised to thyroid dose of 1 Gy

The determination of the change in the excess relative risk normed according to a mean radiation dose (ERR/Dm) in different iodine deficiency in the area of residence will result in the following dependence:

$$ERR/Dm = (27,1\pm2,1)-(1,16\pm0,24)*I, \qquad (2)$$

where I - mean renal iodine excretion in the residence area in mkg/dl. Both coefficients in the formula (2) are determined with a good accuracy. This conclusion is also confirmed by the significance level of these coefficients - 0,005 and 0,04 relatively. The slope in the formula (2) is in 1/Gy*mkg/dl unit . Coefficient errors in the formulas (1) and (2) are determined through the value of so called "general dispersion calculation " which can be calculated either from the range of points in relation to approximated curve, or from errors of single points . The values of "general dispersion" calculated in such a way differ only slightly. This indicates that errors of risk coefficients were calculated correct.

CONCLUSIONS
Our investigation suggests that the development of thyroid cancer in populations exposed to radiation from the Chernobyl accident at the children's and juvenile age depends on both radiation dose and level of iodine deficiency in the residence area within existing thyroid doses. At radiation dose of 1 Gy, ERR of thyroid cancer in populations living under conditions of a severe iodine deficiency is almost by two times higher than in those living in the area without iodine deficiency. The programs of prophylaxe of iodine deficiency in arease suffered following the Chernobyl accident may be a real contribution to the reduction of manifestations of radiation induced effects on the thyroid gland.

Acknowledgements

Authors are very grateful to:
Prof. S. DAVIS, Fred Hutchinson Cancer Research Center, Seattle, Washington, USA, for very useful discussion and comments to the content of this paper.

This work has been supported in part by Grant N N00014-94-1-0049 issued to Georgetown University from the Office of Naval Research in support of the International Consortium for Research on the Health Effects of Radiation. The contents are solely the responsibility of the authors and do not necessarily reflect the views of the Office of Naval Research or Georgetown University.

282

References

1. Abelin T., Averkin J., Egger M. et al. Thyroid cancer in Belarus post-Chernobyl: improved detection or increased incidence. *Soz Praventivmed* 1994; **39**: 189-197.
2. Delange F. *Iodine nutrition and risk of thyroid irradiation from nuclear accidents. Iodine prophylaxis following nuclear accidents.* Oxford, New-York, Frankfurt, Sao Paulo, Sidney, Tokyo, Toronto, 1988.
3. *Endemic goitre.* Geneva: WHO, 1963. Ed. by F.U.Klemens, De Merlous.
4. Nagataki S., Hirayu H., Izumi M. et al. High prevalence of thyroid nodule in area of radioactive fallout. *Lancet* 1989; **v.2**: p.375.
5. Pinchera A., Fenzi G.F., Mariotti S. et al. Iodine and autoimmune thyroid disease. ln:"Iodine prophylaxis following nuclear accidents". Oxford, New York, Frankfurt, Sao Paulo, Sidney, Tokyo, Toronto, 1988; p.39.
6. Ron E,, Moden B. Benign and malignant thyroid neoplasms after childhood irradiation for tinea capitis. *J.Nat.Cancer Ins.* 1980, **v.65**: p.7.
7. Shore R.E. Human thyroid cancer induction by ionizing radiation: summary of studies based on external irradiation and radioactive iodines. *The radiological consequences of the Chernobyl accident,* EUR 16544 EN, 669-676, Luxembourg, 1996.
8. Stepanenko V.F., Tsyb A.F., Parshkov E.M. et al. Retrospective thyroid absorbed doses estimation in Russia following the Chernobyl accident: progress and application to dosimetrical evaluation of childhood thyroid cancer morbidity. *Effects of low-level radiation for residents near Semipalatinsk nuclear test site,* Edited by M.Hoshi, J.Takada, R.Kim and Y.Nitta, 1996.
9. Tsyb A.F., Parshkov E.M., Shakhtarin V.V. et al. Thyroid cancer in children and adolescents of Bryansk and Kaluga region. *The radiological consequences of the Chernobyl accident,* EUR 16544 EN, 691-698, Luxembourg, 1996.

STUDIES ON THE P53 GENE IN CHILDREN WITH THYROID CANCER FROM BELARUS

C. STREFFER[1], S. HILLEBRANDT[1], F. ZÖLZER[1],
E. MILOSLAVSKAIA[1], E.P. DEMIDCHIK[2], J. BIKO[3] AND CHR. REINERS[3]

[1]Institute of Medical Radiobiology, Essen Germany, [2]Center for Thyroid Cancer, Minsk, Belarus, [3]Clinic of Nuclear Medicine, Würzburg, Germany

We report on changes in the p53 gene in a group of 70 thyroid tumours. 9 tumours showed a polymorphism. The same polymorphisms were also found in the blood cells of these patients. Amongst 68 additional blood samples from children with a thyroid cancer a p53 polymorphism was found in 6 patients. Blood samples of 109 healthy children from Belarus showed only 3 polymorphisms. The comparison of all polymorphisms in children with a thyroid cancer with those in children without a thyroid cancer showed a significant difference (p=0.024). In 34 of the 70 tumours the DNA conte nt was measured by flow cytometry. 4 of these 34 tumours showed a polymorphism in the p53 gene and 2 cancers showed aneuploidy. 2 of the 3 aneuploid tumours showed a polymorphism in the p53 gene. The fact that the polymorphisms found in the tumours was also seen in the blood of these patients does not indicate a direct mutagenic effect in the p53 gene by radiation to the thyroid. However, it appears probable that the observed polymorphisms indicate a certain predisposition for radiation induced cancer.

1 INTRODUCTION

In thyroid tumours mutations of the p53 gene occur rarely suggesting that alterations in this gene may not be important for the development of thyroid tumours [1-3]. On the other hand, there are some studies describing a relatively high frequency of mutations in exons 5-8 of the p53 gene in thyroid tumours [4,5]. The reasons for the different results are not known.

Spontaneous thyroid carcinomas in children are rare and their frequency in Belarus before the Chernobyl accident was between one and two cases per year [6,7]. The reports of increasing numbers of childhood cancer cases after the Chernobyl accident. By far the greatest increase was seen in the Gomel region. This region is situated immediately to the north of Chernobyl and is known to have received a high level of radioactivity as fallout after the breakdown of the reactor.

It has been reported that alterations in the p53 gene may be a potential marker for radiation induced cancer[8]. The authors described p53 mutation hotspots in radon-associated lung cancers from uranium miners. Mutations occurring specifically in such tumours may be an indicator for radiation-induced cancer and could help to distinguish those tumours from cancer that developed spontaneously. For this reason, more investigations on tumours derived from patients exposed to ionizing radiation are needed.

2 RESULTS

The p53 gene was analysed from70 thyroid cancers from children of Belarus. Exons 1-9 and the adjacent introns were amplified by PCR and the polymorphisms were identified with the TGGE method. This method based on the principle that heteroduplexes of DNA molecules have a different melting temperature than DNA-homoduplexes, was described in detail by Hillebrandt et al. (1997)[9].

Nine tumours showed a mutation in the p53 gene, eight of these turned out as a polymorphism (change in the DNA without effect on the protein). The distribution of the polymorphic patterns is shown in Table 1. The same polymorphisms were also found in the blood cells of these patients. A mutation which results in a change in the amino acid sequence of the p53 was observed only in 1 cancer (codon 258, exon 7).

Screening of blood cells from 68 additional children with thyroid cancer indicates that 6 patients display a polymorpism in the p53 gene (exon 6: 3, intron 6: 3). Thyroid tumour samples were not available from these children.

Blood samples of 109 healthy children from Belarus showed 3 polymorphisms in intron 6. The comparison of all polymorphisms in children with a thyroid cancer (15/138) with those from children without a thyroid cancer (3/109) showed a significant difference (p=0.024).

In 34 of the 70 tumours the DNA content was measured by flow cytometry. Only 3 cancers showed aneuploidy. This number is lower than in other reports for thyroid cancer (364 aneuploid cancers out of 526 in 7 studies). However, aneuploid cancers are apparently less frequent in patients with an age below 50 (Table 2). 2 cancers of the 3 aneuploid tumours (this study) showed a polymorphism in the p53 gene, whereas only 2 further polymorphisms were found in the 31 diploid tumours.

Table 1. Polymorphisms and mutations in the p53 gene determined in 70 children with papillary thyroid carcinomas as well as in the blood

Case	Area	Intron/exon	Polymorphism	Coding effect	Blood
O7	Gomel	intron 6	G:C->C:G	none	0
A4	Minsk	exon 6/213	A:T->G:C	none	0
A6	Gomel	exon 6/213	A:T->G:C	none	0
A7	Gomel	exon 7/258	G:C->A:T	Glu->Lys	0
A8	Grodno	exon 6/213	A:T->G:C	none	exon 6/A:T->G:C
B3	Brest	intron 6	G:C->C:G	none	intron6/G:C->C:G
D1	Brest	intron 6	G:C->C:G	none	intron6/G:C->C:G
4N	Gomel	exon 1	x	x	0
7N	Grodno	intron 6	G:C->C:G	none	intron6/G:C->C:G
16N	Brest	intron 6	G:C->C:G	none	0

Table 2. Frequencies of diploid and aneuploid thyroid cancers
-Comparison with literature data

	diploid	aneuploid	total
this study			
number of thyroid cancers	31 (91%)	3(9%)	34 (100%)
patients with polymorphisms	2	2	
literature data			
all age groups	162 (31%)	364 (69%)	522 (100%)
patients younger than 50	72 (96%)	3 (4%)	75 (100%)

3 DISCUSSION

Correlations between polymorphic patterns and cancer development have been described by some authors [10,11]. However, the data don't reveal any association between the p53 codon 213 polymorphism described in this work and the development of tumours.

The second polymorphism observed in the group of thyroid tumours analysed here is a G->C substitution in intron 6, 37 bp upstream of exon 7. Intronic point mutations of the gene could lead to abnormal pre-mRNA splicing and defective protein. Mutations at consensus sequences at either the 5'- or 3'-splice site of intron 6 and 7 were found in human hepatocellular carcinomas[12]. The polymorphism found by us in intron 6 is not located at the consensus sequence of the splice sites, but in the region of the branch site also involved in splicing. However, we do not know, whether this polymorphism could be involved in the splicing process.

Sequence alterations in introns could also influence binding of transcription factors to the DNA and thus change the expression of tumour suppressor genes. In particular, a helical distortion as a consequence of intronic sequence alterations could prevent binding of proteins to the DNA. It was suggested, that some intronic polymorphisms may predispose towards coding-region mutations that increase the likelihood of a deleterious phenotype[13].

The differences in the p53 sequence found in the thyroid tumours of children from the regions around Chernobyl are also observed in blood cells (lymhocytes) of the patients.This observation does not indicate a direct mutagenic effect in the p53 gene by radiation exposure to the thyroid. However, it appears probable that the observed polymorphisms indicate a certain predisposition for radiation induced cancer. The fact that most tumours with a polymorphism in the p53 gene also show aneuploidy, can be taken as an indication of a relationship between the observed polymorphisms and a genetic instability which may promote tumour induction. However, the number of observed cases is very small.

References

1. Wright PA, Lemone NR, Goretzki PE, Wyllie FS, Bond J, Hughes C. Mutations of the p53 in differentiated human thyroid carcinomas. Oncogene 1991; **6**: 1693-1697.
2. Dokhorn-Dworniczak B, Schröder S, Dantchewa R, Tötsch M, Stücker A, Brömmelkampf E, Banfalvi A, Böcker W, Schmid, KW. The role of the p53 tumor suppressor gene in human thyroid cancer. Exp Clin Endocrinol 1993; **10**: 39-46.
3. Ito T, Seyama T, Mizuno T, Tsuyama T, Hayashi Y, Dohi N, Nakamura N, Akiyama M. Unique association of p53 mutations with undifferentiated but not with differentiated carcinomas of the thyroid glands. Cancer Res 1992; **52**: 1369-1371.
4. Greenblatt, MS, Bennett WP, Hollstein M, Harris, CC. Mutations in the p53 tumour suppressor gene: clues to cancer etiology and molecular pethogenesis 1994; **54**: 4855-4878.
5. Zou M, Shi Y, Farad NR. p53 mutations in all stages of thyroid carcinomas . J Clin Endocrinol Metab 1993; **77**: 1054-1058.
6. Baverstock K, Egloft P, Pinchera A, Ruchti C, Williams D. Thyroid cancer after Chernobyl. Nature 1992; **359**: 21-22.
7. Williams D, Pinchera A, Karaouglu A, Chadwick KH. Thyroid cancer in children living near Chernobyl, Commission of the European Communities, Radiation Protection Research and Training Programme 1993: 1-108.
8. Taylor JA, Watson MA, Devereux TR, Michels RY, Saccomanno M, Anderson M. p53 mutation hotspot in radon-associated lung cancer. Lancet 1994; **343**: 86-87.
9. Hillebrandt S, Streffer C, Demidchik EP, Biko J, Reiners Chr. Polymorphisms in the p53 gene in thyroid tumours and blood samples of children from areas in Belarus. Mutat Res 1997; **381**: 201-207.
10. Gaidano G, Ballerini P, Gong JZ, Inghirami G, Neri A, Newcomb EW, Magrath IT, Knowles DM, Dalla-Favera R. p53 mutations in human lymphoid malignancies: association with Burkitt lymphoma and chronic lymphocytic leukemia. Proc Natl Acad Sci USA 1991; **88**: 5413-5417.
11. Ilhan I, Erekul S, Atesalp S, Ihan O, Ankar N. p53 codon 213 (A->G) polymorphism in a Turkish population. Pediat Hematol Oncol 1995; **12**:499-501.
12. Lai MY, Chang HC, Li HP, Ku CK, Chen PJ, Shcu JC, Huang GZ, Lee PH, Chen DS. Splicing mutations of the p53 gene in human hepatocellular carcinoma. Cancer Res 1993; **53**: 1653-1656.
13. Malkinson AM, Ming Y. The intronic structure of cancer-related genes regulates susceptibility to cancer. Mol Carcinogen 1994; **10**: 61-65.

THYROID CANCER AND IODINE DEFICIENCY IN CHILDREN OF BELARUS

A.G..MROTCHEK, E.P. DEMIDCHIK, A.N.ARINCHIN, S.V.PETRENKO,
I.M.KHMARA AND K.V.MOSCHIK
*Research and Clinical Institute of Radiation Medicine and Endocrinology,
Ministry of Health, Republic of Belarus; Masherov av.23, Minsk, Belarus*

M.GEMBICKI
University of Medical Sciences, Al. Przybyszewskiego 49, PL-60-355, Poznan, Poland;

K.BAVERSTOCK
*European Centre for Environment and Health, Rome Division, WHO European Bureau, Via
Francesco Crispi, 10, 00187, Rome, Italy.*

As the result of the conducted studies on iodine deficiency among 7777 children and adolescents from Gomel, Minsk and Brest Regions (oblast) within the frame of the joint with WHO European Bureau project as the factor of origin and development of thyroid diseases, it has been ascertained that most pronounced relationship between the level of iodine deficiency and the number of thyroid cancer cases in children was observed in the districts of Gomel and Brest regions most exposed to radioactive contamination with iodine-131.

In the early post-Chernobyl period the main sources of irradiation were short-lived radionuclides of iodine which caused such great contamination that the level of exposure received by the population was estimated as "iodine impact". According to the map of iodine-131 distribution in soil at the territory of the Republic of Belarus for 10.05.1986[1], southern district of Gomel and Brest Regions appeared to be the most contaminated. Iodine-131 intake by inhalation and through the gastrointestinal tract caused the formation of large exposure doses to the thyroid gland in all the children population of the given Regions.

One of the main and serious health effects of the Chernobyl accident is the considerable growth of the incidence of malignant thyroid tumors both among children and adolescents and grown-ups of the Republic. Statistically significant increase in the incidence of thyroid carcinoma in children's population of Belarus was registered 5 years following the accident - in 1992[2]. The highest incidence level is marked in Gomel, Brest and Minsk Regions. The number of children who had fallen ill with thyroid cancer during 1986-1997, made 574 cases, 505 (88%) of which were from Gomel, Brest and Minsk Regions, in particular, 305 - from Gomel Region, 135 - from Brest Region and 65 - from Minsk Region.

At present, in fact of the radiation induced nature of thyroid cancer in children of Belarus is universally recognized. At the same time, the availability of a number of factors contributing to the formation of oncological thyroid pathology is being discussed. Among such factors, iodine deficiency is of particular importance. The Republic of Belarus is the endemic goiter territory which is caused by a low content of stable iodine in soil. This leads to the development of iodine deficiency in the population. Iodine deficiency is most pronounced in the southern districts of Gomel and Brest Regions which can be attributed to the geological and chemical peculiarities of the given regions. Before 1980, iodine prophylaxis was organized at the governmental level through the administration of stable iodine in the form of "antistrumin". The given prophylaxis was conducted both at the individuals and group levels (in kindergardens, secondary schools, institutions and enterprises). This resulted in the decrease of the endemic goiter incidence which was the reason to complete the iodine prophylaxis in 1986.

Radioactive contamination of air and soil with a wide spectrum of radionuclides of iodine during the first weeks after the accident caused the formation of the exposure dose to the thyroid gland which was a "risk" organ at this time. Lack of purposeful iodine prophylaxis and the presence of iodine deficiency caused by the geographical peculiarities of the territory of the Republic, especially of its southern regions were the factors which contributed to radiation damage of the thyroid gland in children.

According to the results of the joint international study of iodine deficiency in 7777 children of Gomel, Brest and Minsk Regions and its role in the development of the observed thyroid pathology in children of Belarus implemented within the frames of the WHO European Bureau Program, it has been ascertained that in Gomel, Minsk and Brest Regions, heterogeneity in the degree of iodine deficiency and goiter expression was observed. At present, the most favorable situation, as to iodine supplementation, was observed in Gomel Region (median of urine iodine excretion made 79.8µg/l (59.2-106.7)).

At the same time, it was just that region where the greatest number of thyroid cancer cases was registered. In the neighboring Minsk and Brest Regions, pronounced iodine deficiency was observed (median of urine iodine excretion - 38.1 µg/l (25.9-73.7) and 27.3 µg/l (16.9-39.9), accordingly. The comparison of data about iodine deficiency and thyroid cancer cases in children are given in the Table 1.

Table 1. Iodine status and number of thyroid cancer cases in children of Gomel, Brest and Minsk Regions of Belarus.

Region	Median of urine iodine excretion, µg/l	Number of children with iodine deficiency (<50 µg/l), %	Number of thyroid cancer cases in children
Gomel	79.8	27.1	305

table 1 (continuation)

Brest	27.3	74.9	135
Minsk	38.1	63.0	65

It is to suppose that before 1986, Gomel, Minsk and Brest Regions had approximately the same degree of iodine deficiency which appeared to be one of the reasons for the enhanced accumulation of radioactive isotopes of iodine by the thyroid gland straight away after the accident and caused the formation of the exposure dose to this organ. Anti-goiter measurements (administration of iodine preparations, consumption of food-stuffs enriched with iodine and polyvitamin complexes with microelements, etc.) conducted in Gomel Region after the accident improved the state of iodine supplementation of children and adolescents at present. Though in Minsk and Brest Regions the situation remained to be the same.

The conducted analysis of the relationship between the number of thyroid cancer cases and the level of iodine deficiency of children's population from all the districts of Gomel and Brest Regions didn't show any significant connection between the studied parameters (Table 2).

Table 2. Comparative characteristics of iodine deficiency and the number of thyroid cancer cases in children from some districts of Gomel and Brest Regions.

District	Median of urine iodine excretion, $\mu g/l$	Number of children with iodine deficiency (<50 $\mu g/l$), %	Number of thyroid cancer cases in children
Gomel Region			
Gomel	79.8	24.4	99
Elsk	85.1	24.5	5
Petrikov	64.0	37.5	3
Octyabrsky	94.1	22.9	0
Zhlobin	106.7	14.3	8
Bragin	59.2	39.6	17
Brest Region			
Brest	39.9	62.6	9
Lyakhovichi	16.9	86.2	1
Stolin	24.7	82.2	26
Pinsk	33.4	68.7	33
Bereza	25.9	75.0	6

It was caused by the fact that not all the districts of Brest Region were exposed to "iodine impact" and the effect of radionuclides of iodine was not significant there. Taking this into account, the relationship between the level of the incidence of thyroid cancer and the iodine status was studied in the districts exposed to the highest level of radioactive contamination with iodine-131 (Fig.1).

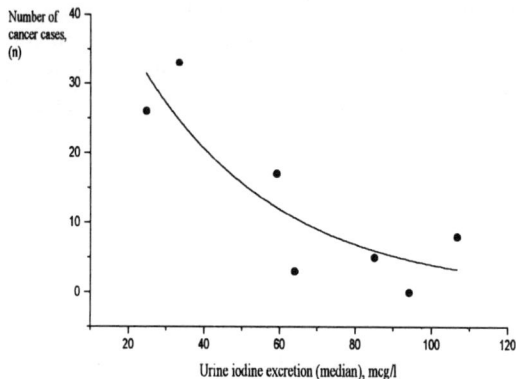

Fig.1. Dependence between the median of iodine excretion and the number of thyroid cancer cases in children residing in the districts of Gomel and Brest Regions exposed to radioactive contamination with iodine-131

The given picture shows that in the districts exposed to "iodine impact", negative exponential dependence is observed between the number of thyroid cancer cases and the iodine status, i.e. the less is the median of urine iodine excretion, the greater number of thyroid cancer cases is observed in children. This confirms the role of iodine deficiency in the occurrence and the development of malignant thyroid tumors in children's population of the Republic exposed to the effect of radionuclides of iodine early after the Chernobyl accident.

Thus, iodine deficiency developed as a result of natural (geochemical) peculiarities of the territory of Belarus and the lack of purposeful system of iodine prophylaxis, appeared to be one of the important etiologic and pathogenetic factors of the increase in malignant thyroid neoplasm in children of the republic following the Chernobyl accident.

References

1. Consequences of the Chernobyl accident in the Republic of Belarus. National report. Edited by Konoplya E.F. and Rolevitch I.V. Minsk, 1996:95.
2. Demidchik E.P. et all Thyroid cancer in children in Belarus *The radiological consequences of the Chernobyl accident* 1996:677-682.

THYROID CANCER IN CHILDREN OF BELARUS AND IMMUNITY

T.VORONTSOVA, E.SHAVROVA, Y.DEMIDTCHIK, E.CHERSTVOY, E.KUTCHINSKAYA and V.POZARSKAYA

Research and clinical institute of radiation medicine and endocrinology, Minsk, Belarus

Minsk state medical institute, Belarus

In the present study we made an attempt to reveal the role of immune system in the pathogenesis of thyroid carcinoma in children. The study group included 162 patients (95 females and 67 males) with papillary thyroid carcinoma diagnosed when they were under 15 years old. Significant difference of distribution of various lymphocytes phenotypes in peripheral blood and fine-needle aspirates was observed: OKT3/OKB19 ratio was higher in blood then in aspirates (5.15 vs 3.1, p< 0,001). At the same time ratio OKT4/OKT8 cells was essentially lower in aspirates then in blood (1,0 vs 2,2 ,p<0,01). Our data indicate that high proportion of children (49,1%) had lymphocytic infiltration of thyroid. Comparison of the autoantibodies levels in groups of children with and without lymphocytic infiltration demonstrated that in the group with LIT the levels of AB-TG as well as were AB-TPO significantly higher (p< 0,01). It was registered that lymphocytic infiltration is more frequent in girls, then in boys(sex ratio 2,2:1,0).

This couldn't be to the fact of autoimmune phenomena since the frequency of antibody positive patients is identical in both groups (sex ratio 1:1). Our results demonstrate that the immune system takes part in the pathogenesis of thyroid cancer in children who were irradiated.

Introduction

It is known that from the moment of its formation and in the process of its development, malignant tissue is in close contact with the immunocompetent cells infiltrating the tumor. Lymphocytic infiltration may be located both within the tumor area and outside it. In separate cases, both intratumorous and peritumorous location of lymphoid infiltration is registered. Though lymphoid infiltration of a number of tumors has been studied long enough, its role, both functional and prognostic, is not absolutely clear. Even with regard to similar tumors, literary data are extremely contradictory [1,2].

The published data show, that morphological and functional characteristics of lymphoid infiltration of a tumor, which reflect the reactions of antitumorigenic immunity, cannot have a definitive interpretation of the tumor's "behaviour" without taking into account the whole complex of complicated and dynamic immunological relations existing between the tumor and different populations of lymphocytes.[3,4,5,6,7]

The aim of our investigation was to evaluate the lymphocytic infiltration of thyroid (LIT) and autoimmune phenomena in pathogenesis of thyroid carcinoma.

Subjects and methods

The study group included 162 patients (95 females and 67 males) with papillary thyroid carcinoma diagnosed when they were under 15 years old. All of them were undergoing fine-needle aspiration before the operation. In 57 of them, a sufficient number of lymphocytes was obtained for further study of the phenotype. At the same time, venous blood was collected in heparinised syringes for the investigation of the lymphocyte phenotype.

Monoclonal antibodies OKT3, OKT4, OKT8, OKT-NK and OKB19 were obtained from Ortho Diagnostic (Germany). Two-colored analysis was carried out on a flow cytometer (Cytoron ORTHO).

Antithyroperoxidase autoantobodies (AB-TPO) and antithyroglobulin autoantibodies (AB-TG) were measured by RIA (Medipan Diagnostica, Germany; normal range <40 U/ml).

Results

As reported in Table 1, a slight decrease of OKT3+ and OKT4+ lymphocyte in the peripheral blood has been shown. The level of OKT8+ was significantly higher and OKT-NK lower ($p<0.01$) than in healthy patients. As it was suggested, the number of lymphocytes in fine-needle aspirates was lower than in blood. The distribution of different phenotypes of lymphocytes in aspirates was distinguished from blood. OKT3/OKB19 ratio was significantly higher in blood than in aspirates (5.15 vs. 3.1; $p<0.01$). The proportion of the OKT4+ and OKT8+ T cell subsets showed a significant reduction (1.04 vs. 2.23; $p<0.001$). Subset of OKT-NK lymphocytes essentially decreased in blood (3.1+0.8%), in aspirates it was practically undetectable (0.3+0.02%).

Table1. Surface phenotype of peripheral blood lymphocytes
and lymphocytes from fine-needle aspirates

| Type of | Sours of cell | |
lymphocyte	Blood	Aspirate
OKT-3 %	65,5 ± 1,8	32,3 ± 4,1
OKT-3 cell/ml	577 ± 121,0	28 ± 4,2
OKT-4 %	46,4 ± 1,1	19,4 ± 1,3
OKT-4 cell/ml	489 ± 48,0	12 ± 2,1
OKT-8 %	20,8 ± 1,1	18,6 ± 3,1
OKT-8 cell/ml	251 ± 34,0	11 ± 1,0
OKT-19 %	12,7 ± 1,0	10,1 ± 1,2
OKT-19 cell/ml	146 ± 26,0	9 ± 1
OKT-NK %	3,6 ± 0,2	0,03 ±0,02
OKT-NK ctll/ml	61 ± 1,4	1 ± 0,5

30 (18.5%) of 162 children with thyroid carcinoma had a positive level of AB-Tg and AB-TPO. A significant difference was still found when analyzing the prevalence of autoantibodies in the group of children whose lymphocytes from aspirates were investigated - 25 (43.8%) of 57 were positive for antithyroid antibodies.

The fact of the presence of a comparatively large amount of lymphocytes in thyroid punctates made it possible to assume the availability of lymphoid infiltration in these patients. To test this assumption, a retrospective analysis of 162 histological preparations from malignant thyroid tumors of children was conducted aimed at revealing of lymphoid infiltration. In histological preparations from 82 children (50.9%), lymphoid infiltration was not revealed. In 49.1% of cases (80 patients), lymphohistocytic thyroid infiltration was marked. Most often, lymphocyte clusters were determined in the thyroid stroma outside the tumor (44 cases) which made 55% of the whole number of cases with lymphoid infiltration . In 14 children (17.5%), LIT was located intratumorously .In 22 children (27,5%), LIT was manifested both in tumorous and intact thyroid tissue .

The comparative analysis of the 4 groups singled out according to age, volume of the performed operation, size of tumor and the extension of tumorous process, revealed no distinctions both among the groups with and without lymphoid infiltration, as well as with different localisation of the infiltration itself. Interesting results were obtained by us during the analysis of the manifestation of lymphoid infiltration and the patients' sex. In the whole of the examined group, the girls/boys ratio made 1.42, but in the group of children without lymphoid infiltration it was 0.95. In children with peritumorous infiltration it was equal to 2.38; in cases with the infiltration outside the tumor, the sex ratio made 3.66; with lymphoid infiltration located both inside and outside the tumor, it corresponded to the average value observed within the whole group, i.e. 1.44.

As to the manifestation of the autoimmune reaction, as it is seen from Fig.1, it made 18.5% for the whole of the group. But it appeared that the frequency of its manifestation depends on the localization of lymphoid infiltration. In the group of patients where the lymphoid infiltration was not revealed, antibodies to thyroid antigenes were observed in 10.9 % of patients. In the group with peritumorous infiltration, antibodies were registered in 16.2% of patients. With intratumorous infiltration, the enhanced level autoantibodies was registered in 28.5% of patients; and with thyroid infiltration, both inside and outside the tumor, antibodies were revealed in 43.4% of patients.

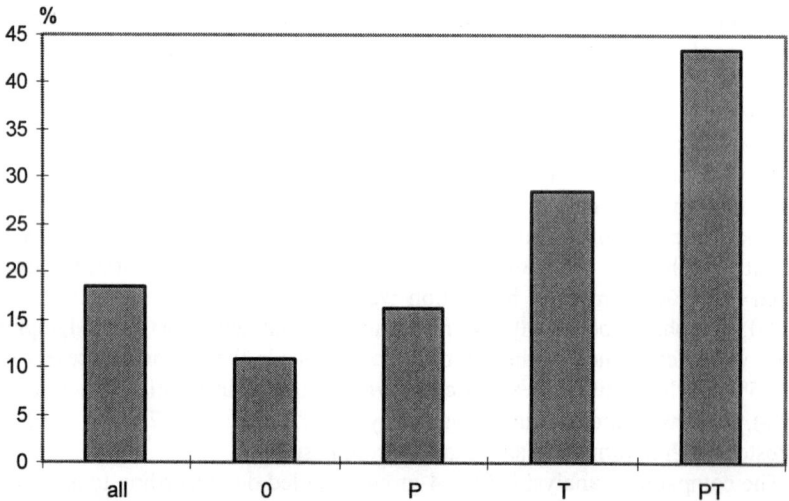

Fig.1. Distribution of children with positive autoantiboolies depending on location of LIT

0 - without infiltration
P - extratumor
T - intratumor
PT - extratumor + intratumor

Discussion

In the present study we made an attempt to reveal the role of immune system in the pathogenesis of thyroid carcinoma in children. Significant difference of distribution of various lymphocytes phenotypes in peripheral blood and fine-needle aspirates was observed: OKT3/OKB19 ratio was higher in blood then in aspirates (5.15 vs 3.1, p< 0,001). At the same time ratio OKT4/OKT8 cells was essentially lower in aspirates then in blood (1,0 vs 2,2 ,p<0,01). According to the some literary data the decrease of OKT4 lymphocytes level in lymphocytic infiltrate is unfavourable prognostic index [8].

Our data indicate that high proportion of children (49,1%) had lymphocytic infiltration of thyroid. Comparison of the autoantibodies levels in groups of children with and without lymphocytic infiltration demonstrated that in the group with LIT the levels of AB-TG as well as AB-TPO were significantly higher (p< 0,01). It was registered that lymphocytic infiltration is more frequent in girls, then in boys(sex ratio 2,2:1,0). This couldn't be to the fact of autoimmune phenomena since the frequency of antibody positive patients is identical in both groups(sex ratio 1:1).

In summary, our results demonstrate that the immune system takes part in the pathogenesis of thyroid cancer in children who were irradiated. The mechanisms involved are not clear , but they include general immunity, as well as local immunity. Undoubtedly, autoimmune reaction is also involved in pathogenesis of the radiation-induced thyroid tumor.

References

1.Ogmundsdottir HM, Peturssdottir I, Gudmundstottir I.Interaction between the immune system and breast cancer. *Acta Oncol* 1995; **34(5)**:647-650.
2. WeiWZ, Heppner GH. Breast cancer immunology. *Cancer-Treat-Res.* 1996; **83**: 395-410.
3. Riemann D, Wenzel K, Schulz T, Hofmann S, Neef H, Lautenschlager C, Langner J. Phenotypic analysis of T lymphocytes isolated from non-small-cell lung cancer. *Int-Arch-Allergy-Immunol.* 1997 Sep; **114(1)**: 38-45.
4. Angevin E, Kremer F, Gaudin C, Hercend T, Triebel F. Analysis of T-cell immune response in renal cell carcinoma: polarization to type 1-like differentiation pattern, clonal T-cell expansion and tumor-specific cytotoxicity. *Int-J-Cancer.* 1997 Jul 29; **72(3)**: 431-440.
5. Goedegebuure PS, Eberlein TJ. The role of CD4+ tumor-infiltrating lymphocytes in human solid tumors.*Immunol-Res.* 1995;**14(2)**: 119-131.

6. Hakansson A,0 Gustafsson B, Krysander L, Hakansson L.Tumour-infiltrating lymphocytes in metastatic malignant melanoma and response to interferon alpha treatment. *Br-J-Cancer.* 1996 Sep; **74(5)**: 670-676.

7. Lee RS, Schlumberger M, Caillou B, Pages F, Fridman WH, Tartour-E. Phenotypic and functional characterisation of tumour-infiltrating lymphocytes derived from thyroid tumours. *Eur-J-Cancer.* 1996 Jun; **32A(7)**: 1233-1239.

8. Bell MC, Edwards RP, Partridge EE, Kuykendall K, Conner W, Gore H, Turbat-Herrara E, Crowley-Nowick PA.CD8+ T lymphocytes are recruited to neoplastic cervix. *J-Clin-Immunol.* 1995 May; **15(3)**: 130-136.

THYROID DOSE ASSESSMENT: AN OVERVIEW OF THE PROBLEMS AND SOLUTIONS

A. BOUVILLE

National Cancer Institute, EPN-530, Bethesda, MD 20892, USA
E-mail: ab76o@nih.gov

Within a few weeks following the Chernobyl accident, about half a million "direct thyroid measurements" (measurements of exposure rate by means of a detector placed against the neck) were made among the populations of Belarus, Russia, and Ukraine that resided in the contaminated areas. The assessment of the thyroid doses received by specified or representative individuals in those countries is based on the results provided by the direct thyroid measurements: (1) doses to the measured individuals are derived from the direct thyroid measurements, using additional information or assumptions on their lifestyle and dietary habits; (2) doses to unmeasured residents of localities where a sufficient number of direct thyroid measurements were made are inferred from the statistical distribution of the measured doses in those localities; and (3) doses to unmeasured residents of localities with no or very few direct thyroid measurements are assessed by means of an environmental transfer model, based on the measurements of activities of ^{137}Cs deposited on the ground and calibrated using information on measured doses from the nearest areas where such data are abundant.

In the U.S. and in Russia, consideration also is currently given to the assessment of thyroid doses from ^{131}I resulting from atmospheric releases of radioactive materials in the early days (1940s and 1950s) of the nuclear weapons complex (fuel reprocessing plants at Hanford and Chelyabinsk; nuclear weapons tests at the Nevada and the Semipalatinsk Test Sites). Because ^{131}I was not measured (with few exceptions) at that time, the thyroid dose assessment is based on the analysis of gross beta or gamma historical measurements, together with environmental transfer models.

The purpose of this paper is to present an overview of the methods used to estimate thyroid doses, as well as of the problems encountered when using those methods. Solutions to some of those problems (or at least possible improvements) also are discussed.

1 INTRODUCTION

The assessment of thyroid doses resulting from substantial releases of radioiodines, especially ^{131}I, in the atmosphere has evolved considerably since the 1940s, as the measurements became closer and closer to the target endpoint, the human thyroid. It is well known now that, under most circumstances, the pasture-cow-milk pathway is the main contributor to the thyroid dose. However, until the mid-1950s, it was thought that inhalation was responsible for the thyroid doses arising from the presence of radioiodines into the environment, and ^{131}I was not singled out as a particular radiological hazard. The environmental radiation programs related to the first nuclear weapons tests conducted in the late 1940s and the early 1950s at Semipalatinsk in Kazakhstan and at the Nevada Test Site in the U.S. consisted essentially of measurements of exposure rates around the site [3,16]. Measurements around the nuclear fuel reprocessing plants of Hanford in the U.S. and of Chelyabinsk in Russia during the early years of operation when the atmospheric releases of ^{131}I were of the order of 1 PBq a^{-1} also were very crude as they included mainly exposure rates and total beta activities of environmental samples [4, 6]. It is only in 1957 that the U.S. Public Health Service initiated a relatively large program of measurement of ^{131}I concentrations in cows' milk [2] and that cows' milk was systematically monitored in England after the Windscale accident [5]. In the 1960s, high-yield nuclear weapons tests were detonated, resulting in substantial radioactive contamination of the environment of the northern hemisphere; the assessment of the thyroid doses from those high-yield tests was based on the results of measurements of ^{131}I concentrations in milk [19]. The same procedure was used when the Chernobyl accident occurred, in April 1986, and ^{131}I was detected in most countries of the northern hemisphere [20]. In addition, for the first time in history, large-scale measurements of exposure rate near the thyroid were made in the most contaminated areas of Belarus, Russia, and Ukraine in order to estimate the ^{131}I content of the thyroid of the affected populations [7, 13, 17].

The main purpose of this paper is to describe how the direct thyroid measurements have been used to estimate thyroid doses, what problems have been encountered, and how the dose estimates could be improved in the future. A description of the manner in which the thyroid doses due to atmospheric releases of ^{131}I in Russia and in the U.S. in the 1940s and the early 1950s are reconstructed is also provided.

A distinction will be made between: (1) personal doses, for which personal information regarding the individuals considered is obtained by means of interviews or questionnaires, and (2) group doses, in which generic values of the whereabouts or dietary habits of the population are used. Personal doses are generally required in epidemiological studies, while group doses are used for the estimation of representative values of the dose levels.

2 ESTIMATION OF THE THYROID DOSES RESULTING FROM THE CHERNOBYL ACCIDENT

Within the framework of this Symposium, the interest is focused on the personal thyroid doses received in Belarus, Russia, and Ukraine, in particular by the residents of the contaminated areas.

The assessment of the thyroid doses from ^{131}I is based on the results of the measurements of external gamma radiation performed within a few weeks after the accident by means of radiation devices placed against the neck of people. These measurements are usually called "direct thyroid measurements". For the individuals who were not measured, but who lived in areas where many persons had been measured, the thyroid doses are reconstructed on the basis of the statistical distribution of the thyroid doses estimated for the people with thyroid measurements, together with the knowledge of the dietary habits of the individuals who are considered. Finally, the thyroid doses for persons who lived in areas with very few or no direct thyroid measurements within a few weeks after the accident are reconstructed by means of relationships using available data on ^{131}I or ^{137}Cs deposition, exposure rates, ^{137}Cs whole-body burdens, or concentrations of ^{131}I in milk.

Even though the presence of ^{131}I in the thyroid accounts, in general, for most of the thyroid dose, there are other pathways of exposure that may need to be taken into consideration: (1) internal irradiation due to the intake of short-lived radioiodines, mainly ^{132}I and ^{133}I, and of ^{132}Te, which is the precursor of ^{132}I, (2) internal irradiation due to the intake of long-lived radionuclides, mainly ^{134}Cs and ^{137}Cs, and (3) external irradiation from radionuclides deposited on the ground and building materials. So far, limited attention has been paid to these additional pathways of exposure.

2.1 Doses from ^{131}I to measured individuals

About half a million "direct thyroid measurements" were made among the populations of Belarus, Russia, and Ukraine that resided in the contaminated areas [7, 13, 17]. Most of the measurements were made in field conditions, sometimes by inexperienced people, by means of many types of devices. Some instruments were collimated, and others were not. Usually, individuals were measured only once, so that only the dose rate at the time of measurement can be readily derived from the measurement. In order to calculate the thyroid dose, the variation of the dose rate with time needs to be assessed. This is done by calculation, and is dependent upon the relative rate of intake of ^{131}I, both before and after the measurement, and upon the metabolism of radioiodine in the body, which may have been modified by the intake of stable iodine for prophylactic purposes. There are therefore two independent steps in the assessment of the "measured" thyroid doses: (1) the determination of the dose rate at the time of measurement, and (2) the estimation of the temporal variation of the thyroid dose rate.

The problems associated with the determination of the dose rate at the time of measurement vary according to the type of device that was used and to the conditions of measurement:

- for all types of devices, large uncertainties may have occurred when the calibration coefficient was not measured, or when the detector was not positioned correctly against the thyroid,
- for non-collimated devices, correct subtraction of the background was not carried out systematically. Errors could have been important for measurements made a few days after the accident if the measured individuals wore contaminated clothes, and also for measurements made a few weeks after the accident, at a time when most of the ^{131}I has decayed and the body burden of radiocesium was relatively important.

The problems associated with the estimation of the temporal variation of the thyroid dose rate result from an incorrect assessment of the environmental conditions or of the individual intakes of ^{131}I and of stable iodine:

- the fallout of ^{131}I was usually assumed to have occurred only in the course of one day. In fact, measurements [14] show that fallout in many locations took place over a number of days, thus affecting the variation of the ^{131}I concentrations in air and in foodstuffs,
- the estimation of the personal thyroid dose depends on the reliability of the answers provided by the individual in a personal interview with regard to many factors, including: (1) the origin of the consumed milk, (2) the length of time during which contaminated milk was consumed, and (3) information on the intake of stable iodine for prophylactic purposes. Most individuals do not remember these factors with accuracy.

2.2 Passport doses from ^{131}I

For the individuals who were not measured, but who lived in localities where at least 10 persons had been measured, the thyroid doses are reconstructed on the basis of the statistical distribution of the thyroid doses estimated for the people with thyroid measurements, stratified according to age. For such localities, group doses are tabulated for 19 age categories (year by year from 0 to 18 adults) and for 5 values of milk comsumption rates, ranging from 0 to 4 Ld^{-1} [7]. Individual doses are then obtained using answers from personal interviews regarding the dietary habits of the individuals who are considered.

2.3 Modeled doses from ^{131}I

The thyroid doses for persons who lived in areas with very few or no direct thyroid measurements within a few weeks after the accident are reconstructed by means of relationships using available data on ^{131}I or ^{137}Cs deposition densities, exposure rates, ^{137}Cs whole-body burdens, or concentrations of ^{131}I in milk. Different empirical approaches have been used in the three Republics of the former Soviet Union with highly contaminated areas (Ukraine, Belarus, and Russia):

- In the Chernigov region of Ukraine, the following empirical relationships were obtained [12]: $D(T) = K \times a^{\exp(-b \times T)}$ [1]
  where: $D(T)$, in cGy, is the thyroid dose for age T (y),
  a (unitless) is a parameter representing the thyroid dose at age 0
  b (y^{-1}) is a parameter describing the age dependence of the thyroid dose
  K (cGy) is a scaling parameter characterizing the radioiodine intake, calculated according to:

$\log (K) = 640 \times (\log (\sigma(^{137}Cs)) / \rho^2) + 2.7 \times \cos(\varphi) + 0.013 \times p \times \sin(\varphi) - 1.6$ [2]

where: σ (^{137}Cs) is the ^{137}Cs deposition at the location considered, ρ (km) and φ are the polar coordinates of that location with respect to the Chernobyl site.

- In Belarus, a relationship has been established between the average thyroid dose received by people in a rural settlements and the ground-deposition density of radionuclides (^{137}Cs or ^{131}I) in the settlement and in the area around the settlement [7]. For the settlements in the Hoiniki in Gomel oblast, and in Kostukovichi and Krasnopolye in the Mogilev oblast:

D_{jr} (adult) $= 3.5 \times 10^{-8} \times \sigma_r (^{131}I) + 1.4 \times 10^{-8} \times \sigma_{jr}(^{131}I)$ [3]

            $= 3.5 \times 10^{-8} \times R_r \times \sigma_r(^{137}Cs) + 1.4 \times 10^{-8} \times R_{jr} \times \sigma_{jr}(^{137}Cs)$ [4]

where: D_{jr} (adult) is the arithmetic mean thyroid dose, in Gy, for the adult population in the settlement, j, in area, r, in the absence of any countermeasures in the settlement and for typical lifestyle and dietary habits,

    $\sigma_r(^{131}I)$, $\sigma_r(^{137}Cs)$ is the average ground-deposition density, in Bq m^{-2}, of ^{131}I or ^{137}Cs, in area, r,

    $\sigma_{jr}(^{131}I)$, $\sigma_{jr}(^{137}Cs)$ is the average ground-deposition density, in Bq m^{-2}, of ^{131}I or ^{137}Cs, in the settlement, j, in area, r,

    R_r, R_{jr} is the average ratio of the ^{131}I to ^{137}Cs ground-deposition densities in area, r, or in the settlement, j, in area, r.

It can be expected that, on average in an area, $\sigma_{jr}(^{131}I) = \sigma_r(^{131}I)$, so that the average relationship between ^{131}I deposition density and the average adult thyroid dose is:

D_r(adult) $= 4.9 \times 10^{-8} \times \sigma_r(^{131}I)$ [5]

Ongoing research may clarify whether equations 3 and 4 are generally applicable to all contaminated areas of Belarus [7] and Russia [17]. It is likely that correction coefficients that take into account the role of fuel particles, and parameters such as the standing crop biomass, the fraction of cow's intake from pasture grass, and the date of the beginning of cow's pasture will need to be factored in [7].

- In Russia, Zvonova and Balonov [22] analyzed the thyroid measurements and radiation survey data for the Bryansk and Tula oblasts. The thyroid doses derived from direct thyroid measurements for 3- to 6-year old children were found to be correlated with the ^{137}Cs ground-deposition density, the kerma rate in air on May 10-12, 1986 (i.e, 14 to 16 days after the beginning of the accident), the mean ^{131}I concentration in milk in the period May 5-12, 1986, and the average radiocesium content in adults in July-August, 1986. With respect to the ^{137}Cs ground-deposition density, the following relationship was obtained:

$$D(3\text{-}6) = (76 \times 10^{-8}) \, \sigma \, (^{137}Cs) \tag{6}$$

where: $D(3\text{-}6)$ is the average thyroid dose for 3- to 6-year old children (Gy), and $\sigma \, (^{137}Cs)$ is the ^{137}Cs ground-deposition density (Bq m^{-2}).

According to Zvonova and Balonov [22], the average ratio of the deposition densities of ^{131}I and ^{137}Cs was approximately 8 immediately after the period of intense deposition, so that:

$$D(3\text{-}6) = (9.5 \times 10^{-8}) \, \sigma \, (^{131}I) \tag{7}$$

The main problem associated with these empirical methods is that they are based on environmental data that are sparse or rather uncertain. However, their development should be encouraged, as: (1) they represent the only feasible technique of dose reconstruction in some areas and can conceptually be used for any affected individual, and (2) they can be used to check that the dose estimates derived from direct thyroid measurements are of the right order of magnitude. It is to early to tell whether these empirical approaches are applicable only to the regions in which they were tested or if they are applicable to all contaminated regions.

It should be noted that the measurement of the gamma radiation emitted by the thyroid with a radiation detector held in the vicinity of the neck is not the only method available to derive the thyroid dose from a direct measurement on man. Measurements of ^{131}I in urine also have been used for that purpose, notably to estimate the thyroid doses received by the Marshallese as a result of the test Bravo in 1954 [11].

2.4 Doses from pathways of exposure other than internal irradiation arising from the intake of ^{131}I

The thyroid dose is not only due to the presence of ^{131}I in the thyroid, but also to: (1) the presence of shorter-lived radioiodines (mainly ^{132}I, ^{133}I, and ^{135}I) in the thyroid, (2) the presence of radionuclides such as ^{134}Cs and ^{137}Cs in other organs and tissues of the body, from where they can irradiate the thyroid, and (3) external irradiation from radionuclides such as ^{134}Cs and ^{137}Cs deposited on the ground. The estimation of the thyroid doses arising from these three components has not received much attention so far as priority was given to the estimation of the thyroid doses resulting from the intake of ^{131}I. For most individuals, the thyroid doses from these additional components is likely to be much lower than that due to the intake of ^{131}I.

The thyroid dose due to the presence of shorter-lived radioiodines (mainly ^{132}I, ^{133}I, and ^{135}I) in the thyroid may prove to be relatively important for those individuals who were exposed essentially through inhalation. This might be the case for the early evacuees who abstained from consuming contaminated foodstuffs after their evacuation. Unfortunately, there are very few measurements of shorter-lived radioiodines, therefore, the estimation of the resulting thyroid dose will have to rely on an accurate assessment of the quantities released during the accident, relative to ^{131}I, and on the use of environmental transfer models. In any case, efforts should be made to estimate carefully the thyroid dose resulting from the intake of shorter-lived radioiodines.

The thyroid doses due to the other two components would be relatively easy to estimate because of the large number of available measurements of ^{137}Cs. Models allowing for the calculation of those doses have been developed. However, they have not been used so far to estimate the doses received by subjects in the epidemiological studies of thyroid disease following the Chernobyl accident.

3 ESTIMATION OF THYROID DOSES RESULTING FROM EARLIER LARGE RELEASES OF IODINE-131 INTO THE ATMOSPHERE

The most reliable method of thyroid dose estimation involves the measurement of ^{131}I in man; this is why direct thyroid measurements were made after the Chernobyl and the Windscale accidents. For the same reason, measurements of ^{131}I in a pooled sample of urine were made following the Bravo shot in 1954 [11] and results of a limited program of measurement of ^{131}I in urine in 1955 was used in the 1990s to validate the thyroid dose estimates related tot he radiation impact of ^{131}I released from the Nevada Test Site [15]. However, for other major releases of ^{131}I, measurements in man were not made, and so could not serve as the basis of the thyroid dose estimation, either because the resulting doses were not expected to be large or because the radiological hazard of ^{131}I had not been recognized when the releases occurred.

3.1 Doses from releases in the 1940s and 1950s (up to 1957)

The importance of the deposition - pasture grass - cow's milk pathway to man as a major dose contributor in the case of an atmospheric release of ^{131}I was not fully recognized until 1957. Therefore, the dose reconstruction efforts related to radioiodine releases prior to 1957 are largely based on measurements of radionuclides other than ^{131}I (or of total beta measurements or exposure rates) as well as on environmental transfer models.

Atmospheric testing of nuclear-weapons-related devices at the Nevada Test Site (NTS) began in 1951; most of the atmospheric releases of radioactive materials, including ^{131}I, took place in test series conducted in 1951, 1953, 1955, and 1957. In the Off-Site Radiation Exposure Review Project of the U.S. Department of Energy, doses were estimated for the "local" populations (less than 800 km from the NTS); the key data used to reconstruct thyroid doses from ^{131}I releases were estimates of ground-deposition densities of ^{131}I at each location of interest and from each important test; these were derived either from the available exposure rates or from contemporary measurements of ^{137}Cs and ^{239,240}Pu in soil, combined with data on the relative abundance of radionuclides produced in each test [1, 10, 18]. Environmental transfer models were then used to calculate the thyroid doses from radioiodine [21]. In the U.S. National Cancer Institute study [15], the basic data are measurements of beta activities on passive collectors, that were exposed to fallout in up to about 100 locations in the U.S. The ^{131}I deposition densities in each county of the contiguous U.S. were estimated after each test. Environmental transfer models together with metabolic models were then used to calculate the thyroid doses from ^{131}I.

Similar methods were used in Russia to estimate the thyroid doses resulting from the early tests detonated at the Semipalatinsk Test Site [16].

Large releases of ^{131}I took place also in the 1940s and the early 1950s in the nuclear fuel reprocessing facilities involved in the manufacturing of nuclear weapons. As environmental monitoring was practically non-existent at the time of the larger releases, thyroid doses are reconstructed using estimated releases and environmental transfer models. For example, the ^{131}I releases from the Hanford Site in the United States during the years 1945 to 1951 were estimated on the basis of the operating histories of facilities on the site and on the knowledge of the effluent control technologies in use at the time of release [9]. Detailed thyroid dose estimates were then prepared for representative individuals at different locations, by means of environmental transfer models and data on milk production, distribution and consumption, among other factors [6]; thyroid dose estimates were made for 12 different representative individuals, distinguished by age and gender, a series of food source scenarios, and 1102 locations around the site [6].

3.2 Doses from releases after 1957 and in the 1960s

During the Windscale accident in 1957 in England and afterwards, measurements of ^{131}I in milk formed the basis of the thyroid dose estimation. For instance, the thyroid doses due to the large releases of ^{131}I that accompanied the program of atmospheric nuclear weapons tests of the 1960s were estimated by UNSCEAR on the basis of the measurements of ^{131}I in milk, that were made in most of the countries affected by the tests. The same method was later used by UNSCEAR to estimate the consequences of the Chernobyl accident in the countries of the Northern Hemisphere where direct thyroid measurements had not been performed [20].

4. DISCUSSION

General information on the major sources of ^{131}I releases into the atmosphere from the nuclear industry, for which either the amounts released or collective thyroid doses are available, is presented in Table 1. Most of these releases occurred more than 30 years ago. The nuclear weapons tests that were conducted in the atmosphere account for most of the ^{131}I that was released into the environment and for most of the resulting collective thyroid dose.

It is only for the Chernobyl accident that thyroid doses are estimated on the basis of direct thyroid measurements. This is the preferred method by far when individual thyroid dose estimates are needed for epidemiological purposes. Following the Chernobyl accident, a very large number of measurements of ^{131}I and other radionuclides was made in the environment and in man. These data provided the opportunity to develop various methods of thyroid dose estimation and to identify problems associated with the use of those methods. These methods are by and large similar in Belarus, Russia, and Ukraine but they were developed almost independently. In order to improve the quality of the thyroid dose estimates, it is recommended to:

- exchange information among specialists of the three Republics in order to review critically the methods that have been used and to prepare unified methodologies of thyroid dose estimation,

- prepare reliable databases of measurements in the environment and in man that can be used, in the short-term to reduce the uncertainties in the current thyroid dose estimates and, in the long-term to allow future generations of scientists to re-evaluate the consequences of the Chernobyl accident under good conditions,

- investigate the feasibility of deriving reasonable estimates of ^{131}I deposition densities in areas where ^{131}I measurements were not made by means of measurements of ^{129}I, which is a long-lived isotope of iodine (half-life of 16 million years) that can be used as a tracer of ^{131}I, as it also was released in substantial amounts during the Chernobyl accident.

Following the Bravo shot of 1954, measurements of ^{131}I were made in a pooled sample of urine. Although pooled samples are not as helpful as individual measurements, it seems reasonable to have used them as a basis for thyroid dose reconstruction for the affected individuals.

For all other major releases of ^{131}I into the environment, thyroid doses are estimated on the basis of ^{131}I concentrations in milk, of ^{131}I deposition densities, or of ^{131}I releases. The resulting thyroid dose estimates are much more uncertain than those based on measurements in man. It may be justified to use them, however, as estimates of group doses.

Table 1. Major sources of ^{131}I releases into the environment.

	Activity released (PBq)	Year(s) of release	Collective thyroid dose (man Gy)	Main basis for thyroid dose evaluation
MILITARY NUCLEAR FUEL CYCLE				
Atmospheric nuclear weapons tests:				
Global fallout	650 000	1962-1963 (mainly)	3.3 x 10^6	^{131}I deposition densities and concentrations in milk
Local and regional fallout (Nevada Test Site)	5 500	1951-1957 (mainly)	4 x 10^6	^{131}I deposition densities
Reactors: Windscale accident	0.7	1957	2 x 10^4	^{131}I release and concentrations in milk
Fuel reprocessing plants (routine releases):				
Hanford	25	1945-1948 (mainly)	2 x 10^5	^{131}I release
Chelyabinsk	About 20	1949-1951 (mainly)	2 x 10^5	^{131}I release
CIVILIAN NUCLEAR FUEL CYCLE				
Reactors:				
Routine releases	0.045	up to 1989	460	^{131}I release
TMI accident	0.00055	1980	Small	^{131}I release
Chernobyl accident	330	1986	1.2 x 10^6	Direct thyroid measurements and ^{137}Cs deposition densities

References

1. Beck HL, Anspaugh LR. *Development of the County Data Base: Estimates of exposure rates and times of arrival of fallout in the ORERP Phase-I area.* USDOE Nevada Field Office DOE/NVO-320/UC-702; 1991.
2. Campbell JE, Murphy JK, Goldin AS. The occurrence of Strontium-90, Iodine-131, and other radionuclides in milk. *Am J Public Health* 1959; 49:186-196.
3. Church BW, Wheeler DL, Campbell CM, Nutley RV. Overview of the Department of Energy's Offsite Radiation Exposure Review Project (ORERP). *Health Phys* 1990; 59:503-510.
4. Degteva MO, Kozheurov VP, Burmistrov DS, Vorobyova MI, Valchuk VV, Bougrov NG, Shishkina HA. An approach to dose reconstruction from the Urals population. *Health Phys* 1996; 71:71-76.
5. Dunster HJ, Howells H, Templeton WL. District surveys following the Windscale accident. *Proc. Second Intern. Conf. Peaceful Uses of Atomic Energy* 1958; 18:296.
6. Farris WT, Napier BA, Simpson JC, Snyder, SF, Shipler DB. *Atmospheric Pathway Dosimetry Report, 1944-1992.* Battelle, Pacific Northwest Laboratories PNWD-2228 HEDR. Richland, Washington; 1994.
7. Gavrilin Y, Khrouch V, Shinkarev S, Drozdovitch V, Minenko V, Shemyakhina E, Bouville A, Anspaugh L. Estimation of thyroid doses received by the population of Belarus as a result of the Chernobyl accident. European Commission 16544 EN; 1011-1020. Luxembourg, 1996.
8. Hartgering JB, Schrodt AG, Knoblock EC, Burstein AG, Melver RD, Roberts JE. *Recovery of radioactive iodine and strontium from human urine – Operation Teapot (S).* Walter Reed Army Institute of Research report WRAIR-IS-55 (AFSWP-893). Washington, D.C.; 1955.
9. Heeb CM. *Iodine-131 releases from the Hanford Site, 1944 through 1947.* Battelle Pacific Northwest Laboratories PNWD-2033 HEDR ; 1993.
10. Hicks HG. Calculation of the concentration of any radionuclide deposited on the ground by offsite fallout from a nuclear detonation. *Health Phys.* 1982; 42:585-600.
11. Lessard ET, Miltenberger RP, Conard RA, Musolino SV, Naidu JR, Moorthy A, Schopfer CJ. Thyroid absorbed dose for people at Rongelap, Utirik and Sifo on March 1, 1954. Brookhaven National Laboratories BNL-51882. Upton, Long Island, New York, 1985.

12. Likhtarev IA, Gulko GM, Sobolev BG, Kairo IA, Chepurnoy NI, Prohl G, Heinrichs K. Thyroid dose assessment for the Chernigov region (Ukraine): estimation based on ^{131}I thyroid measurements and extrapolation of the results to districts without monitoring. *Radiat. Environ. Biophys.* 1994; **33**:149-166.

13. Likhtarev I, Sobolev B, Kairo I, Tabachny L, Jacob P, Prohl G, Goulko G. Results of large scale dose reconstruction in Ukraine. European Commission 16544 EN; 1021-1034. Luxembourg, 1996.

14. Makhon'ko KP, Kozlova EG, Volotokin AA. Dynamics of radioiodine accumulation in soil and reconstruction of doses from iodine exposure on the territory contaminated by the Chernobyl accident. *Radiation and Risk* 1996; 7:140-191.

15. National Cancer Institute. *Estimated exposures and thyroid doses received by the American people from Iodine-131 in fallout following Nevada atmospheric nuclear bomb tests*. U.S. Department of Health and Human Services, 1997.

16. Shoikhet YN, Kiselev VI, Loborev VM, Sudakov VV, Algazin AI, Demin VF, Lagutin AA. *The 29 August, 1949 Nuclear Test. Radioactive Impact on the Altai Region Population*. Barnaul: Institute of Regional Medico-Ecological Problems, 1998.

17. Stepanenko V, Gavrilin Y, Khrousch V, Shinkarev S, Zvonova I, Minenko V, Drozdovich V, Ulanovsky A, Heinemann K, Pomplun E, Hille R, Bailiff I, Kondrashov A, Yaslova E, Petin D, Skvortsov V, Parshkov E, Makarenkova I, Volkov V, Korneev S, Bratilova A, Kaidanovsky J. The reconstruction of thyroid dose following Chernobyl. European Commission 16544 EN; 937-948. Luxembourg, 1996.

18. Thompson CB. Estimates of exposure rates and fallout arrival times near the Nevada Test Site. *Health Phys.* 1990; **59**:555-563.

19. United Nations Scientific Committee on the Effects of Atomic Radiation. Report of the United Nations Scientific Committee on the Effects of Atomic Radiation. General Assembly document, 19th session, Suppl. No. 14 (A/5814). United Nations, New York; 1964.

20. United Nations Scientific Committee on the Effects of Atomic Radiation. Ionizing Radiation: Levels and Effects. United Nations, New York; 1988.

21. Whicker FW, Kirchner TB. PATHWAY: A dynamic food-chain model to predict radionuclide ingestion after fallout deposition. *Health Phys.* 1987; 59:717-737.

22. Zvonova IA, Balonov MI. *The Chernobyl Papers - Vol. I : Doses to the Soviet Population and Early Health Effects Studies, pp. 71-125*. Research Enterprises, 1993.

ESTIMATION OF INDIVIDUAL THYROID DOSES RECEIVED BY THE SUBJECTS OF THE COHORT SCREENED IN THE BELARUSIAN-AMERICAN STUDY

V. MINENKO, E. SHEMYAKINA AND V. DROZDOVITCH
*Research and Clinical Institute of Radiation Medicine and Endocrinology,
23 Masherova Avenue, 220600 Minsk, Belarus
E-mail: dcc@belamir1. Belpak.minsk.by*

Y. GAVRILIN, V. KHROUCH AND S. SHINKAREV
*State Scientific Center "Institute of Biophysics",
48, Jivopisnaya Street, 123182 Moscow, Russia
E-mail: msavkin@rcibph.dol.ru*

A. ULANOVSKY
*Institute of Power Engineering Problems, Sosny, 220109 Minsk, Belarus
E-mail: lab41@sosny.bas-net.by*

A. BOUVILLE
*National Cancer Institute, EPN-530, Bethesda, MD 20892, USA
E-mail: ab76o@nih.gov*

Within the framework of the Belarusian - American joint study of thyroid disease among the children that were exposed to radioiodine fallout as a result of the Chernobyl accident, 1,325 subjects were screened in 1997. The screening procedure included a personal interview aiming at obtaining detailed information on the whereabouts of the subject within a few weeks after the accident, the origin and amount of fresh milk that they consumed, and whether stable iodine preparations were taken for prophylactic reasons. The subjects that were screened were selected from the group of approximately 40,000 children with direct thyroid measurements (measurements of exposure rates against their neck that were performed within a few weeks after the accident in order to provide estimates of the ^{131}I content of their thyroid at the time of measurement). The scientific Protocol of the Belarusian - American joint study calls for repeated examinations of 15,000 subjects for at least 20 years.

Preliminary estimates of thyroid dose are available for all the subjects who were screened. These preliminary estimates, which were made a few years ago, are based on the direct thyroid measurements and on an overall knowledge of the conditions of exposure to radioiodines in the areas where the subjects were located within a few weeks after the accident. A reevaluation of the preliminary estimates of thyroid doses is currently performed for all of the subjects that were screened in light of the answers that they provided during the personal interviews. In a sample of 100 subjects originating from various areas of the country, the revised thyroid dose estimates were found to be within a factor of 2 of the preliminary dose estimates for 90 subjects; for 8 subjects, the correction factor was greater than 2; the remaining subject had not received a direct thyroid measurement and, therefore, was not a member of the cohort.

1. PRESENTATION OF COHORT STUDY

Scientists from Belarus and the United States are conducting a joint study of thyroid diseases among a defined cohort of Belarusian people who were affected by radioactive iodine released as a result of the Chernobyl accident in 1986. The study is planned to continue for at least 20 years, with a biennial medical examination for thyroid function and structure (medical screening) to be performed for individuals whose age at the time of the accident (ATA) was from 0 to 18 years. The most accurate dose estimates are obtained using data on ^{131}I activity in thyroid derived from direct measurements conducted in Belarus during the first weeks after the accident. Direct thyroid measurements were made on approximately 40,000 persons who were children and adolescents ATA, from which group 15,000 were randomly selected to form the cohort of study participants and for medical examination.

Belarusian scientists have made a major effort to identify and to locate cohort subjects and to obtain their consent to participate in the study. By the end of June 1998, more than 2,000 cohort subjects have already passed through an initial medical screening.

2. INITIAL DOSE ESTIMATES

In May-June 1986, radioactivity in the thyroid of more than 200,000 people was measured in areas of Belarus heavily contaminated by the Chernobyl fallout by members of special dosimetry teams. Among the persons measured, approximately 40,000 were children. The measurements were conducted to identify those with higher levels of ^{131}I in the thyroid; in many cases these measurements were performed with a high degree of uncertainty [1]. The absorbed thyroid doses were assessed from the measured ^{131}I thyroidal activities, together with estimated variations with time of the rate of intake of ^{131}I. The estimated variations with time of the rate of intake of ^{131}I were based on the results of interviews conducted in 1988, two years after the accident. The interviews, which were conducted in Belarus in the same areas where the measurements had been made, provided information on population migration, milk and vegetables consumption rates, iodine prophylaxis, and dates on which cows were put on pasture in a specific territory. The results provided average parameter values for population groups, and not for individuals. However, some of the persons interviewed in 1988 also had been measured in 1986 and can be found in the database of direct measurements. For such persons, the results of the interviews of 1988 were used to assess the individual variations with time of the rate of intake of ^{131}I and, subsequently, the thyroid doses [2].

A distribution of the initial estimates of thyroid dose for individuals with ATA of less than 18 years is shown in Table 1.

Table 1. Distribution of the individual thyroid doses (initial estimates) calculated from direct thyroid measurement results for children at the time of the accident.

Dose interval, Gy	Number of persons	Percentage
≤ 0.3	20078	50.8
0.3 – 1.0	11096	28.1
1.0 – 3.0	5917	15.0
3.0 – 10.0	2092	5.3
≥ 10 (max ≈ 50 Gy)	317	0.8
Total	39 500	100.0

3. REVISED DOSE ESTIMATES

Because a) various errors were introduced into direct measurements results, and b) many initial thyroid doses had been estimated with the use of general, rather than individual information on a person's behavior, food consumption, and intake of stable iodine, it was clear that it would be necessary to improve the estimates of thyroid dose for the members of the cohort. The revised dose estimates take into account the information provided during the personal interviews; other improvements, such as the correction and verification of the instruments' calibration factors, and the use of smoothed age-dependent dose factors and metabolic parameters, will be implemented in the near future.

3.1. Individual Interviews

Currently, every individual coming for medical screening is interviewed to obtain the information that is necessary for improvement of the initial thyroid dose estimate. The 'dosimetry' interview is included as a part of the complete medical examination. The interview is designed to obtain detailed information on the location and behavior of the subject during the first weeks after the accident, on the sources and amounts of fresh milk and milk products, as well as leafy vegetables, consumed during that time, and on the intake of stable iodine for prophylaxis. The 'dosimetry' questionnaire, consisting of 25 questions, was prepared in such a way to help the individuals to remember the details of their behavior after the accident. Because most cohort members were children at the time of the accident, a preliminary questionnaire is mailed to their homes to involve their parents in answering the questions. The preliminary questionnaire also helps to prepare the subjects to respond more effectively to the questions at the time of the interview.

The experience acquired so far shows that the persons who were adults at the time of the accident remember that time well, probably because it was an extraordinary event in their life. Reasonably reliable information seems to have been collected by means of the dosimetry questionnaires. Such individual information is then used in the revised assessment of the variation with time of the rate of intake of ^{131}I.

3.2 Direct Thyroid Measurements

The reliability of the manner in which the ^{131}I thyroidal activities were derived from the direct thyroid measurements is being reevaluated. Because of various reasons, such as the non-observance of the protocol for thyroid measurement, the presence of substantial external radioactive contamination on the human body and on clothes, the presence of radionuclides other than ^{131}I in the body, the use of an assumed age-dependence of calibration factors, etc., the initial estimates of the ^{131}I thyroidal activities need to be verified and, when necessary, corrected. An extensive study of the factors that may have resulted in errors in the derivation of the ^{131}I thyroidal activities is being conducted, essentially by means of simulations of the measurement conditions, using appropriate mathematical models of human body and detectors and a Monte Carlo method of calculation [3, 4]. The present knowledge of the influence of some of the factors that affect the initial estimates of ^{131}I thyroidal activities is summarized in Table 2.

Table 2. Range of variation of the correction factors to be applied to the initial estimates of ^{131}I thyroidal activities, as presently estimated on the basis of experiments [1] and Monte Carlo simulations [3, 4].

Source of uncertainty	Range of variation of the correction factor
External radioactive contamination of the human body and/or of clothes	1 − 4
Internal contamination of the human body by $^{134,136,137}Cs$ and other radionuclides	1 − 3
Variation of the calibration factor of the instrument according to the age of the measured person and the measurement conditions (depends on the type of instrument)	1 − 2

3.3 Dosimetric Parameters

The dosimetric quantities and constants used in the assessment of the initial dose estimates were based on [5 - 7] and were interpolated as a function of age on a yearly basis. Such a stepped interpolation procedure was used in the preparation of the revised dose estimates. However, this approach, while reasonable for children over 10 years of age, leads to substantial errors for younger children, reaching a maximum of about 20% for newborns. A smooth interpolation might be used in further revisions of the thyroid dose estimates.

4.   COMPARISON OF REVISED AND INITIAL DOSE ESTIMATES

A comparison of initial and revised dose estimates has been made on a sample of 100 persons taken from the group of more than 2,000 subjects who have already been screened. In the total sample of 100 subjects, one person was found to be misidentified, and therefore the sample size became 99. The geographical (Table 3) and age (Fig.1) distributions of the individuals in that sample are similar to the distributions observed in the database of direct measurements.

Table 3. Geographical distribution of the members of the sample.

Area	Number of persons
Gomel oblast	71
Mogilev oblast	12
Minsk city	16

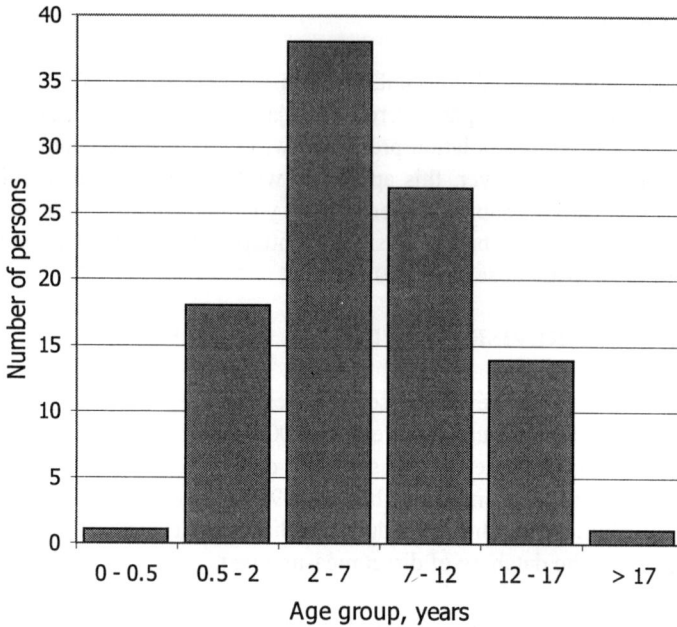

Fig.1. Age distribution of persons in the sample of 99 subjects. Age plotted is at the time of the accident.

Revised and initial dose estimates are shown in Fig.2. In general, there is a rather good agreement between the two estimates. The distribution of the ratio of revised and initial thyroid dose estimates, given in Table 4, shows that the majority of the revised estimates are lower than the initial ones, but that the range of the ratio is from 0.5 to 2 for all but 8 subjects. The maximum ratio (about 7) is observed for a subject who was exposed *in-utero*, but was considered to have been a child in the initial dose estimate.

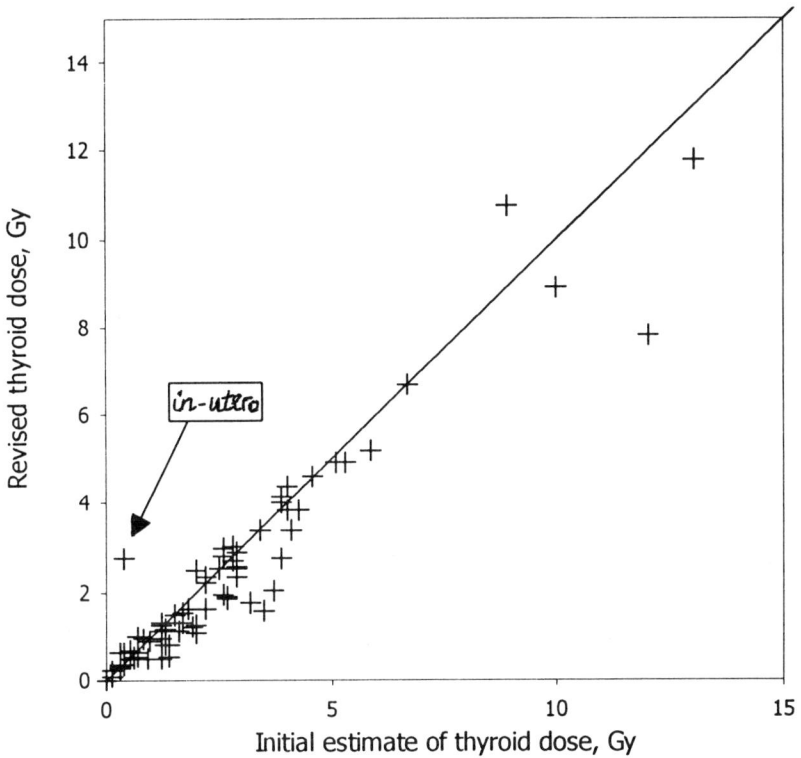

Fig.2. Revised vs. initial thyroid dose estimates for the members of the cohort.

Table 4. Ratio of revised and initial thyroid dose estimates for the sample members.

Range of ratio «revised/initial»	Number of persons
0.25 – 0.5	3
0.5 - 0.67	9
0.67 – 0.9	27
0.9 - 1.0	26
1.0 - 1.1	17
1.1 - 1.5	10
1.5 - 2.0	2
2.0 - 4.0	3
4.0 - 7.0	2

5. DISCUSSION AND CONCLUSION

The observed differences between the revised and the initial dose estimates are mainly caused by:
a) changes in the date of relocation or in the date when the consumption of contaminated milk was stopped;
b) change in the information on iodine prophylaxis;
c) change in the reported birth year; and
d) knowledge of the exact date of birth.

In addition, minor changes would have resulted from the use of improved dosimetric constants and instrument calibration factors.

Special attention was given to a group of four children who reported that they did not drink any contaminated milk. Estimates of thyroid dose that assume an ^{131}I intake by inhalation only seem to be too high. Therefore, it appears that a model accounting for the ^{131}I intake from pathways other than inhalation and ingestion of milk should be considered for such children.

Out of the 99 members of the sample, 34 had already been interviewed in 1988. A comparison of the responses provided in 1988 and in 1997-1998 shows large differences in some cases: (1) The date of relocation differs for 24 subjects, but no difference is found for the children who did not leave the contaminated territories; (2) when iodine prophylaxis was reported, the dates when stable iodine was taken coincide only for one subject. However, there was consistency for the 18 subjects who reported that they did not take stable iodine for prophylactic reasons. It is not clear at the present time whether the highest confidence should be given to answers provided during the 1988 or during the 1997-1998 interviews. A detailed analysis of a larger sample of interview responses will be carried out in order to obtain a better idea of the reliability of the interviews.

It is important to note that the revision of the thyroid dose estimates is still at an early stage, in part because the reevaluation of the ^{131}I thyroidal activities derived from the direct thyroid measurements, in which an extensive set of Monte-Carlo calculations is required, is still in progress. For example, account should be taken of the influence of the cesium isotopes ^{134,136,137}Cs internally distributed in the human body on the gamma radiation received by the detector [4]. Other factors such as the external radioactive contamination of the human body and clothes, the age-dependence of calibration factors, and the variation of measurement conditions also need to be taken into account.

In addition, work is also needed on the estimation of the uncertainties that are attached to the thyroid dose estimates, and on the validation of the thyroid dose estimates, using a radioecological model making use of the environmental radiation data that are available, including the measurements of short-lived radionuclides within a few weeks after the accident and the measurements of long-lived radionuclides, such as ^{129}I.

References

1. Gavrilin YI, Gordeev KI, Ivanov VK, Ilyin LA, Kondrusev AI, Margulis UY, Stepanenko VF, Khrouch VT, Shinkarev SM. The process and results of the reconstruction of internal thyroid doses for the population of contaminated areas of the Republic of Belarus. *News Acad. Med. Sci.* 1992; **2**:35-43.

2. Gavrilin YI, Khrouch VT, Shinkarev SM, Drozdovitch VV, Minenko VF, Shemyakina E, Bouville A, Anspaugh L. Estimation of thyroid doses received by the population of Belarus as a result of the Chernobyl accident. In: *The radiological consequences of the Chernobyl accident. Proceedings of the first international conference, Minsk, Belarus, 18 to 22 March 1996.* EUR 16544 EN. Brussels, Luxembourg, 1996: 1011 - 1020.

3. Ulanovsky AV, Minenko VF, Korneev SV. Influence of measurement geometry on the estimate of ^{131}I activity in the thyroid: Monte Carlo simulation of a detector and a phantom. *Health Phys.* 1997; **71**:34-41.

4. Ulanovsky AV; Drozdovitch VV, Bouville A. Influence of radionuclides distributed in the whole body on the thyroid dose estimates obtained from direct thyroid measurements. *(Manuscript under review).*

5. Cristy M, Eckerman KF. Specific Absorbed Fractions of Energy at Various Ages from Internal Photon Sources. *ORNL/TM-8381/V1-7.* Oak Ridge National Laboratory, Oak Ridge, 1987.

6. International Commission on Radiological Protection. *Radionuclide Transformations: Energy and Intensity of Emissions. ICRP Publication 38.* Oxford: Pergamon Press, 1983.

7. International Commission on Radiological Protection. Age-dependent doses to members of the public from intakes of radionuclides (part 1). *ICRP Publication 56.* Oxford: Pergamon Press; 1989.

RADIOIODINE BIOKINETICS IN THE MOTHER AND FETUS
PART 1. PREGNANT WOMAN

VLADIMIR BERKOVSKI

Radiation Protection Institute, 53 Melnikova Street, Kiev-50, Ukraine

E-mail: rpi@public.ua.net, vlad@rpi.kiev.ua

The epidemiology of prenatally and postnatally irradiated persons necessitates the improvement of dosimetric models for radioiodine. Another aspect of this problem is needs of the radiation protection of pregnant women. A new physiologically oriented biokinetic model has been proposed. The model is applicable both for pregnant and non-pregnant persons. The improvement of the simulation of the stable iodine distribution in maternal extrathyroidal tissues and the introduction of short-term processes to the model has been carried out. For example, the secretion of iodide into saliva and into gastric juice and its subsequent re-absorption represents the gastroenteric iodide cycle. Special attention has been paid to the early kinetics of iodine. This is a most important factor, which influences dose estimation for short-lived radioiodines, such as ^{132}I, ^{133}I, ^{135}I. Time dependence of maternal biokinetics during the course of pregnancy is also a distinguishing feature of the new model for the mother. The first part of this overview paper describes the generic structure of the model and discusses the maternal iodine biokinetics.

1 Introduction

The main aims of this work are to improve the current ICRP iodine biokinetic model for purposes of offspring dosimetry and to introduce into the new model the following features:

- A more realistic distribution of stable iodine in maternal extrathyroidal tissues.

- Short-term processes in maternal extrathyroidal tissues.

- Time-dependencies of the maternal iodine biokinetics during pregnancy.

- An active bi-directional transplacental transport of iodide.

- Improved estimation of the functional activity of the fetal thyroid during the last trimester of pregnancy.

Due to limited space this overview paper describes the generic structure of the model, gives the parameter values and discusses the major input data, which have been used. A more extended article with the detailed description of the model and results of dose calculations is in preparation.

2 Physiological Changes during Pregnancy

In addition to being concentrated in the thyroid gland, iodine is concentrated in the stomach, small intestine, salivary glands, liver, gall bladder, skin, hair follicles and hair, mammary glands, ovaries and the placenta. Because of their large mass, the skeletal muscles contain the largest iodine pool amongst the extrathyroidal tissues [8,10-12,17]. The detailed discussion of iodine metabolism can be found in numerous papers [9-11,14,17].

The physiological changes during pregnancy are accompanied by a rise in basal oxygen consumption, serum protein-bound iodine and thyroid uptake. These changes are often complicated by pregnancy goitre. The parameters of iodine turnover (renal and thyroidal clearance, plasma inorganic iodine concentration and absolute thyroid uptake) during the course of pregnancy has been reported by Aboul-Khair et al. [1]. Berghout et al. determined the levels of thyroid hormones (THs) in the blood at different gestation stages [3].

3   Structure and Parameters of the Model

The diagram of the developed model is presented in Fig. 1. The model contains sets of compartments representing the following processes: the gastroenteric iodine cycle (compartments St, SI, S and J) and the maternal hormonal cycle (I, D, G, g and B). In addition there are compartments for the fetus (FI, FG and FB), the uteroplacental unit (P1 and P2), amniotic fluid (A1 and A2), maternal gonads (O) and excretion pathways (K, UB, ULI, LLI and Br). Parameter values are estimated for the euthyroidal pregnant women, under conditions of optimal intake of stable iodine 150 μg d^{-1} (Tables 1, 2).

4   Gastroenteric Cycle and Iodide Excretion

4.1   Pathways 'Stomach – Iodide in Blood – Salivary Glands – Stomach' and 'Small Intestine – Iodide in Blood – Gastric Secretory Cells – Stomach'

Ingested iodide is absorbed rapidly from the small intestine (SI) and slowly from the stomach (St). The secretion of iodide into saliva (S) and into gastric juice (J) and its subsequent reabsorption represents the gastroenteric iodide cycle. Within three hours after of oral administration, this pool in man contains up to 23% of the intake. The concentration of iodide in gastric juice and saliva can be up to 40 times that in plasma [8,15,17]. The iodide disappearance rate from the gastrointestinal tract is estimated to be in the range 0.01 – 0.05 min^{-1} [8]. Values of 40 d^{-1} and 300 d^{-1} are adopted in this model for iodine absorption from the stomach and SI, respectively.

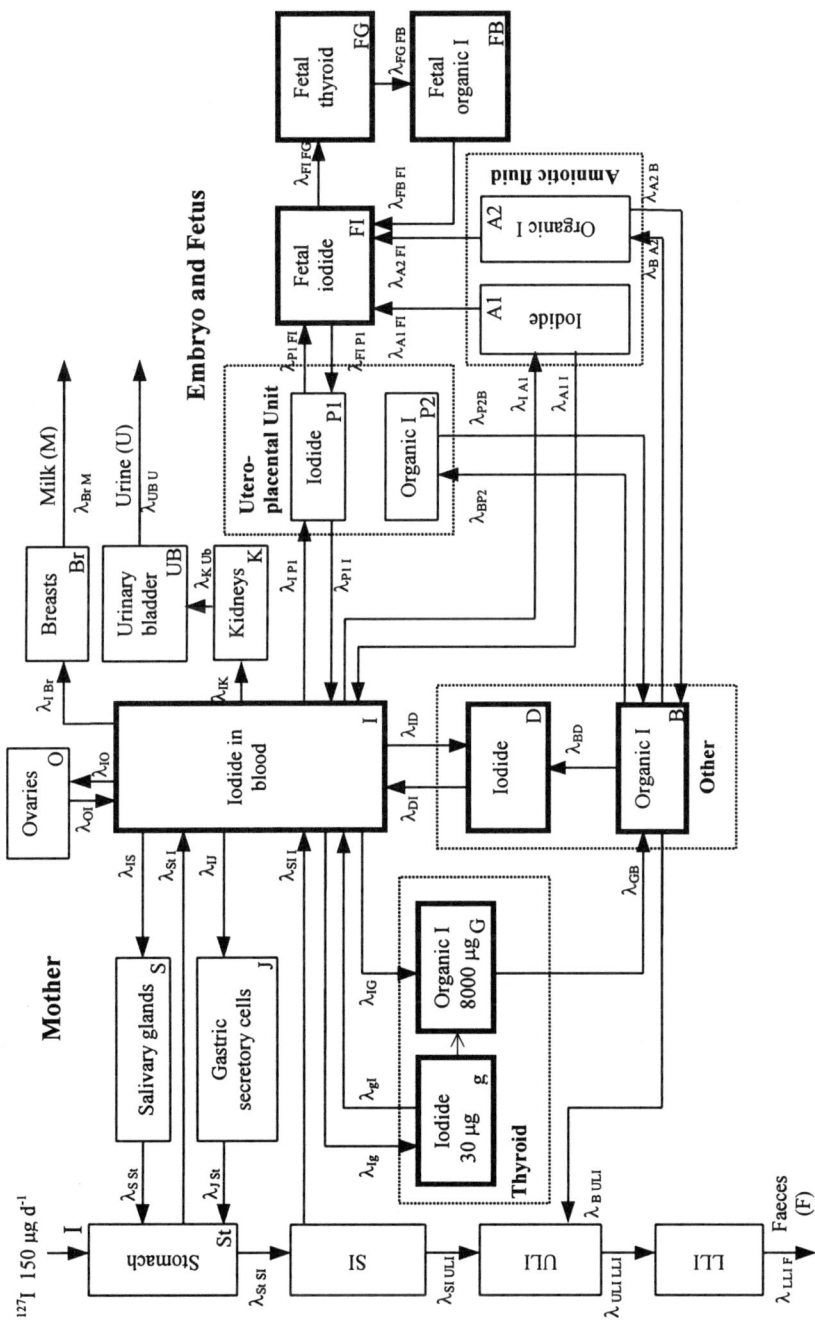

Figure 1. Diagram of the iodine biokinetic model for pregnant women.

Table 1. Time-dependent transfer rates (d^{-1}).

Time,* wk	0	3	8	12	16	24	32	36	38
I→G	2.3E+0	5.1E+0	6.5E+0	7.5E+0	8.4E+0	9.3E+0	9.1E+0	8.8E+0	8.7E+0
I→K	6.4E+0	7.0E+0	8.9E+0	1.0E+1	1.2E+1	1.3E+1	1.2E+1	1.2E+1	1.2E+1
I→P1**	0.0E+0	0.0E+0	3.3E+1	3.3E+1	3.3E+1	3.3E+1	3.3E+1	3.3E+1	3.3E+1
I→A1**	0.0E+0	7.5E-1	7.5E-1	7.5E-1	7.5E-1	7.5E-1	7.5E-1	7.5E-1	7.5E-1
B→D	3.0E-2	3.8E-2	3.8E-2	3.8E-2	3.8E-2	3.8E-2	3.8E-2	3.8E-2	3.8E-2
B→ULI	7.4E-3	9.4E-3	9.4E-3	9.4E-3	9.4E-3	9.4E-3	9.4E-3	9.4E-3	9.4E-3
B→P2**	0.0E+0	0.0E+0	1.8E+1	2.0E+1	2.4E+1	3.1E+1	4.0E+1	4.6E+1	5.1E+1
B→A2**	0.0E+0	5.5E+0	5.5E+0	5.5E+0	5.5E+0	5.5E+0	5.5E+0	5.5E+0	5.5E+0
P1→I**	1.1E+4	1.1E+4	1.1E+4	3.6E+3	1.4E+3	5.1E+2	2.7E+2	1.9E+2	1.6E+2
P1→FI**	0.0E+0	0.0E+0	0.0E+0	3.3E+1	3.3E+1	3.3E+1	3.3E+1	3.3E+1	3.3E+1
P2→B**	1.8E+4	1.8E+4	1.8E+4	7.6E+3	3.9E+3	1.9E+3	1.5E+3	1.5E+3	1.6E+3
FI→P1**	0.0E+0	0.0E+0	0.0E+0	1.0E+2	6.0E+1	3.5E+1	2.0E+1	1.5E+1	1.2E+1
FI→FG**	0.0E+0	0.0E+0	0.0E+0	1.8E+0	3.5E+0	5.0E+0	6.0E+0	6.0E+0	6.0E+0
G→B	6.3E-3	1.3E-2	1.3E-2	1.3E-2	1.3E-2	1.3E-2	1.3E-2	1.3E-2	1.3E-2
A1→I**	1.3E+2	1.3E+2	1.3E+2	4.3E+1	1.7E+1	6.0E+0	3.2E+0	2.2E+0	1.9E+0
A1→FI**	0.0E+0	0.0E+0	0.0E+0	2.5E-1	2.5E-1	2.5E-1	2.5E-1	2.5E-1	2.5E-1
A2→B**	6.4E+3	6.4E+3	6.4E+3	2.3E+3	9.9E+2	3.8E+2	2.3E+2	2.0E+2	1.9E+2
A2→FI**	0.0E+0	0.0E+0	0.0E+0	2.5E-1	2.5E-1	2.5E-1	2.5E-1	2.5E-1	2.5E-1

*Time after conception. **Zero for post-partum.

Table 2. Time-independent transfer rates (d^{-1}).

St→I	4.0E+1	I→S	3.0E+0	O→I	5.9E+2	Br→M*	2.0E+0
St→SI	2.4E+1	I→J	8.6E+0	S→St	1.0E+1	ULI→LLI	1.8E+0
SI→I	3.0E+2	I→Br*	4.3E+0	J→St	2.0E+1	LLI→F	1.0E+0
SI→ULI	6.0E+0	I→O	1.7E+1	K→UB	1.0E+1	UB→U	1.2E+1
I→D	4.8E+1	D→I	1.9E+1	FG→FB	3.5E-2	
I→g	2.3E+0	g→I	1.6E+0	FB→FI**	1.3E-1	

*Non-zero for post-partum. **Zero for post-partum.

4.2 Pathways 'Iodide in Blood – Kidneys – Urinary Bladder'

Renal iodide clearance is remarkably constant at an average 35 mL min^{-1} for non-pregnant euthyroidal persons over all ranges of plasma iodine considered. In the euthyroidal state it is mostly the inorganic iodine component that is excreted in urine. Following [1], renal clearance during pregnancy is increased to 64 mL min^{-1}.

4.3   Pathways 'Iodide in Blood – Iodide in Other Tissues'

Like chloride ions, iodide penetrates into all tissues from the blood. The maximal concentration of ^{131}I is observed at 0.5 – 1 h after giving KI or NaI *per os*. In the model the mother's iodide distribution space is assumed to be 25 L. In order to consider short-term processes of iodide distribution, the iodide space is divided into two compartments: **I** and **D**. Like Colard's model [6], iodide from the alimentary tract enters compartment **I**, which has a volume of 7 L. The homogenisation in **I** is more rapid than the diffusion towards **D**. Brownell [5] estimates a diffusion constant between **I** and **D** of 14 L h^{-1}. For the volume of **D** a value of 18 L is assumed.

5   Maternal Hormonal Cycle

5.1   Pathways 'Iodide in Blood – Thyroidal Iodide' and 'Iodide in Blood – Thyroidal Organic Iodine'

In contrast to renal clearance, thyroid clearance is sensitive to changes in the plasma concentration of iodide and varies greatly with the functional activity of the gland. In normal individuals the thyroid clearance averages 10 – 20 mL min^{-1}. In exophthalmic goitre a clearance of over 100 mL min^{-1} and even over 1000 mL min^{-1} is possible. The organic iodine space in compartment **G** contains 8000 µg of iodine before conception. The time course of maternal thyroid clearance during pregnancy was assessed in the model on the basis of data from Aboul-Khair *et al.* [1]. The initial estimation of the thyroidal uptake rate $\lambda_{I \to G}(\tau)$ at time τ after conception has been calculated by the equation:

$$\lambda_{I \to G}(\tau) = \frac{K_U(\tau)\, S_I(\tau)}{In\, V_I}$$

where $K_U(\tau)$ is the renal clearance. $S_I(\tau)$ is the absolute iodine uptake by the gland. During pregnancy it is increased from 42 to 86 µg d^{-1} [1]. V_I is the volume of the blood compartment (7 L). In is the daily intake of stable iodine (150 µg d^{-1}). Further adjustments of the $\lambda_{I \to G}(\tau)$ value (see Table 1) have been performed to take into account the loss of iodine in faeces.

Analysis demonstrates that the widely used one-compartmental presentation of the thyroid gland gives a substantial error (2 – 3 times) for the early thyroid uptake. The introduction of a compartment **g** with 30 µg of stable iodine adjusts the early thyroid uptake to values observed for euthyroidal persons. After given [131]I *per os*, the predicted 2-hours and 24-hours thyroid uptake constitutes 9% and 25% of administrated dose, respectively. The standard ICRP model gives corresponding values of 3.5% and 25%, respectively. In contrast to existing models with a thyroidal iodide compartment, in our model compartment **G** communicates directly with blood. This refinement gives better agreement with observed accumulation curves and can be justified physiologically.

5.2   Pathways 'Thyroidal Organic Iodine – Organic Iodine – Iodide in Other Tissues'

A detailed discussion of the metabolism of the thyroid hormones thyroxine (T_4), triiodothyronine (T_3), reverse triiodothyronine (rT_3) and other metabolites can be found in numerous papers [2,4,16]. In this model compartment **B** represents the extrathyroidal organic iodine [13]. A volume of 25 L is adopted for **B**. For non-pregnant persons the levels of T_4 and T_3 in serum are about $5 - 6 \ \mu g \ dL^{-1}$ and $0.05 \ \mu g \ dL^{-1}$, respectively.

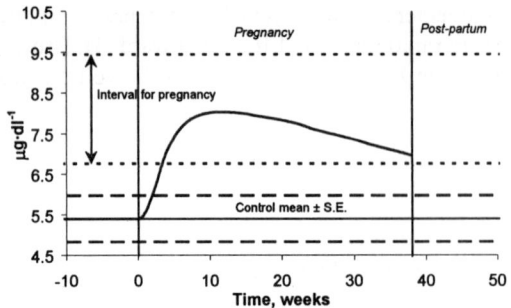

Figure 2. Concentration of organically bound iodine in plasma. Clinical data [3] and model prediction.

Pregnancy is associated with a significant increase in the serum level of the organically bound iodine. As early as the third week the levels rise to the upper part of the normal range or even to levels which, outside of pregnancy, are characteristic of hyperthyroidism [1,3,7]. A comparison of data from Berghout *et al.* [3] and values calculated by the model is depicted in Figure 2.

The description of the fetal part of the model will be given in the second part of this paper.

References

1. Aboul-Khair S. A.,   Crooks J.,   Turnbull A. C.   and   Hytten F. E.,   The physiological changes in thyroid function during pregnancy. *Clin. Sci.* **27** (1964) pp. 195-207.
2. Anbar A., Guttman S., Rodan G. and Stein J. A., The determination of the rate of deiodination of thyroxine in human subjects. *Journal of Clinical Investigation* **44(12)** (1965) pp. 1086-1991.
3. Berghout A.,   Endert E.,   Ross A.,   Hogerzeil H. V.,   Smits N. J.   and Wiersinga W. M., Thyroid function and thyroid size in normal pregnant women living in an iodine replete area. *Clinical Endocrinology* **41** (1994) pp. 275-379.
4. Braverman L. E., Thyroid hormone deiodination. *Thyroid.* **1(1)** (1990) pp. 49-51.

5. Brownel G. L., Analysis of techniques for the determination of thyroid function with radioiodine. *Jorn. Clin. Endocrinol.* **6** (1951) pp. 1095-1105.

6. Colard J. F., Verly W. G., Henry J. A. and Boulenger R. R., Fate of the iodine radioisotopes in the human and estimation of the radiation exposure. *Health Phys.* **11** (1965) pp. 23-35.

7. Danilova E. A., Various iodine metabolism indices and the functional state of the thyroid gland in normal pregnancy. *Zh. Eksp. Klin. Med.* **11(5)** (1971) pp. 61-65.

8. Egoroff P. I. and Cphasman A. Z., Radioactive iodine in diagnostics and treatment of thyroid diseases. (Medgiz, Moscow, 1962).

9. Ekins R. P., Sinha A. K., Pickard M. R., Evans I. M. and Yatama F. Al., Transport of thyroid hormones to target tissues. *Acta Med. Australica* **21(2)** (1994) pp. 26-34.

10. Ilyin L. A., Arkhangelskaya G. V., Konstantinov Y. V. and Likhtarev I. A., Radioactive iodine in the radiation safety problem. (Atomizdat, Moscow, 1972).

11. Mineral metabolism. An advanced treatise. Edited by Comar C. L. and Bronner F. (Academic Press Inc., New York, 1962)

12. Moskalev U. I., The mineral turnover (Medicina, Moscow, 1985).

13. Nicoloff J. T. and Dowling J. T., Studies of peripheral thyroxine distribution in thyrotoxicosis and hypothyroidism. *J. Clin. Invest.* **47** (1968) pp. 2000-2015.

14. Riggs D.S., Quantitative aspects of iodine metabolism in man. Pharmacol. Rev. **4**, (1952) pp. 284-370.

15. Sopliakova N. G., The concentration of common iodine and its hormonal and non-hormonal fractions in serum, saliva and urine. *Paediatrics* **3** (1994) pp. 17-19.

16. Sterling K., Lashof J. C. and Man E. B., Disappearance from serum of [131]I – labelled L-thyroxine and L-triiodothyronine in euthyroid subjects. *J. Clin. Invest.* **33** (1954) pp. 1031-1035.

17. Turakulov Y. H., Iodine turnover and thyroidal hormones. (Tashkent, 1959).

RADIOIODINE BIOKINETICS IN THE MOTHER AND FETUS
PART 2. FETUS

VLADIMIR BERKOVSKI

Radiation Protection Institute, 53 Melnikova Street, Kiev-50, Ukraine
E-mail: rpi@public.ua.net, vlad@rpi.kiev.ua

The second part of the paper presents the model for fetomaternal iodine turnover and fetal hormone production. In contrast with Johnson's model, active bi-directional fetomaternal transport and separate maternal and fetal iodide compartments have been introduced. A higher estimation of thyroxine production by the fetal thyroid has been assumed for the last trimester, which permits substantially faster clearance. These innovations in the model substantially change the dose assessments for the offspring. It was demonstrated that during the first trimester of pregnancy the maternal extrathyroidal radioiodine delivers most of the dose (more than 95%) to the offspring. A detailed description of maternal metabolism is extremely important for correct dose estimation during the early stages of pregnancy, when the fetal thyroid is not fully developed.

1 Introduction

Parameters and the common structure of the iodine biokinetics model have been presented in the first part of this paper. The description of the fetal part of the model will be given here.

The time dynamics of ^{131}I in the human placenta, amniotic fluid, fetal extrathyroidal tissues and thyroid have been measured by Aboul-Khair *et al.* [1]. Fetal thyroid uptake has been reported also by Chapman *et al.* [4], Hodges *et al.* [12], Dyer and Brill [5], Evans *et al.* [7], and Palmer [18]. A comparison of these data and model predictions are given in Figures 1 – 4.

2 Uteroplacental and Fetomaternal Cycles

The placenta plays an active role in the transport and deposition of radioiodine in the fetus. The transfer occurs bidirectionally through the placenta (compartments **P1** and **P2**, see Fig. 1 of Part 1). At even a short time after administration the concentration of radioactive iodide in the fetal serum exceeds that of the maternal serum.

Radioactive iodide accumulates in the fetus before the thyroid starts functioning and is mainly concentrated in liver and intestine. During gestation the concentration of radioactive iodide in the fetal thyroid (**FG**) increases and at the end of gestation it can exceed by 3 – 10 fold that in the maternal thyroid (**G**, **g**) [20]. The concentration of radioiodine in the fetal thyroid is always higher than in the mother's thyroid, which is evident from the data of Aboul-Khair *et al.* and Evans *et al.* [1,7].

For the case when ^{131}I is administered to the fetus, the concentration of fetal blood is as much as 3-5 times more than that in maternal blood and the radioactivity is appearing in the maternal serum very slowly. Therefore, there is a special placental transport mechanism, which transfers iodine against the concentration gradient. The transplacental concentration gradient is inhibited by sodium thiocyanate; this is similar to other extrathyroidal iodide-concentrating mechanisms [14].

2.1 Pathways ' Iodide in Blood – Placental Iodide – Fetal Iodide' and 'Organic Iodine – Placental Organic Iodine'

The large biological half-time assumed for fetal thyroid clearance (more than 1000 days before the 14th week and about 70 days at term) was the main objection to Johnson's model [13]. The separation of maternal (compartment **I**) and fetal iodide (**FI**) compartments and the introduction of bi-directional clearance of iodide in the 'mother – placenta – fetus' (**I – P1 – FI**) chain allows for substantially faster thyroidal clearance **FG→FB** (see Table 2 of Part 1).

The rate of iodine exchange between mother and placenta (**I – P1**, **B – P2**) is derived in the model from the data on uteroplacental blood flow (it reaches the value 900 mL min^{-1} at term [17]) and from the time course of [127]I concentration in the placenta. The latter was established from data on the mass and blood content of the placenta [16,19]. The rate of transplacental iodine transport (**P1 – FI**) is derived from Canning *et al.* [3]. According to Aboul-Khair *et al.* and Palmer [1,18] placental uptake peaks within 0.5 – 3 h of the ^{131}I injection. Figure 1 shows the comparison of the model prediction and the observed concentration of ^{131}I in the human placenta, plotted against 'isotope injection – termination period'.

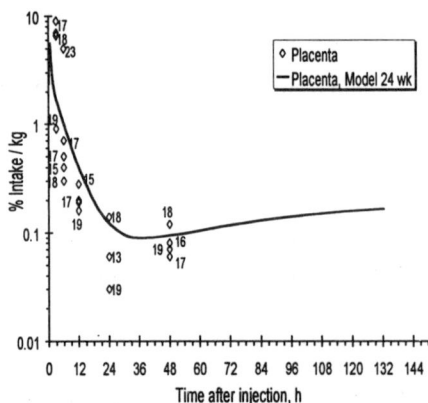

Figure 1. Concentration of ^{131}I in the placenta plotted against 'iodine injection–termination period'. Comparison of clinical data [1] and model prediction. Numbers at data points are fetal age in weeks.

The experimentally observed percentage of ^{131}I uptake in the fetal thyroid (**FG**) [1,4,5,7,12,18] was used to estimate the proportion of stable iodine, which does not return to the mother. Palmer [18] reported the value 1% for ^{131}I placental uptake and 8.9% for fetal uptake in guinea pigs at the third gestation stage. For the human this value corresponds to the fetomaternal concentration (so called C_f/C_m ratio) of about 3 – 4; this value is typical for the human for the last trimester [2].

2.2 Pathways 'Iodide in Blood – Amniotic Iodide – Fetal Iodide' and 'Plasma Organic Iodine – Organic Iodine in Amniotic Fluid – Fetal Iodide'

Tomoda et al. determined the amniotic fluid dynamics and fetal swallowing rate in singleton pregnant sheep [21]. The clearance rate of the labels in 17 ewes on the 5th postoperative day averaged 5% h^{-1}. The rates of fetal swallowing were about 1000 mL d^{-1}. In dead fetuses the disappearance rates were almost zero, suggesting that the labels disappear mainly by swallowing. The absolute volume swallowed and swallowed volume per fetal weight correlated with gestational age. The value of 0.25 d^{-1} is adopted for the fetal swallowing rate (from compartments **A1** and **A2**) in the model. Figure 2 compares the model predictions and the observed concentration of ^{131}I in the human amniotic fluid [1], plotted against 'isotope injection – termination period'.

For a number of years, the consensus amongst endocrinologists was that thyroid hormones (THs) of maternal origin do not transfer to the fetus in significant amounts [8,11]. Recent studies demonstrate that maternal thyroxine (T_4) is transported to the fetus, and is of critical importance in early fetal development [6]. Morreale-de-Escobar et al. [15] evaluated the net contribution of maternal T_4 to the fetal extrathyroidal T_4 pools. In rats, at 21 days of gestation (near term), this represents about 18% of the T_4 in fetal tissues, a value considerably higher than previously estimated.

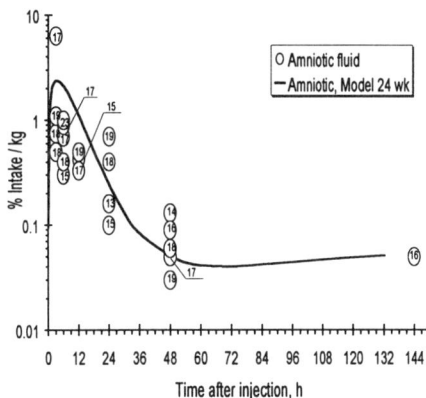

Figure 2. Concentration of ^{131}I in the amniotic fluid plotted against 'iodine injection–termination period'. Comparison of clinical data [1] and model prediction. Numbers in data points are fetal age in weeks.

3 Fetal Hormonal Cycle

A detailed discussion of the iodine metabolism in the fetus can be found in Fisher [11]. The starting point for the estimation of T_4 production by the fetal thyroid (**FG**) was data from Fisher et al. [9-11]. Between mid-gestation and term, the fetal T_4 level may exceed maternal levels. In the sheep, during the last trimester of pregnancy, daily fetal T_4 specific production (per kg body mass) exceeds maternal secretion by 6 to 8 times. Similar values can be expected in the human.

If the maternal secretion of 'iodine in T_4' lies in the range $50 - 90$ µg d^{-1} (or 0.7 $- 1.4$ µg d^{-1} per kg of body mass), than the fetal secretion of 'iodine in T_4' in the last trimester is in the range $4 - 8$ µg d^{-1} per kg of fetal mass. The time course of fetal

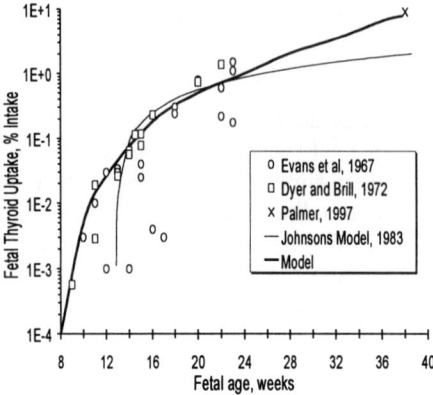

Figure 3. Maximal ^{131}I uptake by fetal thyroid at different gestation stages. Comparison of clinical and experimental data with model prediction.

mass [19] and expert judgements were used to establish the dynamics of the fetal THs production during gestation. It was assumed that the fetal thyroid gland (**FG**) has at term a typical iodine concentration in the range 400 –500 μg g^{-1} and contains at term 600 μg of iodine. Assuming that the organically bound component of iodine occupies 40% of total fetal volume, a value of 150 μg was adopted for the total iodine content in compartment **FB** at term.

The experimentally observed levels of fetal thyroid uptake were used to derive the model transfer rates [1,4,7,18]. The comparisons of these data and calculated curves are shown in Figures 3 – 4. There is good agreement between model and experiment for the absolute thyroid uptake. A 'conservative' data fit was applied at the early stages of gestation in order to prevent underestimation of radiation doses to the fetus.

The substantial dispersion of the experimental data, plotted as the 'uptake per gram of the thyroid gland', (Fig. 4) can be explained by serious problems in the measurements of the small mass of the thyroid gland and by uncertainty in the determination of fetal age. A typical range of uncertainty in the fetal thyroid mass during weeks 8 - 24 of gestation is 2 – 4 times. This statement is confirmed by the data given in [7,19].

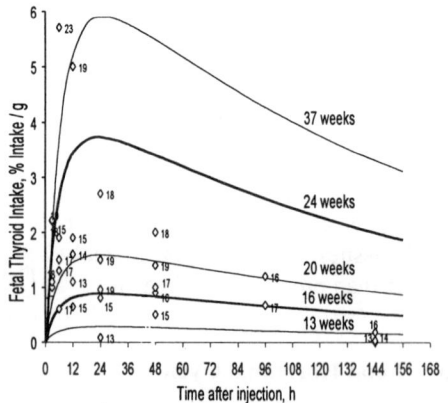

Figure 4. [131]I concentration in fetal thyroid plotted against 'iodine injection–termination period'. Comparison of clinical data [1] and model prediction. Numbers in data points are fetal age in weeks.

4   Discussion

The physiological changes occurring in the mater during pregnancy are important factors, which determine the dose to the offspring as well as the dose to the mother. In the early gestation stages maternal extrathyroidal radioiodine dominates the dose to the offspring. Our calculations demonstrate that during the first 10 weeks the most important sources of the embryo dose are extrathyroidal iodine in the organic and inorganic forms (delivering more than 60% of the dose to the embryo for short-lived radioiodine and more than 98% for ^{129}I) and the urinary bladder content (10-25% of dose to embryo). During late gestation the dynamics in the maternal blood govern fetal thyroid uptake and, therefore, is also a critical factor for correct dose estimations. The contribution of the maternal thyroid to the offspring dose is less than 1% for any of the iodine isotopes. Special attention has been paid in the model to early iodine kinetics. It is a most important factor, which is influences dose estimation for such short-lived radioiodines, as ^{132}I, ^{133}I, ^{135}I. The structure of the model potentially permits the assessment of parameter values also for a non-optimal iodine diet and for non-euthyroidal persons.

Acknowledgements

The author is grateful to Prof. I. A. Likhtarev for fruitful discussions and encouragement throughout the work. The study was closely connected with the preparation of the new ICRP Publication on the embryo and fetus dosimetry. The help of Mr. A. W. Phipps and Mr. T. P. Fell, the collaboration within the framework of the ICRP Task Group on Dose Calculation, chaired by Dr. K. F. Eckerman and discussions with Dr. J. W. Stather were invaluable for this work.

References

1. Aboul-Khair S. A., Buchanan T. J., Crooks J. and Turnbull A. C., Structural and functional development of the human foetal thyroid. *Clin. Sci.* **31** (1966) pp. 415-424.
2. Book S. A., Goldman M., Thyroidal radioiodine exposure of the fetus. *Health Phys.* **29** (1975) pp. 877-871.
3. Canning J. F., Stacey T. E., Word R. H. T. and Boyd R. D. H., Radioiodide transfer across sheep placenta. *Am. J. Physiol.* **250** (1986) pp. R112-R119.
4. Chapman E. M., Corner G. W., Robinson D. and Evans R.D., The collection of radioactive iodine by the human fetal thyroid. *Journal of Clinical Endocrinology* **8** (1948) pp. 717-720.
5. Dyer N.C. and Brill A.B., Maternal-fetal transport of iron and iodine in human subjects. *Adv. Exer. Medicine and Biology* **27** (1972) pp. 351-366.
6. Ekins R. P., Sinha A. K., Pickard M. R., Evans I. M. and Yatama F. Al., Transport of thyroid hormones to target tissues. *Acta Med. Australica* **21(2)** (1994) pp. 26-34.
7. Evans T.C., Kretzschmar R.M., Hodges R.E. and Song C.W., Radioiodine uptake studies of the human fetal thyroid. *Nuclear Medicine* **8** (1967) p. 157.

8. Fisher D. A., Dusault J. K., Sack J. and Chopra I. J., Ontogenesis of hypothalamic-pituitary-thyroid function and metabolism in man, sheep and rat. *Recent Prog. Horm. Res.* **33** (1977) pp. 59-116.
9. Fisher D. A., Fetal maternal thyroid interrelationships. *Excerpta Medica International Congress Series No. 273.* (Amsterdam, 1974) pp. 1045-1050.
10. Fisher D. A., Fetal thyroid hormone metabolism. *Contemp. Obstet. Gynec.* **5** (1974) pp. 47-51.
11. Fisher D. A., Thyroidal function in the fetus and newborn. Medical *Clinics of North America.* **59** (1975) pp. 1099-1107.
12. Hodges R. E., Evans T. C., Bradbury J. T. and Keettel W. C., The accumulation of radioactive iodine by human fetal thyroids. *The Journal of Clinical Endocrinology and Metabolism* **15** (1955) pp. 661-667.
13. Johnson J.R., Fetal thyroid dose from intakes of radioiodine by the mother. *Health Phys.* **43** (1983) pp. 575-582.
14. Mineral metabolism. An advanced treatise. Edited by Comar C. L. and Bronner F. (Academic Press Inc., New York, 1962).
15. Morreale-de-Escobar G., Calvo R., Obregon-M.J., and Escobar-Del-Rey F., Contribution of maternal thyroxine to fetal thyroxine pools in normal rats near term. *Endocrinology.* **126(5)** (1990) pp. 2765-2767.
16. Moskalev U. I., The mineral turnover (Medicina, Moscow, 1985).
17. Munro N.B. and Eckerman K.F., Impact of physiological changes during pregnancy on maternal biokinetic modeling (ICRP/21/95/97).
18. Palmer A.M., Placental transfer of medical radionuclides in the guinea pig and mouse. Abstract. *Intake of Radionuclides. Workshop* (Avignon, 1997) p.91.
19. Reference man: Anatomical and physiological characterization for biokinetic and dosimetric modeling (ICRP/22/69/98; Eckerman K. F. 1998, Private communication).
20. Stieve F. E., Zemlin G. and Griessl I., Placental transfer of iodine and iodine compounds (Gesellschaft fuer Strahlen- und Umweltforschung m.b.H. Muenchen, Neuherberg, Germany. Inst. fuer Strahlenschutz. Contract FE77552, 1985).
21. Tomoda S., Brace R.A., and Longo L. D., Amniotic fluid volume and fetal swallowing rate in sheep. *American Journal of Physiology.* (1985) pp. R133-R138.

NEW RESULTS OF THYROID RETROSPECTIVE DOSIMETRY IN RUSSIA FOLLOWING THE CHERNOBYL ACCIDENT

V. STEPANENKO, A TSYB, V. SKVORTSOV, A. KONDRASHOV,
V. SHAKHTARIN
*Medical Radiological Research Center of RAMS, 4 Korolev Street, 249020
Obninsk, Kaluga region, Russia
E-mail: mrrc@obninsk.ru*

M. HOSHI, M. OHTAKI, M. MATSUURE, J. TAKADA, S. ENDO
*Research Institute for Radiation Biology and Medicine, Hiroshima University,
Kasumi 1-2-3, Minami-Ku, Hiroshima, Japan*

The semi-empirical model was applied for mean and individual thyroid doses reconstruction in contaminated territories of Bryansk region, Russia. A special questionnaire was used to gather data for individual thyroid dose reconstruction, including information about milk consumption, leafy vegetable consumption, and use of thyroid blocking agents. Investigation of the stability of answers according to the applied questionnaires was performed. Individual doses were retrospectively estimated for 26 thyroid cancer cases (0 - 18 years old at the moment of accident) in four of the most contaminated districts of Bryansk region. The results of analysis of available individual dose estimates based on thyroid counting to determine iodine-131 content in May-June 1986 were applied in order to estimate the numbers of young population related to various individual dose ranges. The numbers of thyroid cancer cases corresponding to the different individual dose ranges were referred to the young population of the same dose ranges. The dose dependence of thyroid cancer incidence was found.

BACKGROUND

One of the key questions concerning the health effects of the Chernobyl accident is: is there a correlation between the reported dramatic increase of childhood thyroid cancer and radiation dose? In dosimetry an important task is to develop a method for realistic dose estimation[1]. There are two general approaches: estimation of mean doses for population groups defined by age and location and estimation of individual doses for use in epidemiological studies. Although difficult to achieve, the second approach is quite important.

It has been found that the distributions of individual doses are asymmetric with an extended tail into the high dose region. In the exposed populations there are groups of individuals with relatively high doses. Assigning individual doses is preferable to reliance on mean doses based upon geographic location.

1. DOSE RECONSTRUCTION: MEAN AND INDIVIDUAL DOSES

The results of direct measurements of radioactive iodine content in human thyroid gland (in Bryansk and Kaluga regions, Russia; in Gomel region, Belarus) and also available data on iodine-131 and caesium-137 contamination of the soil were used for investigation of correlations between the mean thyroid doses in settlements and local levels of caesium-137 and/or iodine-131 soil contamination.On the basis of this analysis, a model for retrospective assessment of absorbed doses to the thyroids of individuals in particular areas was developed.[2,3]

Mean doses to population groups in each contaminated Russian settlement were evaluated using the model.[3] New data concerning the beginning of pasture use in different regions as well as the history of radionuclide deposition have been taken into account. As a result, the doses reported here differ from previously published estimates: the collective dose due to the thyroid due to intakes of radioiodine in the most contaminated regions (Bryansk, Tula, Kaluga, and Orel) of the Russian Federation is estimated to be about 100,000 person-Gy. Most of the collective dose (73,000 person-Gy) was received in the Bryansk region.

A special dosimetric questionnaire was developed to aid individual dose reconstruction. The questionnaire addressed the following factors related to the period soon after the accident: age, presence in contaminated areas, time spent indoors and outdoors, migration type of work and activity, protective measures, use of thyroid blocking agents., daily consumption of unskimmed milk with different food products, other kinds of food consumption, the beginning of the pasturing season in the locality, presence or absence of rains during the accident.

The stability of answers given to questions was examined. The results of a second administration of the questionnaire performed 1-3 years after the initial interviews were compared with the first results. These interviews were performed mainly by different teams of specialists. Individuals were first questioned by a team from the Medical Radiological Research Center (MRRC); follow-up interviews were conducted by a team from the Bryansk Diagnostic Center.

Table 1 shows the results of repeated questioning of 16 persons about factors that are quite important to the estimation of thyroid doses. Variations in the two answers about the milk consumption rate varied by not more than 25% in all cases. Identical responses were given in both interviews to yes/no questions about leafy vegetable consumption and about use of stable iodine to block thyroid uptake.

Table 1. Examples of the stability of answers to questions related to thyroid dose estimation

Dates of questioning	milk consumption, l/day	leaf vegetables consumption *)	iodine prophylactic *)
1995/1998	1.2 / 1.1	+ / +	- / -
1996/1996	0.5 / 0.5	- / -	- / -
1994/1998	1.5 / 1.7	+ / +	- / -
1995/1996	0.4 / 0.5	+ / +	+ / +
1994/1996	1.7 / 1.5	+ / +	- / -
1995/1996	0.4 / 0.5	+ / +	- / -
1994/1996	2.0 / 2.0	+ / +	- / -
1995/1996	1.0 / 1.0	- / -	- / -
1995/1997	0. / 0	+ / +	- / -
1996/1997	1.2 / 1.0	+ / +	- / -
1995/1996	0.5 / 0.4	+ / +	- / -
1994/1996	1.7 / 1.5	+ / +	+ / +
1994/1996	0.5 / 0.5	+ / +	+ / +
1994/1996	0.8 / 0.6	+ / +	- / -
1995/1996	0.5 /0.5	- / -	- / -
1994/1996	0.7 / 0.8	- / -	- / -

*) + - "yes"; - "no"

The retrospective individual dose estimations were performed for 26 thyroid cancer cases (17 female and 9 male cases) which had been registered before the end of 1997 in Novozybkovsky, Krasnogorsky, Klintsovsky and Klimovsky districts – the four of the most contaminated territories of Bryansk region. The verification of diagnosis in 18 cases was performed by group of experts at an international level: Prof. D. Williams (Cambridge, UK), Prof. E. Lushnikov (Obninsk, Russia), Prof. G. Frank (Moscow), Dr A. Abrosimov (Obninsk). Other cases were diagnosed and operated in Children Oncology Research Institute of Oncological Scientific Centre (Moscow).

The methodology of individual thyroid dose reconstruction has been described in References. [2,3] Individual thyroid doses for the 26 cases range from 0.004 Gy up to 1.64 Gy (see Table 2). The mean dose for all cases was 0.53 Gy with standard deviation of 0.44 Gy. In Table 3 the values of D and σ_{n-1} are presented for different dose ranges: < 0.25 Gy, 0.25 Gy - <0.5 Gy, 0.5 Gy - <0.75 Gy, 0.75 Gy - 1.0 Gy and > 1.0 Gy.

Table 2. Results of retrospective individual thyroid dose estimation for thyroid cancer cases in four contaminated districts of Bryansk

N	Date of birth	Gender	Thyroid dose, Gy
1	18.02.86	f	0.700
2	25.01.83	f	0.255
3	31.12.80	m	0.200
4	22.12.85	m	0.640
5	12.12.84	f	1.020
6	12.11.85	f	0.650
7	31.10.81	m	0.0040
8	25.01.80	f	0.021
9	09.05.84	m	0.980
10	28.10.83	f	0.051
11	02.04.82	f	0.300
12	28.06.84	f	1.240
13	17.06.85	f	0.805
14	07.09.85	f	0.254
15	04.07.72	m	0.130
16	30.07.72	m	0.0093
17	25.12.74	f	0.320
18	14.09.68	f	0.110
19	22.04.83	m	0.480
20	12.09.84	f	0.700
21	10.03.79	f	0.610
22	22.05.67	f	0.061
23	03.12.85	f	0.830
24	26.04.83	m	0.720
25	26.06.83	m	1.100
26	15.01.86	f	1.640

2. INDIVIDUAL DOSES AND THYROID CANCER INCIDENCE

The results of direct measurements of iodine-131 contents of thyroid glands were used to estimate doses to individuals in the most contaminated areas (Novozybkovsky, Krasnogorsky, Klintsovsky, and Klimovsky districts) of the Bryansk region. The average caesium-137 contamination in these areas was about 470 kBq m^{-2}. Description of the thyroid counting data and the method of dose calculation are given in Reference[3]. The total number of children and adolescents in these four districts (with age less than 18 years old at the time of the accident) was about 58,700. A total of 546 individual doses were computed for children in these areas who were less than 18 years old at the time of the accident. The distributions of calculated doses was analysed in four age groups among children and adolescents and as a result the numbers of persons in different individual thyroid dose ranges were determined for the total young population in investigated districts of Bryansk region[4] (see Table 3). Those numbers were related to the corresponding quantities of thyroid cancer cases in the same individual dose ranges in order to estimate the dose dependence. The "background" level of thyroid cancers for the investigated population during 11.7 years after the accident was taken into account. For calculation of the background level the statistical data of the reference [5] were used. The results of dose dependence estimation are presented in Table 3, in relationships (1), (2) and in Figure 1.

Table 3. Estimation of thyroid cancer incidence dose dependence for population in four contaminated districts of Bryansk region (age group < 18 years old at the moment of accident); see Figure 1 and relationships (1), (2)

Range of individual thyroid doses, Gy	Population in the dose range, persons[4] (n_p)	Number of thyroid cancer cases in the dose range, (n)	"Background" level of thyroid cancers for the population in the dose range (n_b)	Thyroid dose in cancer cases, Gy, (D)	Standard deviation of thyroid dose in cancer cases, Gy (σ_{n-1})	Incidence of thyroid cancer cases in the dose range per 10^4 persons (I)
<0.25	29,316	8	1.53	0.073	0.069	2.21
0.25-<0.5	14,439	5	0.752	0.32	0.096	2.94
0.5-<0.75	9,294	6	0.484	0.67	0.043	5.93
0.75 - 1.0	2,654	3	0.138	0.87	0.095	10.1
> 1.0	2,960	4	0.154	1.25	0.27	13.0

The cancer incidence for each dose range was calculated as follows:

$$I = 10^4 \times (n - n_b)/n_p \qquad (1)$$

where n, n_b, n_p - see Table 3.

Linear regression for cancer incidence (I) Vs thyroid dose (D) is:

$$I = 0.58 (+/- 0.97) + 9.83 (+/- 1.24) \times D \qquad (2)$$

where:

- values in the brackets are standard deviations of the parameters;
- I, D - see (1) and Table 3;

Standard deviation of the linear regression is SD = 1.14; p = 0.0042; r = 0.977. See 95% confidence bands in Figure 1.

338

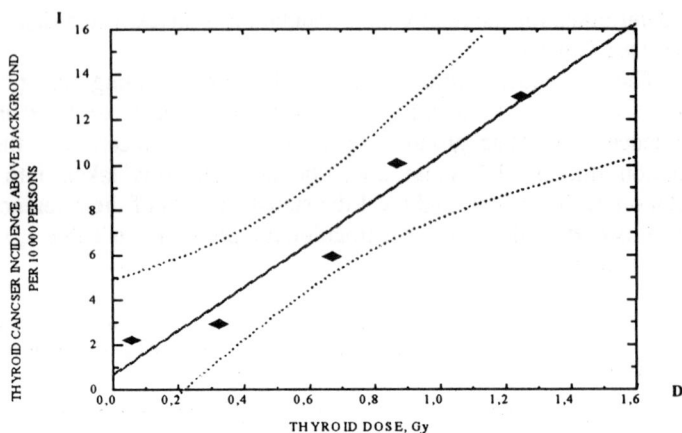

Fig. 1. THYROID CANCER INCIDENCE VS INDIVIDUAL THYROID DOSES
four districts of Bryansk region: 26 cases from 04.1986 till 12.1997).
Only persons of 18 years old by 04 - 05.1986.
Upper and lower curves are 95% confidence bands.
See Table 3 and relationship (1), (2) as well.

This is the example of application of some results in the individual retrospective thyroid dosimetry for the investigation of dose dependence of thyroid cancer incidence in 26 thyroid cancer cases from four contaminated Bryansk districts. To our regret by this moment the verified number of cases is not enough for more detailed analysis: it is clear that we need such kind of analysis for larger number of dose range intervals. This is the subject of our work which in progress now on the basis of individual thyroid dose analysis.

Acknowledgements

Authors are very grateful to:
Dr P. Voilleque,
MJP Risk Assessment, Idaho Falls, ID, USA;
Prof. S. DAVIS and Dr K. KOPECKY,
Fred Hutchinson Cancer Research Center, Seattle, Washington, USA,
for very useful discussion and comments to the content of this paper

This work has been supported in part by Grant N N00014-94-1-0049 issued to Georgetown University from the Office of Naval Research in support of the International Consortium for Research on the Health Effects of Radiation. The contents are solely the responsibility of the authors and do not necessarily reflect the views of the Office of Naval Research or Georgetown University.

The part of this work was supported by Hiroshima University.

References

1. Voigt G, Paretzke HG (eds). Scientific recommendations for the reconstruction of radiation doses due to the reactor accident at Chernobyl. *Radiat Environ Biophys* 1996; **35**: 1-9.
2. Khrousch VT, Gavrilin YuI, Shinkarev SM, Stepanenko VF. *Estimation of thyroid dose due to internal irradiation by Iodine-131 using the results of Iodine-129 determination in the objects of environment.* Moscow: State Committee on sanitary and epidemiological supervision of Russian Federation. MU 2.6.1. 082-96. Official issue; 1996.
3. Stepanenko VF, Tsyb AF, Parshkov EM et al. Retrospective thyroid absorbed doses estimation in Russia following the Chernobyl accident: progress and application to dosimetrical evaluation of childhood thyroid cancer morbidity. In: Hoshi M, Takada R, Kim R, Nitta Y, ed. *Effects of low-level radiation for residents near Semipalatinsk nuclear test site*, Hiroshima, 1997: 31-84.
4. Stepanenko VF, Ohtaki M, Hoshi M et al. *Analysis of individual thyroid dose distributions among population of Bryansk and Kaluga regions with radioactive contamination following the Chernobyl accident.* MRRC of RAMS, Obninsk, 1997.
5. Dvorin VV, Axel EA, Trapesnikov NN. *The statistics of malignant neoplasams in Russia and CIS.* Moscow, 1995.

THYROID DOSE ASSESSMENTS AFTER THE CHERNOBYL ACCIDENT: ACHIEVEMENTS AND PROBLEMS

G. GOULKO AND P. JACOB

GSF-Institut für Strahlenschutz, Ingolstädter Landstr. 1, 85764 Neuherberg, Germany,
E-mail: goulko@gsf.de

I. LIKHTAREV, I. KAYRO, N. CHEPURNY, V. SHPAK AND A. MOSKALYUK

Scientific Center of Radiation Medicine, Melnikova str. 53, 254050 Kiev, Ukraine
E-mail: likh@rpi.kiev.ua

More than twelve years passed after the Chernobyl accident. During this time efforts were made to estimate the thyroid exposure of the population mainly due to [131]I. To reconstruct thyroid doses several population groups were considered. Present estimations of individual thyroid doses are based on ^{131}I activity measurements in thyroids. In the Ukraine this group is amounting of about 150 000 persons with monitoring measurements. It includes people of all ages in rural and urban settlements mainly within a distance of 150 km from the Chernobyl nuclear power plant. In most cases only one single measurement was carried out for each person. Quality and uncertainties of these activity measurements were assessed and the model for the individual dose estimations was developed. This model includes several assumptions about time of deposition, intake functions for the radioiodine, anatomical, metabolic and radioecological parameters. On the basis of the estimated individual thyroid doses, average age-dependent thyroid doses were assessed for settlements with direct measurements. These results were extrapolated to the territories without direct measurements using a correlation with ^{137}Cs deposition and coordinates of the locations. Information about the behaviour during the first month after the accident was used to improve the dose estimates for the people evacuated from Pripyat town. In addition more than 20 000 questionnaires are available for people who lived in the three northern oblasts of Ukraine. On the basis of these data an alternative approach for the dose assessment of people without ^{131}I activity measurements in the thyroid has been developed. To improve present assessments of the thyroid doses and to make them more applicable for the epidemiological study the following tasks should be resolved: reconstruction of individual thyroid doses and estimation of the uncertainties.

1 Introduction

More than twelve years passed after the Chernobyl accident. Increase of the thyroid cancer incidence in exposed children was observed in the most contaminated areas during last 5-8 years [1,4,5]. These results generally confirm first predictions about expected thyroid cancer rate made for the selected areas of the Ukraine in 1991 [6]. Since that time a lot of efforts were made in Ukraine, Belarus and Russia to improve thyroid dose estimates due to [131]I [2,3,7,8,10,12,13]. Increased interest to this problem initiated (stimulated) several epidemiological studies considering different groups of people exposed in childhood due to the Chernobyl accident.

2 Available data and methods

Limited information about concentration of ^{131}I and short-lived isotopes in the environmental media and human thyroids is the main difficulty in the thyroid dose assessment after the Chernobyl accident. Because of this several models were developed to reconstruct radio-iodine concentrations and conditions of exposure for different groups of population [2,3,6,7,8,10,12,13].

Present estimations of thyroid doses are based on:
1. ^{131}I activity measurements in thyroids.
2. ^{131}I activity measurements in milk, air and water and radioecological models.
3. Correlation of the thyroid doses with ^{137}Cs depositions and locations of settlements.
4. Questionnaires.
5. Atmospheric dispersion models.
6. Different combinations of 1. - 5.

In addition, important information about meteorological conditions and beginning of the pasture periods should be taken into account in the development of the model.

To reconstruct thyroid doses several population groups were considered:
- People with short-time period of intake (leaving contaminated area within 5 days).
- People with long-time period of intake (being not evacuated and staying in contaminated area longer than 5 days).
- People evacuated, but staying in contaminated area longer than 5 days.
- People exposed *in utero*.
- People from "non-contaminated" area.
- Liquidators.

These groups of people could have ^{131}I activity measurements in their thyroids or not. They could live in the settlements where such measurements were performed or were not performed. Age is also an important characteristic of the population for the dose reconstruction. Depending from the availability of data the individual or average doses can be estimated for the specific group of people.

Present estimations of individual thyroid doses are based on ^{131}I activity measurements in thyroids. Reliable measurements can be considered as a most important basis for the dose estimations. This group is amounting of about 150 000 persons in Ukraine, about 250 000 (120 000 available at present for the analysis) - in Belarus and about 14 000 - in the most contaminated Bryansk oblast of Russia (additionally some measurements are also available in other low-contaminated areas). It includes people of all ages in rural and urban settlements mainly within a distance of 150 - 250 km from the Chernobyl nuclear power plant. In most cases only one single measurement was carried out for each person. In general, measurements performed in Ukraine considered as a more reliable. Quality and uncertainties of these activity measurements were assessed and the model for the individual dose estimations was developed [3,6,7,8,10]. This model includes several assumptions:

- Deposition on the considered territory occurred during one single day when pasture period is already started (April 27, 1986)
- Intake for the short-time period of stay on the contaminated territories can be represented by a single intake function and for the long-time period - by the time-dependence of milk contamination.
- Reference anatomical, metabolic and radioecological parameters are used.

3   Results and discussion

Dose assessment should proceed at three levels: preliminary, comprehensive and individual dose assessment [11]. Considering situation in the Ukraine, it can be concluded that preliminary dose assessment was done in 1986-1991. During this time-period primary measurements of ^{131}I activity in the thyroids were analyzed and doses in the areas with such monitoring measurements were estimated (individual and average age-specific in the several raions and big towns) [6]. At the next stage of investigation (1991-1993) average age-specific doses in each settlement were assessed in three northern Ukrainian oblasts. This area includes settlements with and without monitoring measurements [3,7,8,10]. At present time more advanced models are applied for the assessment of individual and age-specific doses in different locations. These models are based on more realistic intake functions. To evaluate these functions the results of atmospheric dispersion modeling are used as well as additional information about behaviour factors.

There are two dosimetric tasks which are very important for the epidemiological study: 1) assessment of individual doses for the people under investigation and 2) estimation of the dose uncertainties.

Information about individual behaviour can be applied for the estimation of individual doses. A questionnaire was developed, and 16 250 people (11 766 children up to 18 y at the time of accident) were questioned in the most contaminated areas of Kiev, Zhytomyr, Chernigov oblast and Kiev city. This number includes 2 394 persons with monitoring measurements of the thyroid. Additionally, information about behaviour of approximately 30 000 evacuees is available [9]. These data will be a basis for developing the model of the dose reconstruction based on behaviour factors. From the joint analysis of questionnaires and individual doses based on ^{131}I activity measurements it was established that variability of individual doses in a big areas (one or several raions) due to all important factors is about of 10 000-20 000 times. If age-dependence of doses is taken into account, this variability becomes of 1 500-2 500. Factors characterizing the settlement (area specific factors, such as cesium deposition, distance from Chernobyl and type of settlement) reduce variability of doses to about 20-40 times.

Estimation of the dose uncertainties is another important parameter for the risk assessment. Sensitivity analysis shows that natural variability of the thyroid mass is a main contributor to the final uncertainty of the dose estimated on the basis of ^{131}I activity measurements. Contribution of thyroid mass to the variance of the dose is about 40-60 % depending from age and conditions of measurements. The second important source of uncertainties is error in the measurements of ^{131}I activity in the thyroid. For the good quality measurements this factor can contribute up to about 25-30 % to the variance of the dose. If measurements were performed with non-spectrometric devices and without collimators this factor can become much more important due to variability of contribution of extra-thyroidal activity. Uncertainties due to variability of the thyroid mass or errors of the measurements can not be reduced. Influence of the third important source of uncertainties (15-25%) - unknown date and duration of fallout - can be reduced. Presented sensitivity analysis does not consider another possible contributor to the variance of the thyroid dose - uncertainties due to the modeling of the intake function. Much more additional efforts should be made to solve this problem. It should be mentioned that estimation of the uncertainties for the individual doses based on different correlations methods is even much more complicated.

Further progress in the thyroid dose reconstruction is connected with development of models for the estimation of individual and average age-dependent doses in different locations, as well as with assessments of uncertainties of these estimates.

4 Acknowledgments

This study was supported by the INCO-COPERNICUS project IC15CT960306 of the European Commission.

References

1. Buglova EE, Kenigsberg JE, Sergeeva NV Cancer risk estimation in Belarussian children due to thyroid irradiation as a consequence of the Chernobyl nuclear accident. *Health Phys* 71 (1996) 45-49.
2. Drozdovitch V.V., Goulko G.M., Minenko V.F., Paretzke H., Voigt. G., Kenigsberg Ya.I. Thyroid dose reconstruction for the population of Belarus after the Chernobyl accident. *Radiat Environ Biophys* 36 (1997) 17 - 23.
3. Goulko G.M., Chumak V.V., Chepurny N.I., Henrichs K., Jacob P., Kairo I.A., Likhtarev I.A., Repin V.S., Sobolev B.G., Voigt g. Estimation of ^{131}I thyroid doses for the evacuees from Pripjat. *Radiat Environ Biophys* 35 (1996) 81-87.

4. Ivannov VK, Tsyb AF, Gorsky AI et al. Leukemia and thyroid cancer in emergency workers of the Chernobyl accident; estimation of radiation risks (1986-1995). *Radiat Environ Biophys* **36** (1997) 9-16.

5. Jacob P, Goulko G, Heidenreich WF, Likhtarev I, Kairo I, Tronko ND, Bogdanova TI, Kenigsberg J, Buglova E, Drozdovitch V, Golovneva A, Demidchik EP, Balonov M, Zvonova I, Beral V Thyroid cancer risk to children calculated. *Nature* **392** (1998) 31-32.

6. Likhtarev I.A. Shandala N.K. Goulko G.M. Kairo I.A. Exposure doses to thyroid of the Ukrainian population after the Chernobyl accident. *Health Phys* **64** (1993) p.594-599.

7. Likhtarev I.A., Gulko G.M., Kairo I.A., Los I.P., Henrichs K., Paretzke H.G. Thyroid exposures resulting from the Chernobyl accident in the Ukraine. Part 1: Dose estimates for the population of Kiev. *Health Phys* **66** (1994) p.137-146.

8. Likhtarev I.A., Gulko G.M., Sobolev B.G., Kairo I.A., Chepurnoy N.I., Pröhl G., K. Henrichs. Thyroid dose assessment for the Chernigov region (Ukraine): estimation based on ^{131}I thyroid measurements and extrapolation of the results to districts without monitoring. *Radiation and Environmental Biophysics* **33** (1994) p.149-166.

9. Likhtarev I.A., Chumak V.V., Repin V.S. Retrospectiv reconstruction of individual and collective external γ-doses of population evacuated after the Chernobyl accident. *Health Phys* **66** (1994) 643-652.

10. Likhtarev I.A., Goulko G.M., Sobolev B.G., Kairo I.A., Pröhl G., Roth P., Henrichs K. Evaluation of the ^{131}I thyroid-monitoring measurements performed in Ukraine during May and June of 1986 **69** (1995) *Health Phys* p.6-15.

11. Radiation dose reconstruction for epidemiologic uses. National Academy Press. Washington, D.C. (1995) 138 p.

12. Tsyb A.F.,Stepanenko V.F., Gavrilin Y.I.,Khrouch V.T., Shinkarev S.M., Omelchenko V.N., Ismailov F.G., Peshakov C.Y., Yakubovich N.D., Proshin A.D., Kuzmin P.S. The problems of the retrospective estimation of exposure doses of inhabitants affected by the Chernobyl accident: peculiarities of forming, structure and level of irradiation according to the data of direct measurements. Part 1: Internal thyroid doses. WHO/EOS/94.14, Geneva (1994).

13. Zvonova I.A., Balonov M.I. Radioiodine dosimetry and prediction of consequences of thyroid exposure of the Russian population following the Chernobyl accident. The Chernobyl paper. Vol. 1. Doses to the Soviet population and the early health effects studies, ed. by Mervin S.E., Balonov M.I. Research Enterprises, Richland, Wa., (1993) pp. 71-125.

UNCERTAINTY ANALYSIS OF THYROID DOSE RECONSTRUCTION AFTER THE CHERNOBYL ACCIDENT

ZVONOVA I.A., BALONOV M.I., BRATILOVA A.A. AND VLASOV A.YU.

Institute of Radiation Hygiene, ul. Mira, 8, 197101 St.Petersburg, Russia
E-mail: ira@protection.spb.su

Methodology and some results of reconstruction of group and individual thyroid doses in inhabitants of the areas in Russia contaminated as the result of the Chernobyl accident, and methods of estimations of their uncertainties are presented in the paper. Statistical descriptions of actual distributions of parameters applied for dose calculation were used in stochastic simulation within the Monte Carlo method in the computer code Crystal Ball for estimation of uncertainties of calculated personal and group thyroid dose
Uncertainties in thyroid dose reconstruction were defined, on the one hand, due to statistical errors of measurements and parameters used for dose calculation, on the other hand - to incomplete correspondence of the calculation model to available experimental data. Estimations of uncertainties are presented for different method of thyroid dose reconstruction.

1. Introduction

After the Chernobyl Power Plant accident the most evident consequence of the radioaction influence upon the population of the suffered territories was the increase of thyroid cancers, that is mostly observed in children in 1986. For carrying out epidemiological study among the irradiated population, for calculating risk coefficients for late consequences, for providing and planning medical help to population, it is important not only to have correct dose estimations, but also to understand which are the uncertaities for their distinguishing, and what provokes possible errors.

The basis for all dose assessments were databases of individual measurements of iodine-131 content in thyroid of inhabitants performed in May-June 1986 in the most contaminated regions of Russia [3,4,5,6,7]. Basing on these measurements and using assumed model of radioiodine intake in a human body individual and average for age group doses were estimated.

Individual dose estimations received on the basis of direct measurements, were used for estimating average doses in a settlement for different age groups of the population. The connections of the average "measured" doses with I-131 concentration in milk, with the level of soil contamination with Cs-137, and with Cs-134,-137 radionuclides content in people in June-September 1986 were taken from this data. The received regression equations and age dose dependence were used for reconstructing average thyroid doses due to I-131 in those locations, where the thyroid measurements in population were not done in May-June 1986.

The individual doses for those people for whom I-131 content in the thyroid hadn't been measured, were precised basing on the average dose in the age group in a location using individual interview of population upon the quantity of consumed milk and the regime in May 1986.

Methodology and some results of reconstruction of group and individual thyroid doses in inhabitants of the areas in Russia contaminated as the result of the Chernobyl accident, with primary attention to parameters of their uncertainty are presented in the paper. Statistical descriptions of actual distributions of parameters applied for dose calculation were used in stochastic simulation within the Monte Carlo method in the computer code Crystal Ball [1] for estimation of uncertainties of calculated personal and group thyroid dose

2. Personal thyroid dose reconstruction based on I-131 thyroid measurement

As a rule, a person was measured once, and was not asked about his/her mode of nourishment, behaviour and countermeasures for decrease of radionuclides intake in the body. For each settlement or region, dynamics of iodine-131 intake in the body of inhabitants was assessed on the basis of meteorological conditions of fallout, average food ration for certain age groups, available data on iodine-131 or total beta activity in milk, countermeasures performed in May 1986. We used the models of prolonged intake of iodine-131 in the body of inhabitants with food and air. The simplest among them is the model of uniform intake during 10-15 days after the area contamination, with subsequent intake decrease with the half-period of iodine-131 concentration decrease in milk about 5 days [1, 11,13].

Measurements of I-131 thyroid content in May-June 1986 were performed with two types of devices: radio-diagnostic spectrometers of regional hospitals in the energy selective or integral measurement mode or portable scintillation device SRP-68-01 with the lower registration threshold at the level about 25 keV. Spectrometric measurements of thyroid were accompanied by the second measurement, most frequently of thigh, to take into account contribution from radionuclides distributed in extrathyroid tissues[6, 8].

When the device SRP-68-01 was used, only about 10% of the surveyed people were measured in two body points; however, namely these measurements permitted to calculate the "correction factor" R that took into account contribution of radiation from caesium radionuclides   recorded by the device, for different age groups and dates of measurement. Neglect of contribution from radionuclides in extrathyroid tissues caused overestimation of iodine-131 activity in thyroid by 2-4 times at late periods of measurements (30-40 days after radioactive fallout)[7, 8].

According to results of calculations within the Monte Carlo method, the sources of the uncertainty in assessment of individual thyroid dose on the basis of its I-131 content are the following factors (in order of their significance):

• uncertainty in thyroid mass;
• error of individual determination of iodine-131 activity in thyroid due to variation of detector position, thickness of surface tissues, contribution of extrathyroid radionuclides etc.;
• uncertainty of individual information on food ration and performed countermeasures.

The error of individual dose determination considerably depends on the date of I-131 measurement. Since the difference between counts from neck and thigh is used for calculation of activity in thyroid, its decrease with time due to iodine-131 decay increases the uncertainty. Table 1 presents variation coefficients (the ratio of the standard deviation to the mean value) for individual dose assessments calculated within the Monte Carlo method on the basis of measurements of neck and thigh of patients by means of spectrometric device "Gamma" at the Bryansk cancer hospital in different time periods after the accident. The uncertainty in dose assessment is higher for low values of activity, due to poor statistics of measurements. In this case, the variation coefficient increases almost up to 1 in 40-45 days after the accident. When the thyroid dose is being assessed on the basis of one measurement of neck, with the use of correction factors, the uncertainty increases additionally.

Table 1. Monte Carlo simulation with real ^{131}I in thyroid measurement data: variation coefficient depending on count rate and day of measurement, rel.un.*

Count rate, min^{-1}	Day of measurement		
	20	30	40
100	0,5	0,6	0,8
1000	0,3	0,4	0,5

* Spectrometer; neck and thigh measurements.

To determine individual dose, information about way of life, milk consumption and countermeasures is necessary along with the results of measurement of iodine-131 content in thyroid. Since no such questions were put usually during wide-scale measurements, individual assessments were often based on average (for a settlement or region) parameters of the dosimetric model. This fact could be the main source of systematic uncertainty in dose estimation both individual and average. For example, the error may arise with neglect of pointed on interrupting the of ecological transfer of iodine-131 along the chain "pasture - grass - cow - milk - man". These were: delay in beginning of cattle pasturing, temporary halting of cattle pasturing, refusal from consumption of local contaminated milk, and intake of stable iodine preparations by inhabitants.

3. Average thyroid dose based on personal measurements

The results of measurements of iodine-131 content in thyroid ensure the best assessment of average dose of thyroid exposure. As a rule, the dose distribution was asymmetric, close to lognormal one with $K_{var} = 0.8 - 1.0$. However, as we discussed above, the use of such data does not guarantee the absence of systematic error connected with incorrectly set function of radioiodine intake in the body.

Group assessments of thyroid doses showed clear dependence of the average dose on age. These dependencies were different for rural and urban inhabitants[5,6]. For example, in towns with food products provision through shops the dose in thyroid of children below 2 years of age was 10-12 times higher than in adults. In rural settlements with private production of milk, the dose in these age groups differed by 5-7 times. The age factor was the main in assessment of average group thyroid doses in population of different settlements.. Using the obtained age relations, we reconstructed the mean dose in all age groups, if reliable results of measurements were present for at least one age group in the settlement [5,6].

The uncertainty in assessment of the average thyroid dose for an age group on the basis of measurements of iodine-131 content in thyroids of inhabitants is attributed to the following main reasons: uncertainty in determination of individual thyroid doses and limited number of measurements.

4. Average thyroid dose for settlement without direct measurements

Among methods for average thyroid dose reconstruction with empirical equations of regression of thyroid dose on parameters of environmental contamination, the most preferred is to use data on contamination of milk with iodine-131[5,6]. But such data are available only for Tula region where regular spectrometric measurements of I-131 concentration in milk began May 14, 1986. Linear correlation of thyroid dose with I-131concentration in milk was shown for this data[7].

Correlation with the average content of caesium radionuclides in the body of inhabitants in June-September 1986 has the second priority. Since the regularities of intake of iodine and caesium radionuclides in the body of man during the initial time period after the area contamination were alike, the correlation of thyroid dose with Cs-134,-137 content in human body formed during the period of surface contamination of vegetation with radionuclides is rather high. Actually, we most frequently used the dependence of thyroid dose on the surface soil contamination with Cs-137 in a settlement, because this database is the most extensive.

If the average dose has been assessed by means of regression equations, the error of the parameter used for the dose reconstruction (iodine-131 concentration in milk, content of caesium radionuclides in the body of inhabitants, soil contamination with caesium-137) is added to the uncertainties enumerated above.

5. Individual thyroid dose in persons without thyroid measurements

Individual dose of thyroid exposure depends on the amount of milk consumed in 1986. A special work was performed in 1986 for studying influence of milk consumption on thyroid dose[2]. A group of about 200 inhabitants of the Bryansk region was asked about consumption rate of locally produced milk along with measurements of iodine-131 content in their thyroids. The results of regression analysis showed that the accumulated iodine-131 activity in thyroid significantly correlates with the amount of consumed milk[2]. The obtained regularities were used for assessment of individual dose on the basis of the average thyroid dose in the age group and data of individual poll about amount of consumed milk as compared with the average consumption in the settlement.

Individual thyroid dose reconstruction for about 60 thousands of residents of Bryansk region was made in 1987-1988 with using this method. For special epidemiological studies (case-control, etc.), retrospective interviewing of persons displaying thyroid diseases along with control groups. and subsequent dose reconstruction has being performed since 1990.

For such method the main sources of error were uncertainties in average dose estimations and milk consumption and inaccuracy of people's answers. If empirical distributions of the aged thyroid dose and milk consumption rate are used in stimulating the dose counting with the Monte Carlo method, the variation coefficient becomes equal to 1,2-1,5.

In all these cases, uncertainties of the used intake function influence most strongly on the average dose assessment. The intake function is strongly influenced by social factors and sometimes unknown countermeasures performed in a settlement to reduce internal exposure of inhabitants.

At this stage of work, the standard geometrical deviation of individual dose assessments obtained on the basis of direct measurements of iodine-131 in thyroid was estimated in range from 1.5 to 2.0, and when radioecological models were used - within the range 2 to 4.

6. Conclusions

1.Review of thyroid dose reconstruction methodologies used for population suffered after the Chernobyl accident and analysis of possible sources of its uncertainties are presented in the paper.
2. Uncertainties in thyroid dose reconstruction were attributed, on the one hand, to statistical errors of measurements and parameters used for dose calculation, on the other hand - to incomplete correspondence of the calculation model to available experimental data. In particular, such social feature as the time of stopping local milk consumption, the time of beginning of cows pasturing with respect to the moment of area radioactive contamination could be the reason of the second sort uncertainty .
3. Main sources of the uncertainty for individual estimations of thyroid dose are biological variability of thyroid mass, errors in definition of I-131 content in thyroid gland due to contribution of extrathyroidal radionuclides etc.; poor statistics at the late dates of measurements, variation of detector position, thickness of surface tissues, etc.
4. Uncertainty of calculated methods of dose estimation based on empirical correlation equations is defined mainly with errors in determination "measured" average thyroid dose and parameters used in correlation equations.

The work on reconstruction of thyroid dose in exposed population after the Chernobyl accident is in progress and associated uncertainty analysis is also continued.

References

1. Crystal Ball: User's Guide. Decisioneering, Inc., Denver, Colorado, 1994.
2. Korelina N.F., Bruk G.Ya., Kaidanovsky G.N., Konstantinov Yu.O., and Porosov N.V. Control and interpretation of radiometric survey data for determination of personal doses of internal exposure of the thyroid after the Chernobyl accident. In: Proc. Russian-Hungarian seminar on Radiation Protection, St.-Petersburg, 1992. pp.23-29.
3. .Pitkevich V.A., Hvostunov I.K., Shishkanov N.G. Influence of I-131 dynamic due to the Chernobyl accident on absorbed doses in thyroid of inhabitants of Bryansk and Kaluga regions of Russia. *Radiation and Risk* 1996; 7: 192-215.
4. Tzyb A.F., Stepanenko V.F., Matveenko E.G., et.all, The structure and levels of thyroid exposure in inhabitants of the contaminated areas of the Kaluga region. *Radiation and Risk,* 1994, 4: 87-93 (In Russian).
5. Zvonova I.A. and Balonov M.I., Radioiodine Dosimetry and Forecast for Consequences of Thyroid Exposure of the RSFSR Inhabitants Following the Chernobyl Accident. In: The Chernobyl Papers. V.I: Doses to the Soviet Population and Early Health Effects Studies. Ed. by S.Merwin and M.Balonov. Research Enterprises, 1993, pp. 71-125.
6. Zvonova I .A., Balonov M.I., and Bratilova A.A.. Thyroid Dose Reconstruction for Population of Russia Suffered after the Chernobyl Accident. *Radiat. Prot. Dosim.,* 1998, in print.
7. I.A.Zvonova, M.I.Balonov, A.A.Bratilova, G.E.Baleva, S.A.Gridasova, M.A.Mitrohin, V.P.Sazhneva. Thyroid absorbed dose estimations for population of the Bryansk, Tula, Orel regions according to results of radiometry in 1986. *Radiation and Risk,* 10, 1998, in print. (In Russian)

ASSESSMENT OF THE SOURCES OF CONTAMINATION OF THE RIVER GARONNE, FRANCE, BY IODINE-131

S. GAZAL

Groupe de Recherche Pluridisciplinaire en Environnement, Université de Toulouse
Commission Locale d'Information auprès du CNPE de Golfech, Tarn-et-Garonne,
BP 783, 82013 Montauban Cedex, France

Aquatic plants are known to concentrate radionuclides and hence constitute a good bio-indicator of a radioactive contamination of water.

Measurements of radioactivity in aquatic plants is part of the monitoring protocol carried out by the Laboratoire Vétérinaire Départemental de Tarn-et-Garonne (Conseil Général de Tarn-et-Garonne) to assess the environmental impact of the Golfech nuclear power plant radioactive releases.

Measurements from the river Garonne revealed significant levels of gamma contamination of *Myriophyllum spicatum* L. samples by [131]I (up to 13701 ± 1443 BqKg^{-1} dry weight). The highest levels occurred immediately downstream from Toulouse (population 350,000), but were undetectable upstream. The source of the contamination was thus from within Toulouse itself and not from the Golfech nuclear power plant.

Following investigations at the medical centres within Toulouse carried out by the local authorities, contamination levels measured in *Myriophyllum spicatum* L. by the Laboratoire Vétérinaire Départemental were observed to decrease by one order of magnitude.

Few data are available concerning ^{131}I activity in water samples. All measurements were below the detection levels (ranging from 0.1-3.7 Bql^{-1}).

An attempt is made to assess the health consequences of this contamination.

1 SOURCES OF RADIOACTIVE POLLUTION OF RIVERS

Radioactive pollution of rivers has three pathways : migration from soils, dry and wet deposition from the atmosphere, and direct releases in the river. It has both a natural and anthropogenic origin. A possible contribution is from radioactive iodine, sources of which include :

- atmospheric nuclear weapons tests,
- liquid and gaseous releases from nuclear facilities such as research centres, NPPs ([129]I, [131-135]I)[1] and reprocessing facilities, both routine and accidentally,
- research and analysis laboratories (^{125}I)[3,9],
- departments of nuclear medicine (radioanalysis: [125]I, *in vivo* diagnosis and therapy: [131]I, ^{123}I).

The management of risk generally and river quality in particular has many aspects including:

- planning/accident stages,
- the sources/ the consequences of the risk, identification and minimization,
- diffuse/accidental risk management.

It relies on regulations and control by both the responsible agencies and the operators.

2 MANAGEMENT OF SOURCES OF RADIOACTIVE POLLUTION FROM CIVIL NUCLEAR FACILITIES AND DEPARTMENTS OF NUCLEAR MEDICINE

Although they differ in nature and mission, these two types of sources operate on the same basic principles:
• an establishment procedure including several major stages (authorization, compliance control, various licencing steps including the holding and use of radioisotopes),
• regulations concerning the management of radioactive wastes, including liquid and gaseous releases to the environment,
• the responsibility of the operator and user,
• the control of facility and releases by regulating bodies.
They rely on separate national regulations.

However the regulations concerning waste management from nuclear power plants (NPPs) and nuclear medicine departments are not comparable. Those for NPPs govern the volumetric and total annual activities of the effluents released (either gaseous or liquid) and the resulting activities in the receiving medium. They also accurately define the configuration of the facilities, as well as monitoring protocols for the releases and the environment for both operators and regulating bodies . The regulations concerning nuclear medicine departments include some prescriptions about the waste storage and release facilities, and the volumetric activities of releases. Some of these are not clearly established and rely on questionable data and concepts.

Concerning the actual iodine releases by NPPs, a typical 1300 MWe NPP such as Golfech released in 1997 4.45 MBq (111μCi) of ^{131}I in the river Garonne (data for other isotopes not available) and 81 MBq (2mCi) of halogens and aerosols in the atmosphere. More generally, Table 1 shows that the total liquid activity (^{3}H, ^{40}K, Ra excluded) released by 1300 MWe NPPs (iodine in a ratio about 10^{-2}) decreased by a factor of 12 between 1984 and 1997, whereas the total activity released in halogens and aerosols (mainly iodine) increased by a factor of 10 with a peak c. 1993 (factor 30).

Table 1. Mean activities released per 1300 MWe reactor between 1984 and 1997[2]
(*: the number of operating 1300 MWe NPPs for the year considered)

Type of Release	1984 (2 x 1300 MWe)*	1990 (14 x 1300 MWe)*	1993 (20 x 1300 MWe)*	1997 (20 x 1300 MWe)*
Liquids (excl ^{3}H, ^{40}K, Ra)	177 GBq	24 GBq	2.7 GBq	1,4 GBq
Halog. & aerosols	0.076 GBq	0.106 GBq	0.196 GBq	0,08 GBq

No data are available concerning iodine activities released to the environment by nuclear medicine departments.

3 THE RADIOLOGICAL QUALITY OF THE RIVER GARONNE

Regulations on radioactive sources do not stand in the framework of any general regulation of the radiological quality of drinking and freshwaters, either French or European. Consequently no systematic monitoring is carried out on water bodies.

In the framework of the independent environmental monitoring of the Golfech NPP by the Conseil Général de Tarn-et-Garonne, a radiometric monitoring protocol has been defined by the Laboratoire Vétérinaire Départemental, which includes a monthly monitoring of water bodies: drinking water, surface and ground waters, sediments and bioindicators (aquatic plants). Since the beginning (May 1990), measurements in aquatic plants from 16 locations in the river Garonne revealed significant and variable levels of contamination of *Myriophyllum spicatum* L. samples by ^{131}I, increasing from the furthest downstream station (below the NPP) up to near Toulouse (~130 km upstream, population 350,000), below which there was a maximum value of 13701 ± 1443 Bq kg⁻¹DW. No significant contamination was detected upstream of Toulouse[6] (Figure 1).

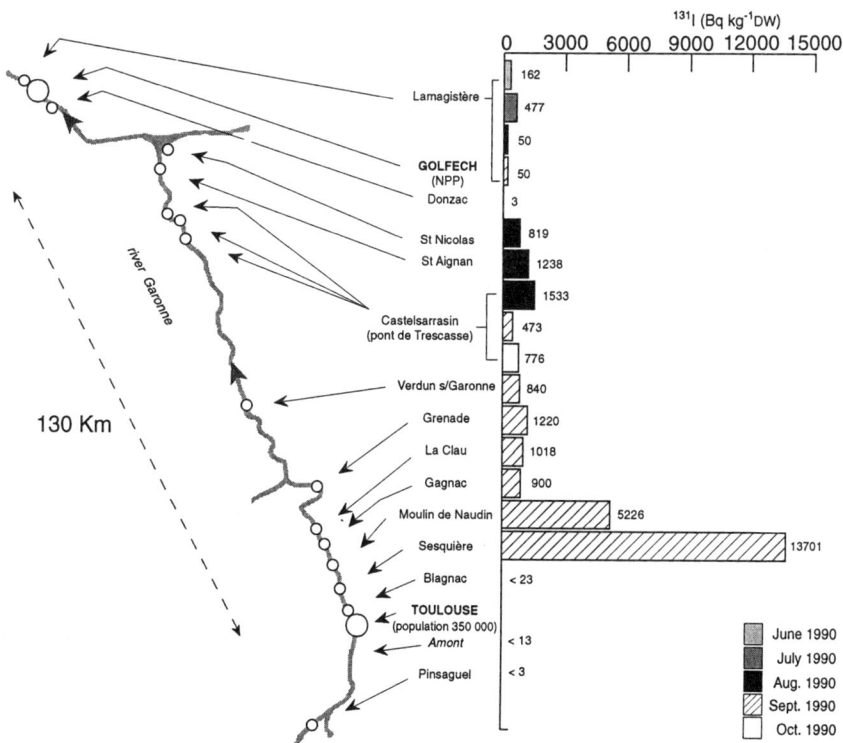

Fig. 1. Contamination of *Myriophyllum spicatum* L. by ^{131}I in the river Garonne (1990). The values indicated are monthly means.

Investigations were carried out by the national health authorities and by the Regional Council between 1991-5. They confirmed that these contaminations originated in medical centres in Toulouse. The contamination of waste waters from these centres ranged from < 0.2 to 34961 ± 2074 Bq l^{-1} after dilution of the radioactive releases, ^{131}I concentrations in the waste waters at the entrance and exit of the municipal sewage work being 3 ± 0.7 and 2 ± 0.4 Bq l^{-1} respectively. They also pointed out:
- the disregard of the limits for the release of radioactive effluents from some of the nuclear medicine departments,
- the non-conformity of some facilities (capacity of storage tanks, modalities of release),
- the part played by the waste waters from non-protected rooms either in the nuclear medicine department or possibly from non-nuclear medical departments where people examined or treated in the nuclear medicine department may stay,
- the low part played by home releases (people examined or treated with radioactive iodine back from hospital).

Since 1994, the contamination of *Myriophyllum spicatum* L. measured by the Laboratoire Vétérinaire Départemental is lower by about one order of magnitude than the 1990, 1991 values (31 ± 4 to 83 ± 21 Bq kg^{-1}DW in the NPP's environment).

4 HEALTH IMPACT OF RIVER GARONNE CONTAMINATION BY ^{131}I

The biological effects of radiation commonly separate into deterministic and stochastic effects (cancers and genetic effects).

The risk factor for stochastic effects have been estimated to be 5×10^{-2} lethal cancers and 1×10^{-2} severe genetic effects per sievert received [4]. An increase of cancer risk by several times that for an adult is also pointed out for infants exposed *in utero*. Consequently, the recommended limits for radiation exposure of 1 mSv a^{-1} for the population[4] entails 50 lethal cancers and 10 severe genetic effects (plus the corresponding non-lethal cancers and non-severe genetic effects) per million people exposed to 1 mSv a^{-1}. An age dependant evaluation of doses from intake of radionuclides (the evaluation of the irradiation caused by the intake of one unit of activity, i.e 1 Bq) for ingestion of radioisotopes for the population leads to the following IEDC (Ingestion Effective Dose Coefficient) for ^{131}I : 1.8×10^{-7} Sv (<1 year olds), 1×10^{-7} Sv (5 year olds), 5.2×10^{-8} Sv (10 year olds), 3.4×10^{-8} Sv (15 year olds) and 2.2×10^{-8} Sv (adults)[5]. Consequently, a 1 year old child (the critical group) ingesting 15 Bq d^{-1} of ^{131}I over one year will receive an irradiation of 1 mSv. This corresponds to a daily consumption of 70 cc or 1 litre of water contaminated by 21.4 Bq l^{-1} or 15 Bq l^{-1} respectively.

A few measurements of water samples were carried out. But the values were all below detection thresholds (<0.1 to 3.7 Bq l^{-1}). Moreover, an extrapolation from *Myriophyllum spicatum* L. activity to running waters is not feasible. The only data available are the activities measured at the municipal sewage work. Their dilution rate is a function of river flow (ranging from a few tens to 2×10^3 m^3 s^{-1}, mean flow 4×10^2 m^3 s^{-1}) and of the river conditions. So one can expect a water contamination after dilution of about 10^{-2} to 10^{-1} Bq l^{-1}, which stands below the limits stated above by 2-3 orders of magnitude. This is in good compliance with three measurements by the health authorities downstream from Toulouse (0.032 to 0.056 Bq l^{-1})[7]. Consequently, the expected stochastic effects of the water contamination of the river Garonne for critical groups might be 0.5 lethal cancer (mainly thyroid cancer) and 0.1 severe genetic effect (plus the associated non lethal cancers, about 19 times more for thyroid cancers, and non severe genetic effects) for 1 million infants consuming such water.

But even this is not possible to assess, IEDC for iodine being seriously questionned in the aftermath of the Chernobyl accident [10,11].

5   CONCLUSION

It was demonstrated that *Myriophyllum spicatum* L. is a sensitive indicator of radioactivity. Beyond this, it appears that the sources of contamination by ^{131}I must be carefully investigated, identified, regulated and controlled. Regulations must be particularly improved for nuclear medicine departments using unsealed sources, and for drinking and fresh waters concerning limitations as well as monitoring and control. More generally, it is urgent that derived limits for food products and media be assessed on the basis of the relevant IEDCs, of the different routes of exposure and of life habits, c.f. NRPB[8], and that the questions of cumulative exposure (such as ^{99m}Tc or ^{125}I measured together with ^{131}I up to 1×10^6 and 1×10^3 Bq l^{-1} respectively), cumulative sources and synergetic effects with other pollutants be considered.

358

References

1. EDF. *Centrales Nucléaires du palier 1 300 MWe - Textes du Rapport de Sûreté communs à toutes les tranches du palier*, Edition publique. Paris : EDF, 1985 : II 5.3.23, 24.
2. EDF. *Rapports d'Activité - Environnement* 1993, 1997 : 33,41.
3. Gambini D, Granier R. *Manuel Pratique de Radioprotection.* Paris : Editions Médicales Internationales, 1992.
4. ICRP. *1990* Recommendations of the International Commission on Radiological Protection. *Annals of the ICRP* 1991 ; Publication 60 : 11-25, 43-49.
5. ICRP. Age dependent doses to members of the public from intake of radionuclides : Part 2. Ingestion dose coefficents 1993. *Annals of the ICRP*, 1994 ; Publication 67 : 153.
6. Laboratoire Vétérinaire Départemental de Tarn-et-Garonne. *Rapports d'Activité* 1990-1997.
7. SCPRI / OPRI. *Tableaux Mensuels de Mesures* 1990-1997.
8. NRPB Revised generalised derived limits for radioisitopes of strontium, iodine, caesium, plutonium, americium and curium. *GS* 1987 ; 8.
9. Moretti J.L, Rigo P, Bischof - Delaloye A, Taillefer R, Caillat - Vigneron N, Karcher G. *Imagerie Nucléaire Fonctionnelle.* Paris : Masson, 1991.
10. Shore R.E. Human thyroid cancer induction by ionizing radiation : summary of studies based on external irradiation and radioactive iodines. In : Karaoglou A, Desmet G, Kelly G.N, Menzel H.G, ed. *The Radiological Consequences of the Chernobyl Accident.* Luxembourg : Office for Official Publications of the European Communities, 1996 : 669 - 675.
11. Sobolev B, Likhtarev I, Kairo I, Tronko N, Oleynik V, Bogdanova T. Radiation risk assessment of the thyroid cancer in Ukrainian children exposed due to Chernobyl. In : *The Radiological Consequences of the Chernobyl Accident.* Luxembourg : Office for Official Publications of the European Communities, 1996 : 761 - 748.

THYROID DOSIMETRY, POST-CHERNOBYL THYROID IRRADIATION AND EPIDEMIOLOGY IN LITHUANIA

T. NEDVECKAITE AND V. FILISTOVIC
Institute of Physics, Radiation Protection Department, Savanoriu 231, 2028 Vilnius
LITHUANIA
E-mail: Vitfil@julius.ktL.mii.Lt

A. KRASAUSKIENE
Lithuanian Institute of Endocrinology, Laboratory of Thyroid Disorders
Eiveniu 2, Kaunas 3007

K. KADZIAUSKIENE
Lithuanian National Nutrition Center, Kalvariju 153, Vilnius 2048
E-mail: rmc@post.omnitel.net

Aim of the study was the evaluation of the equivalent doses to thyroid and investigation of thyroid disorders in Lithuania after the Chernobyl accident. The evaluation of doses to thyroid was performed by mean of mathematical model, including radioiodine terrestrial pathway and modified ICRP three-compartment cyclic model together with software APSVITA. These calculations applied Monte Carlo method and consideration of regional stable iodine deficiency. After the Chernobyl accident the highest adult thyroid doses range up to 28 mSv and infant's doses - up to 280 mSv in the most contaminated area of Lithuania. Cancer register data demonstrate that there are no significant trend changes of thyroid disorders in Lithuania. The results of thyroid disorders investigation provide support to the view that one decade after the Chernobyl accident such doses and the middle stable iodine deficiency offer no significant threat to the health of general public and rightly emphasises the importance and relevance of social, ecological and economic factors.

1. INTRODUCTION

Global exposure due to Chernobyl accident can be assessed on the bases of the extensive information available from international and national groups that have collected and analysed these data. Assessment of routine and accident releases have identified ^{131}I as the nuclide liable to cause the highest radiation doses because of its abundance and volatility, rapid transfer to milk, and accumulation in the thyroid. The aim of this study was the evaluation of post-Chernobyl equivalent doses to thyroid and the analysis of thyroid pathology data in Lithuania.

2. MATERIALS AND METHODS

Iodine radionuclides may be transferred through various environmental media before being taken into the human body, e.g. air-grass-cattle milk-man pathway. General description of the experimental radioiodine pathway data has been published previously [6]. Major parts of the measured data are presented on Fig. 1.

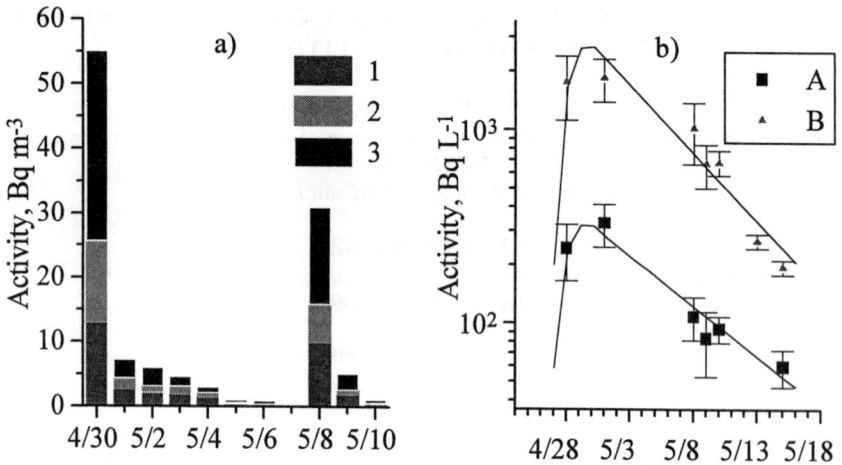

Fig. 1. ^{131}I activity concentration after the Chernobyl accident: a) atmospheric air activity in Vilnius (1-aerosol fraction; 2-3 – gaseous fractions; b) milk activity in different areas (A,B) of Lithuania

In addition, the estimation of equivalent doses to thyroid should consider the biokinetic of stable iodine metabolism in the human body and regional prevalence of iodine deficiency. Augmentation of iodine trapping is the fundamental adaptive mechanism by which the thyroid gland maintains the possibility to accumulate sufficient amount of iodide. The experimental data on the concentration of iodide in urine (Fig. 2) allows including Lithuania into region of mild iodine deficiency[4].

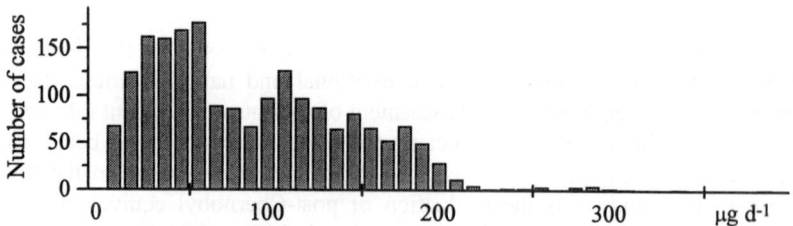

Fig. 2. Daily urinary excretion of stable iodine

Thyroid doses were estimated using the modified ICRP three-compartment cyclic model with consideration of stable iodine deficiency and Monte Carlo method to generate frequency distribution of thyroid doses to infant, children and adult thyroid gland by mean of computer program APSVITA [1-3] (Fig.3). The probabilistic dose assessment method was used in conjunction with more realistic estimates of equivalent doses to thyroid.

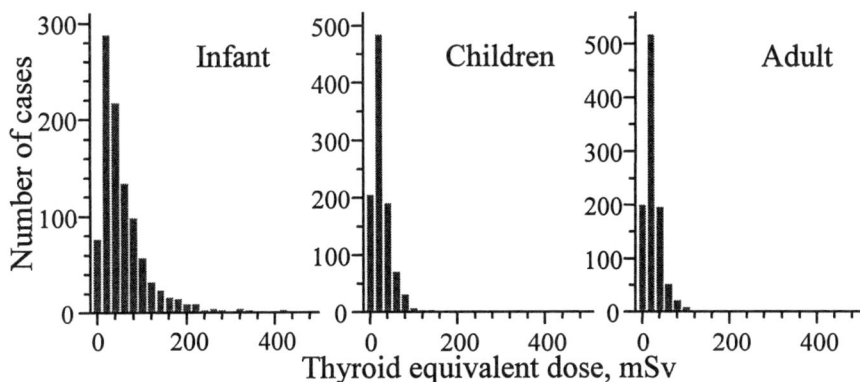

Fig. 3. Thyroid equivalent doses frequency distribution in (B) region of Lithuania (according to Fig. 1b) after the Chernobyl accident

3. RESULTS AND DISCUSSION

The results of thyroid dose evaluations in two (A, B) regions with different contamination levels are presented Table 1.

Table 1. Equivalent doses to thyroid in Lithuania after the Chernobyl accident

Age	Area	Equivalent doses to thyroid (mSv)					
		Determ.	Stochastic				95th
		mean	mean	s.d.	Median	Mode	percent.
Infant	A	21±4	22	10	20	16	39
	B	158±20	164	70	150	127	280
Adult	A	2.7±0.4	2.8	1.0	2.6	2.3	4
	B	20±2	21	7.5	20	17.7	28

As is evident the highest adult doses range up to about 28 mSv and infant's doses - up to 280 mSv in the most contaminated area of Lithuania. The consideration of regional stable iodine deficiency resulted in increase of thyroid equivalent doses as compared with calculations free of these considerations.

A rapid increase of thyroid disorders in Lithuania made physicians and scientists of various fields unit in solving this problem. Endocrinologist and pediatrian-endocrinologist have performed the screening of thyroid disorders. Collection, accumulation and evaluation of medical data have been performed according WHO standard. The results of adult thyroid examination[5] (Table 2) demonstrate high abnormal thyroid (up to 30 %) and thyroid with nodes (up to 16%) amongst adult Lithuanian inhabitants.

Table 2. Prevalence of adult thyroid gland pathology in Lithuania (1992-1996)

Region	Pers. exam.	Abnorm. thyr., %	Nodules/ cancer	Hypo- thyr., %	Hyper- thyr., %	Micr. Antib., %	Auto imun. thyrd.
Kaunas	239	25.6	12 / 0	10.3	7.1	15.8	-
Varena	336	26.8	15 / 2	7.3	6.2	15.0	22
Klaipeda	294	27.5	10 / 0	2.1	2.6	22.5	34
Joniskis	338	29.8	16 / 3	3.9	4.3	21.7	31

In the most contaminated region of Lithuania 362 children born in 1985-1986 has been examined. Thyroid palpation and ultrasonografy were performed. Thyroid nodules were found in 1.1 % of children. The results of fine-needle aspiration biopsy of nodules did not show any signs of malignisation. According these results, there is no increase in prevalence of childhood thyroid nodules[5].

4. SUMMARY AND CONCLUSIONS

Risk of radiation at low doses has been increasingly studied in recent year. The consequences of Chernobyl accident in Lithuania have presented scenario of thyroid disorders at low irradiation level and moderate degree of stable iodine deficiency. In an explicit form clear increase of induction of thyroid diseases over the spontaneous rate can not be established during one decade after the Chernobyl accident. Cancer register data demonstrate that there are no significant trend changes of thyroid disorders in Lithuania. These investigations are under a way and are useful for evaluating the future health effects.

REFERENCES

1. Dunning DE, Schwarz G. Variability of human thyroid characteristics and estimates of dose from ingested ^{131}I. *Health Phys* 1981; **40**: 661 - 675.
2. Johnson JR. Radioiodine dosimetry. *J. Rad. Chem* 1981; **65**: 223 – 238.
3. Nedveckaite T, Filistovic V. Estimates of thyroid equivalent doses in Lithuania following the Chernobyl accident. *Health Phys* 1995; **69**: 265-268.
4. Nedveckaite T, Filistovic V, Krasauskiene A, Kadziauskiene K. Relation between post-Chernobyl low level thyroid irradiation, stable iodine deficiency and thyroid disorders in Lithuania. *IAEA-TECDOC-976* Vienna, 1997: 299-302.
5. Sidlauskas V, Krasauskiene A, Aukstuolyte A, Masanauskaite D, Nedveckaite T. Chernobyl accident and thyroid disorders in Lithuania. *Acta Medica Lithuanica* 1997; **2**: 73-76.
6. Styra B, Nedveckaite T, Filistovic V. *Iodine isotopes and radiation safety.* Sankt-Peterburg: Gidrometeoizdat, 1992 (in Russian).

MEASURES TO REDUCE EXPOSURE OF THE THYROID GLAND TO RADIATION

Martin J. SCHLUMBERGER
Institut Gustave-Roussy 94805, Villejuif, France
Furio PACINI
Institute of Endocrinology,Ospedale Cisanello, Via Paradisa, 2, 56124 Pisa, Italy
E-mail f.pacini@endoc.med.unipi.it

If potassium iodine prophylaxis is combiçned with prompt protection and control of food sources, human exposure to 131I can be reduced by a factor of 1000 ; this will probably eliminate the risks of 131I exposure after a severe nuclear power plant accident. The protection of young children should be a priority.

1. INTRODUCTION

Large amounts of radioiodine isotopes released into the atmosphere can expose the thyroid to harmful levels of radiation.

Evidence acquired through studies on victims of radioactive fallout in the wake of the atomic bombs in Japan, of test detonations in the Marshall Islands and more recently of the Chernobyl power plant accident, now establishes, beyond doubt, that such exposure increases the incidence of benign and malignant thyroid tumors (1, 2, 3).

Three measures can be implemented to reduce exposure to radioiodine isotopes. Firstly, the population should be instructed to remain indoors. Secondly, consumption of contaminated food (milk) should be totally restricted. Thirdly, administering a large amount of potassium iodide will decrease radioiodine uptake by the thyroid gland.

The protection of young children should be a priority given their milk requirements, their small thyroids and their high susceptibility to the carcinogenic effects of ionizing radiation on the thyroid gland (4, 5).

2. REDUCTION OF RADIOIODINE INTAKE

The major routes of radioiodine intake are oral and respiratory. It has been estimated that contaminated food was responsible for more than 90 % of the total 131I intake in the populations living in the Marshall Islands and in the Chernobyl area. Respiratory intake is likely to be considerable and concerns both short-lived isotopes and 131I in individuals living very close to a nuclear reactor accident.

Instructing the population to remain indoors and to keep their doors and windows closed may reduce or at best delay body contamination through inhalation.

Restricting the consumption of contaminated food is a an imperative prophylactic measure to decrease total 131I intake. In most communities, fresh milk, obtained from cows that grazed on exposed pastures, is believed to be the chief source of 131I intake. Restrictive dietary measures would have to be maintained for up to 3 to 4 weeks because contamination of some food would be at a maximum after 5 to 20 days (6).

The maximal level of radioiodine tolerated in milk is 500 Bq/l, and 2000 Bq/kg in fresh vegetables (7, 8).

3. BLOCKADE OF RADIOIODINE THYROID UPTAKE

3.1 Background

As the thyroid actively concentrates iodine (and therefore its radioactive isotopes), the dose of radiation to the thyroid is 1000 to 10.000 times greater than that received by other organs after exposure to 131I (9). Uptake in the thyroid 24 hours after the administration of 131I depends on dietary intake of iodine which is 20-30 % when the iodine diet is normal and 60 % or more when the iodine diet is low. The dose delivered to the thyroid gland after oral administration of 3.7×10^7 Bq (1mCi) is 1300cGy in an adult with 25 % uptake in the thyroid at 24 hours. Thus, when radioiodine contamination occurs, the thyroid gland is the critical organ which should be protected imperatively.

A marked reduction has been demonstrated in radioiodine uptake after the administration of a large amount of stable iodine. A rapid effect is achieved because radioiodines are diluted in large amounts of stable iodine, the iodine-transport mechanism is then saturated and intrathyroid organification of iodide is rapidly inhibited (acute Wolff-Chaikoff effect). Such a decline in the level of uptake is particularly important since beta radiation delivered to thyroid follicular cells continues after radioiodine has been concentrated in the thyroid, while radioiodine is being organified and incorporated in thyroid hormones and precursors.

Radioiodine uptake at 24 hours can be decreased by more than 98 %, if 3 measures are implemented.

3.2 Administration of a large amount of potassium iodide

In adults, a single dose of 100 mg of iodide (130 mg potassium iodide) given with 131I reduces uptake in the thyroid to less than 1 % at 24 hours ; lower doses (30 or 50 mg) are as effective in subjects with a normal or high iodine diet, but may be significantly less effective in subjects with a deficient iodine diet ; larger doses (200 mg or more) are not significantly more effective (10). Lower doses are required in children to achieve optimal blockade.

3.3 Speed for KI administration

The effectiveness of a dose of 100 mg iodine in blocking thyroid uptake decreases rapidly, the longer ingestion is delayed. When this dose is administered shortly before (1 or 2 hours) contamination occurs or concurrently, thyroid blockade ensues rapidly, in less than 30 minutes and the 24 hour thyroid uptake is reduced by more than 98 %. A 90 % decrease is achieved when KI is administered 1 hour after contamination, 84 % after 2 hours and only 60 % after 3 hours. This was the rationale underlying the decision to distribute KI to populations living in the vicinity of nuclear power plants in France.

Even if iodine uptake is only partially decreased when iodide is not given immediately after contamination, iodide prophylaxis still reduces uptake by half, even after a delay of 3 hours, and should prove beneficial in case of prolonged exposure.

3.4 Repetition of KI administration

Thyroid radioiodine uptake will increase significantly within 1 or 2 days following a single dose of KI. The thyroid will also continue to concentrate a small amount of radioiodine generated peripherally from released radioiodinated hormones and large quantities from continued exposure. Daily administration of KI is therefore advisable in case of prolonged contamination. Treatments exceeding 1 or 2 weeks may however increase the side effects of KI.

3.5 Side effects of KI

Allergic reactions to the doses of iodine likely to be employed under these circumstances are rare and occur at a rate of 1 in a million to 1 in 10 million doses (12). KI was administered prophylactically to 10.5 million children and to 7 million adults in Poland, following the Chernobyl accident. Extra-thyroid side effects (nausea, vomiting, abdominal pain, skin rash) which were mild and transient occurred in 0.35 % of children and in 0.2 % of adults. Only 2 patients with a history of allergy were hospitalized (13).

Large amounts of iodide can give rise to adverse effects on thyroid function and especially in patients with underlying disease. Indeed, hypothyroidism or goiter or both may be induced in euthyroid patients previously treated with 131I or surgery for Graves' disease, Hashimoto's thyroiditis or benign nodules. Hypothyroidism and goiter have also been reported in neonates whose mothers ingested large quantities of iodine during pregnancy ; these findings indicate the enhanced sensitivity of the fetal and neonate thyroid to the inhibitory effect of iodide on hormone synthesis. On the other hand, the fetal and neonatal thyroid is very sensitive to radiation from radioactive iodine isotopes which readily cross the placenta and iodide prophylaxis in pregnant women is indicated. Finally, iodine-induced hyperthyroidism rarely occurs in patients who do not have a known underlying thyroid disease (12).

Abnormalities in thyroid function generally occur after more prolonged iodide therapy than that recommended as prophylaxis against thyroid exposure to radiation. In the Polish report, no iodine-induced hyperthyroidism occurred ; the incidence of congenital hypothyroidism did not increase in 1986, and 12 of the 3212 neonates who received potassium iodine during their first day of life had a transient and moderate increase in their blood TSH level with a moderate decrease in their blood T4 level during the following 3 to 5 days. Two to 3 years later, thyroid function and the development of these children were normal (13).

4. INDICATIONS

KI prophylaxis is decided by the authorities if a nuclear power plant accident occurs. Doses from radioiodine can also be reduced by evacuating and sheltering populations, restricting access to contaminated food and controlling farming practices.

International organizations have recently reviewed the intervention levels recommended for the administration of stable iodine (14, 15). For the IAEA : The intervention level for iodine prophylaxis for an advertable dose to the thyroid is 100 mGy (15).

KI is available in tablet form (130 mg KI per tablet, i.e. 100 mg iodide). Tablets are chemically stable for 3 years. The recommended doses are 100 mg iodide for adults (including pregnant women), 50 mg iodide for children under 13 years of age and 25 mg iodide in children under 3 years of age. A single dose should suffice. Whether this is repeated will depend upon the predicted doses to the thyroid and the duration of the contamination.

Since 1997, KI tablets have been distributed in France to the population living less than 5 km from a nuclear power plant. They are available at the chemist for the population living 5 km from a nuclear power plant (16, 17). Evaluation of the efficacy of predistribution of KI tablets was satisfactory.

In case of an accident priority should be given to the protection of children and pregnant women with KI prophylaxis. The inocuity of a single dose of KI in pregnant women and neonates has been demonstrated by the Polish report, but repeated administrations should be avoided, as they may cause hypothyroidism in neonates. After KI administration, pregnant women should be submitted to stringent follow-up by an obstetrician, and neonates to screening for hypothyroidism.

The benefits of KI prophylaxis in adults have yet to be shown, because the risk of radiation-induced thyroid tumors is low and furthermore there is a risk of iodine-induced hyperthyroidism after the age of 45.

Acknowledgements

This work was supported in part by a grand from the European Commission, Directorate General XII, Radiation Protection Research Unit. The author is grateful to Lorna Saint-Ange for editing.

References

1. THOMPSON DE, MABUCHI K, RON E, et al. Cancer incidence in atomic bomb survivors. Part II : solid tumors, 1958-1987. Radiat Res 1994; 137: S17-S67.
2. DOBYNS BM, HYRMER BA. The surgical management of benign and malignant thyroid neoplasms in Marshall islanders exposed to hydrogen bomb fallout. World J Surg 1992; 16: 126-140.
3. KARAOGLOU A, DESMET G, KELLY GN, et al. The radiological consequences of the Chernobyl accident. Publication EUR 16544 EN of the Commission of the European Communities, Brussels, Luxembourg, 1996.
4. RON E, LUBIN JH, SHORE RE, et al. Thyroid cancer after exposure to external radiation : a pooled analysis of seven studies. Radiat Res 1995; 141: 259-277.
5. PACINI F, VORONTSOVA T, DEMIDCHIK EP. et al. Chernobyl thyroid carcinoma in Belarus children and adolescents : comparison with naturally occurring thyroid carcinoma in Italy and France. J Clin Endocrinol Metab 1997; 82: 3563-3569.
6. VAN MIDDLESWORTH L. Nuclear reactor accidents and the thyroid. Thyroid Today 1987; 10: 1-5.
7. EURATOM. Règlement n° 3954/87 du Conseil du 22 Décembre 1987. JO des Communautés Européennes 1987; 30: L371/11-13.
8. EURATOM. Règlement n° 2218/89 du Conseil du 18 Juillet 1989 modifiant le règlement (EURATOM) n° 3954/87. JO des Communautés Européennes, L221/1-2.
9. LOEVINGER R, BUDINGER TF, WATSON EE. MIRD primer for absorbed dose calculations. New York : the Society of Nuclear Medicine, 1988.
10. STERNTHAL E, LIPWORTH L, STANLEY B, ABREAU C, FANG SL, BRAVERMAN LE. Suppression of thyroid radioiodine uptake by various doses of stable iodine. N Engl J Med 1980; 303: 1083-1088.
11. BLUM M, EISENBUD M. Reduction of thyroid irradiation from 131I by potassium iodide. JAMA 1967; 200: 112-116.

12. ROTI E, VAGENAKIS AG. Effect of excess iodide : clinical aspects. In : Braverman LE, Utiger RD (ed) : The Thyroid, 7th edition, Lippincott-Raven, Philadelphia,1996, pp. 316-327.

13. NAUMAN J, WOLFF J. Iodide prophylaxis in Poland after the Chernobyl reactor accident : benefits and risks. Am J Med 1993; 94: 524-532.

14. INTERNATIONAL COMMISSION ON RADIOLOGICAL PROTECTION (ICRP). Principles for intervention for protection of the public in a radiological emergency. Annals of the ICRP, vol. 22, n° 4.

15. International Atomic Energy Agency (IAEA). Intervention criteria in a nuclear or radiation emergency. Safety Series n° 109, IAEA, Vienna, 1991.

16. France. Ministère de l'Intérieur et Ministère de la Santé. Circulaire DGS/92-45 relative à l'administration d'iode stable en cas d'accident nucléaire, 18 Août 1992.

17. Direction Générale de la Santé, Direction de la Sécurité Civile. Circulaire relative à la distribution et mise à disposition d'iode stable aux habitants voisins des installations nucléaires ; 30 Avril 1997.

MONITORING AND PREVENTION OF THE DEVELOPMENT OF THYROID CARCINOMA IN A POPULATION EXPOSED TO RADIATION

SHUNICHI YAMASHITA, MASAHIRO ITO, KIYOTO ASHIZAWA, YOSHISADA SHIBATA, SHIGENOBU NAGATAKI AND KENZO KIIKUNI

Atomic Bomb Disease Institute, Nagasaki University School of Medicine, Radiation Effects Research Foundation, Hiroshima, Sasakawa Memorial Health Foundation, Tokyo, Japan

E-mail: shun@net.nagasaki-u.ac.jp

Since an accurate estimation of basal incidence of thyroid disease around Chernobyl is needed before discussion of relationship between radiation and thyroid carcinoma, we have screened and monitored the childhood thyroid disease within the framework of the Chernobyl Sasakawa Health and Medical Cooperation Project. Early detection of thyroid abnormalities by an ultrasound examination revealed a high incidence of thyroid nodules and carcinomas around Chernobyl, especially in Gomel region, Belarus. Malignant potential of thyroid nodules was also evaluated, introducing the fine needle aspiration biopsy and cytological diagnosis. Characteristic features of childhood thyroid disease are clarified and compared to those of radiation non-exposure group in Japan. The largest number of patients subsequently developed thyroid carcinomas were less than 1 year of age at the time of accident. The histological differences between childhood thyroid carcinoma in Belarus and Japan might be reflected in a different process of carcinogenesis. On a basis of established diagnostic centers around Chernobyl, intensive screening and careful follow-up for children and even now adolescence who have thyroid abnormalities are essentially needed. Only early detection and early treatment with an appropriate surgery for malignant thyroid nodules are the best way to prevent the development and worsening of thyroid carcinoma.

1. CHERNOBYL SASAKAWA HEALTH AND MEDICAL COOPERATION PROJECT

1.1. Subjects and methods

Territories radiocontaminated by the Chernobyl accident are vast, and , more than 4 million people resided in these contaminated areas. The subjects of study are children born between April 26, 1976 and April 26, 1986 (age at the time of accident: 0-10 years old), and examined in the period from May 15, 1991 to April 30, 1996. The data obtained from 120,000 children were analyzed and used for further evaluation. The course of health examination, either at the mobile diagnostic laboratory or at the center (Gomel and Mogilev in Belarus, Klincy in Russia, Kiev and Korosten in Ukraine), included the following; (1) collection of disease history and biographical information; (2) anthropometric data; (3) measurement of whole body Cs-137 radiation count; (4) ultrasonography of the thyroid; and (5) blood sampling for further analysis. Although we have all the health examination data, this presentation is focused on thyroid-related examination and the necessity of continuous screening and follow-up for these children will be discussed. The whole body Cs-137 counting data has been described elsewhere [1, 2]. The summary of the 5-year examination and procedures of thyroid examination has already been published[3]. Diagnosis of thyroid disease was established on the basis of the following criteria of thyroid images: (1) position, (2) structure, (3) echogenicity, (4) presence of nodules and cysts and (5) thyroid volume: The children were divided in to two groups according to thyroid volume; normal and goiter. The criterion for goiter has been previously described[3]

Table 1 Number of study subjects by region, sex and year of examination

Region	Sex	Year of examination						Total
		1991	1992	1993	1994	1995	1996	
Gomel	Boys	1035	1573	1603	2679	1963	632	9485
	Girls	1131	1708	1774	2840	2090	634	10177
	Total	2166	3281	3377	5519	4053	1266	19662
Megilev	Boys	636	2350	3069	2749	1876	983	11663
	Girls	680	2443	3184	2836	2010	965	12118
	Total	1316	4793	6253	5585	3886	1948	23781
Bryansk	Boys	373	1411	4320	2588	841	459	9992
	Girls	332	1552	4226	2576	1075	417	10178
	Total	705	2963	8546	5164	1916	876	20170
Kiev	Boys	692	971	3367	4028	3249	955	13262
	Girls	719	1094	3789	4400	3456	973	14431
	Total	1411	2065	7156	8428	6705	1928	27693
Zhitomir	Boys	645	1827	2668	3719	3328	1503	13690
	Girls	844	2175	3169	4067	3491	1597	15343
	Total	1489	4002	5837	7786	6819	3100	29033
Total	Boys	3381	8132	15027	15763	11257	4532	58092
	Girls	3706	8972	16142	16719	12122	4586	62247
	Total	7087	17104	31169	32482	23379	9118	120339

The serum-free thyroid thyroxine (FT4) and thyroid stimulating hormone (TSH) levels were determined with Amerlite hormone analyzer. Titers of anti-thyroglobulin antibody (ATG) and anti-microsome antibody (AMC) were determined by the reaction of indirect hem agglutination(Fujirevio). Determination of iodine and creatinine content in the urine was carried out with a BRAN+LUBBE automatic Analyzer II[4]. Four hundred and forty-six children showing echographic thyroid abnormalities were selected for fine-needle aspiration (FNA) biopsy, and a sample was successfully obtained for cytological diagnosis from 399 cases. Despite the presence of sampling bias of nodular lesions, cystic lesions and abnormal echo findings over 5mm in diameter, were chosen as targets for FNA. The diagnostic criteria for each disorder were described elsewhere [5, 6].

1.2. Thyroid ultrasound

The 11 ultrasonograms taken from each subject (not just those with abnormal findings) are preserved semipermanently on optic disks. According to common diagnostic criteria, a prevalence of childhood goiter in the different districts of the five region has been described elsewhere[3]. The incidence of goiter in the Mogilev region varied from 3 to 33% by district. The average goiter incidence was 22%. In contrast to the Mogilev region, there was a high prevalence of goiter in the Kiev region, Ukraine, with an average goiter incidence of 54%, which suggests that one of two children has an increased thyroid gland size. A large inter-regional variation was observed in the prevalence of goiter and it was highest in children from Kiev. A further investigation of geographical variation is needed in addition to the monitoring of iodide supplementation in school. The number of subjects with thyroid ultrasound abnormality is summarized in Table 2. The average frequency of thyroid nodules was 0.6%, and although FNB has not been performed in all cases, most of whom are thought to be either adenomatous goiter or adenoma. The highest incidence of thyroid nodule (1.64%) was observed in the Gomel region, Belarus. The frequency of abnormal echogenicity was also high in the Gomel region (4.09%), meanwhile Korosten was observed in the low frequency of abnormal echogenicity despite the high frequency of auto-antibody positive subjects.

Table 2 Incidence of thyroid diseases at the five centers around Chernobyl

	Belarus		Russia	Ukraine	
	Mogilev	Gomel	Klincy	Kiev	Korosten
Total number	23.531	19.271	19.918	27.5	28.958
Goiter (%)	22	18	41	54	8
Nodules (%)	0.18	1.64	0.52	0.2	0.26
Abnormal echogenecity (%)	1.09	4.09	2.37	2.37	0.66
Hyperthyroidism (%)	0.16	0.18	0.05	0.08	0.07
Hypothyroidism (%)	0.06	0.25	0.08	0.05	0.22
Positive autoantibodies					
ATG(%)	1.2	1	1.3	1.4	2.4
AMC(%)	2	2.5	1.9	2.5	3.2

The incidence of goiter, nodule(s) and abnormal echogenicity was analyzed by ultrasound imaging. ATG: antithyroglobin antibody, AMC: antimicrosomal antibody

1.3. Thyroid function

The results obtained, although within normal range (FT4, 10-25 pmol/l; TSH, 3-5μIU/ml) showed an uneven distribution, suggesting that the values exceeding the normal limits may be reflected not only by inaccurate measurement but by the age-dependent alteration of normal ranges. Based on the hormonal data and clinical findings, the incidence of thyroid dysfunction was also summarized in Table 2, all of these patients need to be treated. The high incidence of hyperthyroidism, including exogenous hyperthyroidism which is thought to have been treated with an inappropriate medication of thyroid hormone, has been discussed separately[7]. After excluding these artifacts corrected incidence of hyperthyroidism in Mogilev region was 0.1% and there were no differences in the data among the five centers. Positive thyroid auto-antibody titers were found most frequently in Korosten (3%). The average among the five centers was 1.5% for ATG and 1.8% for AMC. Investigations are also being conducted to determine whether or not the frequency of auto-antibody-positive children in the Chernobyl region is reasonable on the basis of a comparison with other reports. The age-dependent increase of positive thyroid autoantibodies was also noticed, all of which data indicate the similar incidence of childhood chronic thyroiditis in the world.

1.4. FNA biopsy and cytological diagnosis

The results of cytological examinations performed in 446 children are summarized in Table 3; these subjects were selected by the local staff based on abnormal ultrasound findings in the thyroid. The percentage and distribution of the various diseases were demonstrated and 34 cases of childhood thyroid cancer were discovered. Other diseases, such as adenomatous goiter, cyst and chronic thyroiditis, were also confirmed by cytology or in combination with other laboratory data. A high incidence of cancer was observed in Gomel, which was supported by the evidence that the prevalence of thyroid nodules and abnormal echogenicity findings in children were highest in this area. Table 4 shows the classification of the 446 subjects by FNA cytological diagnosis in comparison with ultrasonographic findings. Most cases of papillary carcinoma and follicular neoplasm were found in subjects showing nodular pattern by ultrasonography, while chronic thyroiditis was detected mainly in subjects showing abnormal echogenicity.

Table 3 Childhood thyroid disease around Chernobyl (1991, May-1996, March)

	Cases	Papillary carcinoma	Medullary carcinoma	Follicular neoplasm	Adenomatous goiter	Cyst	Chronic thyroiditis	Unclassified
Belarus								
Mogilev	32	1	0	1	7	11	7	5
Gomel	111	22	0	14	20	27	24	4
Russia								
Klincy	102	4	2	7	39	25	20	5
Ukraine								
Kiev	30	1	0	1	4	8	7	9
Korosten	171	4	0	23	30	31	59	24
Total	446	32	2	46	100	102	117	47
%	100	7.2	0.4	10.3	22.4	22.9	26.2	10.5

Table 4 Classification of 446 subjects by ultrasonographic and fine-needle aspiration (FNA) cytological diagnosis (1991 May - 1996 March)

	Ultrasonographical findings			
FNA cytology	Nodule	Cyst	Abnormal echogenecity	Total
Papillary carcinoma	30	1	1	32
Medullary carcinoma	1	0	1	2
Follicular neoplasm	44	2	0	46
Adenomatous goiter	46	50	4	100
Cyst	16	80	6	102
Chronic thyroiditis	10	7	100	117
Unclassified	7	19	21	47
Total	154	159	133	446

1.5. Urinary iodine concentration

As the incidence of goiter differed widely in the Mogilev and Kiev regions, urinary iodine secretion was measured in some children in the different districts. In Mogilev, about 20% of children had less than $10\mu g/dl$ urinary secretion of iodine. In Kiev, 85% of children had a concentration of less than $10\mu g/dl$ urinary iodine, where the deficiency was not correctly compensated by iodine supplementation. These results support the evidence of different degrees of endemic goiter around Chernobyl[8].

2 CHARACTERISTIC FEATURES OF CHILDHOOD THYROID CARCINOMA AROUND CHERNOBYL

2.1. Malignant potential of thyroid nodule(s)

Thyroid nodules are common in adult, but rare in children in general. Around Chernobyl, however, the average frequency of childhood thyroid nodules was 0.6% and the highest 1.6% in Gomel region. According to the results of FNA biopsy and cytological diagnosis, 7% of thyroid nodules detected by ultrasound images was confirmed as malignant thyroid nodules. Although sampling biases and false-negative cytological diagnosis for follicular carcinoma involved, it is very important to follow-up carefully the children who have thyroid nodule(s) around Chernobyl. Now these centers can apply on-site cytological diagnosis using the thyroid ultrasound echo-guided FNA biopsy. Preliminary, but important data appeared which among these patients with thyroid nodule(s), two cases of papillary carcinoma were newly diagnosed, suggesting the importance of follow-up of these patients as a high risk group for development of thyroid cancer around Chernobyl.

2.2. Comparison of Belarus and Japan

To clarify the clinical and histological characteristics of childhood thyroid cancer in Belarus, we therefore compared these patients to a radiation non-exposed control series in Japan[9]. In Belarus, 26 thyroid cancers in subjects aged 15 or younger were analyzed and compared to 37 childhood thyroid cancers in Japan diagnosed between 1962 and 1995. The age distribution at operation in Belarus showed a peak at 10 years old, with a subsequent fall in numbers. In contrast, the age distribution at operation in Japan showed a smooth increase between the ages of 8 and 14. The mean tumor diameter was smaller in Belarus than that in Japan (1.4 ± 0.7 vs. 4.1 ± 1.7 cm, $P<0.001$). The sex ratio, regional lymph node metastasis, extension to surrounding tissues or lung metastasis did not differ significantly. Histologically, all cases in Belarus were papillary and in Japan 33 cases were papillary and 4 cases were follicular carcinomas. Among papillary carcinomas, the frequency of a solid growth pattern, a criteria for classifying a tumor as poorly differentiated, was higher in Belarus than that in Japan (61.5 vs. 18.2%, $P<0.001$)[10].

The difference between the features of childhood thyroid cancer in Japan and Belarus may be due to the difference in the process of carcinogenesis[11]. However, despite of the screening effort for early detection of malignant thyroid nodule(s), the rate of metastasis and local invasion is highly observed in Belarus cases, suggesting the difficulty of prediction of early development of childhood thyroid carcinoma. Therefore it should be emphasized that children who have observed abnormal thyroid ultrasound images must be followed up carefully and the application of FNA biopsy is deeply considered during the follow-up period. The incidence of ret/PTC gene rearrangement may support the characteristic findings of post-Chernobyl childhood thyroid carcinoma[12-16], however, careful analysis is needed[17].

3. SUMMARY

It is widely accepted that clear evidence of the public health impact of radiation exposure as a result of the Chernobyl accident is a highly significant increase in the incidence of thyroid cancer among those persons in the affected areas who were children in 1986. The Chernobyl Sasakawa Health and Medical Cooperation Project have now completed under the same protocol and procedure which demonstrated the comparable data of childhood thyroid diseases around Chernobyl, indicating the highest number of thyroid nodules and cancer in Gomel region, Belarus. Practically there are handicap of remoteness and inadequate supply of medical knowledge and experience on radiation medicine and endocrinology around Chernobyl. To assist these remote-area medical problems, we need to cooperate each other at the different levels, nationally and internationally. Especially the following cooperation is needed to improve the monitoring and prevention of the development of thyroid carcinoma; (1) double check of thyroid disease diagnosis screened by ultrasound images, (2) quality control of medical data, (3) appropriate guidance of cytological diagnosis, medical treatment and follow-up and (4) promotion of exchange of medical knowledge and experience. The cooperative studies are directed to standardize the diagnostic criteria and procedure of thyroid cancer, to identify a high risk group of thyroid cancer and to establish the most effective follow-up system of operated thyroid cancer patients, especially in Gomel region. Therefore, a novel approach of Chernobyl Sasakawa Project is now going to establish a remote area medical assistance, especially assistance of thyroid image diagnosis and cytological diagnosis. Based on our valuable data bank established in the past 5 year-project, more effective monitoring and diagnosis system will be established near in the future.

Acknowledgments

We greatly appreciate the following counterparts; Ministries of Health and diagnostic centers in 3 NIS countries (Belarus, Russia, Ukraine): Gomel Specialized

Dispensary, Mogilev Regional Medical Diagnostic Center, Belarus; Klincy City Children's Hospital, Russia; Kiev Regional Hospital No. 2, Korosten Inter-Area Medical Diagnostic Center, Ukraine.

References

1. Hoshi M, Yamamoto M, Kawamura H, Shinohara K, Shibata Y, Kozlenko MT, Takatsuji T, Yamashita S, Yokoyama N, Izumi M, Fujimura K, Danilyuk VV, Nagataki S, Kuramoto A, Okajima S, Kiikuni K, Shigematsu I: Fallout radioactivity in soil and food samples in the Ukraine: measurement of iodine, plutonium, cesium, and strontium isotopes. Health Phys 1984; 67: 187-191.
2. Hoshi M, Shibata Y, Okajima S, Takatsuji T, Yamashita S, Namba H, Yokoyama N, Izumi M, Nagataki S, Fujimura K, Kuramoto A, Krupnik TA, Dolbeshkin NK, Danilchik SA, Derzhitsky VE, Wafa KA, Kiikuni K, Shigematsu I: Cesium-137 concentration among children in areas contaminated with radioactive fallout caused by the Chernobyl accident: the results in Mogilev and Gomel oblasts, Belarus. Health Phys 1994; 67: 268-271.
3. Yamashita S, Shibata Y (eds): Chernobyl; A Decade, Excerpta Medica, Amsterdam ICS 1997; 1156: pp1-613.
4. Tsuda K, Namba H, Nomura T, Yokoyama N, Yamashita S, Izumi M, Nagataki S: Automated measurement of urinary iodine with use of ultraviolet irradiation. Clin Chem 1995; 414. 581-585.
5. Ito M, Yamashita S, Ashizawa K, Namba H, Hoshi M, Shibata Y, Sekine I, Nagataki S, Shigematsu I: Childhood thyroid diseases around Chernobyl evaluated by fine needle aspiration cytology. Thyroid 1995; 5. 365-368.
6. to M, Kotova L, Panasyuk GD, Ashizawa K, Nishikawa T, Nagataki S, Yamashita S: Cytological characteristics of pediatric thyroid cancer around Chernobyl. Acta Cytol, 1997; 41: 1642-1644.
7. Ashizawa K, Krupnik T, Nagataki S, Yamashita S: Transient thyrotoxicosis around Chernobyl. Thyroid (in press)
8. Ashizawa K, Shibata Y, Yamashita S, Namba H, Hoshi M, Yokoyama N, Izumi M, Nagataki S: Prevalence of goiter and urinary iodine excretion levels in children around Chernobyl. J Clin Endocrinol Metab 1997; 82: 3430-3433.
9. Shirahige Y, Ito M, Ashizawa K, Nishikawa T, Yokoyama N, Namba H, Ishikawa N, Mimura T, Fukata S, Yokozawa T, Yamashita S, Sekine I, Kuma K, Ito K, Panasyuk G, Demidchik EP, Nagataki S: Characteristic features of childhood thyroid cancer in Japan and Belarus. Endocrine J 1998; 45: 203-209.
10. Ito M, Yamashita S, Ashizawa K, Hara T, Namba H, Hoshi M, Shibata Y, Sekine I, Kotova L, Panasyuk G, Demidchik E, Nagataki S: Histopathological characteristics of childhood thyroid cancer in Gomel Belarus. International J Cancer 1996; 65: 29-33.

11. Nagataki S, Ashizawa K, Yamashita S: Cause of childhood thyroid cancer after Chernobyl accident. Thyroid 1998; 8: 115-117.

12. Klugbauer S, Lengfelder E, Demidchik IP, Rabes HM: A new form of RET rearrangement in thyroid carcinomas of children after the Chernobyl reactor accident. Oncogene 1996; 13: 1099-1102.

13. Fugazzola L, Pierotti MA, Vigano E, Pacini F, Vorontsova TA, Bongarzone I: Molecular and biochemical analysis of RET/PTC 4, a novel oncogenic rearrangement between RET and ELE 1 genes, in a post-Chernobyl papillary thyroid cancer. Oncogene 1996; 13: 1093-1097.

14. Klugbauer S, Demidchik EP, Lengfelder E, Rabes HM: Detection of a novel type of RET rearrangement (PTC5)in thyroid carcinomas after Chernobyl and analysis of the involved RET-fused gene RFG5. Cancer Res 1998; 58: 198-203.

15. Nikiforoz YE, Rowland JM, Bove KE, Monforte-Munoz H, Fagin JA: District pattern of ret oncogene rearrangements in morphological variants of radiation-induced and sporadic thyroid papillary carcinomas in children. Cancer Res 1997; 57: 1690-1694.

16. Bongarzone I, Butti MG, Fugazzola L, Pacini F, Pinchera A, Vorotosova TV, Demidchik EP, Pierotti MA: Comparison of the breakpoint resions of ELE1 and RET genes involved in the generation of RET/PTC 3 oncogene in sporadic and in radiation-associated papillary thyroid carcinomas. Genomics 1997; 42: 252-259.

17. Motomura T, Nikiforov VE, Namba H, Ashizawa K, Nagataki S, Yamashita S, Fagin JA: Ret rearrangements in Japanese pediatric and adult papillary thyroid cancers. Thyroid (in press)

PRACTICAL EXPERIENCE OF PROPHYLAXIS FOR LARGE SCALE EXPOSURE AFTER A NUCLEAR ACCIDENT

JANUSZ A. NAUMAN

Department of Medicine & Endocrinology, University Medical School of Warsaw and Department of Endocrinology, Medical Research Center of Polish Academy of Sciences, Warsaw, Poland.

The objectives which during Chernobyl accident led to the Potassium Iodide (KI) prophylaxis in Poland , the model of prophylaxis approved and its implementation are described. Epidemiological studies (MZ-XVII Research Programme) shown that although this protective action (single dose of KI) was only mandatory for children 16 years old or under substantial number of adults also took the single dose of iodide. All together KI was given to about18 milion of Poles .Single dose of KI taken on April 29 reduced thyroid radioiodine burden by 40%, while the same dose taken on April 30 reduced thyroid committed dose by about 25%. Maximal thyroid doses in children living in 12 provinces where radioioiodines contamination was high, varied without protection from 55.1 to 136.2 mSv. The transient, and mild intrathyroidal side-effects were only seen in 0.37% of newborns. The extrathyroidal side-effects were developed by 4.6% of children and 4.5% of adults. They represented supersensitivity to iodine and all were mild. It is concluded that the single dose of KI given in Poland reduced thyroid dose below 50 mSv. It is also concluded that this prophylaxis proven to be safe procedure

INTRODUCTION

It is now established that internal radiation can be tumorogenic for the thyroid [1,2], therefore in case of nuclear accident, thyroid dose especially in such risk groups as pregnant women, newborns and children should be kept as low as possible. The accumulation of radioiodines by the thyroid gland can be effectively decreased by administration of stable iodine [3]. The thyroid radioiodines uptake can be either almost totally blocked if sufficient and repeated doses of stable iodine are given immediately before, or soon after exposure [3,4].Moreover, the final thyroid dose can be reduced if a single dose of stable iodine is given in time of prolonged radioiodines contamination [5].The Chernobyl accident was the first in which different prophylactic measures were undertaken to protect the health of a large population. The aim of the present paper is to describe the objectives which led to the decision to implement KI prophylaxis in Poland, to discuss the model of prophylaxis, , its effiacacy, and side-effects of KI given to different age groups. Part of the data which will be presented were already published [5,6].

1. OBJECTIVES FOR DECISION TO IMPLEMENT KI PROPHYLAXIS IN POLAND

In time of the Chernobyl accident reliable information about its size and possible effects on public health were not available from former Soviet Union authorities. In Poland increased air radioactivity and external radiation was first identified in the night of April 27 and 28. In the early hours of April 28 all Polish monitoring stations were placed on permanent emergency alert. Because of environmental findings showing radiological contamination, mostly by radioiodines in the whole country on early hours of April 29, children at different age received neck measurments at the Center for Radiological Protection in Warsaw. Although at that time Warsaw area was only moderately contaminated thyroid counts amounted from 500 to 1300 Bq. A governmental commission which was called to assess damage potential and protect public health made several decisions. First, it accepted the scenario of the accident (presented by members of the Center for Radiological Protection) which stated that the accident was very serious and would lead to a prolonged release of radionuclides including radioiodines. Second, it recommended the following intervention levels:

(1) whole body committed dose should not exceed 5mSv;

(2) thyroid committed dose should not exceed 50 mSv in children and 500 mSv in adults;

(3) thyroid 131-I content in children at any moment should not exceed 5700 Bq.

Third, the commission defined the population at risk as about 11 million of children and adolescents. The commission also realized that due to relative iodine deficiency in Polish diet, the thyroid uptake of radioiodines, especially in children might be higher than in other European countries. At 10 AM of April 29 monitoring stations were reporting continuing and growing radiological contamination especially in eastern and central Poland. **It was then concluded that at least in 11 Voivodoships (Provinces) the thyroid committed dose in children might well exceed the 50 mSv limit**. It was felt that although some thyroid radioiodines uptake already occurred it is necessary to protect the gland against continuing radioiodine contamination coming from the damaged Chernobyl power station reactor. At that moment Poland had no sufficient supply of KI tablets, however, the Central Pharmacy Organization (CEFARM) had stores of KI in substance which were sufficient to prepare the KI solution containing about 90 millions doses of 100 mg of KI each.

1.1 Potassium iodide prophylaxis adopted in Poland

Evidence from literature [7] shows that mean effect of 70 mg of iodide on radioiodine uptake in thyroid is similar to that produced by 100 mg of iodide and the only difference is 30-60 min latency until the smaller dose starts its action upon thyroid. Information about side effects of iodide was also published elsewhere [3,4] although it came from observation of small groups of patients. Nevertheless, it was obvious, that intrathyroidal and extrathyroidal side-effects depend on the KI dose and the number of such doses taken by the same person [3]. When the final model of KI prophylaxis was formulated in Poland it was realized that on April 29 total block of thyroid radioiodines uptake is not possible any more. On the other hand, members of the commission felt that final burden to the thyroid should be reduced to a level relatively safe in terms of prospective tumorogenic effects of internal radiation. It was also expected that a single dose of iodide would not lead to serious side-effects. At noon hours of April 29 after discussing all aspects of prophylaxis the Minister of Health ordered to preparation and distribution of KI solution in all hospitals, public health care centers, drug stores, schools, kindergardens and so forth. The KI prophylaxis was ordered to be mandatory to all under 16 years old and voluntary to all others. Pregnant and lactating women were advised to take prophylaxis. The following protocol was used: 15 mg of iodide for newborns(the dose of 30 mg was given on the first day), 50 mg for children 5 years or under and 70 mg for all others. The prophylaxis was first introduced in 11 eastern Voivodoships. On April 30 As situation on April 30 deteriorated further the prophylaxis was ordered for all Poland. It was also decided that a second dose of KI would be distributed if radiological air contamination would continue to be high.. Fortunately by May 3 and 4 ,due to the change in the meteorological situation, air contamination decreased at least fourfold and in the next days further decrease of radioactivity was observed. Therefore distribution of the second dose of KI was not necessary.

1.2 Follow-up programmes (Research projects MZ-XVII and PBZ 38-08)

After radioiodines contamination caused by the Chernobyl accident and the protective phase in Poland was over it was clear that a research follow - up programme should be initiated with the following objectives:

1. To evaluate thyroid 131-I committed doses in children and adults living in different regions of Poland and to investigate possible effects of thyroid irradiation;

2. To estimate the degree of thyroid protection achieved by administration of KI and to obtain estimates of the incidence of intrathyroidal and extrathyroidal side effects;

3. To evaluate thyroid function in newborns who were exposed to the radiation and KI administration while *in utero* or soon after delivery;

4. To evaluate possible detrimental effects of a single dose of KI on subjects with past history of thyroid diseases.

The implementation of MZ-XVII research programme (1987-1990), was previously described in details [5,6]. Briefly 52092 persons were questioned and 34491 completed the study. The sample studied representing approximately 0.09% of the population of Poland and its distribution (age, sex, living in towns and villages) was typical for Poland as a whole.

The research programme PBZ 38-08 started in the middle of 1997 and will be completed at the end of 1999. The population under the study will be the same as that investigated within the MZ-XVII programme. This time, however, it was decided to reexamine only these who were 25 years old or under at the time of the Chernobyl accident and who lived in Voivodoships (provinces) where radioiodines contamination was described as high or average. The population considered this time to be *the sample* consists of about 21000 subjects. It is expected that at least 15000 subjects will complete the study. The PBZ 38-08 research programme has the following objectives:

1. To obtain more accurate thyroid burden estimates for children, adolescents and adults in randomly selected regions of Poland, using for thyroid dose reconstruction the results of population study on iodine intake in diet which was carried on between 1993 and 1994 in specified Polish provinces;

2. To evaluate possible functional and morphological effects of thyroid irradiation and compare them with findings obtained in the same subjects during implementation of MZ-XVII programme (studies performed 2-4 years after the accident);

3. To evaluate hormonal and immunological status of approximately 1000 relatively young patients referred for thyroid surgery with cytologically confirmed diagnosis of thyroid tumors (adenomas and cancers) and to preserve the tissue not only for pathological but also for molecular studies.

1.3 Thyroid committed doses for 131-I in Poland

As already described [5] thyroid burden was evaluated in 1500 subjects by the direct method in 5 study regions between April 29 and May 16 1986. The thyroid burden in population was also evaluated in each Voivodoship (province) by an indirect method developed by Johnson [8] This method is based on the 5 compartmental model of iodine metabolism using values of 131-I measured in air, milk, other foods, standard value for inhalation rate and milk and food consumption, and such parameters as age, sex, thyroid size, and iodine uptake. Table 1 presents minimal and maximal 131-I thyroid committed doses in 12 highly contaminated provinces as evaluated during MZ-XVII programme and most recently in the course of PBZ-38-08 programme where more appropriate iodine uptake was used in dose calculation.

Table 1: Predicted minimal and maximal 131-I thyroid committed doses (mSv) in 12 highly contaminated voivodoships (provinces)

Age of inhabitants	doses estimated[*]	
	minimal	maximal
< 1 year old	15.5 (26.4)	68.1 (136.2)
< 2-5 years	11.3 (19.2)	48.1 (69.4)
< 6-10 years	10.9 (17.2)	32.4 (55.1)
Adults	7.1 (12.1)	18.1 (30.8)

[*]Data in parenthesis represent the dose reconstruction performed within PBZ 38-08 Research Programme

From preliminary data on thyroid dose reconstruction (Table 1) it can be suggested that about 17% of children of all age groups in 12 highly contaminated voivodoships (provinces) who reached maximal 131-I thyroid committed doses all exceeded 50 mSv limit without protective action. It should be also added that in all Poland including the above mentioned voivodoships there were a number of „hot spots" wherein the thyroid doses could have been approximately 6 - 10 times that of the surrounding areas. More comprehensive data on thyroid committed dose reconstruction will be available at the end of 1999 after PBZ-38-08 Programme will be completed.

1.4   Potassium Iodide prophylaxis in Poland

As previously described [5,6] approximately 95.3% of Polish children (about 10.5 millions) and 23.2% of adults (7.5 millions) took KI prophylaxis. Evidence obtained in the MZ-XVII Programme also shows that over 6% of children were given diluted tincture of iodine by their parents before the start of protective action in the afternoon hours of April 29. Inquired parents stated later, that their action was a result of enormous stress and fear that the health and even life of their children were at risk. It was also estimated that for the same reason about 3% of children   reason were given two or more doses of KI. As already stated the protective action was first ordered on April 29 only for 12 voivodoships which were highly contaminated. Very strong pressure from the authorities and these living in the rest of Poland as well as further deterioration of the weather leading to higher contamination of provinces which up to early morning hours of April 30 were only mildly contaminated resulted in the extension of the protective action to the whole country on April 30. In the 12 provinces where prophylaxis started on April 29 the bulk of KI distribution occurred during the next two days, however in areas bordering with former Soviet Union almost 75% of children were reached within 24 hours The protective action ordered on April 30 was less efficient and the bulk of children from these provinces received prophylaxis on May 2nd. Predicted thyroid burden reduction in children living in 12 highly contaminated voivodoships and who took KI prophylaxis is summarized in Table 2. On the basis of Johnson model it was assumed that prophylaxis given on April 29 reduced thyroid burden by about 40% and prophylaxis given on April 30 by about 25%[5].

Table 2: Predicted thyroid burden reduction by a single dose of KI in children who received maximal thyroid doses in 12 highly contaminated voivodoships (provinces)

Age of inhabitant	Maximal thyroid doses (mSv) reconstructed within PBZ 38-08 Programme		
	without prophylaxis	KI on April 29	KI on April 30
< 1 year old	136.2	81.7	102.1
< 2-5 years	69.5	41.6	52.1
< 6-10 years	55.0	33.1	41.2

When the thyroid burden and effect of KI protection was investigated by direct method [5] the dose reduction in subjects leaving around Ostroleka province who took KI on April 29 was estimated to be 45% and in those who took KI on April 30 to be 41% respectively. Nevertheless there is no doubt that early KI administration is more effective. In our previous study assumed that if there were prompt warning from the Soviet Union authorities and if KI prophylaxis were implemented in Poland on April 27 the thyroid burden reduction would have been close to 67% [5].

1.5 Side effects of single dose of Potassium Iodide Intrathyroidal

The protective measures undertaken in Poland were the first to permit an evaluation of possible side effects after a known intake of KI in a large population. The comparison of serum TSH, T4 and T3 of children who took prophylaxis with those who were unprotected in all age groups showed no significant difference. Similar conclussions were drawn from screening studies for congenital hypothyroidism for 1985,1986 and 1987. Neither there were statistical difference in results of thyroid evaluation between adults who took prophylaxis and those who did not. The acute intrathyroidal side effects of single dose of KI were seen in 0.37% of newborns who received either 30 mg or15mg of KI on the second day of life. Apart from the fact that this dose was 5 times higher on the basis of KI mg/kg of body mass only few infants showed the transient increase of serum TSH and transient decrease of free T4. This Wolff - Chaikoff phenomenon disappeared after 10 days without any treatment. The representative randomly selected group of newborns who took KI was carefully examined on the 3rd year of life and their thyroid status was similar to that of the group of children who were born one year after Chernobyl accident. This group is again carefully investigated within the PBZ 38-08 Program. Preliminary results confirm the conclusion that administration of the single dose of KI in the early stage of life and even transient Wolff-Chaikoff phenomenon remain without effect upon further thyroid function.

1.6   Extrathyroidal

As already reported [5,6] the number of extrathyroidal side effects identified after the single dose of KI were more common than expected and this reaction was seen in about 4.6% of children and 4.5% of adults. All of those side- effects were of hypersensitivity type and all were mild and transient. Vomiting which was most common was never previously described as a extrathyroidal side-effect of KI administration. It is likely that this effect e depended more on the formula of prophylaxis than on the effect of iodide itself. Two adults with chronic obstructive lung disease and well documented allergy to iodides took the prophylaxis because they felt that radioiodines might be detrimental to their life. Both promptly developed acute respiratory distress which was released by hydrocortisone administration. Besides these two patients such reaction was not described in other subjects.

2.   COMMENTS AND CONCLUSIONS

At the time of the Chernobyl accident there were no international regulations on early warning in case of nuclear disaster and the first official information of Soviet TASS Agency published on April 28 said that „the accident was of limited size and that there is no risk for public health". As an international agreement is now in power, it should be expected that if a severe nuclear accident with a risk to thyroids of public happend, sufficient information would be available for all countries and KI prophylaxis, if needed, would be introduced very early; therefore being more effective than that in Poland. The growing evidence that even relatively low thyroid doses of radioiodines can lead to significant rise in the incidence of thyroid cancer among those exposed in childhood [9] strongly support the need for such a protective action for pregnant women, newborns and children. Increased incidence of thyroid cancer in children and more recent estimate of risk for thyroid cancer in children [10] suggest to national authorities that intervention levels for pregnant women and children should be below 20 mGy radiation dose to the thyroid therefore lower that those approved in Poland in 1986 which at that time seemed to be very conservative.. The Polish experience shows that in time when in our opinion public health was at risk, KI solution could be rapidly prepared and quite efficiently distributed. It should however be remembered that in 1986 the power in Poland was centralized and the Minister of Health could order immediate and country-wide action. It is of open question how much the Minister of Health could do at a situation when the power would be in part distributed to local communities. Our findings that at the time of Chernobyl accident parents gave to their children tinctura of iodine demonstrate how strong was fear and stress may become in time of nuclear accident. In addition, desperate decision to administer the drug with the warning,, poison, only for external use" to one own children shows that in case of nuclear disaster the confidence that official communication would calm the fear might be doubtful. On the other hand it is likely that stress and fear of coming danger was instrumental in the fast delivering the KI to majority of children living in voivodoships bordering with former Soviet Union. The results of studies completed within MZ-XVII research programme and preliminary results of PBZ 38-08 research programme show that even the single dose of KI might limit thyroid burden to that relatively safe for the gland. Although non-complited evaluation suggests some increase in the incidence of thyroid cancer in children and adults living in areas bordering with the Belarus it is still very limited. In 1999 with PZB 38-08 programme completed, it will be possible to say whether this increase is significant or non-significant. As already published [5,6] and shown again in the present paper single dose of KI is a safe procedure. We believe that the intrathyroidal side effect seen in newborns was related to the dose of KI given on the first day (30 mg) which was next day reduced to 15 mg, while some of extrathyroidal side-effects (especially vomiting) were related to the formula of KI and not to KI itself. The KI tablets available at present on the market have quite long shelf- time and their price could probably be reduced. It is suggested that their pre-distribution is a crucial issue for effective prophylaxis in case of nuclear accident.

In conclusion we suggest that the decision to block the thyroid uptake of radioiodines by repeated doses of KI or the decision to reduce final committed thyroid burden by single KI depend on the evaluation of radiological contamination, approved intervention levels, size of population at risk, and preparedness (including pre-distribution of KI tablets and education of the population).

We also proved that in the situation which prevailed in Poland during Chernobyl accident even a single dose of KI if given on time significantly reduced the final thyroid committed dose and was a safe procedure.

References

1. Williams ED, Pacini F, Pinchera A. Thyroid cancer following Chernobyl. J. Endocrinol Invest 1995; 18: 144-146.

2. Likhtarew IA, Sobolev BG, Kairo IA, Chepurny NI. Thyroid cancer in Ukraine. Nature 1995; 375: 365.

3. Crocker DG. Nuclear reactor accidents-the use of KI as a blocking agent against radioiodine uptake in the thyroid-a review. Health Physics 1984; 46: 1265- 1279.

4. Becker DV, Braverman LE, Dunn JT, Gaitan E, Gorman C, Maxon H, Schneider AB, Van Middlesworth L, Wolff J. The use of iodine as thyroidal blocking agent in the event of a reactor accident. JAMA 1984; 252: 659-661.

5. Nauman J, Wolff J. Iodide prophylaxis in Poland after the Chernobyl reactor accident: benefits and risks. Am J Medicine 1993; 94:524-532.

6. Nauman J. guest editor. Results of studies performed within MZ-XVII Programme (Chernobyl, iodide, thyroid). Pol J Endocrinol 1991; 42: 153-367.

7. Sternthal E, Lipworth L, Stanley B, Abreau C, Fang SL, Braverman LE. Supression of thyroid radioiodine uptake by various doses of stable iodide. N Engl J Med. 1980; 303: 1083-1088.

8. Johnson JR. Radioiodine dosimetry. J Radioanalitical Chem 1981; 65:223-231.

9. Nikiforow Y, Gnepp DR Pediatric thyroid cancer after the Chernobyl disaster. Cancer 1994; 74: 748-751.

10. Ron E.Thyroid cancer after exposure to external radiation: a pooled analysis of seven studies. Rad Res 1995; 141: 259-277

CLINICAL FEATURES AND TREATMENT OF THYROID CARCINOMA FOLLOWING RADIATION

Furio Pacini, Eleonora Molinaro, Laura Agate, Rossella Elisei, Aldo Pinchera
Department of Endocrinology, University of Pisa, via Paradisa 2, 56124, Pisa, Italy
E-mail:endo@endoc.med.unipi.it

Eugeni P. Demidchik, Tatiana Vorontsova , Elena Shavrova, Eugeny D. Cherstvoy, Yuriy Ivashkevitch, Elvira Kuchinskay
Institute of Radiation Medicine and Oncology- Pathology Department, State Medical University, Minsk, Belarus

Martin Schlumberger,
Institute Gustave Roussy, Villejuif, France

Giuseppe Ronga,.
Medicina Nucleare, Clinica Medica II, Università La Sapienza, Roma, Italy

An increased incidence of papillary thyroid carcinoma has been observed several years after external irradiation to the head and the neck in subjects treated for various non-thyroidal disorders, in atomic bomb survivors in Japan, and in residents of the Marshall Island exposed to radiation during the testing of hydrogen bombs. The Chernobyl nuclear reactor accident, has clearly shown that exposure to radioactive fall-out was the cause of an enormous increase in the prevalence of childhood thyroid carcinoma observed in Belarus, Ukraine and, to a lesser extent, in the Russian Federation starting from 1990. About 800 thyroid cancers have been observed in children less than 15 years old living in the most contaminated areas. A comparison between clinical and epidemiological features of thyroid carcinomas, diagnosed in Belarus after the Chernobyl accident and naturally occurring thyroid carcinoma of the same age group observed in Italy and in France, shows that the post-Chernobyl thyroid carcinomas were much less influenced by gender, were virtually always papillary (solid and follicular variants), had higher aggressiveness at presentation, and were more frequently associated with thyroid autoimmunity. Gene rearrangements, involving the RET proto-oncogene (less frequently TRK), have been demonstrated as causative event specific for papillary cancer. Much higher rates of RET activation (nearly 70%) have been found in post-Chernobyl papillary thyroid carcinomas. The prevalence of specific types of rearrangement differs in sporadic tumors (mainly RET/PTC 1) with respect to radiation-induced neoplasm (mainly RET/PTC 3). The initial treatment of differentiated thyroid cancer is surgery. Four-six weeks after surgery all patients should be treated with radioiodine for ablation of any post-surgical residual thyroid tissues. The other essential step in the treatment of childhood differentiated thyroid cancer is hormonal therapy (thyroid hormone suppressive therapy). The drug of choice is L-thyroxine (LT4). When appropriately treated, differentiated thyroid cancer is a curable disease, with very high cure rate even in the presence of distant metastases.

Introduction

Both external and internal ionizing radiations are recognized as one of the main risk factors for developing thyroid carcinoma especially when radiation exposure occurred during childhood. An increased incidence of thyroid carcinoma, mainly of the papillary histotype, has been observed several years after external irradiation to the head and the neck in subjects treated for various non-thyroidal disorders (1-3), in atomic bomb survivors in Japan (4), and in residents of the Marshall Island exposed to radiation during the testing of hydrogen bombs (5).

The Chernobyl nuclear reactor accident has clearly shown that exposure to radioactive fall-out was the cause of an enormous increase in the prevalence of childhood thyroid carcinoma (6-10). The size of this increase, the geographical and the temporal distribution of the cases strongly suggest that the increased incidence of thyroid cancer is due to radiation exposure and, most likely, to the huge amount of iodine radioisotopes released by the damaged Chernobyl reactor, which includes 131-I and other short-lived iodine isotopes (11). A state of endemic iodine deficiency and the absence of immediate iodine prophylaxis might have further contributed to high radiation exposure of the thyroid, expecially in children, in whom the final radiation dose per gram of tissue is much more important with respect to adults (12).

Following diagnostic or therapeutic administration of radioiodine isotopes (131-I), no evidence of an increased relative risk of thyroid carcinoma has been detected (13,14), at least in adults. No evidence of an increased risk was observed in children, but admittedly the relatively low number of children submitted to these treatment modalities does not allow to exclude a risk albeit small.

Clinical features of post-Chernobyl thyroid carcinomas

An increase in the number of thyroid carcinomas in children and adolescents after the Chernobyl accident has been observed in the south of Belarus, in the north of Ukraine starting from 1990 and in the regions of Briansk and Kaluga (south of Russian Federation) since 1994. A relative increase in the number of thyroid cancers has been observed even in adults from Belarus and Ukraine. This increase is much less important than that observed in children and it is likely due to the greater attention at thyroid diseases after the nuclear accident.

About 800 thyroid cancers have been observed in children less than 15 years old living in the most contaminated areas. Such data correspond to an increase from 0.03 to 3 thyroid cancers per 100,000 children per year. About 98% of these thyroid tumors have been observed in children less than 10 years of age and 65% in children less than 5 years at the time of the accident. Thyroid cancer cases were also registered in some children who were already generated, but still in the uterus, at the time of the accident.

The yearly distribution of new cases shows that the increase in children reached its peak in 1993, with a trend to a "plateau" in the following years (15). It is also apparent that the patients of the 5-years-or-less age group at the time of the accident, accounted for the majority of the cases in each year of observation, while a decreasing trend in the number of thyroid cancer cases was observed in the subjects who were 9 years old or more at the time of the accident, with no new cases being observed in 1995.

The mean latency period between radiation exposure and diagnosis is about 9-10 years, with a similar trend in children and adolescents, shorter than that found after external thyroid radiation (2,3).

A comparison between clinical and epidemiological features of thyroid carcinomas, diagnosed in Belarus after the Chernobyl accident and those of 369 children and adolescents that in the past 20 years were followed for thyroid carcinoma in Italy and in France, shows that the post-Chernobyl thyroid carcinomas were much less influenced by gender, the female-to-male ratio being significantly higher in Italy and in France (2.5/1) compared with Belarus patients (1.6/1). Furthermore, most of the Belarussian cases (87.9%) were diagnosed before the age of 15, while the distribution of cases in Italy and France increases progressively with the age, the majority (57.4%) of the patients being diagnosed after the age of 14.

Morphological analysis of post-Chernobyl childhood thyroid carcinomas showed that the large majority of them are papillary carcinomas, very few being of the follicular histotype (15,16,17). Among the papillary type, many (33%) are of the solid and follicular variants (17). Focal micropapillary hyperplasia is frequently found in post-Chernobyl thyroid glands (18). Post-Chernobyl thyroid cancers showed a great aggressiveness since the presentation of the disease. A comparison with naturally occurring thyroid carcinomas in Italy and France showed a significantly higher extrathyroidal extension in Belarussian children (49.1 %) with respect to age-matched cases in Italy and France (24.9%). A frequent association of post-Chernobyl tumors with lymphocytic infiltration and humoral thyroid autoimmunity has also been reported (15).

Molecular biology investigation shows some peculiarities. Ras and p53 genes are not involved in the pathogenesis of these tumors while rearrangements of the RET proto-oncogene (Table 1) are found in nearly 70% of the cases, a percentage higher than that observed in non-irradiated papillary thyroid carcinomas (19-22).

Tab. 1 Ret/PTC rearrangements in post-Chernobyl childood papillary thyroid cancer

	RET Activation	RET/PTC Rearrangements
TAKAHASHI	4/7 (57.1%)	not done
KLUGBAUER	8/12 (66.6%)	2/12 PTC2 (16.6%) 6/12 PTC3 (50.0%)
FUGAZZOLA	4/6 (66.6%)	1/6 PTC2 (16.6%) 3/6 PTC3 (50.0%)
NIKIFOROV	33/38 (86.8%)	6/38 PTC1 (15.7%) 1/38 PTC2 (2.6%) 22/38 PTC3 (57.8%)
TOTAL	45/56 (80.3%)	6/56 PTC1 (10.7%) 4/5 PTC2 (7.1%) 31/56 PTC 3 (55.3%)

The type of RET rearrangements differs in post-Chernobyl cases and in spontaneous tumors (23). RET/PTC3 is the form more frequently expressed in radiation-induced tumors, particularly in the solid variants, while RET/PTC1 is predominant in spontaneous tumors and in the classical papillary variant (22). These findings suggest that RET/PTC3 mutation could be specifically related to the radiation effect, although the young age of affected subjects *per se* might be a contributing factor, as demonstrated by the higher incidence of RET rearrangements found in children and adolescents with papillary thyroid cancer not exposed to radiation (24).

Treatment of radiation-induced differentiated thyroid cancer

The initial treatment of differentiated thyroid cancer in adults, children and adolescents, is surgery. Although some controversy still exists on the extent of thyroid surgery to be performed, we are in favour of the so called "near-total thyroidectomy", a procedure intended to leave no more than 2-3 gr. of thyroid tissue. Surgery should be performed by an experienced surgeon who can perform this operation with minimal morbidity. Both permanent hypoparathyroidism and vocal cord palsy are almost absent in the hands of an experienced surgeon, and should not be advocated as reasons against total or near-total thyroidectomy. The reasons for total thyroidectomy are:

a) to allow the diagnosis and treatment of metastatic lesions with radioactive iodine;

b) to use serum thyroglobulin as a sensitive indicator of recurrent or persistent disease;

c) to remove multifocal disease, thus decreasing the rate of local recurrence (25, 26).

Four-six weeks after surgery all patients should be treated with radioiodine for ablation of any post-surgical residual thyroid tissues. A 131-I Whole Body Scan (WBS) is performed 3-5 days after the administration of this ablative dose, in order to search local or distant metastases. Serum thyroglobulin (Tg), a specific marker of residual or metastatic thyroid tissue in differentiated thyroid cancer, is also measured at this stage. The positivity of WBS and/or the finding of elevated serum Tg levels are the indications to treat the patient with a therapeutic dose of 131-I (usually 1 mCi/Kg of body weight in children). In case of persistent disease after surgery and residue ablation, WBS and 131-I therapy are repeated at intervals of 8-12 months. The aim of this therapy is to achieve a definitive cure, demonstrated by negative WBS and undetectable serum Tg concentrations off L-thyroxine.

The other essential step in the treatment of childhood differentiated thyroid cancer is hormonal therapy. Cancer cells of the follicular thyroid epithelium are, at least in part, TSH dependent for their function and growth. Thus, suppression of TSH (thyroid hormone suppressive therapy) is part of the therapeutic strategy. The drug of choice is L-T4 and the effective dosage needed to suppress endogenous TSH in children is between 2.2-2.8 µg/Kg of body weight. To avoid overtreatment (subclinic hyperthyroidism) an attempt should be made to use the smallest dose of L-T4 necessary to suppress TSH secretion, while determining a normal level of circulating thyroid hormones (FT4, FT3). Monitoring of the effectiveness of the therapy is performed by measuring serum TSH, FT4 and FT3 every six months. Following these indications L-T4 suppressive therapy is safe in children and adolescents, and does not affects the normal growth and development. When appropriately treated, differentiated thyroid cancer is a curable disease, with very high cure rate even in the presence of distant metastases.

References

1) Schneider AB, Shore-Freedman E, Weinstein RA. Radiation induced thyroid and other head and neck tumors: occurrence of multiple tumors and analysis of risk factors. *J Clin Endocrinol Metab* 1986; **63**: 107-112.

2) Favus MJ, Schneider AB, Stachura ME, et al. Thyroid cancer occurring as a late consequence of head-and-neck irradiation. Evaluation of 1056 patients. *N Engl J Med* 1976; **294** : 1019-1025.

3) Shore RE. Issues and epidemiological evidence regarding radiation-induced thyroid cancer. *Radiat Res* 1992; **131** : 98-111.

4) Nagataki S, Shibata Y, Inoue S, Yokoyama N, Izumi M, Shimaoka K. Thyroid disease among atomic bomb survivors in Nagasaki. *JAMA* 1994; **272**: 364-370.

5) Conrad RA, Pegia DE, Larson PR, et al. Review of medical findings in a Marshallese population twenty-six years after accidental exposure to radio-active fallout. BNL 51261, NTIS, January 1980; 1-138.

6) Baverstock K, Egloff B, Pinchera A, Ruchti C, Williams D. Thyroid cancer after Chernobyl. *Nature* 1992; **359**: 21.

7) Demidchik E, Kazakov VS, Astakhova LN, Okeanov AE, Demidchik YuE. Thyroid cancer in children after the Chernobyl accident: clinical and epidemiological evaluation of 251 cases in the Republic of Belarus. In: Nagataki S, ed. Nagasaki Symp., Chernobyl: Update and Future. Amsterdam 1994: Excerpta Medica, Elsevier Press; 21-30.

8) Kazakov US, Demidchik E, Astakhova LN. Thyroid cancer after Chernobyl. *Nature* 1992; **359** : 21.

9) Sobolev B, Likhtarev I, Kairo I, Tronko N, Oleynik V, Bogdanova T. Radiation risk assessment of the thyroid cancer in Ukrainian children exposed due to Chernobyl. In: Karaoglou A, Desmet G, Kelly GN, Menzel HG, eds. The Radiological Consequences of the Chernobyl Accident. ERU 16544 EN. Luxembourg 1996: European Commission: 741-748.

10) StSjazhko VA, Tsyb AF, Tronko ND, et al. Childood thyroid cancer since accident at Chernobyl. *Br Med J* 1995; **310** : 801.

11) Williams D, Pinchera A, Karaoglou A, Chadwick KH, eds. Thyroid cancer in children living near Chernobyl. Report EUR 15248 EN, Office for Official Publications of the European Communities, Luxembourg 1993; 1-108.

12) Dumont JE, Corvilain B, Coclet J,Raspe E, Reuse S. Recent progress in fundamental thyroidolgy with rilevance to the prevention of medical consequences of a nuclear accident. In: Rubery E, Smales E, eds. Iodine prophylaxis following nuclear accident. WHO/CEC Workshop, July 1988; 33-37.

13) Globel B, Globel H, Oberhausen E. Epidemiologic studies on patients with iodine-131 diagnostic and therapy. In: Kaul A., Neider R., Pensko

J. at al., eds. Radiation Risk Protection, vol. II°. International Radiation Protection Association. Koln: Fachverband fur Strahlenschutz e. v., 1984; 565-568.

14) Hall P, Mattsson A, Boice JD, JR. Thyroid cancer after diagnostic administration of iodine-131. *Radiat Res* 1996; **145** : 86-92.

15) Pacini F, Vorontsova T, Demidchik E.P, et al. Post-Chernobyl thyroid carcinoma in Belarus children and adolescents: comparison with naturally occurring thyroid carcinoma in Italy and France. *J Clin Endocrinol Metab* 1997; **82** : 3563-3569.

16) Williams ED, Cherstvoy E, Egloff B, et al. Interaction of pathology and molecular characterization of thyroid cancers. In "The radiological consequences of the Chernobyl accident", (Eds: A. Karaoglou, G. Desmet, GN Kelly, HG. Menzel), ERU 16544 EN, Luxembourg 1996; 699-714.

17) Nikiforov Y and Gnepp DR. Pediatric thyroid cancer after the Chernobyl disaster. Pathomorphologic study of 84 cases (1991-1992) from the Republic of Belarus. *Cancer* 1994; **74** : 748-766.

18) Nikiforov Y, Gnepp DR, Fagin JA. Thyroid lesions in children and adolescents after the Chernobyl disaster: implcations for the study of radiation tumorigenesis. *J Clin Endocrinol Metab* 1996; **81**: 9-14.

19) Fugazzola L, Pilotti S, Pinchera A, et al. Oncogenic rearrangements of the RET proto-oncogene in papillary thyroid carcinomas from children exposed to the Chernobyl nuclear accident. *Cancer Res* 1995; **55**: 5617-5620.

20) Klugbauer S, Lengfelder E, Demidchik EP, Rabes H.M. High prevalence of RET rearrangement in thyroid tumors of children from Belarus after the Chernobyl reactor accident. *Oncogene* 1995; **11:** 2459-2467.

21) Takahashi M, Ritz J, Cooper GM. Activation of a novel human trasforming gene, ret, by DNA rearrangement. *Cell* 1985; 42: 581-588.

22) Nikiforov YE, Rowland JM, Bove KE, Monforte-Munoz H, Fagin JA. Distinct pattern of ret oncogene rearrangements in morphological variants of radiation-induced and sporadic thyroid papillary carcinomas in children. *Cancer Res* 1997; **57**: 1690-1694.

23) Santoro M, Carlomagno F, Hay ID, et al. Ret oncogene activation in human thyroid neoplasms is restricted to the papillary cancer subtype. *J Clin Invest* 1992; **89**: 1517-1522.

24) Bongarzone I, Fugazzola L, Vigneri P, et al. Age-related activation of the thyrosine kinase receptor protooncogenes RET and NTRK1 in papillary thyroid carcinoma. *J Clin Endocrinol Metab* 1996, **81**: 2006-2009.

25) Witt TR, Meng RL, Economou SE, Southwick HW. The approach to the irradiated thyroid. *Surg Clin North Amer* 1979; **59** : 45-63.

26) Harness J, Thompson NW, McLeod MK, Pasieka JL, Fukuuchi A. Differentiated thyroid carcinoma in children and adolescents. *World J Surg* 1992; **16**: 547-554.

OBSERVED AND PREDICTED THYROID CANCER INCIDENCE FOLLOWING THE CHERNOBYL ACCIDENT EVIDENCE FOR FACTORS INFLUENCING SUSCEPTIBILITY TO RADIATION INDUCED THYROID CANCER

E. CARDIS, E AMOROS AND A. KESMINIENE,

IARC, Unit of Radiation and Cancer, 150 cours Albert Thomas, 69 372 Lyon Cedex 08, France. E-mail: cardis@iarc.fr

I.V. MALAKHOVA, S.M. POLIAKOV, AND N.N. PILIPTSEVITCH

Belorussian Centre for Medical Technologies, Information, Computer systems, Health Administration and Management, 7-a Brovki st. 220600 Minsk, Belarus E-mail: belcmt@belcmt.belpak.minsk.by

E.P. DEMIDCHIK,

Republican Scientific and Practical Center for Thyroid Tumours, 64, Skoriny Av., 220600 Minsk, Belarus

L.N. ASTAKHOVA,

BELMED, Medical Centre of Thyroid Pathology, 54 Sourganov Street, Minsk 220100, Belarus

V.K. IVANOV, A.P. KONOGOROV, E.M. PARSHKOV AND A.F. TSYB

Medical Radiological Research Center RAMS, 4, Korolev st., 249020 Obninsk, Kaluga region, Russia; E-mail: mrrc@obninsk.ru

Data on thyroid cancer incidence in children exposed to radiation from the Chernobyl accident in Belarus and Russia are analysed using different models of risk over time. The best fitting model at this time is a constant relative risk model, which is consistent with results of follow-up of other exposed populations. Over the time period 5-11 years after the accident, a constant absolute risk model is strongly rejected.

Predictions of thyroid cancer incidence over time in the Belarus and Russian exposed populations are made using different scenarii. Using risk estimates derived from other populations of children exposed, there is an important discrepancy between predictions in the first 10 years following the accident and the substantial numbers of cases observed until now in CIS countries following the Chernobyl accident. Lifetime predictions using these risk estimates are also quite different from those based on our own analyses of the observed patterns of risk among children exposed in Belarus and Russia. This suggests that there may be factors either environmental (iodine status), host (age and sex) and/or genetic which modify the risk of radiation induced thyroid cancer.

The identification of these factors and the characterization and quantification of their effect therefore has important public health implications for the affected CIS populations. It is also important for the protection of patients treated with radiotherapy, of radiation workers and of the general population exposed to enhanced levels of environmental radiation around the world.

1 INTRODUCTION

The dramatic increase in thyroid cancer observed among those who were children and lived in territories contaminated by fall-out from the Chernobyl accident has been well documented and is discussed in details in other papers in this workshop. Figure 1 shows the yearly incidence of thyroid cancer among those who were children in Belarus at the time of the accident. The incidence in this population does not, over the period studied (1987-1997), show an indication of declining.

Figure 1: Incidence of childhood cancer in Belarus among persons exposed in childhood

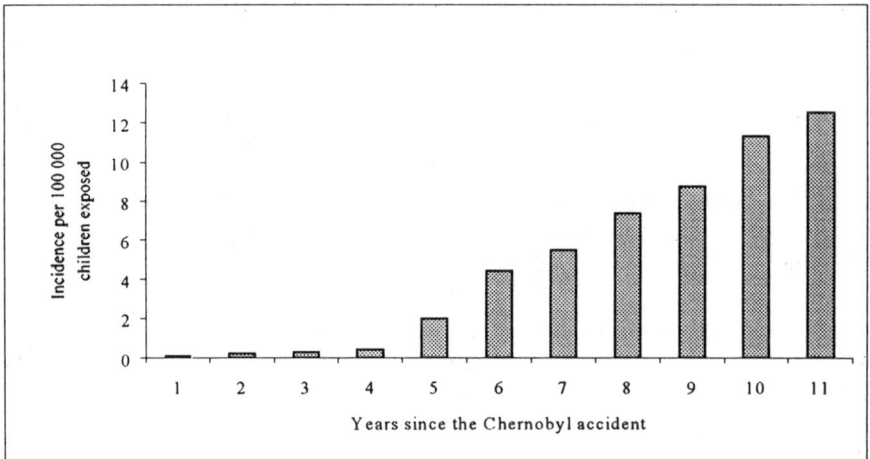

The future of this increase is of great concern to public health authorities in the affected countries and to radiation protection authorities worldwide. In the affected countries, health resources need to be adequately planned to diagnose and treat an unknown number of thyroid cancer cases in coming years. Planning at this time can only be based on uncertain predictions. In this paper, predictions are carried out based on two main approaches: extrapolation from other exposed populations and analyses of the observed patterns of risk among children exposed in Belarus and Russia.

2 MATERIALS AND METHODS

All cases of thyroid carcinoma diagnosed between 1990 and 1997 in Belarus and in three contaminated regions of Russia (Kaluga, Orel and Tula) among persons who were children (below the age of 15) at the time of the Chernobyl accident were identified from cross-checking of cancer registries and the records of medical institutions treating these tumours. The one-year age and sex distribution of the children population in 1986 was obtained for each of the oblasts (regions) under study from the relevant department of statistics. Age at accident-, attained age-, sex-, year- and region specific incidence rates were calculated as the ratio of the number of cases to the population at risk. Analyses were restricted to a 6 full years of follow-up from 1991 (to allow for a five-year lag between exposure from the Chernobyl accident and diagnosis of disease) to 1997.

The effects of age at exposure, sex, region, attained age and time since the accident were analyzed in multivariate models with Poisson regression, using age- and sex-specific rates for England and Wales as a comparison. Risk was modeled both on an absolute risk (AR) and on a relative risk (RR) scale. The significance of factors was assessed using the likelihood ratio statistic.

Predictions of risk over life were made for populations of children exposed before the age of 5 — using age- and sex-specific thyroid cancer rates from England and Wales as baseline and age- and sex-specific mortality rates for the period 1986-90 and 1992-93 for Belarus — under different scenarii as follows:

- using the risk estimates from Ron and collaborators[6]. Three alternatives were used: model 1 corresponds to a constant ERR of 7.7 per Gy over life; model 2 to the same ERR over 40 years; model 3 to the constant ERR model over life with sex and time since exposure modifiers
- using the estimates obtained from fitting constant and time-varying RR and AR models to Belarus and Russian data, as described above (assuming the observed risk continues throughout life or for a period of 40 years).

3   RESULTS

3.1   Modeling the risk of radiation induced thyroid cancer after the Chernobyl accident

Table 1 shows the number of thyroid cancer cases which were available for analysis. Table 2 shows the estimated RR and associated 95% confidence intervals by age at exposure compared to the UK population. Although the confidence intervals of the RR are wide, one notes very high RR's both in Gomel region and in Belarus as a whole. These RR decrease markedly with age at the time of accident.

Table 1. Number of cases observed in 1987-1997, by age at accident and region

		Belarus		Russia
	Whole	*Gomel*	*Mogilev*	3 oblasts
0-4	323	*157*	*16*	21
5-14	270	*108*	*15*	58
Total	593	*265*	*31*	79

398

Table 2. RR of thyroid cancer in Belarus compared to UK population

Age at accident	Belarus Number of cases	RR	95% CI	Gomel oblast Number of cases	RR	95% CI
<1	73	237	164-343	31	576	365-908
1	75	186	132-261	40	582	390-869
2	75	138	101-191	38	407	276-600
3	53	84	60-118	25	230	148-357
4	47	59	42-82	23	166	107-259
5	61	47	36-62	30	137	94-199
6	43	26	19-36	19	120	67-214
7	31	16	11-23	13	144	50-412
8	32	14	10-20	15	38	22-63
9	20	8	5-12	9	20	11-39
10	19	6	4-9	7	12	6-26
11	14	4	2-6	3	5	1.5-15
12	8	2	1-4	0	-	0-∞
13	22	4	2-7	5	6	2-15
14	20	4	2-6	7	7	1-50

Various forms of RR models were fit to the data from Belarus and Russia. Strong significant associations were found between relative risk of thyroid cancer and age at exposure, sex and region. When adjusted for age at exposure and sex, there was no evidence for a modifying effect of age at operation. Over the period of observation (5 to 11 years since the accident), the best fitting relative risk model was found to be constant over time. Resulting RR estimates are shown in Table 3.

Table 3. Estimated RR and 95% CI for Belarus as a whole, for the oblasts of Gomel and Mogilev and for contaminated oblasts of Russia, age at exposure, compared to UK age-specific rates *(constant RR model)*

Age at accident	Belarus Number of cases	RR *(95% CI)*	Gomel Number of cases	RR *(95% CI)*	Mogilev Number of cases	RR *(95% CI)*	Russia (Kal.+Orel+Tula) Number of cases	RR *(95% CI)*
<1	73	237 *(164-343)*	31	576 *(365-908)*	2	51 *(13-213)*	2	11 *(1.5-78)*
1-2	203	159 *(126-201)*	103	481 *(364-636)*	11	78 *(40-153)*	10	25 *(12-55)*
3-4	47	70 *(55-86)*	23	194 *(142-265)*	3	28 *(11-68)*	9	9 *(3-24)*

Various forms of AR models were also fit to the data from Belarus and Russia. Strong significant associations were found between absolute risk of thyroid cancer and age at exposure, sex, region and time since exposure or attained age. When adjusted for age at exposure and sex, there was very strong evidence for a modifying effect of time since exposure or age at operation. Over the period of observation (5 to 11 years since the accident), a constant absolute risk model was found to provide a very poor fit of the data and was rejected with strong statistical significance ($p<0.00001$).

The AR estimates by age at exposure and region are shown in Table 4 both for the poor fitting constant AR model and for the best AR model, i.e. a time varying AR model. For the time varying AR model, estimated AR are shown for two distinct years – 5 years and 15 years after the accident –. It is noted that a very important increase in AR is predicted over time, which is very similar to the increase expected if the risk followed a constant RR model.

Table 4. Estimated AR per 100 000 children exposed and 95% CI for Belarus as a whole, compared to UK age-specific rates *(constant and time varying models)*

Age at accident	Number of cases	Constant AR[1]		Time-varying AR	
		AR	95% CI	AR at 5 years	AR at 15 years
<1	73	3.34	2.19-4.50	2.70	21.70
1-2	203	7.42	6.23-8.62	2.47	14.80
3-4	47	5.29	4.24-6.34	0.81	8.61

Results of these analyses indicate that the best fitting model at this time is a constant relative risk model. This is consistent with results of follow-up of other exposed populations[6,8]. Over the time period 5-11 years after the accident, a constant absolute risk model is strongly rejected. The risk estimates presented are, however, uncertain (with wide confidence intervals).

3.2 Predictions of risk

Table 5 shows the number of cases predicted over life – as well as over the first 10 years after the accident – using the risk estimates of Ron et al[6] under 3 different scenarii (see materials and methods above) for children below the age of 5 at the time of the accident. The spontaneous number of cases corresponds to the numbers

---

[1] Note: these results are given as an indication and should be interpreted with caution as there is very significant departure from a constant AR over time

400

of cases expected in these populations in the absence of an effect of exposure from the accident.

Table 5. Number of cases predicted from RR estimates of Ron et al[6] *(children 0-4 at exposure)*

Age at exposure	Populat. in 1986	Dose[2] (Gy)	First 10 years Cases	Sponta neous cases	Model 1 Cases	AF%[3]	Model 2 Cases	AF%	Model 3 Cases	AF%
Gomel										
<1	28 888	1.30	0.6	26	293	91	97	74	258	90
1-3	85 341	1.23	3.8	80	837	91	319	75	761	89
4	26 839	0.97	1.2	25	212	88	87	72	194	87
0-4	141 068		5.6	131	1 342	90	503	74	1213	89
Mogilev										
<1	20 661	0.61	0.2	19	109	83	44	57	97	80
1-3	60 927	0.42	1.1	57	245	77	116	51	222	74
4	19 358	0.35	0.4	18	68	74	34	47	62	71
0-4	100 946		1.7	94	422	78	194	52	381	75
Russia (Kaluga+Tula+Orel)										
0-4	247 899	0.06	1.4	234	333	30	275	15	291	20

It is notable that the total number of cases predicted in the first 10 years after the accident is very small (respectively 5.6, 1.7 and 1.4 for Gomel, Mogilev and the three regions of Russia) compared to the numbers actually observed up till now (157, 16 and 21 – see Table 1), particularly in Gomel.

For predictions over life, the model incorporating sex and time since exposure modifying factors (Model 3) gives results which are fairly close to the constant RR model over life (Model 1). The predicted number is, however, less than half if the ERR is assumed to be 0 after 40 years since exposure (Model 2).

Table 6 shows the number of cases predicted over life using the RR and AR estimates derived from our analyses of the Belarus and Russian data (Tables 3 and 4) for children below the age of 5 at the time of the Chernobyl accident. The predicted numbers of cases are considerably greater than those predicted using the

[2]Average thyroid dose from ^{131}I in this age group in the most contaminated districts of the region – note: this is likely to be a substantial overestimation of the average dose in the region
[3] AF%: attributable fraction %: percentage of total number of predicted cases attributed to the radiation exposure

ERR estimates of Ron et al. and should be interpreted with caution, as the risk estimates are very uncertain. Although there is, at present, no indication of a departure from a constant relative risk pattern over time, the follow-up of the exposed populations is still quite short and the pattern of risk will most likely change with time. It should be noted, however, that even under a time varying AR model, a substantial proportion of those who were 0-4 at the time of the accident may develop thyroid cancer.

Table 6. Number of cases predicted over life from estimates derived from analyses of Belarus and Russian data *(children 0-4 at exposure)*

Country /region	Population in 1986	Spontaneous	Constant RR over life		Constant RR over 40 years		Time varying AR model	
			Cases	%.	Cases	%	Cases	%
Belarus	815 146	472	66 198	8	17 710	2	25 990	3
Gomel	141 068	131	51 345	36	15 263	11	n.d.[4]	
Mogilev	100 946	94	5 023	5	1 569	2	n.d.	
Russia	247 899	234	3 699	1	1 279	1	n.d.	

4   DISCUSSION

The analyses shown above indicate that the number of thyroid cancer cases observed up till now, particularly in the region of Gomel, among those who were very young at the time of the Chernobyl accident is considerably greater than that which is predicted from the experience of other populations exposed in childhood.

The lifetime predictions shown in the previous sections are extremely uncertain and must be taken with great caution. They are presented only as an indication that, if current trends of risk continue, a considerable number of cases is to be expected among those exposed as very young children. It is most probable – and very much hoped – that current trends of risk will change over time and that the actual numbers of cases will be much less than indicated here.

The reasons for uncertainties in the predictions are various. They include:

- *The short duration of follow-up*: 11 years of follow-up is a very short time on which to base lifetime predictions and the pattern of risk may well change over time. It is surprising to note that over such a short follow-up period, a constant AR model is very strongly rejected and that the data are most consistent with a

---

[4] n.d.: not defined – due to convergence problems when fitting the model on the relative small numbers of cases in these regions

constant RR model (the model supported by analyses of other populations exposed in childhood).

- *The uncertainty of the baseline rates used in the analyses*: analyses were based on incidence rates from England and Wales, the only population for which one-year age-specific incidence rates of childhood thyroid cancer were available. Thyroid cancer rates in that population are similar to pre-accident rates from the Belarus cancer registry. They are lower, however, than those of other western populations. As a result, the RR estimates shown in Tables 2 and 3 may be overestimated (by as much as a factor of 2 or 3). This should not affect predictions very much, however, since UK rates were also used for the lifetime predictions and hence the overestimation of the RR is compensated by the underestimation of the baseline incidence.

- *The effect of screening for thyroid cancer*: a considerable amount of screening for thyroid disease has taken place in the contaminated regions. The effect of screening on the incidence of thyroid cancer can be very important – resulting in up to 10 fold increases of incidence[7]. Screening can also change the apparent pattern of risk over time – by advancing the detection time of tumours. It is difficult to evaluate the effect of screening in young people, as little information is available on occult tumours of children and adolescents.

  Despite the uncertainties of the results presented here, the number of cases observed to date is much greater than that which would have been expected over 11 years, based on the experience of other populations exposed as children. The reasons for this discrepancy may be the existence of modifying factors, including;

- *age at exposure*, which is the only established modifying factor for radiation induced thyroid cancer[8]. There is little data from other studies on children who were very young at the time of exposure, and it is possible that the risk in these is even higher than previously estimated and that the pattern of risk over time differs from a constant relative risk model.

- *genetic predisposition*: there is evidence for genetic predisposition to papillary thyroid carcinoma both in irradiated and non-irradiated populations[1,2,4]. Among the cases which we studied in Belarus and Russia, 10 families were found in which two siblings were affected. Given the rarity of this disease in children, this observation strengthens the assumption that genetic predisposition – perhaps related to ethnic origin – may be increasing the susceptibility to radiation induced thyroid cancer.

- *iodine status*: as indicated by a number of speakers in this workshop, some of the contaminated areas of Belarus, Russia and Ukraine were (and continue to be) areas of moderate iodine deficiency. Experimental studies indicate that iodine deficiency could be an important modifier of the risk of radiation induced thyroid cancer[3,5], while results of epidemiologic studies are inconsistent.

- other short lived isotopes: little is known about the carcinogenic potential of isotopes of iodine other than [131]I. Exposure has occurred among Marshall Islanders but epidemiological and experimental studies to date do not permit a conclusive evaluation of their carcinogenic potential.

- other factors: both diet and reproductive factors may play a role in thyroid cancer and could modify the risk of radiation induced thyroid cancer. Little is known about the effect of hormonal factors in radiation induced thyroid cancer. If thyroid stimulation at menarche and during pregnancy increases the risk of thyroid cancer in general, it is likely that it also plays a role in the expression of radiation induced thyroid cancer. If this is so, young women who were children at the time of the Chernobyl accident may have an even greater increased risk as they become young adults and start to have children.

5 CONCLUSIONS

The current paper has reviewed the current status of our knowledge concerning risk factors and modifying factors for radiation induced thyroid cancer and, through analyses of the data from Belarus and Russia, raised the hypothesis that the observed thyroid cancer increase following the Chernobyl accident is much greater and may have greater public health consequences than predicted from the experience of other populations. In particular, analyses of 11 years of follow-up of the accident have shown that the observed pattern of incidence is not consistent with a constant absolute risk model. As a result, two types of actions are needed.

1. *Public health actions* to prevent or limit the radiological consequences of the accident in the contaminated territories. They include:

- Primary prevention of thyroid cancer through iodine supplementation of the diet of populations residing in iodine deficient areas

- Secondary prevention through focused screening of the "highest risk groups": those who were youngest at exposure in the most contaminated areas.

2. *Research* to further elucidate the effects of the accident:

- Continued monitoring of rates in the contaminated areas: this will allow better planning of public health actions. It will also allow the characterization of the pattern of risk over time and thus help make better predictions in the case of future accidents for the purpose of radiation protection

- Studies of possible modifying effects: the increase in thyroid cancer following the Chernobyl accident is a unique opportunity to learn about possible modifying factors for radiation induced thyroid cancer. Finding a genetic predisposition or elucidating the role of iodine deficiency and of reproductive factors will have important implications both for radiation protection of patients and the general population in the case of future accidents. It will also allow more focused public health actions among exposed populations, helping to further identify the high risk groups which need to be screened.

Acknowledgements

This work was supported by contracts ICI5-CT96-0308 and F14C-CT96-0014 with the INCO-Copernicus and Nuclear Fission Safety Programs of the European Commission.

References

1. Goldgar, DE, Easton, DF, Cannon-Albright, LA, Skolnick, MH. Systematic population-based assessment of cancer risk in first- degree relatives of cancer probands. *J Natl Cancer Inst* 1994; **86**: 1600-1608.

2. Harach, H.R. and Williams, E.D. Solitary, multiple and familial oxyphil tumours of the thyroid gland. J Pathol. (in press)

3. Kanno, J, Onodera, H, Furuta, K, Maekawa, A, Kasuga, T, Hayashi, Y. Tumor-promoting effects of both iodine deficiency and iodine excess in the rat thyroid. *Toxicol Pathol* 1992; **20**: 226-235.

4. McTiernan, A, Weiss, N, Daling, J. Incidence of thyroid cancer in women in relation to previous exposure to radiation therapy and history of thyroid disease. *J Natl Cancer Inst* 1984; **73**: 575-581.

5. Ohshima, M, Ward, J. Dietary iodine deficiency as a tumor promoter and carcinogen in male F344/NCr rats. *Cancer Res* 1986; **46**: 877-883.

6. Ron, E, Lubin, J, Shore, RE, Mabuchi, K, Modan, B, Pottern, LM, Schneider, AB, Tucker, MA, Boice, JD, Jr. Thyroid cancer after exposure to external radiation: a pooled analysis of seven studies. *Radiat Res* 1995; **141**: 259-277.

7. Schneider, A et al. Dose-response relationships for radiation induced thyroid cancer and thyroid nodules: evidence for the prolonged effects of radiation on the thyroid. *J Clin Endocrinol Metab* 1993; 362-369.

8. Shore, RE. Issues and epidemiological evidence regarding radiation-induced thyroid cancer. *Radiat Res* 1992; **131**: 98-111.

RESULTS OF RADIOIODINE TREATMENT IN 158 CHILDREN FROM BELARUS WITH THYROID CANCER AFTER THE CHERNOBYL ACCIDENT

CHR. REINERS , J. BIKO AND J. FARAHATI

Clinic and Policlinic for Nuclear Medicine,
University of Würzburg, Josef-Schneider-Straße 2, D-97080 Würzburg, Germany
E-mail: reiners@nuklearmedizin.uni-wuerzburg.de

ST. DANILOVNA , V.DROZD AND E. P. DEMIDCHIK

Republican Centre for Thyroid Tumors, Skorina Av.54, 220600 Minsk, Belarus

The incidence of thyroid cancer in children increased considerably in the three republics afflicted by radioactive fallout from the Chernobyl Reactor Accident in 1986. In a joint Belarussian-German project, 158 children with advanced stages of thyroid cancer have been selected out of 574 cases diagnosed in Belarus between 1986 and 1997. With the exception of 2 cases, all of the 158 cancers were papillary tumors staged clinically in 82 % of the cases as pT4, in 96 % as pN1 and in 48 % as pM1. Totally 530 courses of radioiodine treatment have been applied in those children between April 1, 1993 and March 31, 1998. In 75 % of children complete remissions could be achieved. In the remaining 25 % of the cases, partial remissions have been observed up to now. In some of the cases without complete remissions further courses of radioiodine treatment are applicable. In spite of the clinical signs of aggressiveness of childhood cancers from Belarus treated in Germany, the prognoses seems to be fairly good.

1 INTRODUCTION

After the Chernobyl Reactor Accident in 1986, the frequency of thyroid cancer in children from the most contaminated parts of Belarus, the Ukraine and Russia increased considerably since 1990 (1, 2). Totally, in the 3 republics afflicted by radioactive fallout from the Chernobyl accident more than 1000 cases of thyroid cancer in children and adolescents have been diagnosed between 1990 and 1997 as compared to approximately 100 cases diagnosed between 1986 and 1989. The most reliable epidemiological data are available from Belarus (1,2). The relative incidence of thyroid cancer per 100.000 children below age of 15, which amounted to 0.1 - 0.3 between 1986 and 1989 increased to 1.2-3.5 between 1990 and 1995. In the region of Gomel, which has been most heavily contaminated after the Chernobyl accident by radioactive fallout, the relative incidence increased from

0.3 - 1.0 between 1986 and 1989 to 3.3 - 13.5 between 1990 and 1997. On the whole, 574 cases of childhood thyroid cancer have been diagnosed and operated by the Centre for Thyroid Tumors in Minsk between 1986 and 1996 (1, 2).

Between April 1st, 1993 and March 31st, 1998 a joint German-Belarussian project "Scientists help Chernobyl Children" has been carried out by the Joint Committee for Radiation Research (3). This committee consists of 7 German scientific societies which are active in the field of radiation research. The project has been supported by the German Minister of the Environment, Radiation Protection and Reactor Safety as well as by the Minister of Health of the Republic of Belarus. Generous funds for this project amounting to more than 5 Million German Marks could have been raised from German Electricity Suppliers.

2   PATIENTS AND PROTOCOL

Surgical resection of thyroid tumors and removal of lymph nodes has been performed by the surgical team of the Centre for Thyroid Tumors in Minsk. In selected children with most advanced tumor stages, radioiodine treatment followed at the Clinics for Nuclear Medicine in Essen and later Würzburg. Between April 1st, 1993 and the March 31st, 1998, 158 children from Belarus with most advanced stages of thyroid cancer have been selected for repeated treatment with radioiodine in Germany (Tab. 1).

The diagnostic protocol included ultrasonography and scintigraphy of the neck, thorax X-ray or spiral CT, computer tests of pulmonary function, determinations of thyroglobulin, TSH, free T4 and free T3 in serum as well as measurements of calcium, phosphate and differential blood cell counts. For elimination of thyroid remnants 50 MBq of I-131 per kg of bodyweight have been applied. For ablation of metastases, 100 MBq of I-131 per kg of bodyweight were given. Simultaneously, antiemetica and emulsions for the protection of gastric mucosa were administered to reduce gastrointestinal side effects. 2 days after treatment, replacement therapy with levothyroxine which had been withdrawn 4 weeks before treatment was restarted. The mean dose amounted to 2.5 μg of levothyroxine per kg of bodyweight. For staging, wholebody scans were performed 4-5 days after the application of radioiodine.

Table 1: **Children with advanced thyroid cancer from Belarus: [131]I therapy at the universities of Essen and Würzburg (1.04.93 - 31.03.98)**

Number	158 Children 530 Treatment Courses
Origin	71 Gomel Area 87 Other Parts of Belarus
Sex	95 Girls 63 Boys
Age	7 - 18 Years (11.9 ± 2.5) at the Time of Diagnosis
Histology	156 Papillary Cancers 2 Follicular Cancers
Stage	pTx - 4 pN0 - 5 pM0 - 82 pT1 - 3 pT2 - 17 pN1 - 152 pM1 - 76 pT3 - 4 pulm 74 pT4 - 130 oss 2
Pretreatment	37 x I-131 Treatment in Minsk 5 x I-131 Treatment in Italy 19 x Percutaneous Irradiation 6 x Chemotherapy

3   RESULTS

In 134 out of 158 children more than one course of radioiodine treatment has been performed in Germany up to now. In those cases, the results of treatment could be checked by follow-up with I-131 scintigraphy, ultrasonography of the neck, X-ray or spiral CT of the thorax and determinations of thyroglobulin in serum.

In 101 out of 134 children (=75 %) complete remissions of thyroid cancer could be achieved up to now. In the remaining 25 % of the cases, we were able to recognize partial remissions defined as decreases of tumor volume, tumor marker serum level or intensity of radioiodine uptake for at least 50 %. Fortunately, in no single case progressive disease has been observed. It is important to mention that the results given here are not the final results of treatment since in some of the cases without complete remission further courses of radioiodine are applicable.

Table 2: Children from Belarus with advanced thyroid cancer treated with
^{131}I-in Essen and Würzburg 1.04.93 - 31.3.98
Results of scintigraphy after more than 1 course of ^{131}I therapy

N = 134		Complete Remission	
pT1-3	N0M0	1/1	
	N1M0	6/6	(100%)
	N0-1M1	3/9	(33%)
pT4	N0M0	1/1	
	N1/M0	50/52	(96%)
	N0-1M1	40/65	(62%)
Total		101/134	(75%)

References

1. Demidchik EP, Demidchik YU: Thyroid Cancer Promoted by Radiation in Children of Belarus. In: *Radiation Research 1895-1995*, Proceedings of the 10th International Congress of Radiation Research, Würzburg 27.08.-01.09.1995.
2. Demidchik EP: Personal Communication 1998
3. Reiners C, Biko J, Kruglova N, Demidchik EP. Therapy of thyroid carcinoma in children from Belarus after the Chernobyl accident. In: Nauman I, Glinoer D, Braverman LB, Hostalek U, eds. *The Thyroid and Iodine*. Stuttgart - New-York: Schattauer 1996: 89-97

GONAD EFFECTS OF RADIOIODINE-131 IN PATIENTS TREATED FOR DIFFERENTIATED THYROID CANCER

C. Ceccarelli, F. Pacini, D. Morciano, R. Bonacci, A. Pinchera
Dipartimento di Endocrinologia e Metabolismo, Sezione di Endocrinologia;
University of Pisa, Italy
E-mail: claudiac@endoc.med.unipi.it

M. Schlumberger
Institut Gustave Roussy; Paris, France

P. Battisti
Italian Agency for New Technologies, Energy and the Environment (ENEA AMB PRO IRP), Bologna

Following I-131 therapy for ablation of thyroid remnant in Differentiated Thyroid Cancer (DTC) the dose to ovaries was found to be 2 - 5 times greater than that reported in the ICRP tables for euthyroid women, while testes dose was similar to the reported values for euthyroid men. After I-131 therapy a transient ovarian failure has been demonstrated by the increased levels of FSH and LH. In males, I-131 therapy may be followed by a transient increase of FSH and reduction of normokinetic sperm. After large cumulative activities, permanent impairment of the male reproductive capability has been demonstrated by permanent increase of FSH levels. In large series of females with DTC, recent studies failed to show fertility impairment or effect on pregnancies and offspring except for an increase of miscarriages in the year after I-131 administration. There are no such studies on I-131 irradiated men.

INTRODUCTION

Differentiated thyroid cancer (DTC) may affect subjects in any age group, including children and young adults. When appropriately treated, DTC is compatible with normal life, including fertility. I-131 is used for ablation of the post-surgical thyroid remnant and for destruction of metastases. The I-131 activity administered in a single dose ranges from 1110 to 5500 MBq and may be given repeatedly in the presence of metastases. Thus, large cumulative amounts of I-131 may be administered and give a radiation dose to the gonads that could impair fertility, influence the outcome of pregnancies and the offspring. Aim of the present work was to review the information on the effects of I-131 on fertility.

1. RADIATION DOSE TO GONADS

The radiation dose delivered from I-131 is approximately 4.2×10^{-2} mGy/MBq to the ovary and 3.7×10^{-2} mGy/MBq to the testis in euthyroid subjects[3]. In subjects with DTC the radiation dose to the gonads may be increased by the hypothyroid status because of the reduced iodine renal clearance and subsequent prolonged exposure to relatively high I-131 levels in blood and urine. I-131-iodoproteins released in blood from damaged thyroid tissue may also contribute to augment the radiation dose.

1.1 Radiation dose to the ovaries

In a previous work the mean radiation dose to the ovaries were evaluated retrospectively by the MIRD method in 48 females with DTC following the administration of very large amounts of I-131 (8700 ± 224 MBq) for ablation of thyroid remnant[4]. The dose to ovaries was 1140 ± 340 mGy and was poorly related to the administered activity and more to the body mass. The dose per administered MBq ranged from 9.85 to 20.27 x 10^{-2} mGy/MBq, thus 2 - 5 times higher than that indicated by ICRP tables for normal women.

1.2 Radiation dose to the testes

We evaluated the radiation dose to the testes in three men after I-131 administration for ablation of thyroid remnant. In this study the beta dose was calculated by the MIRD method from blood activity and the gamma dose was directly measured by TLDs applied close to the lower poles of the testes by an athletic supporter. In the studied patients the total dose absorbed by the testes resulted 3.0 - 4.2 x 10^{-2} mGy/MBq. These values were close to those reported by ICRP for euthyroid men, indicating that at least in these cases metabolic status of patients could not significantly influence the dose to the testes. There were some differences in I-131 kinetic in the subjects, who had different remnant uptake (0, 18 and 40%, respectively) and different degrees of hypothyroidism. The subject with a more severe hypothyroidism and no uptake in thyroid bed received the largest part of the gamma dose to the testes in the first 3 days of the study, while the subject with a milder degree of hypothyroidism and a large uptake in the remnant (40%) still received a significant dose to the testes at the day 14 of the study. This was in keeping with the higher and prolonged levels of I-131 due to the release of I-131-iodoproteins from the damaged remnant.

2.   GONAD EFFECTS OF I-131 THERAPY

2.1 Effects of I-131 therapy on the ovaries

Following large I-131 activities administered for ablation of thyroid remnants short periods of amenorrhea were reported in 18/66 women starting from the second to the fourteenth month[6]. This is in keeping with the fact that intermediate oocytes are more radiosensitive than mature and small oocytes. Patients who experienced interruption of cycles had increased levels of FSH and LH, indicating that amenorrhea was due to the primary ovarian failure. The interruptions of cycles were mainly reported in older women and were not related to the absorbed dose in the ovaries, thyroid uptake, thyroid autoimmunity. No permanent effects on female fertility was observed in a large epidemiological study[1].

2.2 Effects of I-131 therapy on the testes

A transient increase of FSH was found after the I-131 administration for DTC[2,5]. A small but significant transitory increase of FSH levels was found 60 days after 1850 MBq of I-131[2]. In a large series of male subjects with DTC the increased levels of FSH after I-131 administration were related to the cumulative administered activity[5]. The sperm analysis showed a reduction of normokinetic sperm. Four patients receiving cumulative activities ranging from 18500 to 29600 MBq in repeated doses showed FSH levels permanently high. There was not an effect on Leydig cells and testosterone levels remained unchanged.

3.   EFFECTS OF I-131 ON PREGNANCY AND OFFSPRING

The evidence of mutagenic effect of radiation is based mainly on experimental studies on animals; scanty data are available in humans. In survivors of atomic bombing - the largest irradiated population studied until now - no mutation surely related to the radiation was found. Sparse reports on offspring of subjects treated with I-131 failed to show any increase of congenital malformation. In a recent work[9] we assessed the mutagenic effect of I-131 by untoward pregnancy outcomes, such as miscarriages, congenital anomalies and malignancies in offspring from a large series of women with DTC. In the pregnancies conducted after cancer diagnosis and treatment (only surgery or surgery +I-131) there was no change in the number of stillbirth, prematurely low weight at birth, congenital anomalies and death during the first year of life with respect to the pregnancies conducted before cancer. An increase of miscarriages after diagnosis and treatment of cancer was observed, not related to the cumulative received activity (20% after cancer v/s 11% before). However, the miscarriages were significantly increased (40%) in the pregnancies started in the first year after a large dose. Of the eight pregnancies started in the first 6 months after a large therapeutic dose, 6 ended in abortion and 2 in miscarriage. A possible explanation for miscarriages after I-131 therapy could be the failure to correct rapidly the hypothyroidism. No definitive studies on offspring of male subjects with DTC treated with I-131 are available in the literature.

4.   CONCLUSIONS

I-131 therapy for DTC gives an irradiation dose to the ovaries 2 - 5 fold higher than that reported from the ICRP tables for euthyroid women, while the dose to testes is in the same range than that reported in the ICRP tables for men. After I-131 therapy temporary ovarian and testes failure are observed. High cumulative activities permanently impair the testicular function, while permanent ovarian damage is not documented. No effect on offspring has been observed in irradiated women. Pregnancy is influenced only in the first year after I-131 therapy.

References

1. Dottorini ME, Lomuscio G, Mazzucchelli L, Vignati A, Colombo L. Assessment of female fertility and carcinogenesis after Iodine-131 therapy for differentiated thyroid carcinoma. *J Nucl Med* 1995; **36**:21-27.
2. Handelsman DJ, Turtle JR. Testicular damage after radioactive iodine (I-131) therapy for thyroid cancer. *Clinical Endocrinol* 1983; **18**: 465-472.
3. ICRP Publication 53. *Radiation dose to patients from radiopharmaceutical.* New York: Pergamon Press, 1987; 259-278.
4. Izembart M, Chauvadra J, Aubert B, Vallée G. Retrospective evaluation of the dose received by the ovary after radioactive iodine therapy for thyroid cancer. Eur J Nucl Med 1992; **19**: 243-247.
5. Pacini F, Gasperi M, Fugazzola L, Ceccarelli C, Lippi F, Centoni R, Martino E, Pinchera A: "Testicular function in patients with differentiated thyroid carcinoma treated with radioiodine" *J Nucl Med* 1994; **35**: 1418-1422.
6. Raymond JP, Izembart M, Marliac V, Dagousset F, Merceron RE, Vulpillat M, Vallèe G. Temporary ovarian failure in thyroid cancer patients after thyroid remnant ablation with radioactive iodine. *J Clin Endocrinol Metab* 1989; **69**: 186-190
7. Schlumberger M, DeVathaire F, Ceccarelli C, De Lisle MJ, Francese C, Couette JA, Pinchera A, Parmentier C. Exposure to radioactive Iodine-131 for scintigraphy or therapy does not preclude pregnancy in thyroid cancer patients. *J Nucl Med* 1996; **37**:606-612.

BIOKINETIC AND CYTOGENETIC STUDIES IN THYROID CANCER PATIENTS AFTER ^{131}I TREATMENT

ANA CRISTINA DE H. NASCIMENTO , JOYCE L. LIPSZTEIN,
ÉDER A. LUCENA AND BERNARDO M. DANTAS*

Instituto de Radioproteção e Dosimetria - Av Salvador Allende s/no.
Recreio dos Bandeirantes, Rio de Janeiro CEP 05422-970
Brasil
E-mail: acris@ird.gov.br

ROSSANA C. MELLO AND EDUARDO R. OLIVEIRA

Instituto Nacional do Câncer - Praça Cruz Vermelha, 23.
Centro, Rio de Janeiro CEP28630-050
Brasil

BERDJ A. MEGUERIAN

Hospital dos Servidores do Estado -Rua Sacadura Cabral, 178.
Centro, Rio de Janeiro CEP28630-050
Brasil

Thyroid cancer patients have significant irradiation of body tissues when submitted to an oral administration of ^{131}I in order to eliminate residual thyroid tissue after near-total thyroidectomy. The average activity administered in this treatment is very high (3.7 GBq of Na[131]I for ablative dose, approximately) and there are no conclusive results on the literature about radiation absorbed dose of these patients. Radioiodine metabolic behaviour in four patients submitted to this treatment was studied through measurements of ^{131}I in total body, in remnant thyroid tissue and in urine samples. In addition, cytogenetic analysis was performed in peripheral blood lymphocytes. Our results suggest that ten days after ablative dose administration, almost all residual thyroid tissue will be eliminated and, since then, ^{131}I will be less heterogeneously distribuited through patients' body. The retention of radioiodine after the first ten days following the ablative dose administration may be mathematically represented by the sum of two exponential terms: the first and shorter one with a biological half-life of, approximately, 3.2 days (effective half-life = 2.3 days) and the second one, with a biological half-life of, approximately 26 days (effective half-life = 6.2 days). Whole body radiation absorbed dose estimates by cytogenetics ranged from 0.3 to 0.4 Gy.

1 INTRODUCTION

In nuclear medicine, ^{131}I have been used to treat differentiated thyroid carcinoma for 50 years: thyroid cancer patients are submitted to an oral administration of the radionuclide in order to ablate the remnant thyroid tissue, after near-total thyroidectomy.

However, there is, as yet, no conclusive information in the literature about the radiation absorbed dose owing this procedure. There is also no fixed policy on the dosage of radioiodine needed to be effectively, so the activity of ^{131}I administered has been largely empirical and most clinicians give a fixed activity for ablation and for therapy (approximately 3.7 and 7.4 GBq, respectively). This lack of tumour dosimetry contrasts sharply with planning for external-beam radiotherapy where precise tumour-dose prescription is mandatory [1,2].

The aim of this investigation is to study biokinectics and detect biological damage from internally deposited radioiodine for thyroid cancer treatment. These data may help in the elaboration of a metabolic model for this specific case.

1.1 Significance of This Study

The biokinetic moldels for iodine available in scientific literature can not be applied to thyroidectomized patient's studies [3,4,5,6]. For a realistic evaluation of risks, it is necessary to make biokinetics analysis of these patients, aiming a specific metabolic model elaboration, which will permit absorbed dose-assessment. The possibility of a correlation of these data with results from a biological indicator of dose, certainly, would be very usefull.

The methods adopted in this study are the most reliable and developed for radionuclides intake measurements and for biological dosimetry: bioassay analysis and chromosome aberration analysis, respectively [7].

2 PATIENTS AND METHODS

2.1 Patients Characteristics

Four thyroid cancer patients without metastases, one man and three females, between 25 and 60 years old, who had never have undergone treatment with ionizing radiation or mutagenic chemicals agreed to contribute to this study. They were monitored periodically in the whole body counter and donated urine and blood samples for bioanalysis and chromosome aberration analysis, respectively. Measurements for the first three patients started just after ^{131}I ablative dose administration. For the fourth patient, measurements started after ^{131}I diagnosis dose administration and following ^{131}I ablative dose administration. All measurements proceeded until body burdens lowered to background levels, in terms of bioanalysis.

2.2 Bioassay Analysis

For the *in vitro* monitoring, urine samples were collected in polyethylene bottles which were positioned over the surface of a 20.3 x 10.2 cm Na I (Tl) detector. Patients were instructed to collect the first urine in the morning. The amount of ^{131}I excreted per liter was determined. Calibration was performed using different volumes with known activities of [131]I.

For the *in vivo* bioassay, whole body monitoring was performed using the chair geometry and a 20.3 x 10.2 cm Na I (Tl) detector. Thyroid burden was also measured using a 7.6 x 7.6 Na I (Tl) collimated detector positioned directly over the gland location region. For the calibration of the "in vivo" system, an anthropomorphic phanton [8] filled with bags containing known activities of radioactive solution was used for simulating whole body; the thyroid phanton consisted of two picnometers containing a known amount of activity of the radionuclide.

2.3 Cytogenetic Methods

Heparinized venous blood samples were collected from the first three patients and, for each lymphocyte culture, aproximately 2 mL of whole blood were inoculated into 10 mL of complete culture medium (71% HAM F-10 media [CULTILAB], 25% v/v heat-inactived fetal bovine serum [CULTILAB] and 3.6% reconstituted phytohemagglutinin [PHA; Burroughs-wellcome]. After incubation at 37° C for 46 h, colchicine was added to culture to arrest mitosis and 2 h later all cultures were harvested. Slides were prepared by standard procedures and stained by Giemsa. During microscopic analysis it was scored dicentric chromosome and centric ring.

3   RESULTS

3.1   Bioassay Analysis

After ablative dose administration, monitoring data by *in vitro* bioassay analysis of patients 1, 2 and 3 suggest that the biokinetics of ^{131}I could be represented by two exponential terms, one of them with a half-life very short (shown in Fig. 1, 2, and 3, respectively). It was decided to follow another patient up (patient 4) and compare with biokinetics data of the radionuclide after diagnosic dose administration, approximately 0.18 GBq (shown in Fig. 4), and after ablative dose administration (shown in Fig. 5 and 6). The two half-times are well depickted in those two pictures.

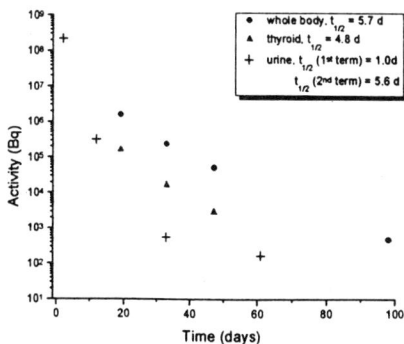

Fig. 1. Activity of ^{131}I on Patient 1 after Ablative Dose Administration.

420

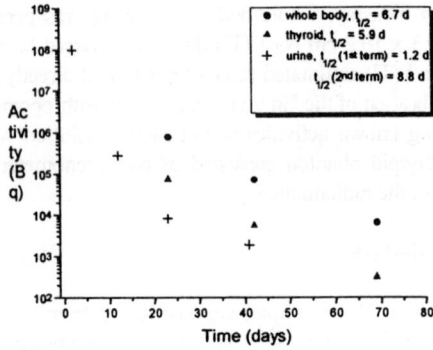

Fig. 2. Activity of ^{131}I on Patient 2 after Ablative Dose Administration.

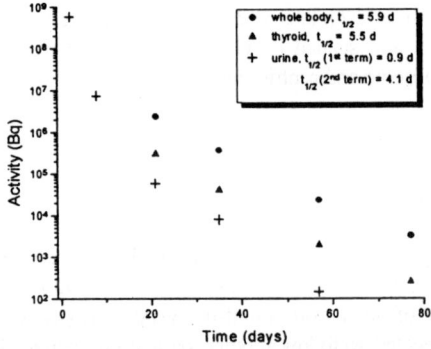

Fig. 3. Activity of ^{131}I on Patient 3 after Ablative Dose Administration.

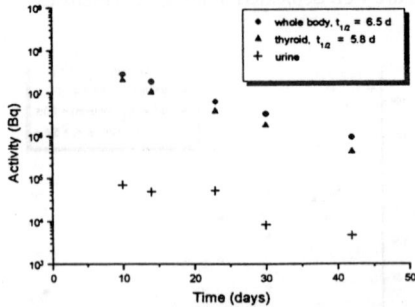

Fig. 4. Activity of ^{131}I on Patient 4 after Diagnosis Dose Administration.

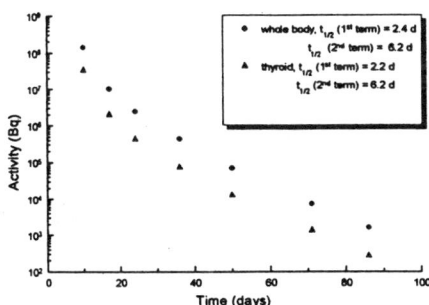

Fig. 5. Activity of ^{131}I on Patient 4 after Ablative Dose Administration.

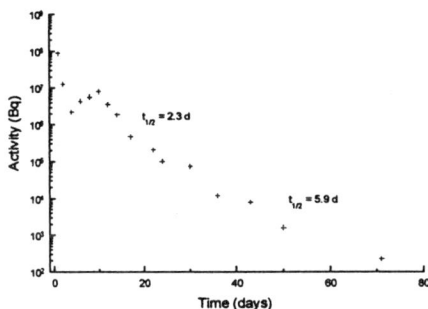

Fig. 6. Activity of ^{131}I on Urine of Patient 4 after Ablative Dose Administration.

Retention curves obtained from measurements of patients 1, 2 and 3 show that while thyroid burdens approached to background levels, there was still a significant corporal residual activity. Since the thyroid's ability to concentrate iodide is shared with other tissues of endodermal nature, principally sallivary and gastric glands [9], it was decided, for each monitoration, to make a screening in order to investigate the possibility of detection of a preferencial concentration of radioiodine in any other tissue of patients' body, i. e., to perform a qualitative analysis of ^{131}I distribuition in thyroidectomized patients' body.

3.2 Cytogenetics

It was not observed any dicentric chromosome or centric ring during chromosome aberration analysis of control samples (blood samples collected from patients, imediatelly before ablativedose administration). Table 3 shows the results of chromosome aberration analysis of blood samples periodically collected after ablative dose administration.

TABLE 1. Count Rate Relationship (CRR) Between Thyroid Regionand Interest Area Observed on Patient 4, After Diagnosis Dose Administration

Interest Area	Time After I-131 Administration (Days)				
	10	14	23	30	42
			CRR		
Skull	4.9	4.7	2.8	6.5	3.1
Salivary glands	1.5	1.5	1.5	1.5	1.2
Thyroid	1.0	1.0	1.0	1.0	1.0
Breast	11.5	5.4	2.1	1.4	2.7
Stomach	57.6	28.3	10.1	8.3	8.9
Liver	99.2	62.2	28.8	26.1	14.9
Intestine	133.9	103.2	52.2	40.7	19.2
Bladder	199.0	143.2	76.4	60.2	22.3
Upper thigh	140.9	270.2	139.1	96.3	26.9
Lower thigh	560.0	359.0	152.4	104.1	31.0
Knee	691.8	418.3	171.3	115.1	31.0

TABLE 2. Count Rate Relationship (CRR) Between Thyroid Region and Interest Area Observed on Patient 4, After Ablative Dose Administration

Interest Area	Time After I-131 Administration (Days)				
	10	17	24	36	50
			CRR		
Skull	5.8	3.4	3.3	2.3	2.3
Salivary glands	1.7	1.3	1.2	1.1	1.2
Thyroid	1.0	1.0	1.0	1.0	1.0
Breast	1.4	0.8	0.7	0.6	0.8
Stomach	2.0	0.7	0.7	0.6	1.0
Liver	2.6	0.7	1.1	0.8	1.4
Intestine	4.4	1.3	1.8	1.3	1.7
Bladder	7.0	2.2	2.6	1.7	1.7
Upper thigh	13.3	3.5	4.4	3.0	3.3
Lower thigh	18.7	5.1	5.5	3.9	3.6
Knee	24.8	6.9	6.5	4.9	4.5

TABLE 3. Statistics Uncertainty of Chromosome Aberrations Yields Observed

Patient n°	[a]T	[b]N	[c]Y	[d]sd	[e]VC (%)	D (Gy)
	12	600	0.005	0.003	60	
	33	410	0.012	0.005	42	
1	47	475	0.010	0.005	50	
	61	480	0.009	0.004	44	
	103	500	0.010	0.004	40	
Total		2465	0.009	0.002	22	0.27
	12	540	0.009	0.004	44	
2	42	460	0.011	0.005	45	
	69	490	0.010	0.004	40	
	92	500	0.008	0.004	50	
Total		900	0.010	0.002	20	0.30
	8	500	0.018	0.005	33	
	35	480	0.015	0.006	40	
3	57	450	0.016	0.006	37	
	77	470	0.015	0.006	40	
	98	475	0.015	0.006	40	
	126	450	0.013	0.005	38	
Total		2825	0.015	0.002	13	0.41

a. Time after ablative dose administration b. Number of analised cells
c. Chromosome aberration yield d. Standard desviation e. Variation coefficient

4 CONCLUSIONS

. Our results suggest that ten days after ^{131}I ablative dose administration, almost all remnant thyroid tissue will be eliminated and the radionuclide will have a tendency to be less heterogeneously distributed through the patients' body.

. Since the tenth day after the ablative dose administration, the retention of ^{131}I in the body may be mathematically represented by the sum of two exponential terms: the first and shorter one, with a biological half-life of aproximately 3.2 days and an effective half-life of 2.3 days; and the second one with a biological half-life of aproximately 26 days and an effective half-life of 6.2 days.

. It was not observed any dicentric chromosome or centric ring after diagnosis dose administration (control blood samples).

. The estimated absorbed dose by cytogenetics was in the range of 0.3 to 0.4 Gy. Radiation absorbed dose assessment for these patients was based on the equivalence with external and uniform irradiation of gamma and X radiation, for whole body.

. It is necessary to continue this study following more patients and in earlier points, aiming to generate subsidy to develop a specific mathematical metabolic model and evaluate the risks which come along ^{131}I incorporation for thyroid cancer treatment purposes.

REFERENCES

1. O'Connell, MEA, Flower, MA., Hinton, PJ, Harmer, CL, McReady, VR. Radiation dose assessment in radioiodine therapy. Dose-response relationships in differentiated thyroid carcinoma using quantitative scanning and PET. *Radiotherapy and Oncology* 1993; **28:** 16-26.

2. International Atomic Energy Agency (IAEA). Practical radiation safety manual. Manual on therapeutic uses of iodine-131. Incorporating applications procedures basic guides. Vienna: IAEA, 1992: 7.

3. International Commission on Radiological Protection (ICRP). Limits for intakes of radionuclides by workers (Publication 30) . Oxford: Pergamon Press, 1979.

4. International Commission on Radiological Protection (ICRP). Radiation dose to patients from radiopharmaceuticals (Publication 53). Oxford: Pergamon Press, 1987.

5. International Commission on Radiological Protection (ICRP). Age-dependent doses to members of the public from intakes of radionuclides (Publication 56, part 1). Oxford: Pergamon Press, 1989.

6. International Commission on Radiological Protection (ICRP). Age-dependent doses to members of the public from intakes of radionuclides: part 3: Ingestion dose coefficients (Publication 69). Oxford: Pergamon Press, 1995.

7. International Atomic Energy Agency (IAEA). Biological dosimetry: Chromosomal aberration analysis for dose assessment (STI/DOC/10/260). Vienna: IAEA, 1986.

8.Dantas,B.M., Lourenço, M.C.R. & Lucena, E.A., **Manual de procedimentos da Unidade de Contador de Corpo Inteiro,** Instituto de Radioproteção, CNEN, Rio de Janeiro,1995.

9. Ingbar, S.H. & Woeber, K.A., **The thyroid gland In: Textbook of Endocrilology,** Academic Press, N. Y., 1981.

EARLY DIAGNOSIS OF RADIATION INDUCED THYROID CANCER IN CHILDREN OF BELARUS BY ULTRASOUND

V.M. DROZD V.M., E.P. DEMIDCHIK, L.N. HARABETS AND A.P. LYCHTCHIK
Research and Clinical Institute of Radiation Medicine and Endocrinology, 23 Masherova Av., Minsk, Belarus
E.D. CHERSTVOY
Minsk State Medical Institute, 83 Dzerzhinsky Av., Minsk, Belarus
Chr. REINERS AND J. TEREKHOVA
Klinik und Poliklinik fur Nuklearmedizin Universitat Wurzburg, Josef Schneider Str.2, Wurzburg, Germany

The studies of medical consequences after the Chernobyl accident have shown that there is a need for solving specific tasks how to use ultrasound: performing mass ultrasonic screening for early recognition of pathology; following up patients for early nosologic diagnosis, and conducting differentiatede diagnosis between benign and malignant pathology of the thyroid. The purpose of the study was to explore ultrasonic visualisation of thyroid carcinoma for its early diagnosis.

We have studied particularities of thyroid cancer ultrasonic pictures in 97 patients before the surgical removal (female-male ratio 1.6:1). The ultrasonic picture of thyroid carcinoma can be distinguished into two forms: nodular and diffuse. The nodular variant can be divided into nodes with limited spread (which have either regular or rather regular outlines) and nodes with a vast spread (with an irregular outline). More frequently the tumour is visualised as a hypoechogenic node. However, isoechogenic character of the node might indicate either the dissemination or multifocal growth of tumour within the thyroid gland. Isoechogenic character of visualised cervical lymph nodes is likely to indicate the presence of malignancy in the thyroid. Thyroid carcinoma is frequently followed by metastases in the area of regional lymph nodes. Location of the node next to the thyroid capsule might cause extracapsular invasion of the tumour (pT4). Signs of "node ageing" -cystic degeneration and calcification- are rarely visible.

1. INTRODUCTION

Initial information on ultrasonic visualisation of the thyroid occurred in 1966-1967. Yamakawa and Naito et al. and Fujimoto et al. published ultrasonic images of the thyroid which were made in A and B- mode.[1,3] At present due to the ultrasonic method we can distinguish diffuse pathological processes from focal ones, cystic formations from solid ones; conduct topic and, in some cases, nosology diagnosis; measure thyroid volume for the control of hormone therapy and estimate the radiation dose for radioiodine therapy; and conduct fine needle aspiration more precisely.[2,3,4]

The studies of medical consequences after the Chernobyl accident have shown that there is a need for solving specific tasks how to use ultrasound: performing mass ultrasonic screening for early recognition of pathology; following up patients for early nosologic diagnosis and conducting differentiatede diagnosis between benign and malignant pathology. The purpose of this study was to explore ultrasonic visualisation of thyroid carcinoma for its early diagnosis.

2.   MATERIALS AND METHODS

Thyroid ultrasound investigation was performed with the ultrasonic real-time scanner, "Toshiba" SSA 240A 7.5 MHz probe, and Hewlett Packard Image Point scanner with colour and power Doppler imaging in the hospital of Research and Clinical Institute of Radiation Medicine and Endocrinology.

3.   RESULTS AND DISCUSSION

The early recognition of thyroid carcinoma has become now possible because of conducting mass ultrasonic screening and following up patients from the risk group exposed to radiation. For example, due to control by follow-up a case of nodular goitre, which was found in 1993, was diagnosed as thyroid cancer and operated on in 1996.(Fig. 1) We have studied particularities of thyroid cancer ultrasonic picture in 97 patients before the surgical removal (female-male ratio 1.6:1). According to TNM classification the cases of thyroid carcinoma were distributed in the following stages: T1-50%, T2-21%, T3-2% and T4-27%; metastases in the regional lymph nodes were found in 59% cases.

A visualisation of carcinoma is possible into two forms: nodular (90 patients - 92.8%) and diffuse (7 patients - 7.2%). The nodular variant of thyroid carcinoma is visualised as a node that is located within the enlarged gland. The enlargement of the gland can be up to 1.5 times compared with the normal size of the thyroid. Average diameter of the node was 1.6 cm. A single node was registered in 88% cases; two or more nodular formations were visible in 12% cases.(Fig. 2)

The node was topically located next to the thyroid capsule in 95.5% patients (Fig. 3). The nodular formation looked more frequently like an inhomogeneous structure (84%) with irregular outline (63%) (Fig. 4). A "Halo", a hypoechogenic margin, was observed in 12.4% children with thyroid cancer (Fig. 5.). Nodes of the thyroid were hypoechogenic in the majority of patients (62%), isoechogenic in 24% and mixed in 14% cases (Fig. 6). In general, regional lymphatic nodes were visible in 66% children with the nodular form of thyroid cancer.

The diffuse variant is characterised by essential volume enlargement of the thyroid (more than 2 times) with a diffuse structure modification, hypo- or mixed, inhomogenous echogeneicity. Enlarged lymphatic nodes were visible in all cases. Although a hypoechogenic character of the thyroid was found in 3 out of 7 children, mixed echogeneicity occurred more frequently (in 4 children). Inhomogeneous and hypoechogenic character of the enlarged thyroid in children with the diffuse form of carcinoma looked like an ultrasonic picture of autoimmune thyroiditis, so diagnosis only could a male by fine needle aspiration biopsy (Fig. 7).

Microcarcinomas (n=47) were characterised by the following ultrasonic picture: irregular outline (51.5%), hypoechogenic (92.3%) and mixed echogenic nodes in several cases. A visualisation of lymph nodes was seen in 54% microcarcinomas.

A comparison of ultrasonic data on thyroid carcinoma with histology data showed that an isoechogenic character of the node might indicate either the dissemination of neoplastic process or multifocal growth of tumour within the thyroid gland.

In patients with suspected thyroid cancer it is important to assess regional lymph nodes. More frequently we found enlarged isoechogenic lymph nodes on both sides of the neck. By fine needle biopsy we managed to show that isoechogenic lymph nodes were always metastases of thyroid carcinoma (Fig. 8). On the other hand, hypoechogenic lymph nodes can indicates both specific and non-specific character.

Six children with thyroid carcinoma were examined by a colour Doppler-imaging system. Hypervasculasisation of the node itself was diagnosed in three children where as in other three patients hypervascularity was seen in the node periphery. Additional information on the node architecture and its interaction with surrounding tissues can be received by the three dimensional reconstruction.(Fig.9)

We observed the diffuse sclerotic variant of thyroid carcinoma in seven children. All these cases were revealed at more advanced stage than pT1, and this variant was more frequently visible as multiple lesions with irregular outlines in both lobes of the thyroid (4 out of 7). Also, lymph nodes were bilaterally enlarged. However, it is impossible to differentiate morphological variants of papillary thyroid carcinoma with ultrasound.

4. CONCLUSION

Ultrasonic particularities of thyroid carcinoma in children exposed to radionuclides could be characterised as following:

1. The ultrasonic picture of thyroid carcinoma with respect to spread can be distinguished into two forms: nodular and diffuse. The nodular variant can be divided into nodes with the limited spread (which have either regular or rather regular outlines) and nodes with a vast spread (with an irregular outline).

2. More frequently the tumour is visualised as a hypoechogenic node. However, isoechogenic feature of the node might indicate either the dissemination or multifocal growth of tumour within the thyroid gland.

3. Thyroid carcinoma is frequently followed by metastases in regional lymph nodes. Isoechogenic character of visualised cervical lymph nodes is likely to indicate the presence of malignancy in the thyroid.

4. Location of the node next to the thyroid capsule might cause extra capsular dissemination of tumour (T4).

5. Ultrasonic signs of "node ageing" - cystic degeneration and calcification- are rarely visible.

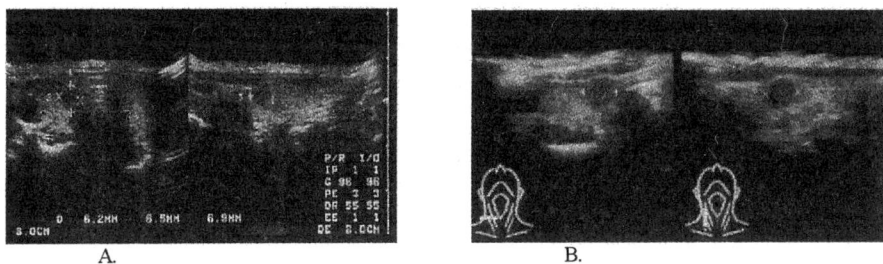

Fig. 1. (A., B.) A. Papillary carcinoma (6x6 mm) in the right lobe (T1N0M0), 1993. B. The size of the nodule has increased more than 2 times for the three year follow-up (12x12 mm), 1996.

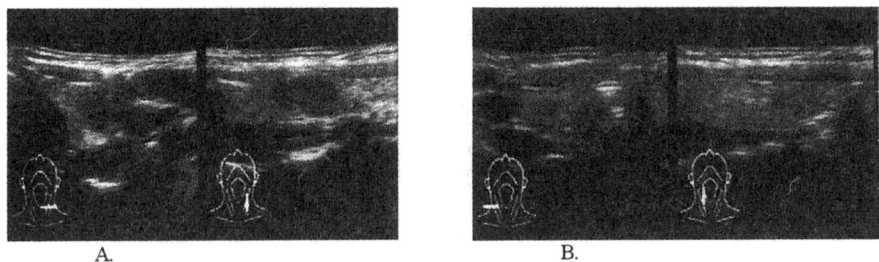

Fig 2. (A., B.) Multiple papillary carcinoma in both lobes of the thyroid, the left (A.) and the right lobes (B.).(T2BN1AM0).

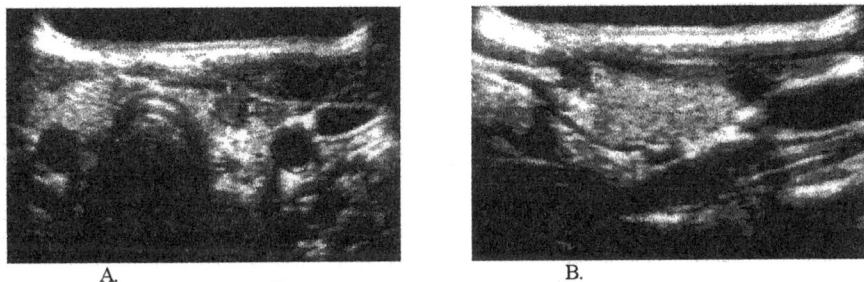

Fig. 3. (A., B.) A. Papillary carcinoma next to the thyroid capsule in the transverse scan (T4N1AM0). B. The same nodule in the longitudinal scan.

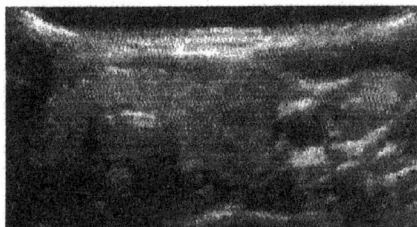

Fig. 4. Papillary carcinoma with inhomogeneous structure in the left lobe in transverse scan. (T4N1BM0).

430

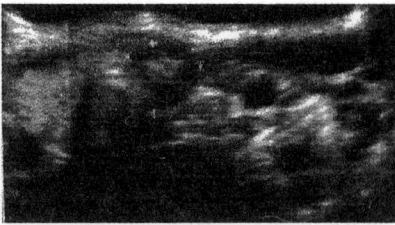 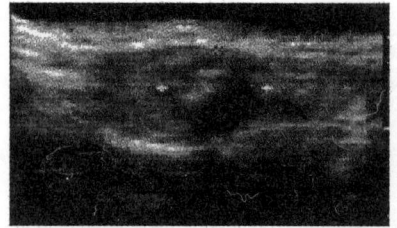

A.   B.

Fig. 5. (A., B.) A. Papillary carcinoma with "halo" sign in the left lobe in transverse scan (T2N1BM0). B. The nodule in longitudinal scan.

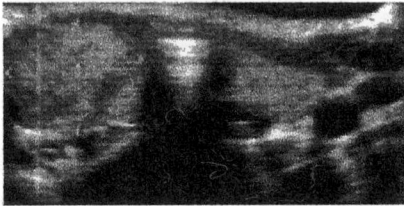 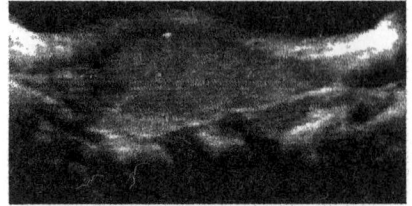

A.   B.

Fig. 6. (A., B.) A. Papillary carcinoma as the isoechogenic node in the right lobe in transverse scan. (T4N1AM0) B. The node in longitudinal scan.

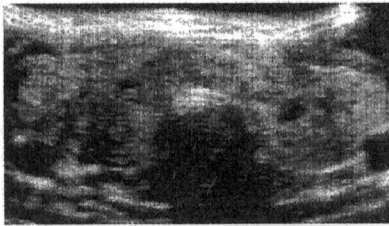 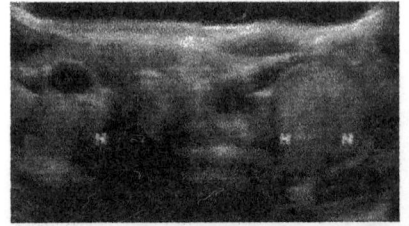

Fig. 7. Papillary carcinoma diffuse variant in transverse scan- diffuse variant. (T4N1BM0).

Fig. 8. Papillary carcinoma (T4N1BM1). Multiple metastasises in lymph nodes after second surgery.

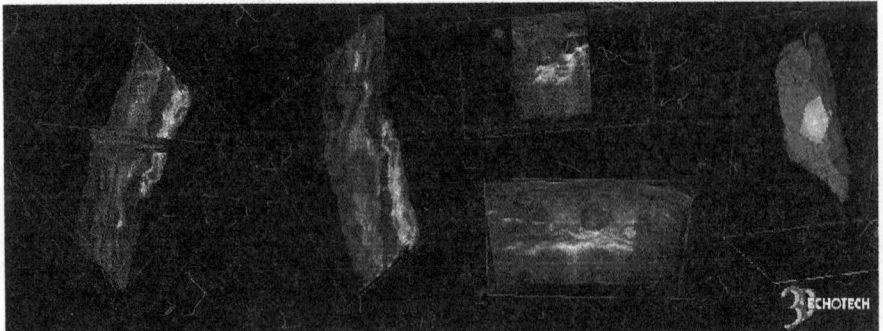

Fig. 9. Three dimensional reconstruction of the node in the left lobe of thyroid gland.

References

1. Fujimoto Y, Oka A, Omoto R et al. Ultrasound scanning of the thyroid gland as a new diagnostic approach. *Ultransonics* 1967; **5**: 177-180.
2. Garcia CJ, Daneman A, McHugh K et al. Sonography in thyroid carcinoma in children. *Br J Radiol* 1992; **65**: 977-982.
3. Maier R. *Ultraschalldiagnostik der Schilddruse*. N. V. : Schattauer, 1989: 224
4. Reiners Chr, Sieper I, Simons G. *Schilddrusendiagnostik*. Behringwerke AG, 1994: 143.
5. Yamakawa K, Naito S. Ultrasonic diagnosis in Japan. Application for the disease of the thyroid: 1st Int Conf Diagn. Pittsburgh 1966: 27-41

POTASSIUM IODIDE PROPHYLAXIS AND THE
UNITED STATES GOVERNMENT: A CASE STUDY

PETER G. CRANE[1]
4809 Drummond Avenue, Chevy Chase, MD 20815
Tel :301-656-3998
E-mail : pgcrane@erols.com

On July 1, 1998, the U.S. Nuclear Regulatory Commission (NRC) announced that it had voted to grant a petition for rulemaking that will require states to consider potassium iodide (KI) prophylaxis, along with evacuation and sheltering, in emergency planning for nuclear power plant accidents. This decision, by a 3-1 vote of the Commissioners, represents a major step in the U.S. Government's 20-year consideration of the KI issue. A review of the NRC's actions over this 20-year period points up serious deficiencies in the handling of the issue by the NRC and its technical staff, with the result that the United States is now far behind other developed countries in ensuring comprehensive protection for its citizens, especially its children, in the event of a major release of radioiodines. The review suggests that in governmental decision making concerning public health effects of nuclear power plant emergencies, the views of public health agencies and emergency management agencies should be given dominant weight.

On July 1, 1998, the U.S. Nuclear Regulatory Commission (NRC) announced that it had granted a petition for rulemaking, filed by me, that would require states to consider the drug potassium iodide (KI) as part of their emergency plans for radiological mishaps at nuclear power plants2. In voting to begin rulemaking, NRC Chairman Shirley A. Jackson and Commissioners Nils J. Diaz and Edward McGaffigan, Jr., rejected the recommendation of the NRC's own technical staff that the petition be denied3. KI stockpiling is also bitterly opposed by the U.S. nuclear power industry. The rule change will be coupled with a new U.S. policy, not yet final, under which stocks of KI will be given to any U.S. state that requests it.

---

1 Counsel for Special Projects, Office of the General Counsel, U.S. Nuclear Regulatory Commission; former Member, Nuclear Claims Tribunal, Republic of the Marshall Islands. This paper, submitted in the author's private capacity, represents his personal views only.

2 See NRC Press Release of July 1, 1998.

3 The vote was 3-1. Commissioner Greta J. Dicus, whose term expired June 30, 1998, sided with the NRC staff.

The grant of the petition did not bring an instant change in the NRC's rules. Before that can happen, the NRC must publish a proposed rule, receive and analyze comments from the public, and issue a final rule. Thus the three Commissioners' commendable decision represents not the end, but perhaps the beginning of the end, of the U.S. Government's protracted consideration of the KI issue, a process that began some 20 years ago.

To the international community, it is well known by now that KI stockpiling is routine throughout the developed world; that some nations, notably France and Switzerland, go further, with house-to-house predistribution4; that KI has long had the backing of the World Health Organization5 and the American Thyroid Association; that it is an element of the International Basic Safety Standards6 sponsored by the International Atomic Energy Association and other organizations; and that its safety in actual use was proved in Poland, as Drs. Janusz Nauman and Jan Wolff described in their seminal 1993 paper7. The question that an international audience may be asking is how the United States could contrive to spend 20 years resolving an issue so straightforward and obvious that 20 weeks should have been more than enough time for a reasoned decision.

I will try to offer an answer to that question, through a case study of the handling of the KI issue by the United States Government. My purpose is to suggest the problems that can arise when public health decisions relating to radiation are placed in the hands of an agency whose primary expertise is not health, but nuclear technology.

I should interject that I am a lawyer, not a physician or a scientist. I make no pretensions to medical expertise, except insofar as I have gained it as a patient with thyroid cancer, presumably radiogenic.[8] My 15-year involvement in the KI issue stems from my conviction, born of experience, that thyroid cancer is a disease well worth preventing, especially if prevention can be achieved easily and cheaply.

---

4 Electricité de France and the Swiss Government both publicize their KI policies through Internet sites.

5 World Health Organization, EUR/ICP/CEH 102(S), § 4.3.3. (1991).

6 International Basic Safety Standards for Protection Against Ionizing Radiation and for the Safety of Radiation Sources (interim edition), International Atomic Energy Agency (Vienna, 1994).

7 J. Nauman & J. Wolff, "Iodine Prophylaxis in Poland after the Chernobyl Reactor Accident: Benefits and Risks," American Journal of Medicine, Vol. 94, p. 524 (May, 1993).

8 I was part of the cohort of some 5000 children who, some 50 years ago, received head and neck radiation -- in my case, 750 rads of x-ray to my enlarged tonsils and adenoids -- at Michael Reese Hospital in Chicago, Illinois. In 1973, I had a partial thyroidectomy for papillary thyroid cancer; in 1983, had the thyroid remnant ablated; in 1988, was diagnosed with a recurrence; and in 1992, after five courses of radioiodine therapy, totaling 700 millicuries of I-131, was given a clean bill of health.

Benjamin Franklin once wrote, "A child thinks that 20 shillings and 20 years can never be spent." Let me offer now a brief chronology of where the last 20 years went in the U.S. Government's consideration of KI.

-- 1978: The U.S. Food and Drug Administration (FDA) declares KI "safe and effective" for use in nuclear power plant emergencies, and approves its over-the-counter sale.[9]

-- 1979: During the Three Mile Island accident, federal and state officials, fearing a major release, search for supplies of KI and discover none exist. Later, the President's Commission investigating the TMI accident castigates the Government's failure to stockpile KI and recommends stockpiling for the public and radiation workers.[10] A month later, the NRC announces its agreement, declaring its intent to make the availability of KI a "necessary part of an acceptable State emergency response plan."[11]

-- 1982: The NRC technical staff recommends that the Commissioners approve an interagency U.S. Government policy endorsing the use of KI as a "useful ancillary protective action."[12] Nineteen days later, without explanation, the NRC technical staff withdraws that recommendation, saying that it plans to prepare a new paper that will recommend against stockpiling and distribution of KI on cost-benefit grounds.[13]

-- 1983: The NRC technical staff briefs the Commission in a public meeting on its new, anti-KI position. The gist of the NRC staff's argument is that though KI is cheap, it will be even cheaper in the long run to treat radiation-caused illnesses after an accident than to spend even a small amount to prevent them with

9 Food and Drug Administration, "Potassium Iodide as a Thyroid-Blocking Agent in a Radiation Emergency," 43 Federal Register 58798 (Dec. 15, 1978).

10 Report of the President's Commission on the Accident at Three Mile Island ("Kemeny Commission"), at 41-42.

11 NUREG-0632, "NRC Views and Analysis of the Recommendations of the President's Commission on the Accident at Three Mile Island" (November, 1979).

12 SECY-82-396, "Development of a Federal Policy Statement on the Distribution and Use of Potassium Iodide for Thyroidal Blocking in the Event of a Nuclear Power Plant Accident" (September 27, 1982), Attachment 3, at 3-4.

13 SECY-82-396A, "Withdrawal of SECY-82-396 (Federal Policy Statement on Use of Potassium Iodide)" (October 15, 1982). The memorandum notes that the Federal Emergency Management Agency (FEMA) has just dropped plans to buy a large amount of KI for stockpiling. Unlike the NRC, which is an independent regulatory agency, FEMA is part of the Executive Branch, *i.e.*, under Presidential control.

KI. The comparison is exclusively in dollar terms: dollars for KI pills vs. dollars for medical treatment, as though illness had no burdens other than the expense involved. The briefers mention neither cancer nor the possibility of fatalities.[14]

-- 1985: The U.S. Government issues a national policy on KI.[15] Referring to the NRC's "cost-benefit analysis," it dismisses the idea of requiring KI as "not worthwhile."

-- 1989: As NRC internal rules allow, I file a "Differing Professional Opinion," challenging the agency's KI policy. I argue that new information warrants reconsidering the KI issue, and that existing policy was tainted from the start by NRC staff misinformation to the Commissioners and the public.

-- 1994: The NRC staff, while not addressing the issue of misinformation, recommends to the Commissioners that stockpiling KI in the vicinity of nuclear plants "appears prudent."[16] It proposes a new federal policy to buy KI and encourage states to establish stockpiles. The staff estimates that it would cost less (a few hundred thousand dollars) to buy a national stockpile of KI than go on studying whether to do so. But the Commissioners then in office tie 2-2, so the old policy remains in place.

-- 1995: Acting as a private citizen, on my own time, I file a petition for rulemaking, asking the NRC to require that KI be among the "range of protective actions" included in state emergency plans. I also write to the Director of the Federal Emergency Management Agency, which chairs the interagency committee responsible for overall KI policy.

-- 1996: At a public meeting called by FEMA, several state officials describe KI stockpiling as undesirable and unnecessary. An Illinois official explains, "Loss of the thyroid is not life-threatening."[17] Several months later, the

---

14 The briefers refer instead to "nodules." They convey the impression that any thyroid illness resulting from an accident would be trivial: "There's a few days loss from -- it's a relatively simple operation that's involved in removing the thyroid or removing the nodules." Transcript of November 22, 1983 meeting, at 52-53. When the NRC Chairman suggests that if he survives an accident because of KI, he will think the $.20 cost of the pills to be money well spent, the NRC staff corrects him, telling him that "the surviving question is not the question." Transcript at 63.

15 "Federal Policy on Distribution of Potassium Iodide Around Nuclear Power Sites for Use as a Thyroidal Blocking Agent," 50 Federal Register 30258 (July 24, 1985).

16 SECY-94-087, "Addendum to SECY-93-318 Re-evaluation of Policy Regarding Use of Potassium Iodide After a Severe Accident at a Nuclear Power Plant" (March 29, 1994), at 2.

17 The identical sentence appears in a separate statement filed by a South Carolina official. Later, the Illinois Department of Nuclear Safety, offended by my criticism of it, writes to the NRC that the State of

interagency committee headed by FEMA calls for a new federal policy that would give KI at federal expense to any state requesting it.[18]

-- 1997: The NRC staff proposes a draft federal policy statement on KI to the Commissioners.[19] While the policy would make KI available to states requesting it, the notice includes no recommendation that they do so. It does not refer to Chernobyl or the Polish experience with KI; states that there is "no new information" warranting a change in existing policy; and mentions only near the end of the notice that the purpose of using KI is to prevent cancer. After a protest from FEMA, the NRC staff apologizes in a public Commission meeting for having "misrepresented" FEMA's position on KI in its June 1997 paper.[20]

-- 1998: The NRC staff recommends to the Commission that it deny my petition.[21] It offers a 40-page "technical assessment" of KI, offering its own highly equivocal judgment of the drug's safety. Although the obvious starting point for any such analysis by a U.S. Government agency is the Food and Drug Administration's finding that KI is "safe and effective," the NRC staff "technical assessment" omits even to mention it.

The "technical assessment" appears calculated to raise alarm that KI will have severe side effects, and that these side effects will expose state governments to legal liability. For example, it warns: "In the U.S., the implementation of a protective action *may entail litigation and liability for long after the accident.* The TMI accident is a case in point. One can expect that *administration of KI on a*

Illinois "stands firmly behind its contention that hundreds of thousands of people live normal, healthy lives without functioning thyroid glands." Letter from Thomas W. Ortciger, Director, January 8, 1998.

18 Despairing of persuading the Government to provide the states and the public with accurate and up-to-date information on KI, I decided in early 1996 to try to reach the public directly through newspaper articles. The first, in the New York Times, was designed to coincide with the tenth anniversary of Chernobyl. Other articles followed. (I did not accept payment for them.) They helped stimulate citizen action at the state level, which in turn led to state meetings, in which I participated, in Maine, Ohio, and New York. Maine and Ohio have decided in favor of stockpiling, and the issue remains under active consideration in New York State. In each of these states, great weight has been given to the advice of thyroid cancer experts from the American Thyroid Association.

19 SECY-97-124, "Proposed Federal Policy Regarding Use of Potassium Iodide After a Severe Accident at a Nuclear Power Plant," June 16, 1997.

20 At this meeting, believing that I did not have the votes to gain approval of my petition as written, I stated that I would be satisfied if states are required by rule to "consider" KI in developing their emergency plans. At the Commission's request, I submitted an amended petition a week later.

21 SECY-98-061, "Staff Options for Resolving a Petition for Rulemaking," March 31, 1998.

mass basis would certainly entail litigation in this country, whereas the government of Poland, which administered KI on a mass-basis, did not appear to be faced with such litigation." [Emphasis added.][22]

The authors of the "technical assessment" evidently recognize that the strongest empirical evidence for the safety of KI is the very low incidence of adverse medical reactions observed in Poland. Accordingly, in an apparent effort to disparage Nauman and Wolff's report, the NRC "technical assessment" says of it in passing, "to the extent that we believe the report...."[23] The authors of the "technical assessment" cast this aspersion upon two internationally renowned medical experts without offering any evidence to support the insinuation that the report should not be believed.[24]

While the staff's paper is pending before the Commission, a FEMA official writes to the NRC to point out an erroneous statement about FEMA's position on KI by the NRC staff and "misleading" comments by a nuclear industry lobbying group and an Illinois state agency.[25] Her letter refers to the FDA's 1978 approval of KI, and adds pointedly, "This FDA approval was empirically reinforced by the experience in Poland with KI, subsequent to the Chernobyl accident." It appears to be an implicit warning to the NRC that FEMA will not be a party to withholding key information on the safety of KI from the public.

---

22 Technical assessment, at p. 22. Why a legal judgment of this kind has any place in what purports to be a technical assessment of a particular medication, and what qualifications the authors have to offer any legal opinion -- particularly one as sweeping as that just quoted -- are unexplained. The authors' effort to invoke the specter of legal liability may help explain the absence from the "technical assessment" of any reference to the Food and Drug Administration's finding on KI. If state governments were made aware that the FDA had approved KI as "safe and effective," that fact would be doubly reassuring to them. First, it would indicate that the drug was safe. Second, it would mean that even if, as the NRC staff confidently predicts, use of KI in a radiological emergency were to lead to lawsuits over side effects, states could defend themselves by showing that they had relied on the FDA's finding. The NRC staff "technical assessment" is careful not to address the point, often made by supporters of KI stockpiling, myself included, that states concerned about possible exposure to lawsuits relating to KI should probably worry most about a different type of lawsuit: those that would be brought if an accident occurred and children developed thyroid cancer because KI had *not* been stockpiled.

23 *Id.* at 11.

24 The NRC, which has made the "technical assessment" public, should withdraw the document and offer Drs. Nauman and Wolff a deep and contrite apology.

25 Letter from Kay C. Goss, FEMA Associate Director, April 9, 1998.

As I mentioned at the outset, the Commissioners rejected the staff recommendation and directed the NRC staff to begin a rulemaking that would incorporate into the NRC's rules a requirement that states "consider" iodine prophylaxis as a part of radiological emergency planning. This requirement would be coupled with an offer of free KI from the Federal Government. As of late July, 1998, Commission action on the draft policy statement was expected shortly.

Thus in the end, the Commissioners decided wisely, and the United States may no longer be at odds with the rest of the civilized world on whether it is "worthwhile" to protect children from thyroid cancer. In such cases, it is common to declare that "the system worked." But did it? To be sure, it speaks well for the American democracy that the citizen's right to seek redress of grievances is not an empty phrase. Likewise, it reflects no small credit on the NRC that it tolerated with such good grace the campaign that an NRC employee was conducting in his spare time.

By any other measure, however, the system did *not* work. First and foremost, there is no excuse for American children still to have second-class protection, so many years after the recommendations of the WHO. When nations rich and poor, from Japan to Armenia, can afford to buy KI, surely the U.S. can do the same. It is or should be a reproach to the richest nation on earth that its policy on protecting children from cancer should be based on the notion -- a fallacious notion at that -- that cure is cheaper than prevention.

The safety of American children should also not depend on citizens hammering on their Government to do what it promised to do almost 20 years ago. Moreover, a system for allowing interested citizens to seek regulatory change that takes nine years even to approach fruition cannot be said to be working satisfactorily. Finally, the record shows too many instances in which the NRC staff provided information to the Commissioners and the public that lacked balance, accuracy, and completeness.[26] I have offered examples of the way in which facts that did not support the desired result have disappeared down the "Memory Hole," in George Orwell's well-known phrase. The NRC staff's treatment of pro-KI comments, including those from internationally known medical experts representing the American Thyroid Association, is another example. The

---

26 FEMA is to be commended for having brought some of these lapses to the NRC Commissioners' attention.

opportunity to submit views to a federal agency is of little value if the technical staff ignores those comments it finds difficult to rebut.[27]

I have high confidence in the NRC staff to make sound, well-supported and intellectually honest judgments about nuclear safety hardware, conditions of reactor operation, and the like. Sadly, the record does not permit a similar statement about the NRC staff's past handling of the KI issue.[28]

One can speculate that part of the underlying problem may be that the technical experts involved in nuclear safety decisions do not in their hearts view major accidents as credible, at least in the United States, and therefore regard all emergency planning as no more than a political concession to the public's irrational fears of nuclear power. If one starts from the premise that emergency planning is a pointless charade, then any upgrading of planning, even one as inexpensive as KI, may seem worth resisting. By the same token, it may seem unnecessary to be overly punctilious in how one analyzes a health issue that one believes will never arise.

The cause of the phenomenon is beside the point, however; the issue is what to do about it. I believe that one part of the answer is to ensure a proper division of governmental responsibilities among different agencies. The primary responsibility for radiological emergency planning must be placed (or kept) in the hands of agencies whose mission is emergency preparedness, not nuclear regulation. In the U.S. context, this means FEMA. Such agencies know from experience that accidents can happen and can develop unpredictably, and they plan accordingly.

Likewise, decisions affecting human health should be made in the first instance by health agencies and health professionals. It seems unlikely, for example, that any medical doctor, answerable to his or her peers, would ever discuss the consequences of radiation-caused thyroid disease in a public meeting without mentioning cancer. Nor would medical doctors presume to discuss the safety of a drug without reference to the Food and Drug Administration's judgment that it is "safe and effective." The line between nuclear regulation and nuclear

---

27 The NRC staff's recent memoranda to the Commissioners on the KI issue illustrate how essential it is that Commissioners and their personal staffs read the actual comments that are submitted to the NRC on controversial issues, rather than relying on the NRC staff to summarize the comments for them.

28 Now that the Commissioners have voted, it is reasonable to expect that the highest levels of NRC staff management will loyally accept the direction they have received. The more problematic issue concerns NRC staff management below the highest levels. Suffice it to say that the deficiencies of the "technical assessment" are of such a nature that it would be prudent to excuse the individuals principally responsible for that document from any further involvement with the KI issue.

promotion is not an easy one to maintain, and needs to be guarded vigilantly, as must the line between science and propaganda. Here, something went seriously wrong, not once but repeatedly.

Thanks to the three NRC Commissioners now in office, the U.S. Government's long mishandling of the KI issue may now be nearing its end. Nevertheless, it should be an object lesson within the U.S. and for authorities in other countries as well.

442

References

1. *Journal Article:*
2. Nauman J, Wolff J. Iodine Prophylaxis in Poland after the Chernobyl Reactor Accident: Benefits and Risks. *Am J Med* 1993; Vol. 94, p. 524.
3. *Publications of International Organizations:*
4. International Basic Safety Standards for Protection Against Ionizing Radiation and for the Safety of Radiation Sources (interim edition), International Atomic Energy Agency (Vienna, 1994).
5. World Health Organization Report EUR/ICP/CEH 102(S) (1991).
6. *U.S. Nuclear Regulatory Commission Publications:*
7. NUREG-0632, "NRC Views and Analysis of the Recommendations of the President's Commission on the Accident at Three Mile Island" (November, 1979).
8. SECY-82-396, "Development of a Federal Policy Statement on the Distribution and Use of Potassium Iodide for Thyroidal Blocking in the Event of a Nuclear Power Plant Accident" (September 27, 1982).
9. SECY-82-396A, "Withdrawal of SECY-82-396 (Federal Policy Statement on Use of Potassium Iodide" (October 15, 1982)
10. SECY-94-087, "Addendum to SECY-93-318 Re-evaluation of Policy Regarding Use of Potassium Iodide After a Severe Accident at a Nuclear Power Plant" (March 29, 1994)
11. SECY-97-124, "Proposed Federal Policy Regarding Use of Potassium Iodide After a Severe Accident at a Nuclear Power Plant" (June 16, 1997)
12. SECY-98-061, "Staff Options for Resolving a Petition for Rulemaking" (March 31, 1998)
13. *Other U.S. Government Publications:*
14. "Federal Policy on Distribution of Potassium Iodide Around Nuclear Power Sites for Use as a Thyroidal Blocking Agent," 50 Federal Register 30258 (July 24, 1985)
15. "Potassium Iodide as a Thyroid-Blocking Agent in a Radiation Emergency," (U.S. Food and Drug Administration), 43 Federal Register 58798 (Dec. 15, 1978)
16. Report of the President's Commission on the Accident at Three Mile Island (1979)

DETERMINATION OF IODINE KINETICS IN LUNG METASTASES DURING RADIOIODINE THERAPY OF BELARUSSIAN CHILDREN WITH THYROID CARCINOMA

MICHAEL LASSMANN, LUTZ SCHELPER, HERIBERT HÄNSCHEID,
JOHANNES BIKO AND CHRISTOPH REINERS
Clinic for Nuclear Medicine, University of Würzburg, Germany
Josef-Schneider-Str.2, D-97080 Würzburg
E-mail: lassmann@nuklearmedizin.uni-wuerzburg.de
HERWIG PARETZKE
Institute for Radiation Protection, GSF - Research Center for the Environment and Health,
Ingolstädter Landstr.1, D-85764 Neuherberg, Germany
CORNELIS HOEFNAGEL
Department of Nuclear Medicine, The Netherlands Cancer Institute, Plesmanlaan 121,
1066 CX Amsterdam, The Netherlands
SUSAN CLARKE AND SARAH ALLEN
Department of Nuclear Medicine, Guy's Hospital, St.Thomas Street, London SE1 9RT, UK

For the determination of iodine kinetics in lung tissue in children from Belarus mostly with a disseminated miliary form of thyroid cancer a dedicated measuring device has been constructed for the determination of uptake in lung tissue and metastases in order to optimize radioiodine therapy. With this device a series of measurements has been started immediately after the application of a therapeutic activity of I-131 in order to register the iodine kinetics during the first days of the therapy. Using a collimator with adequate shape and aperture either a point target or the whole lung can be quantitatively evaluated with a dynamic range from 1 to 0.0003 of the activity administered. First investigations with 37 children from Belarus treated in Würzburg show good agreement between measurements with a calibrated gamma camera and the new probe 24h-48h after application if I-131. The device is well suited to extend the uptake measurements to the first two days p.a.

1   INTRODUCTION

The frequency of thyroid cancer in children from Belarus is increasing since 1990[1, 3]. On the whole, 508 cases of childhood thyroid cancer have been diagnosed and operated by the Centre for Thyroid Tumors in Minsk between 1986 and 1996[1, 3].

In selected children with most advanced tumor stages, radioiodine treatment followed. In half of these children distant metastases had been present with most of the secondaries localized as disseminated miliary spread in the lungs. The conventional way of I-131-treatment with fractionated activities is less effective for the treatment of these metastases than it is for ablation of thyroid remnants or lymph node metastases, resulting in higher numbers of therapy courses with the risk of radiation induced pulmonary fibrosis. Neither for lung metastases nor for the surrounding lung tissue the dose from I-131-treatment has been investigated quantitatively. The knowledge of the iodine kinetics is therefore a prerequisite for dosimetry and the optimization of tumor treatment and lung tissue protection.

2   MATERIALS AND METHODS

2.1   Construction of the measuring device

For the purpose of this study we constructed a measuring device which is dedicated to the estimation of the activity in areas of different size such as focal or disseminated pulmonary metastases and well suited for a wide range of incorporated activity particularly for the determination of the first 48h after administration of therapeutic activities of I-131.

In the following a detailed description of the system components is given:

Bed: For measurement we used the pallet of a gamma camera. This pallet has variable height for bed-detector distances and therefore allows variable measuring field sizes and system sensitivity. For optimal positioning of the patient the lucite pallet can be moved in and perpendicular to the patients long axis.

Detector: As a detector we used a high purity germanium detector with a relative efficiency of 35 %[1]. The germanium detector was chosen due to its superior quality in terms of energy resolution and dead time and for the simplicity to introduce attenuation correction algorithms[2,4,5].

Shielding and collimators: The detector is mounted in an iron box filled with lead with the exception of an opening which is well suited to put in different collimator inserts as shown in the cross-section in figure 1. Radiation of the 360 keV photons of I-131 is attenuated to a factor of 4×10^{-9}. After preliminary investigations we manufactured collimators with cylindrical holes of 2, 8, 13 and 18 mm diameter and cone collimators with diameters of 2, 4, 8 and 14 mm. For a constant measurement geometry with high reproducibility we integrated a commercial laser pointer into an insert fitting into the collimator opening of the lead shielding.

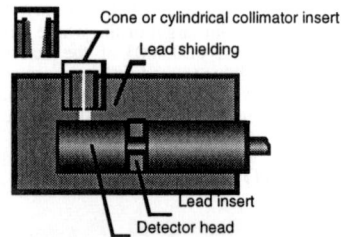

Fig. 1. Schematic drawing of the detector and the shielding

Processing device: The signals from the preamplifier of the detector are processed through a PC based spectroscopy card. The areas of the 364 keV peaks in the measured spectra are evaluated using commercially available software[2].

Torso phantom: With a commercial heart-thorax phantom[3] with integrated inserts for heart, liver and perfusable and non-perfusable lungs the activity calibration

---

[1] Canberra-Packard, D-63303 Dreieich, Germany

[2] Aptec Nuclear Inc., North Tonowanda, N.Y., USA

[3] Radiology Support Devices Inc., Long Beach, California 90810, USA

of the measuring device was performed. If the phantom lungs are filled with water and/or calibration solution an anatomic correct mass density for lung tissue of 0.4 g/cm^3 is reached. To simulate inhomogeneous activity distributions such as focal metastases refillable markers with a volume ranging from 0,5 to 2 cm^3 can be put in the lungs. These markers can be placed in different regions of the lungs.

3   RESULTS

3.1   Spatial resolution

For determining the spatial resolution of the system we measured the relative efficiency of the system as a function of the distance from the center of the measured area at three detector to bed surface distances. With these data we calculated the full width at half maximum (FWHM) and the useful field of view of the detector defined as the diameter at which the counts at the peak maximum drop to 5%. For the cylindrical collimator the FWHM ranged from 4 cm for a collimator diameter of 2 mm to 280 mm for a detector-to-patient distance of 760 mm and a collimator diameter of 18 mm.

The function for the cylindrical collimator is nearly gaussian with a width of 12 cm FWHM and shows a steep decrease of the efficiency around the central area of high efficiency. These collimators were constructed to measure single focal metastases with negligible background activity from surrounding tissue.

The cone collimators show a narrow plateau with an almost constant efficiency and a diameter of the field of view of 28 cm and were designed to provide a larger central area of constant efficiency in the case of homogeneously distributed metastases. In addition, the use of the cone-shaped collimators allows the direct comparison of uptake values obtained with the device and the gamma camera. The diameter of the measured area for the conically shaped collimators is almost constant for each bed height and ranged from 26 cm to 36 cm.

3.2   Calibration and activity range

For quantification of lung uptake an efficiency calibration of the detector system is essential. We calibrated the device for three different positions of metastases within the torso phantom (upper quadrant of the lung in front of the breast, in front of the back area and in the lower lung quadrant in the center of the coronal lung axis) and for homogeneously distributed activity in lung tissue. In table 1 an estimation of the optimal activity ranges of the different collimators is given.

Furthermore we calibrated a planar dual-headed gamma-camera (Siemens Bodyscan[4]) for the determination of the activity retention of the upper part of the

---

[4] Siemens Medizinsysteme, D-91052 Erlangen, Germany

446

body, lung and lung metastases with the same heart-thorax phantom with the same activitiy levels of I 131 which were used for the probe calibration.

Table 1. Estimation of activity range for the use of different collimators for I-131.

Cylindrical Collimators		Conical Collimators	
Diameter [mm]	Activity range [MBq]	Diameter [mm]	Activity range [MBq]
18	556 – 0,2	14	831 – 0,2
13	1150 – 0,3	8	2550 – 0,7
8	3050 – 0,8	4	5940 – 1,6
2	45000 – 12	2	19400 – 5,2

Measurements of children from Belarus treated in Würzburg show good agreements between measurements with the camera and the new probe as can be seen from the example in figure 2. The device is well suited to extend the uptake measurements to the first two days p.a., which is the most important phase for the iodine kinetics in lung tissue and disseminated metastases due their short effective halflives. Up to now the iodine kinetics in 37 patients from Belarus was measured with good agreement between gammacamera measurements after 48h and probe measurements.

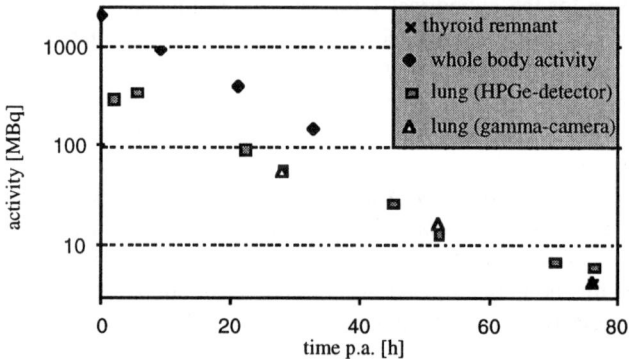

Fig. 2. Iodine kinetics in one patient up to 72h after administration of I-131 determined with a whole body probe, gamma-camera and the new detector system

4. CONCLUSION

The newly constructed device is well suited for uptake measurements after the first two days p.a. of high activities of I-131. In this phase approximately 80-90% of the tumor dose is reached. The determination of the I-131 kinetics in lung tissue in the 37 patients measured so far must be combined with computed results on the energy deposition of I-131 in lung metastases to give resulting doses as the combination of biological and physical data.

Acknowledgment

This work was sponsored by the EC (Contract: FI4CT-CT96-0009)

References

1. Demidchik EP, Demidchik YU: Thyroid Cancer Promoted by Radiation in Children of Belarus. In: *Radiation Research 1895-1995*, Proceedings of the 10th International Congress of Radiation Research, Würzburg 27.08.-01.09.1995.
2. Hänscheid H, Lassmann M, Reiners, C. Berücksichtigung der Tiefe der Aktivitätsverteilung bei der Speicherungsmessung vor der Therapie der Schilddrüse. In: G. Heinemann, H. Pfob, eds. *Strahlenbiologie und Strahlenschutz: Moderne Entwicklungen und Tendenzen in der Strahlenbiologie*, Fachverband für Strahlenschutz, 1996: 256-260.
3. Reiners C, Biko J, Kruglova N, Demidchik EP: Therapy of thyroid carcinoma in children from Belarus after the Chernobyl accident. In: I Nauman, D Glinoer, LB Braverman, U Hostalek, eds, *The Thyroid and Iodine*. Schattauer Stuttgart - New-York 1996: 89 - 97
4. Schelper L, Lassmann M, Hänscheid H, Reiners, C. Tiefenkorrektur bei Messungen im Ganzkörperzähler mittels Gammaspektrometrie. In: . H. Leitner, G. Stücklschwaiger, eds. *Medizinische Physik 1996*, Deutsche Ges. f. Med. Physik, 1996: 375-376.
5. Schelper L, Lassmann M, Hänscheid H, Reiners, C. Schwächungskorrektur bei gammaspektroskopischen Ganz- und Teilkörpermessungen durch Analyse der Energiespektren. In: P. Sahre, ed. *Hochauflösende Gamma-Spektrometrie an Ganz- und Teilkörperzählern*, VKTA-47, 1997: 77-90.

REACTOR ACCIDENTS AND THYROID CANCER RISK:
USE OF THE CHERNOBYL EXPERIENCE
FOR EMERGENCY RESPONSE

E. BUGLOVA AND J. .KENIGSBERG

Research and Clinical Institute of Radiation Medicine and Endocrinology,
Masherov ave 23, Minsk 220600, Belarus
E-mail: risk@rcirme.belpak.minsk.by

T. MCKENNA

Nuclear Regulatory Commission, MS 4A43 Washington DC, 20555, USA
E-mail: TJM2@nrc.gov

In addition to exist experience the Chernobyl data could provide a new information to protect the human thyroid in the case of the reactor accident. The paper presents the registered and prognosed number of radiation-induced thyroid cancer cases among population of Belarus. The data about distribution of the cases in Belarussian children and adolescents as a function of distance from the Chernobyl NPP is given. Importance of thyroid blocking for the people living on the different distances from the site is brought out. The system to protect the thyroid for the inhabitants of the Belarussian territories located close to the Ignalina NPP is described. The Chernobyl experience was used in the development of new draft guidance by the IAEA, the main principles of which are also presented.

Nuclear power reactors have a large inventory of radioiodine and other radionuclides. Typically total inventory of radioiodine in the reactor core is about 27×10^{18} Bq. In the event of an accident in an operating nuclear reactor involving a release of radioactivity, the iodine isotopes will be among the first fission products to be released. The isotopes of iodine are metabolically active and once inhaled or ingested by the person are retained in the thyroid. Exposure of the thyroid in low doses can lead to thyroid cancer. Risk of this consequence can be reduced by intervention early during an accident.

In response to the Chernobyl accident several types of protective actions to decrease exposure of the thyroid were taken in Belarus. The effectiveness of these protective actions was assessed by analysis of registered thyroid cancer cases. Among persons less than 18 years old who were evacuated from the 30-km zone of Belarussian territory 4 thyroid cancer cases were observed. All these cases were registered after the end of latent period for the radiation induced thyroid cancer. Taking into account spontaneous rate of the disease in this age group and number of evacuated persons, all these cases can be considered as accident-induced. There have also been about 790 thyroid cancer cases among the Belarussian population under 18 years old at the time of the accident.[1] The vast majority of these thyroid cancers are considered accident-induced. Based on the prognosis more than 6000 excess thyroid cancers are expected among all exposed Belarussian population during their lifetime as a result of the accident. It has been suggested that most of these excess cancers could have been prevented by timely administration of stable iodine and effective restriction of the locally produced milk and vegetables.

Low efficiency of thyroid gland protection performed in Belarus stipulated the formation of thyroid doses and, as a consequence, development of radiation-induced thyroid cancer case not only among the population of the nearby territories but also among the population of the long-distance territories (Table 1).

Table 1. Number of thyroid cancers in Belarus during 1986-1996 among those 0-18 years old at the time of the Chernobyl accident.

Distance from the Chernobyl NPP, km	Number of cases		
	1986-1996	1986-1989	1990-1996
0-30	4	0	4
31-50	26	1	25
51-100	72	2	70
101-150	177	8	169
151-200	66	2	64
201-250	84	2	82
251-300	68	3	65
301-350	136	9	127
351-400	45	2	43
> 400	77	6	71

The data of the table shows that the vast majority of the thyroid cancers were diagnosed among those living more than 50 km from the site. Distribution of the registered thyroid cancer cases among inhabitants of the territories located at the different distances from the Chernobyl NPP is an important proof of the necessity of iodine prophylaxis for the inhabitants of the territories located far from the site.

A system is created in Belarus to protect the thyroid of the inhabitants of the Belarussian territories located close to the Ignalina NPP (Lithuania). More than 20,000 people are living at the Belarussian side of the 30-km zone. Among this population the distribution of stable iodine was performed in advance. Tablets of stable iodine along with instruction of use are located in the family first-aid sets. Additional stocks of the tablets are in local medical services. In every local medical service there is special prepared person and transport to go along the known route to distribute additional tablets of stable iodine when necessary. Combination of such availability of stable iodine in families and local medical services is a strong guarantee of possibility to take first dose of iodine during first hours after making the decision to perform iodine prophylaxis. The decision is made by the head of medical service at the district level based on the criterion of gamma dose rate.

Efficacy of this system was tested during exercises at the territory of the Belarussian side of the 30-km zone. The results of the exercises showed that during 3-6 hours after the warning signal iodine prophylaxis was performed for 95% of the population.

Emergency plan makes provisions not only for iodine prophylaxis but also for sheltering and evacuation if criteria of gamma dose rate are exceeded.

One of the important actions to reduce ingestion of radioiodine is the grounded restriction of consumption for the potentially contaminated local foods (in particular, milk and leaf vegetables). At the territory of Belarus close to the Ignalina NPP radiation survey teams with all necessary equipment to collect samples were organized. The analyses are performed in laboratories. In-situ gamma spectroscopy is not available that build a background for some delay to obtain a results. For the territories that are far from the NPP the possibilities for collection and analyzing of samples also exist. As for the thyroid blocking among the population of the long-distance territories, there are centralized stocks of stable iodine in medical services and pharmacies without predistribution of the tablets. After the decision about thyroid blocking the distribution of the tablets will be performed through the medical system.

One of the crucial points in the performance of the thyroid blocking is the time when the person takes the pill. It is well known that to obtain the maximum reduction of the radiation dose to the thyroid, stable iodine should be administrated before any intake of radioactive iodine; otherwise, as soon as practicable thereafter. If stable iodine is administrated orally within the six hours preceding the intake of radioactive iodine, the protection provided is almost complete; it is about 90% if stable iodine is administered at the time of inhalation of radioiodine. [3]

The results of the protective actions, which were performed in Belarus and other countries after the Chernobyl accident, gave the possibility to extend our knowledge in this field. The experience of thyroid blocking in Poland showed that after the accident no cases of thyroid cancer were registered among persons for whom the thyroid blocking was performed. [4,5] However this action was done in several days after the accident. This experience showed that in relatively low thyroid doses the late performance of thyroid blocking gave certain effect.

As for Belarus we have confirmed information about late use of stable iodine. Taking into account that doses for thyroid in Belarus are higher than in Poland, it is necessary to access the efficacy of late use of stable iodine among population of Belarus. Preliminary assessment did not bring out the thyroid cancer cases among children with confirmed information of dates and doses of stable iodine.

The Chernobyl accident has been extensively studied. These studies have included a reassessment of the actions taken to protect the population from thyroid cancer. The result has been the development of new draft guidance by the IAEA. [2] The IAEA guidance for responding to a severe reactor accident includes the following elements. The power plant will immediately notify states within 1000 km of any accident with the potential for a major trans-boundary release. This would include any accident involving actual or projected core damage. This notification should occur before the release. The population within 5-10 km of the site will be immediately evacuated or be provided with substantial shelter. Stable iodine will be distributed 100 km or more from the plant. For practical reasons distribution of stable iodine may be done in advance inside of the 25-km zone as the zone with the greatest risk and shortest period of time for making the decision. Effective thyroid prophylaxis will require blocking of the thyroid before or shortly after the release.

Care must be taken to be sure that the distribution of stable iodine will not delay evacuation or sheltering.

In the case of major release following core damage, the people within about 300 km will be instructed not to drink milk from cows that have been grazing on potentially contaminated pasture and not to eat fresh vegetables, fruit or other food that could have been contaminated. These restrictions will continue for several weeks after a release or until sampling determine that food or milk are not contaminated beyond the established limits. Extensive environmental monitoring and laboratory analysis will also be conducted to identify areas where additional actions are needed. The members of the population with high doses to thyroid will be registered and monitored throughout their life. The IAEA guidance includes detailed procedures and operational criteria. The Belarussian experience was a major consideration in developing this strategy of intervention for protection of the thyroid gland.

References

1. Buglova E, Demidchik E, Kenigsberg J, Golovneva A. Thyroid cancer in Belarus after the Chernobyl accident: incidence, prognosis of progress, risk assessment. International Conference. Low Dosses of Ionizing Radiation: Biological Effects and Regulatory Control. 1997: 280-284.
2. Generic Assessment procedures for determining protective actions during a reactor accident. IAEA - TECDOC - 955. 1997: 227p.
3. Intervention Criteria in a Nuclear or Radiation Emergency. IAEA. Safety Series N 109. 1994: 118p.
4. Nauman J, Wolff J. Iodine prophylaxis in Poland after the Chernobyl reactor accident: benefits and risks *Am.J.Med* 1991; **94:** 524-532.
5. Wolff J. Iodide prophylaxis for reactor accident. Nagasaki Symposium. Radiation and Human Health: Proposal from Nagasaki. Elsevier, 1996: 227-237.

PUBLIC HEALTH IMPLICATIONS OF IODINE PROPHYLAXIS IN RADIOLOGICAL EMERGENCIES

J. R. HARRISON

National Radiological Protection Board, UK, WHO Collaborating Centre,
E-mail: johnr.harrison@nrpb.org.uk

WENDLA PAILE

STUK-Radiation and Nuclear Safety Authority, Helsinki, WHO Collaborating Centre
E-mail: wendla.paile@stuk.fi

and

K. F. BAVERSTOCK

WHO Rome
E-mail: keith.baverstock@stuk.fi

Abstract

The increase in childhood thyroid cancer around Chernobyl indicates that significant thyroid doses occurred from radioiodine uptake at distances of several hundred kilometres from the accident site. Dose reconstruction suggests the bulk of iodine uptake resulted from ingestion of contaminated milk and leafy vegetables. Experience from Poland where stable iodine was taken by ten and a half million children and seven million adults in the aftermath of the accident, shows that the side effects of administration can be ignored. The maximum public health benefit from inhalation of radioiodine is obtained by taking stable iodine before exposure or as soon as possible afterwards, particularly if a rapid release occurs. Late administration has little health value to protect against inhaled or ingested radioiodine. In this situation the control of the supply of foodstuffs is the preferred intervention, but if this is not possible then iodine prophylaxis is essential. The protective effect of stable iodine needs to be ranked against other interventions such as shelter, evacuation and particularly the control of contaminated foodstuffs.

Introduction

Radioactive iodine released to the environment after a reactor plant accident poses a health threat to those exposed due to its affinity for the thyroid gland and the effective transmission to individuals through the food chain, primarily in fresh cows' milk. The principal hazard to the public is from inhalation in the plume or ingestion of contaminated foodstuffs. One specific method exists to protect the thyroid gland from excessive uptake of radioiodine and this is rapid prophylaxis with stable iodine (as a tablet or fluid). Ideally this should be taken before the release occurs. This may be possible where the release occurs after a warning period. In catastrophic accidents occurring without warning, such as the Chernobyl accident, this is not feasible.

Measurements of activity in the thyroids of those close to the Chernobyl accident[8] and the increased incidence of childhood thyroid cancer indicates that significant thyroid doses occurred from radioiodine uptake, principally iodine - 131 (^{131}I), at distances of several hundred kilometres(km) from the accident site.[18] These findings suggest that the control of contaminated foodstuffs and the institution of iodine prophylaxis were not effectively implemented. This paper concentrates on the public health hazards from the uptake of radioiodines and reviews the case to improve the distribution of stable iodine as an intervention in contingency plans.

Background

Nuclear plant emergency plans are in place to protect public health utilising a number of interventions: sheltering, control of foodstuffs, evacuation, and stable iodine prophylaxis. These would be employed on the basis of averting the dose to individuals, thereby reducing the risk of stochastic effects. The "averted dose" concept aims at ensuring that interventions result in a net benefit to public health. Most interventions entail some degree of hazard and also costs, both economic and social. No single intervention should be seen in isolation and their relative merits depend on the actual threat to public health, which may vary with according to the circumstances of the emergency. For distribution of stable iodine the relevant factors to be considered are the:

- extent to which thyroid disease can be averted by administration of stable iodine
- risks of side effects from stable iodine
- costs, social and economic, entailed in administration

Factors relevant to the first consideration are the:

- likelihood of further releases of ^{131}I of public health significance
- size of population likely to be subject to a significant public health risk from such a release
- relationship between any exposure to the release and thyroid disease.

Factors relevant to the second and third consideration are the:

- hazards associated with the administration of stable iodine
- costs of providing, maintaining and distributing stocks of stable iodine to the population potentially at risk

Risk of future accidents

Most commercial power generating reactors have been designed to high safety standards so that failures entailing reactor core damage and releases are rare (typically of the order of one in ten to one hundred thousand reactor years of operation). World wide, two major accidents have occurred, Three Mile Island and Chernobyl, during some 8000 reactor years of operation. In both accidents the reactor core was destroyed but in only one, Chernobyl, was there a significant release of radioiodine to the environment. Considering this past experience the maximum likelihood estimate of the probability of another serious accident in the decade following the Chernobyl accident was estimated to be not less than 0.25[6]. For the current decade the estimate is not less than 0.15.[4] The disparity between the design risk of a technical failure leading to core damage and actual experience may be due to "human error", which was a feature in both accidents. Risks based on past experience do not necessarily apply to the future as important lessons have been learned.

Thyroid doses after a release

Radioiodine in the atmosphere is carried by prevailing winds mainly as a gaseous cloud, and deposits by absorption on to foliage, including the grass. Precipitation will considerably enhance the deposition process. There are thus two main routes by which radioiodine may enter the body, inhalation from the cloud and through the food chain, principally from drinking milk from cows that have eaten contaminated pasture and, to a lesser extent, from the consumption of contaminated vegetables

Close in to a plant accident doses to the thyroid would arise from inhalation of radioiodine, with contributions from tellurium -132 (^{132}Te) (which decays rapidly to ^{132}I). Further afield inhalation ceases to be important and ingestion of ^{131}I, primarily from fresh milk, dominates dose. External irradiation from the cloud from other isotopes can also contribute to thyroid dose. At Chernobyl estimates suggest radioiodine and ^{132}Te could have accounted for up to 50% of the thyroid dose by inhalation close to the plant during the first day, but only about 10% of the total dose if the intake occurred by both inhalation and the later ingestion of contaminated foodstuffs.[10] Indeed dose reconstruction in Belarus,[6] the Russian Federation[22] and the Ukraine[11] even at considerable distances from the source suggest that the bulk of iodine uptake resulted from ingestion of contaminated milk and leafy vegetables. This is a general feature of iodine releases and has been seen at the Windscale pile accident[1] and following the Nevada US weapons testing programme.[12]

Risks of thyroid cancer resulting from exposure to radioiodine

X-rays have been used to treat a number of childhood conditions, such as tinea capitis, enlarged thymus and tonsillitis; follow-up of these populations has indicated the sensitivity of the child's thyroid to external radiation. A pooled analysis of these studies shows the combined absolute risk for all childhood exposure is 4.4 per 10000 person-year-Gray (PYGy).[16] A strong age dependency of risk was noticed, small children being at higher risk. Conversely, external radiation has not been shown, with certainty, to cause thyroid cancer in adults. In the Japanese Life Span Study the risk for thyroid cancer in persons exposed between age 20 and 40 was not significant, and no risk was identified in those over 40.[19]

[131]I has been extensively used in the treatment and diagnosis of thyroid disorders. Follow-up of the exposed groups has shown little or no induced disease.[17] However, the majority of treated people have been adults. Before the Chernobyl accident, there were very few data upon which to determine the effect of ^{131}I in children.

Thus, what has generally been believed to be an essential difference in carcinogenic potential between external radiation and ^{131}I is, in reality, an age effect. The sensitivity in adults to both external radiation and ^{131}I seems to be minimal or even absent in some age groups, while the sensitivity in small children is high. Indeed experience from the follow-up of the Chernobyl accident,[2,8] suggests that there is little difference in the risks associated with exposure to x-rays and [131]I. Thus, for public health purposes equivalence of carcinogenic effect between x-rays and ^{131}I may be assumed.

Lessons from the increase in childhood thyroid cancer after Chernobyl

In the period 1990-95 more than 600 childhood thyroid cancer cases have been reported.[21] This increase has been observed up to 500 km from the accident site, well beyond typical emergency planning zones. This emphasises the need to protect children in locations remote from the sites of potential accidents. Also, while small children in the most severely contaminated areas close to the accident received mean thyroid doses of several Gy, (and the cancer incidence in these areas has been correspondingly higher) the majority of cases have occurred in children who received less than 300 mGy. This was true for almost 80% of the cases in Ukraine.[20] The public health significance of low doses is illustrated by the fact that in Belarus, among 300000 children under the age of six exposed to an average thyroid dose as low as 60 mGy, 84 cancer cases have been recorded.[5] Only two cases would have been expected in the same time without radiation exposure.

A recent dose-response-analysis for all children based on data from the three affected countries reported that the combined risk for those born 1971-1986 was 2.3 per 10000 PYGy.[9] Besides being subject to a greater risk per dose, small children can also receive thyroid doses several times higher than adults in case of a release of radioiodine due to the smaller size of their thyroid gland and their higher intake of radioiodine from contaminated milk in relation to their body mass. So in the countries affected by the Chernobyl accident the highest incidence of thyroid cancer has been observed in children less than six years old at the time of exposure. If the risk per year is assumed to persist unchanged for 40-50 years, this means a lifetime risk for those exposed as children of the order of 1-2 % per Gy.

On the other hand, from earlier experience cited above the risk for thyroid cancer in those exposed as adults is low, and it may well be almost zero in persons over 40 years of age. Although data from Belarus has been presented, indicating an increase in thyroid cancer in adults,[5] the increase started well before the accident, and it is evident that any possible real increase in young adults is likely to be masked by a more efficient registration of cases. In later years, increased ascertainment from an improved thyroid screening effect leading to detection of clinically indolent, or occult, tumours may also have contributed to the apparent increase.

Administration of stable iodine

There is only one published record of widespread administration of stable iodine and this was in Poland, where stable iodine was distributed as a single dose to 10½ million children; no serious side effects were seen.[13] In 7 million adults, taking iodine against recommendation, two cases of serious allergic reaction were observed. On this basis, the frequency of serious side effects was less than 10^{-7} in children and less than 10^{-6} in adults. Minor side effects, such as, mild skin rash or gastrointestinal complaints, were not uncommon. In some new-born children, who were given 30 mg potassium iodide in the first few days of life, a reversible rise in thyroid stimulating hormone (TSH) was seen. This has been confirmed in chimpanzee experiments which show that daily doses of stable iodine over a ten day period leads to a reversible rise in TSH but had no effect on thyroid function.[14] Similar results were also found in pregnant chimpanzees in protection of the fetal thyroid.[15] These experiments also confirm the effectiveness of stable iodine as a blocking agent.

The costs of stable iodine administration

The principal costs of stable iodine administration are in the planning, production, storage and maintenance of stocks and the arrangements for distribution.[3] Since, to be effective stable iodine must be distributed before or as soon after exposure as possible some form of pre-distribution or stock piling is required together with a method of rapid distribution and the provision of public information in the event of an emergency.

Finding the balance between risk and benefit

Using a lifetime cancer risk for childhood thyroid cancer of 1% per Gy and the risk of serious side effects from a single dose of stable iodine of 10^{-7}, a risk-benefit analysis gives a balance between the risk and the benefit, based on health consequences, of 0.01 mGy thyroid dose. This would suggest that the risk of side effects can be ignored when deciding on an intervention level for stable iodine prophylaxis as a single dose to children. So decisions would not be based on health considerations but social and economic costs. An important and very relevant issue for contingency planning, however, is to further balance the undoubted benefits from iodine administration and the effectiveness of other interventions, such as shelter and control of contaminated foodstuffs.

For children a mean thyroid dose of 10 mGy would give rise to 20-30 cases of thyroid cancer per million children over ten years; this increase would be measurable against the natural incidence of childhood thyroid cancer. Protecting children from thyroid cancer is important. It is not usually fatal but requires long term therapy leading to impairment of their quality of life and the costs of treatment may be considerable. Even if "avertable dose" was grossly overestimated no net harm to health would result from stable iodine administration.

For adults, because of the low risk of cancer and of side effects the balance is probably in favour of iodine administration, however, in people over 40, the cancer risk is probably close to zero. In that case, the administration of stable iodine has no benefit, unless predicted doses approach levels that pose a threat to thyroid function, that is several grays.

If it is not possible to control foodstuffs stable iodine may need to be given daily for several weeks. The frequency of side effects from repeated doses in humans is not known. Generally, agricultural measures to prevent uptake of ^{131}I in milk and food, with milk controls and provision of milk powder, are the preferred interventions.

Summary

Interventions to protect public health from exposure to radioactive iodine should not be seen in isolation. The benefits for children of the administration of stable iodine seen against the low risk of side effects, and the need for rapid implementation argue in favour of robust plans so that, if indicated, early distribution can be effectively carried out. Prevention of exposure through control of foodstuffs is the preferred intervention but if this is not possible then iodine prophylaxis is essential. There is a need for greater public awareness of the implication of such releases and their mitigation by stable iodine. When informing the public, it should be stressed that small children are at greatest risk from radioiodine uptake, while the risk for young adults is low and for the elderly probably very low.

References

1. Baverstock, K F and Vennart J. Emergency reference levels for reactor accidents: A re-examination of the Windscale reactor accident. *Health Phys* 1976; **30**: 339-344.
2. Baverstock, K F. Thyroid cancer in children in Belarus after Chernobyl. *World Health Stat Q*. **46(3)**: 204-208. 1993.
3. Becker DV and Zanzonico P. Potassium iodide for thyroid blockade in a reactor accident: administrative policies that govern its use. *Thyroid* 1997; **7(2)**: 193-197.
4. Blomquist L. Personal communication. 1996.
5. Buglova, E, Demidchick, E, Kenigsberg, I, and Golovneva, A. Thyroid cancer in Belarus after the Chernobyl accident: incidence, prognosis of progress, risk assessment. In: *Low doses of ionizing radiation: biological effects and regulatory control. Contributed papers*. International conference. Seville, Spain, 17-21 November 1997. IAEA-TECDOC-976. IAEA, Austria. 1997.
6. Edwards, A W F. How many reactor accidents? *Nature* 1986; **324**: 417-8
7. Gavrilin Yu, V Krouch, S Shinkarev et al. Estimation of thyroid doses received by the population of Belarus as a result of the Chernobyl accident.: in: Karaoglou, A. et al. (eds): *The radiological consequences of the Chernobyl accident. Proceedings of the first international conference*. Minsk, Belarus, 18-22 March 1996. ECSC-EC-EAEC, Brussels-Luxembourg. 1996: 1011-1020.
8. Goulko GM, Chepurny NI, Jacob P, et al. Thyroid dose and thyroid cancer incidence after the Chernobyl accident: assessments for the Zhytomyr region (Ukraine). *Radiat Environ Biophys* 1998; **36(4)**:261-273.
9. Jacob P, Goulko G, Heidenreich WF, et al. Thyroid cancer risk to children calculated. *Nature* 1998; **392**:31-32.
10. Krouch V T, Yu Gavrilin Yu O Konstantinov et al. Characteristics of the radionuclides inhalation intake. In: Medical Aspects of the Accident at the ChNPP. *Proceedings of the International Conference*, Kiev, May 1988. Zdorovie Publishing House. 1988.
11. Likhtarev, I A, N K Shandala, G M Gulko et al. Ukrainian thyroid doses after the Chernobyl accident. *Health Phys* 1993; **64(6)**: 594-599.
12. National Cancer Institute. Estimated exposures and thyroid doses received by the American people from iodine-131 in fallout following Nevada atmospheric bomb tests. National Cancer Institute, Washington DC. 1997

13. Nauman, J, Wolff, J. Iodide Prophylaxis in Poland After the Chernobyl Reactor Accident: Benefits and Risks. *Am J Med* 1993; **94**: 524-32.

14. Noteboom J L, Hummel WA, Broerse JJ,et al. Protection of the infant thyroid from radioactive contamination by the administration of stable iodide. An experimental evaluation in chimpanzees. *Radiat Res* 1997;**147(6)**:698-706.

15. Noteboom JL, Hummel WA, Broerse JJ, et al. Protection of the maternal and fetal thyroid from radioactive contamination by the administration of stable iodide during pregnancy. An experimental evaluation in chimpanzees. *Radiat Res* 1997; **147(6)**: 691-697.

16. Ron E, Lubin JH, Shore RE et al. Thyroid cancer after exposure to external radiation: a pooled analysis of seven studies. *Radiat Res* 1995; **141(3)**: 259-277.

17. Ron, E. Cancer risk following radioactive iodine 131 exposure in medicine. *Proceedings of the thirty-second annual meeting of the National Council on Radiation Protection and Measurements*. Arlington, VA National Council on Radiation Protection and Measurements. 1996.

18. Stsjazhko VA, Tsyb AF, Tronko ND, et al. Childhood thyroid cancer since accident at Chernobyl. *Br Med J* 1995; **310**: 801.

19. Thompson, D.E., Mabuchi, K., Ron, E., et al. Cancer incidence in atomic bomb survivors. Part II: solid tumors, 1958-1987. *Radiat Res* 1994;**137**: S17-S67.

20. Tronko, N, Bogdanova T, Komissarenko, I, etal. Thyroid cancer in children and adolescents in Ukraine after the Chernobyl accident (1986-1995) pp 683-690. In: Karaoglou, A. et al. (Eds): *The radiological consequences of the Chernobyl accident. Proceedings of the first international conference.* Minsk, Belarus, 18-22 March 1996. ECSC-EC-EAEC, Brussels-Luxembourg. 1996.

21. Williams, E D, Becker, D, Dimidchik, E P, et al. Effects on the thyroid in populations exposed to radiation as a result of the Chernobyl accident. In: *International Atomic Energy Agency, International Conference on One Decade After Chernobyl: Summing Up the Consequences of the Accident.* Proceedings. Vienna, Austria. 1996. 207-230.

22. Zvonova, I A And M I Balonov. Radioiodine dosimetry and prediction of consequences of thyroid exposure of the Russian population following the Chernobyl accident. In: *The Chernobyl Papers. Doses to the Soviet Population and early Effects Studies, Vol 1* (S E Maerwin and M I Balonov, Eds) Research Enterprises Inc., Richland, Washington. 1993. 71-125.

CHERNOBYL AID PROGRAMMES AS A BASIS OF AN INTEGRATED SYSTEM OF THYROID CANCER DIAGNOSIS AND THERAPY FACILITIES AND RESEARCH IN BELARUS

E. LENGFELDER[1], CH. FRENZEL[1], E. P. DEMIDCHIK[2], J. E. DEMIDCHIK[3], V. J. REBEKO[4], J. D. SIDOROV[4], L. W. BIRUKOVA[5], T. I. PRIGOSCHAJA[6] AND D. V. OKOUNZEV[6]

[1]*Ludwig-Maximilians-University and Otto Hug Radiation Institute, Munich; Germany;*
[2]*Belarussian National Thyroid Centre, Minsk;* [3]*Chair of Oncology, Medical Institute, Minsk;*
[4]*Oncological Dispensary, Minsk;* [5]*Endocrinological Dispensary, Gomel;* [6]*Oncological Dispensary, Gomel, Belarus*

The unexpected serious increase in the incidence of thyroid cancer in children following the reactor accident in Chernobyl lead to considerable efforts from abroad to support Belarus in order to mitigate these health problems. It is preferable and more effective to install and equip suitable diagnosis and treat-ment facilities inside the country instead of taking selected patients for medical procedures abroad. Following these principles, the Otto Hug Strahleninstitut - MHM (Otto Hug Radiation Institute - Medical Relief Measures), a German non-governmental medical-scientific charity organisation, started several interrelated long term treatment and research projects on thyroid cancer and other diseases of this organ in 1991. Since 1993, the project „Thyroid Centre Gomel" had more than 50 000 patients from this oblast for diagnosis and treatment of thyroid diseases including cancer. The project of the „Pathological Anatomical Laboratory", starting in 1995, is situated in the clinic, where all childhood and juvenile thyroid cancers of Belarus are operated. More than 4 100 thyroid tumours were diagnosed preparing over 17 000 pathological slides according internationally accepted standards. During the last weeks in 1997, the new project of „Radioiodine Therapy" started in Gomel. The offer of some western countries to give a selected group of patients radioiodine treatment abroad, unfortunately leaves the fundamental problem of long term aftercare unresolved.

1 Introduction

Among the CIS countries, the republic of Belarus has received the biggest part of the radioactive releases after the reactor accident in Chernobyl. Belarus has not the capacity to face up to the enormous costs of remedying the Chernobyl effects on its own. The diagnosis and treatment of diseases associated with the Chernobyl desaster as well as the creation of the public health infrastructure capable of combating the future development of Chernobyl-related health disorders have been supported by aid prorammes from international governmental and non-governmental organisation. The three CIS countries affected, in particular Belarus, experienced dramatic increases in the incidence of thyroid cancer in children and, with respect to the absolute number of cases, in the meantime also in adults.

2 The Medical Programmes of the Otto Hug Strahleninstitut - MHM in Belarus

After studying the health system and the available possibilities under the situation of the post-sovjet time, it became clear that it would be preferable and more effective to install and equip suitable diagnosis and treatment facilities inside the country instead of taking selected patients for medical procedures abroad. Following these principles, the Otto Hug Strahleninstitut - MHM, a German non-governmental medical-scientific charity organisation, started several long term medical and research projects on cancer and other diseases of the thyroid in 1991. At that time the incidence of thyroid cancer in children in Belarus had already risen 30-fold over the mean incidence of the ten years period before Chernobyl.

List of the long term programmes of the Otto Hug Strahleninstitut - MHM in Belarus, with the year of the programme start and the institutions beeing supported

1. Radiometric Control of Food and Territories (1991)
   Centres of Hygiene and Epidemiology, Public Health Departments
2. Prenatal Diagnostics - Genetic Consultation (1994)
   Oblast Centre of Genetic Consultation, Gomel
3. Equipping of Hospitals (1991)
   Hospitals and Dispensaries
4. Thyroid Centre in Gomel (1992)
   Endocrinological Dispensary of Oblast Gomel
5. Pathological Anatomical Laboratory (1992)
   Oncological Dispensary of the City of Minsk, Medical High School, National Thyroid Centre of Belarus
6. Nuclear Medicine Treatment of Patients with Thyroid Tumours(1996)
   (in collaboration with the Luxembourg Foundation „Help for children having cancer")
   Oncological Dispensary of Oblast Gomel
7. Further Education (Medicine, Medical Technology, Radioecology) (1991)
   Health authorities of all levels, University and Medical High School of Minsk, International Sakharov Institute od Radioecology, Minsk
8. Thyroid Endocrinology Laboratory in Minsk (1997)
   Oncological Dispensary of the City of Minsk, Medical High School, National Thyroid Centre of Belarus

According its statute, the Otto Hug Strahleninstitut - MHM has the task after events or in situations with radiological exposure to give the people affected humanitarian aid and to protect their health. The relief measures have to be accompanied by qualified scientific investigation of the radiological situation and the examination of the health disorders in order to increase the knowledge of the processes of the development of radiation induced diseases and to get the knowledge for adaption and improvement of the measures to the actual needs. It is a principle of all medical aid programmes of the Otto Hug Strahleninstitut that the medical care has priority over scientific investigation.

Four out of eight programmes in Belarus serve the direct purpose of diagnosis, treatment and after-care of thyroid diseases including thyroid cancer in children, juveniles and adults. The iterrelated programmes are also basis of international scientific collaboration including scientists of the institutions in Belarus beeing supported and several research groups in the West.

Since 1993, the project „Thyroid Centre Gomel" had more than 50 000 patients from this oblast for diagnosis, treatment of thyroid diseases including cancer, and medical after-care and performed more than 100 000 thyroid status blood tests. The work of the hormone laboratory of this project is regularly tested for its quality through the participation in an international quality test programme. The project of the „Pathological Anatomical Laboratory", starting in 1995, is in collaboration with the Belarussian National Thyroid Centre and situated in the clinic, where all childhood and juvenile thyroid cancers of Belarus are operated. Until spring in 1998, more than 4 100 thyroid tumours were diagnosed preparing over 17 000 pathological slides for the differential diagnosis of various types of thyroid tumours according internationally accepted standards. During the last weeks in 1997, the new project of „Radioiodine Therapy" started in Gomel. This is of particular importance for Belarus, because it includes also the long term aftercare and controlled medication of the patients with L-thyroxine, taking advantage of the possibilities of the Gomel Thyroid Centre. About 50 % of the children with thyroid cancer in Belarus come from the district of Gomel.

Until spring 1998, goods and services to the value of 18 millions Deutsche Mark have been spent for the programmes and projects of the Otto Hug Strahleninstitut - MHM in Belarus.

3 Thyroid Cancer after Chernobyl: Some Aspects Concerning Apropriate Treatment, Humanitarian Aid and Scientific Investigation

There is a controversy about the question whether in cases of unifocal cancer nodes in the thyroid of children, the total gland should be removed or merely the unilateral lobe affected. Even with patients in the west, where levothyroxine medication and hormone control after-care is available without limitations, this question is not answered generally unequivocally. However, regarding the situation in Belarus (and the other CIS countries), one has to bear in mind that totalectomy of the thyroid also means lifetime supply of levothyroxine for the patient. If this cannot be guaranteed - and this is the reality of the situation in Belarus for the next future - the lack of adequate thyroid hormone levels in the blood of the patients results in elevated levels of TSH, which is known to have also tumour promoting activity, not only with respect to thyroid tumours, but also to others. On the other hand, remaining thyroid tissue in the body prevents the testing for thyreoglobulin beeing released from thyroid tumour metastases.

Medical aid was offered from abroad inviting children from Belarus, suffering from thyroid cancer and beeing already operated in Minsk, to western countries for nuclear medicine radioiodine and other treatment. But it happened that with about 40 of these children from Gomel oblast, during their holidays in the west, diagnose and treatment procedures were undertaken in a western clinic, including after-operation and radioiodine treament in some cases. Questions about the motivation of these activities rise, if one faces the fact that the Belorussian thyroid experts and the health authorities in Belarus became informed only afterwards, that the complete health records of the young patients concerning all steps of pretreatment were not available abroad, and that only a few weeks after this all, a scientific paper about the diagnoses and the treatment of interesting thyroid cancer cases in Belorussian children was proudly presented in a big scientific congress.

In such aid projects, where patients having thyroid cancer are treated in the west, a high percentage of the money available flows in general expenses such as for repeated transportation of children and accompanying persons, lodging, high basic hospital costs of „bed per night", which then is lost for pure treatment expenses. For the money which has been already spent in this way by some organisations, a treatment centre located in Belarus could have been equipped with all necessary instrumentation and could have been supplied with radioiodine and other drugs and consumables for the benefit of many more patients than had the opportunity to be chosen for the trip to the west. Another important point of the treatment abroad is that as a rule there are no concepts or measures offered to the patients returning home, where and how to get the essential after-care in Belarus (frequent hormone analyses, regular levothyroxine medication etc.).

The Otto Hug Strahleninstitut follows strictly the principle, to make all efforts to improve the diagnostic and treatment capacity for patients with thyroid diseases including cancer (and for other diseases) in Belarus. By this, the money available is used in a very effective way and the collective therapeutic gain is maximal. In order to follow this way, experts from the west come frequently to Belarus to train the staff, and own logistics makes the regular direct supply of the clinics possible.

The Chernobyl aid programmes of the Otto Hug Strahleninstitut serve also as a basis for many international research activities and fruitful scientific collaboration. This improves the knowledge on radiogenic carcinogenesis as well as the chance of an earlier diagnosis and treatment of patients in Belarus, who will develop thyroid cancer in the future.

REVERSE TRANSCRIPTASE POLYMERASE CHAIN REACTION FROM FINE NEEDLE ASPIRATION BIOPSIES: A POTENTIAL NEW DIAGNOSTIC TOOL FOR THYROID GLAND DISORDERS

C. SCHMUTZLER, R. WINZER AND J. KÖHRLE

Medizinische Poliklinik, Abteilung Molekulare Innere Medizin, Universtät Würzburg,
Röntgenring 11, D-97070 Würzburg, Germany
E-mail: C.Schmutzler@mail.uni-wuerzburg.de

J. RENDL AND C. REINERS

Klinik und Poliklinik für Nuklearmedizin, Universtät Würzburg, Josef-Schneider-Str. 2,
D-97070 Würzburg, Germany

Cytological examination of fine needle aspiration biopsies (FNAB) of the thyroid gland is an important diagnostic technique bringing a minimum of discomfort for the patient. We wanted to expand the amount of information obtained from an FNAB by combining it with the sensitive method of RT-PCR. To constitute practicable protocols, we used 10 - 10,000 cells of the thyroid carcinoma line FTC-133 to simulate a FNAB. Afterwards, established methods were applied to biopsies from four thyroid nodules and a lymph node metastasis; material remaining in the syringe after the preparation of cytological smears was used for RT-PCR. Total RNA was extracted by the aid of commercially available kits and reverse transcribed. 1/20 (cell samples) or 1/40 (FNABs) of the cDNA was utilised for PCR. After 35 to 45 cycles of amplification, products specific for Tg, TSH-receptor, type I and II 5′-deiodinase, β-actin and glyceraldehyde phosphate dehydrogenase were detectable; amplicons derived from the sodium/iodide symporter mRNA were seen after a "nested PCR". We conclude that FNAB provides sufficient material for cytology and the parallel detection of multiple diagnostically relevant mRNAs by RT-PCR. Combination of cytology and RT-PCR may become a valuable new diagnostic tool for the evaluation of thyroid disorders.

1   INTRODUCTION

Cancer is a complex, multistep process, which, in the case of thyroid carcinogenesis, is not yet completely understood.[1] The follicular cell of the thyroid gland gives rise to a spectrum of tumours, ranging from the benign adenoma, two forms of differentiated carcinomas, termed "follicular" and "papillary", to the highly malignant anaplastic variant.[2] It is not yet proven that benign nodules develop into differentiated carcinomas, but differentiated carcinomas may progress to an anaplastic form, with a dismal prognosis.[3,4,5]

Cytological examination of fine needle aspiration biopsies (FNAB) is a highly reliable diagnostic technique in the evaluation of thyroid nodules, bringing about minimal discomfort for the patient.[6] The sensitivity of this procedure varies from 83 % to 99 % and the specificity from 70 % to 90 %.[7] However, the diagnosis of follicular neoplasm still presents a problem.[8] This leads to an increased demand of sensitive preoperative diagnostic techniques. It would be of great value, if the cytological diagnosis obtained by FNAB could be strengthened by a molecular analysis, e. g. the detection of diagnostically relevant thyroid markers by RT-PCR.

2 MATERIALS AND METHODS

The human follicular thyroid carcinoma cell line FTC-133 was grown as described previously.[9] Samples of 10 - 10,000 cells were prepared by serial dilution of cell suspensions.

Four patients with thyroid nodules detectable by ultrasound imaging and one patient with a swollen cervical lymph node underwent FNAB, which was performed using a 22 G x 1¼ " needle. For cytological examination three smears were prepared and the remaining material was used for RNA preparation.

RNA isolation was carried out with the PUREscript kit (Gentra, Minneapolis, USA) from FTC-133 cells or with the RNeasy kit (Quiagen, Hilden, Germany) from FNABs according to the recommendations of the manufacturers. Reverse transcription (final volume 20 µl) was performed with Superscript Reverse Transcriptase and Oligo-dT$_{(12-18)}$ as a primer (Life Technologies, Eggenstein, Germany) following the protocol recommended by the manufacturer. The cDNAs from the five FNABs were diluted to 40 µl.

PCR amplification was carried out with 1 µl of the cDNA mixture and 3 U of Taq DNA Polymerase (USB, Cleveland, Ohio, USA) in a buffer provided by the manufacturer (final volume 50 µl). PCR conditions and primers for β-actin, glyceraldehyde phosphate dehydrogenase (GAPDH), Thyroglobulin (Tg), TSH-receptor (TSHr), sodium/iodide symporter (NIS), type I (5′DI), and type II (5′DII) 5'-deiodinase are described elsewhere.[10] In the case of NIS and 5′DI, a "nested" PCR was done, with 1/50 of the PCR product of the first amplification as the template for reamplification. 1/10 (5 µl) of each PCR reaction was analysed on a 1 % agarose gel stained with ethidium bromide (EtBr) or SYBR-green (Molecular Probes, Leiden, Netherlands).

FNABs were obtained with the informed consent of the patients and experiments were done according to the regulations of the local ethics committee.

3 RESULTS

FNABs of thyroid nodules usually contain 100 - 1,000 cells. To establish practicable protocols for RT-PCR with such small cell numbers, we used dilutions

(10,000 - 10 cells) of the follicular thyroid carcinoma line FTC-133 to simulate FNABs. After 45 cycles of amplification and using 1/20 of the cDNA isolated from the small cell samples, products specific for β-actin and the thyroid-typical markers NIS, Tg, TSHr, and 5′DI were detected in 10,000 or less cells on an agarose gel stained with EtBr or SYBR-green (not shown). This data demonstrated that in minimal numbers of thyroid carcinoma cells, RT-PCR can detect expression of multiple tissue-specific markers in parallel and suggested that a similar approach was applicable to FNABs.

Table. Clinical data of four FNABs from thyroid nodules and RT-PCR detection of thyroid-specific mRNAs

sample	1	2	3	4
cytological diagnosis	*degenerative colloid goitre*	*goitre nodule*	*follicular neoplasm* DD*: goitre nodule follicular adenoma	*goitre nodule*
signs of malignancy	no	no	suspected	no
^{99m}Tc-Pertechnetate scan	cold	hot	cold	hot
amplicon and conditions of detection	**observed in the respective sample ?**			
β-actin: 35 PCR cycles, EtBR-staining	yes	yes	yes	yes
GAPDH: 35 PCR cycles, EtBr-staining	yes	yes	yes	yes
Tg: 45 PCR cycles, SYBR-green-staining	yes	yes	yes	yes
TSHr: 45 PCR cycles, SYBR-green-staining	yes	yes	yes	yes
NIS: 2 x 45 cycles ("nested" PCR), SYBR-green-staining	weak	yes	no	yes
5′DI: 35 PCR cycles, EtBr-staining	no	yes	yes	yes
5′DI: 35+45 cycles ("nested" PCR), EtBr-staining	yes	yes	yes	yes
5′DII: 35 cycles, EtBr-staining	weak	yes	yes	yes

*DD: differential diagnosis

472

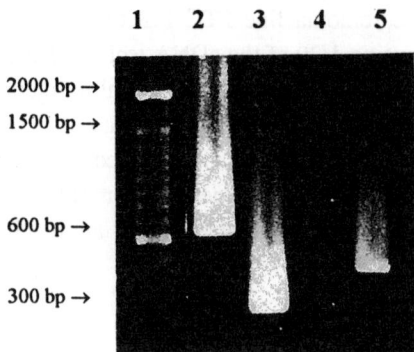

1 2 3 4 5

2000 bp →
1500 bp →

600 bp →

300 bp →

Figure. RT-PCR with a FNAB from a lymph node metastasis of an undifferentiated thyroid carcinoma. Lane 1: length standard; lane 2: GAPDH-, lane 3: Tg-, lane 4: TSHr-, lane 5: NIS-specific PCR products. The gel was stained with EtBr.

Four patients underwent ultrasound guided FNAB as it is routinely performed for the diagnosis of thyroid nodules. In all four FNAB samples, β-actin- and GAPDH-specific products were detectable, proving successful RNA isolation and adequate reverse transcription. Also, Tg-, TSHr-, 5′DI-, and 5′DII-specific products were detected, with the exception of 5′DI in the degenerative colloid nodule, where a reamplification of 45 cycles was required. To observe NIS-specific products, a nested PCR was necessary; products were obtained in all samples, except for the suspicious follicular neoplasm. Clinical data of the four FNABs and details concerning RT-PCR detection of thyroid-specific mRNAs in the cDNAs prepared therefrom are summarised in the Table.

A patient with a palpable lymph node metastasis of an undifferentiated thyroid carcinoma was subjected to FNAB. Using 1/40 (1/200 for GAPDH) of the corresponding cDNA, products specific for Tg and GAPDH were observed after 35 cycles of amplification, for TSHr after 40 cycles, and for NIS after a nested PCR of 40 cycles followed by a reamplification of 30 cycles (Figure).

4 DISCUSSION

In an attempt to expand the amount of information obtained from a FNAB by combining it with the highly sensitive technique of RT-PCR, we found that one single FNAB gives enough material for RT-PCR and the detection of multiple thyroid-specific markers in parallel after smears for cytological evaluation had been prepared from the content of the same needle. For this purpose, the method of RNA preparation is the most critical step. It must guarantee that the minute amounts of RNA expected from a FNAB (about 100 to 1000 cells) can be quantitatively isolated without major losses. This problem was solved by taking advantage of the selective binding properties of a silica gel-based membrane. This method avoided the troublesome centrifugation and precipitation steps required in other current protocols for RNA preparation. It allows adaptation to variations of contaminating fluid volumes (e. g. blood) and is sensitive enough to isolate small amounts of RNA. Approaches comparable to ours have been described by Weiss et al.[11] and Arturi et al.[12] who detected mucin 1 mRNA in a FNAB from the thyroid and Tg, TSHr, and GAPDH mRNAs in a FNAB from a lymph node metastasis, respectively. However, both groups used two different samples for cytological and molecular analysis, which may have the consequence that different cell populations are examined with the two techniques.

Further experiments will have to establish whether there is a correlation between the cytological diagnosis and the expression pattern of various thyroid-specific or other diagnostically relevant genes in thyroid diseases as observed by RT-PCR. A first hint that such a correlation may be detected is the result that NIS mRNA was not detected in the suspicious follicular neoplasm (Table). With a loss of function and/or progressive dedifferentiation, a decrease of mRNA levels of gene products required for normal thyroid function is observed, and a reduced expression of NIS mRNA has been shown for follicular and anaplastic thyroid tumours and cell lines,[9,13,14] although some exceptions have been described for papillary thyroid carcinomas.[15] On the other hand, the two goitre nodule samples show a similar pattern of all thyroid typical markers analysed.

Though FNAB is a highly reliable diagnostic test in the cytological evaluation of a thyroid nodule, especially the diagnosis of "follicular neoplasm" presents a problem. The procedure described allows to control the expression of several, in this case up to seven, different genes in parallel. Other recently described tumour markers, like glucose transporter type I,[16] telomerase,[17] vascular endothelial growth factor,[18] and E-cadherin,[19] may also be detectable. The analysis of several differentiation markers in parallel to the cytological diagnosis may help to distinguish (follicular) neoplasms at a preoperative state. However, prognostic relevant differences in gene expression have still to be found. This protocol may also open the possibility to follow complex changes in gene expression during an intervention. For example it could be used to follow up the effects of a redifferentiation therapy with 13-*cis* retinoic acid applied to patients with differentiated thyroid carcinomas by control, among others, of the NIS mRNA levels; it has been shown that retinoic acid increased NIS mRNA in follicular thyroid carcinoma cell lines.[9] Furthermore, in a clinical study performed to evaluate the feasibility of a re-differentiation therapy in the case of thyroid cancer, 8 of 16 patients examined responded with an increase in iodide uptake.[20] However, the method does not need to be confined to carcinomas: e. g. FNAB followed by

RT-PCR might be employed to analyse the pattern of cytokines expressed by lymphocytes infiltrating the thyroid gland during the autoimmune process.[21] Finally, with products of special interest even semi-quantitative analysis, which requires a higher amount of cDNA aliquots because of multiple calibration and competition reactions,[22] may be feasible.

In summary, we present evidence for the clinical suitability of the molecular analysis of FNABs. It allows to get two different results from the same FNAB, the cytological diagnosis and information on diagnostically relevant marker gene expression. A more differentiated diagnosis could be performed in the preoperative state, and may lead to a more specific therapeutic regimen.

Acknowledgements

The authors would like to thank Prof. H. Griesser, Institute of Pathology, University of Würzburg, for the cytological diagnosis of the four FNABs. This work was supported by grants from the Deutsche Forschungsgemeinschaft (Wi 231/9-2, TP1) and Wilhelm Sander Foundation.

References

1. Wynford-Thomas, D. Origin and progression of thyroid epithelial tumours: cellular and molecular mechanisms. *Horm Res* 1997; **47:** 145-157.
2. Williams DW, Williams ED. The pathology of follicular thyroid epithelial tumours In: Wynford-Thomas D, Williams ED ed. *Thyroid tumours: Molecular basis of pathogenesis.* Churchill Livingstone1989, Edinburgh, p 57.
3. Williams ED. The aetiology of thyroid tumours. *Clin Endocrinol Metab* 1979; **8:** 193-207.
4. Moore JH Jr, Bacharach B, Choi HY. Anaplastic transformation of metastatic follicular carcinoma of the thyroid. *J Surg Oncol* 1985; **29:** 216-221.
5. Venkatesh YS, Ordonez NG, Schultz PN, Hickey RC, Goepfert H, Samaan NA. Anaplastic carcinoma of the thyroid: a clinicopathologic study of 121 cases. *Cancer* 1990; **66:** 321-330.
6. Greenspan, FS. The role of fine-needle aspiration biopsy in the management of palpable thyroid nodules. *Am J Clin Pathol* 1997; **108:** S26-S30.
7. Ridgeway EC. Clinical evaluation of solitary thyroid nodules In: Braverman LE, Utiger RD, ed. *Werner and Ingbar's: The thyroid,* Philadelphia: Lippincott-Raven Publishers, 1996: p 966.

8. Yokozawa T, Miyauchi A, Kuma K, Sugawara M. Accurate and simple method of diagnosing thyroid nodules by the modified technique of ultrasound-guided fine needle aspiration biopsy. *Thyroid* 1995; **5**: 141-145.

9. Schmutzler C, Winzer R, Meissner-Weigl J, Köhrle J. Retinoic acid increases sodium/iodide symporter mRNA levels in human thyroid cancer cell lines and suppresses expression of functional symporter in non-transformed FRTL-5 rat thyroid cells. *Biochem Biophys Res Com* 1997; **240**: 832-838.

10. Winzer R, Schmutzler C, Jakobs TC, Ebert R, Rendl J, Reiners C, Jakob F, Köhrle J. RT-PCR analysis of thyrocyte-relevant genes in fine-needle aspiration biopsies of the human thyroid. (submitted to Thyroid).

11. Weiss M, Baruch B, Keydar I, Wreschner DH. Preoperative diagnosis of thyroid papillary carcinoma by reverse transcriptase polymerase chain reaction of the muc 1 gene. *Int J Cancer* 1996; **66**: 55-59.

12. Arturi F, Russo D, Giuffrida D, Ippolito A, Perrotti N, Vigneri R, Filetti S. Early diagnosis by genetic analysis of differentiated thyroid cancer metastases in small lymph nodes. *J Clin Endocrinol Metab* 1997; **82**: 1638-1641.

13. Robbins R, Ghossein R, Rosai J, Levy O, Carrasco N. Localization of immunoreactive Na$^+$/I$^-$ symporter (ir-NIS) in normal and neoplastic human thyroid cells. Prog. & Abstr. Endocrine Society Meeting 1997, Minneapolis, MN, USA, p 292.

14. Smanik PA, Kwon-Yul R, Theil KS, Mazzaferri EL, Jhiang SM. Expression, exon-intron organization, and chromosome mapping of the human sodium iodide symporter. *Endocrinology* 1997; **138**: 3555-3558.

15. Saito T, Endo T, Kawaguchi A, Ikeda M, Katoh R, Kawaoi A, Muramatsu A. Increased expression of the sodium/iodide symporter in papillary thyroid carcinomas. *J Clin Invest* 1998; **101**: 1296-1300.

16. Haber RS, Weiser KR, Pritsker A, Reder I, Burstein DE. GLUT1 glucose transporter expression in benign and malignant thyroid nodules. *Thyroid* 1997; **7**: 363-367.

17. Meyerson M, Counter CM, Ng Eaton E, Ellisen LW, Steiner P, Dickinson Caddle S, Ziaugra L, Beijersbergen RL, Davidoff MJ, Liu Q, Bachetti S, Haber DA, Weinberg RA. hEST2, the putative human telomerase catalytic subunit gene, is up-regulated in tumor cells and during immortalization. *Cell* 1997; **90**: 785-795.

18. Soh EY, Duh QY, Sobhi SA, Young DM, Epstein HD, Wong MG, Gracia YK, Min YD, Grossman RF, Siperstein AE, Clark OH. Vascular endothelial growth factor expression is higher in differentiated thyroid cancer than in normal or benign thyroid. *J Clin Endocrinol Metab* 1997; **82**: 3741-3747.

19. Huang-Vu C, Cetin Y, Scheumann GFW, Behrends J, Horn R, Von zur Mühlen A, Dralle H, Brabant G. Expression of cellular adhesion molecule, E-cadherin,

in normal human thyrocytes, and in differentiated and undifferentiated thyroid carcinomas. *Exp Clin Endocrinol* 1993; **101** (Suppl. 3): 78-82.

20. Simon D, Köhrle J, Reiners C, Boerner A, Schmutzler C, Mainz K, Goretzki PE, Röher HD. Redifferentiation therapy with retinoids - a therapeutic option in advanced follicular and papillary thyroid carcinoma? *World J Surgery* 1998; **22**: 569-574.

21. Heuer M, Aust G, Ode-Hakim S, Scherbaum WA. Different cytokine profiles in Graves'disease, Hashimoto's thyroiditis, and nonautoimmune thyroid disorders determined by quantitative reverse transcriptse polymerase chain reaction (RT-PCR). *Thyroid* 1996; **6**: 97-106.

22. Köhler T. Quantitation of absolute numbers of mRNA copies in a sample by competitive PCR. In: Köhler T, Laßner D, Rost AK, Thamm B, Pustowoit B, Remke H: Quantitation of mRNA by polymerase chain reaction. Berlin: Springer-Verlag, 1995: p 143.

L-THYROXINE TREATMENT OF CHILDREN WITH THYROID CARCINOMA IN MINSK

E.P. DEMIDCHIK, V.M. DROZD, T.V. VORONTSOVA, S.S. KORYTKO,
I.M. KHMARA, O.A. LAVNICHUK, L.L. LEONOVA, M.Y. DZIAUHO,
N.M. GRITSEVITCH, N.M. LIKHORAD, T.Y. PLATONOVA,
*Research and Clinical Institute of Radiation Medicine and Endocrinology, 23
Masherova Av., Minsk, Belarus*
M. SCHLUMBERGER,
Institute Gustave-Roussy, Paris, France
C. SEIDEL,
Medipan Diagnostica, Rotberger Street 18, Selchow, Germany

411 patients exposed to radiation during the Chernobyl accident and operated in the childhood (3-14 years of age) were under observation; among them, 158 boys and 253 girls. All the children were observed with the interval of 3-6 months. During their first visit to the medical establishment, the dose of thyroxine was administered according to the body mass, i.e. 2.8-3 mcg/kg a day, with subsequent 25 mcg correction in the direction of decrease or increase.

Thus, the obtained data showed that thyroxine suppressive therapy combined with RIT contributes to a more effective treatment of children with thyroid cancer.

1. INTRODUCTION

The initial treatment of patients with thyroid cancer is surgical ablation of the tumor. Taking into account the high aggressiveness of the thyroid cancer, especially in children and adolescents, metastases to different organs often occur in the postoperative period. Rational for the use of radioiodine therapy (RIT) and suppressive therapy with thyroxine.

Experimental and clinical practice showed convincingly that a stable increase of the thyroid-stimulating hormone (TSH) in blood is an important factor in the grows of thyroid tumors[1, 2].

The aim of the study was to specify the influence of the suppressive therapy on the course of thyroid carcinoma in children of Belarus.

2. SUBJECTS AND METHODS

411 children (3-14 years of age) exposed to radiation during the Chernobyl accident were under observation; among them, 158 boys and 253 girls. All the children were observed with the interval of 3-6 months. During their first visit to the medical establishment, the dose of thyroxine was administered according to the body mass, i.e. 2.8-3 mcg/kg a day, with subsequent 25 mcg correction depending on their TSH levels.

The patients underwent clinical and laboratory examination with the determination of serum TSH and Tg levels using kits from "Medipan Diagnostica",

Selchow (Germany) kits provided together with L-thyroxine, "Merck", within the frame of the Electricity de France humanitarian programme.

3. RESULTS AND DISCUSSION

Fig.1 (a,b) gives the data about 411 patients (239 of them underwent clinical examination twice, 105 patients - three times). During the first visit, only in 45% of the examined individuals a sufficiently suppressive TSH level was observed (TSH<0.3 IU/l). The second visit revealed 57 % of such patients and the third - 49%. The state of hypothyroidism was registered in 13 %,9% and 6% of the patients, respectively (Fig.1a).

On the background of the reached suppression Tg level was above 1 ng/l in 37% of the cases during the first visit, in 32.8% - during the second and in 30% - during the third consultation (Fig.1b).

To determine the reasons for the lack of the suppressive effect in a larger number of cases, all the patients were divided into three groups: 1st group - patients who underwent total thyroidectomy without radioiodine therapy (55 patients); 2nd group - patients who underwent total thyroidectomy with radioiodine therapy (183 patients); 3d group - patients who underwent less then total thyroidectomy (169 patients).

In the first group of patients (Fig.2a, b), the number of individuals with the achieved suppressive effect was growing from visit to visit (34.5%, 50.0%, 71.4% respectively). Tg

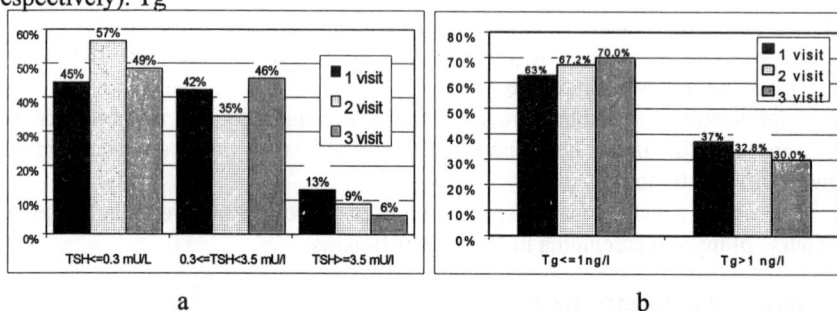

a   b

Fig. 1(a,b). a. TSH-levels in 1-st, 2-nd, 3-d visit in all children.

b. Tg-levels during complete TSH suppression in all children in 1-st, 2-nd, 3-d visit.

The frequency of hypothyroidism decreased from 40 to 0%. At the same time, the number of patients with detectable Tg (>1 ng/l) did not decrease indication persistent disease.

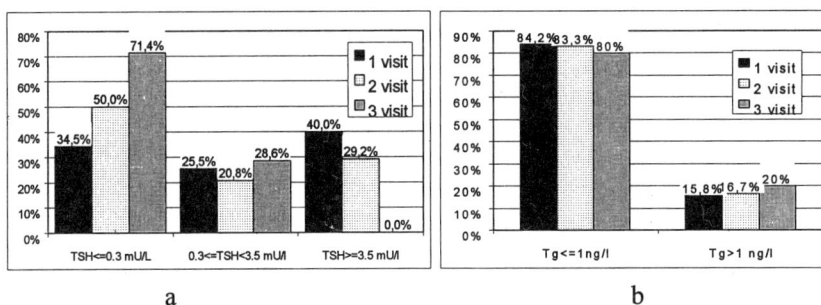

a

b

Fig. 2(a,b).a. TSH-levels in 1-st, 2-nd, 3-d visit in children after total thyroidectomy without RIT.

b. Tg-levels during complete TSH suppression in children after thyroidectomy without RIT in 1-st, 2-nd, 3-d visit.

In the second group (Fig.3a, b), TSH suppression was reached depending on the patients' visit, in 50.6%, 61.1% and 54.8% of cases, respectively. The frequency of hypothyroidism was insufficiently decreasing insufficiently (12.6%-9.5%). However in contrast to the previous group, elevated Tg levels (>1 ng/l) under TSH suppression, was registered more rarely (16.3%, 9.5%, 8.7%).

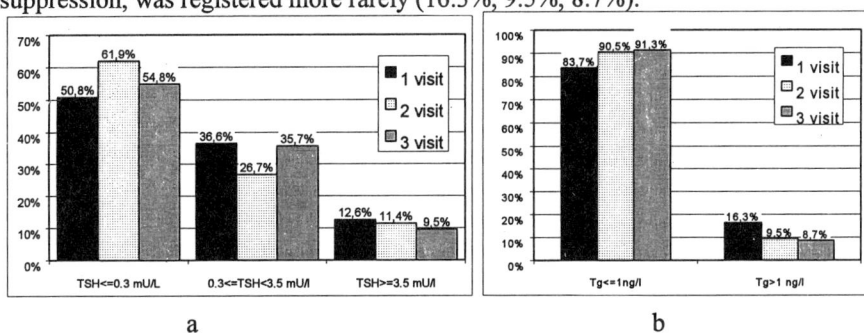

a

b

Fig. 3(a,b). a. TSH-levels in 1-st, 2-nd, 3-d visit in children after total thyroidectomy with RIT.

b. Tg-levels during complete TSH suppression in children after thyroidectomy with RIT in 1-st, 2-nd, 3-d visit.

In the third group of patients (Fig.4a, b) with partially remained thyroid tissue, it was most difficult to achieve a sufficient level of TSH suppression (41.4%, 52.3%, 40.0%), also hypothyroidism occurred relatively rare, too (5.3%-3.6%). With the achieved TSH suppression (<0.3 IU/l), the percentage of patients with the detectable Tg level (>1ng/l) was more frequent than in the two previous groups (70.0%, 62.5%,

54.5%), indicating either insufficient extend of surgery and /or the need of radioiodine treatment.

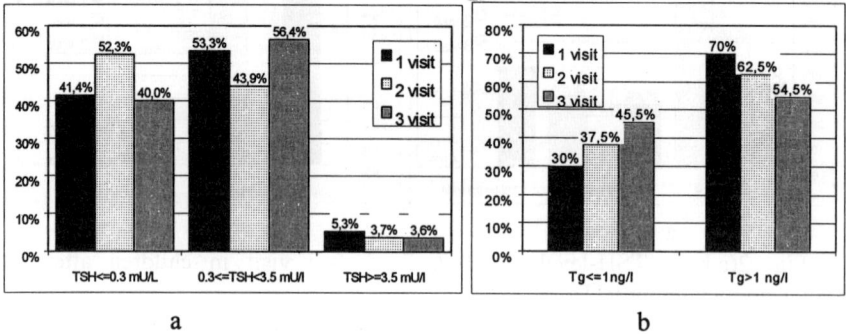

a   b

Fig. 4(a,b). a. TSH-levels in 1-st, 2-nd, 3-d visit in children after nontotal thyroidectomy.

b. Tg-levels during complete TSH suppression in children after nontotal thyroidectomy in 1-st, 2-nd, 3-d visit.

The continuation supply of thyroxine individually tailored on the basis of respective TSH measurements has significantly improved the situation of the thyroid cancer patients in Belarus. Introduction of continues serum Tg determination lead too more clarify separation between those patients actually at lower risk and those with persistent and progressive disease. Furthermore it is demonstrated that radioiodine, not available in the required capacity at the moment in Belarus would significantly contribute to a more effective therapy and follow-up of the patients.

REFERENCES

1. Pujol P, Daures J, Nskala et al. Degree of thyroid suppression as a prognostic determinant in differentiated thyroid cancer. *Journal of clinical endocrinology and metabolism* 1996; **81**, 12: 4318-4323.
2. Schlumberger MJ. Papillary and follicular Thyroid carcinoma. *The New England Journal of Medicine* 1998; **338**: 297-306.

OUTCOME OF POST-CHERNOBYL PAPILLARY THYROID CARCINOMAS TREATED BY SURGERY, RADIOIODINE AND TSH-SUPPRESSIVE THERAPY.

M. Ferdeghini, G. Boni, M. Grosso, R.C. Bellina, R. Bianchi
Dipartimento di Oncologia, Divisione di Medicina Nucleare;

P. Miccoli, C. Spinelli
Dipartimento di Chirurgia;

F. Massei, P. Macchia
Dipartimento di Medicina della Procreazione e della Età Evolutiva;

A. Antonelli
Dipartimento di Medicina Interna;

M. Lazzeri
U.O. Fisica Sanitaria;

F. Pacini, E. Molinaro, L. Agate, F. Lippi, R. Elisei, A. Pinchera
Dipartimento di Endocrinologia e Metabolismo, Sezione di Endocrinologia;
All from the University of Pisa, Italy.

G. Panasiuk
Gomel Regional Specialized Dispensary Gomel, Belarus

Eugeni P. Demidchik
Research and Clinical Institute of Radiation Medicine and Endocrinology,
Minsk, Belarus

The association between exposure to radiation and increased frequency of thyroid carcinoma has been reported in populations exposed to radioactive fallout after the Chernobyl nuclear accident. Thyroid carcinoma occurred mainly in children and adolescents, it was of the papillary histotype, and showed more aggressive histological features compared to naturally-occurring papillary thyroid carcinoma. Very few data are available regarding the outcome of these tumors and their response to treatment. We studied the outcome of 64 Belarus children with radiation-induced papillary thyroid carcinoma, who received post-surgical treatment and follow-up in Pisa. Initial treatment consisted of total thyroidectomy in all patients. Post-surgical treatment consisted in all cases of ^{131}I therapy for ablation of any thyroid residue and/or for treatment of functioning local or distant metastases and l-thyroxine suppressive therapy. The result of treatment was analyzed according to serum thyroglobulin (Tg) levels and results of 131-I whole body scan (WBS). After a mean follow-up of 38.6±25.8 months, 33 (58.9%) patients were free of disease and 23 (41.1%) had persistent disease including 14 with lymph node metastases, and 9 with lung metastases. According to the staging classification proposed by DeGroot et al. (1), complete remission was observed in 100% of Class I, in 57.1% of Class II, in 65.3% of Class III, and in 38.5% of Class IV patients. Two patients (one in Class II and one in Class III) developed lung metastases during follow-up. The longitudinal behavior of serum Tg paralleled the scintigraphic evolution. Serum Tg, at the last control, became undetectable in 27 (48.2%), decreased with respect to post-surgical levels in 7 (12.5%), was unchanged in 9 (16.1%) and was not reliable because of positive anti-Tg antibodies in 12 (21.2%). The results of this study indicate that patients with radiation-induced papillary thyroid carcinoma treated with the combination of surgery, radioiodine and hormonal therapy, have a successful response to treatment not different from that observed in age-matched series of patients with naturally-occurring papillary thyroid carcinoma.

Introduction

Differentiated thyroid cancer is relatively uncommon in the general population, and is particularly rare in childhood. In several published series (2,3) thyroid cancer in children is usually more advanced at presentation than in adults. Nevertheless, when appropriately treated, with the combination of total thyroidectomy, l-thyroxine (l-T4) suppressive therapy and radioiodine treatment, the outcome of childhood thyroid cancer is very good, with high rate of definitive cure.

The post-Chernobyl outbreak of thyroid cancer observed in Belarus, Ukraine and the Russian Federation, affected mainly children and adolescents exposed to the radioactive fallout (4,5). The epidemiological features of these radiation-induced thyroid carcinomas have been the object of extensive studies, showing that the post-Chernobyl thyroid carcinomas are mainly of the papillary histotype, and show more aggressive histological features compared to naturally-occurring papillary thyroid carcinomas (6). However, very few data are available regarding the outcome of these tumors and their response to treatment. In this study we report the outcome of a group of Belarus children with radiation-induced papillary thyroid carcinoma, who received post-surgical treatment and follow-up in Pisa in the last 4 years.

Patients and methods

The study group included 20 males and 44 females (F/M ratio: 2.2/1). The epidemiological data of these patients are reported in Table 1: mean (±SD) age at the time of diagnosis was 10.7±2.9 (range 4-17 years); mean (±SD) age at the time of the nuclear accident was 4.0±2.2 (range 1-10 years).

Tab. 1 Epidemiological and clinical data

Studied Subjects	64
Males	20
Females	44
Mean (±SD) age at diagnosis (yrs)	10.7±2.9
Range	4-17
Mean (±SD) age at accident (yrs)	4.07±2.2
Range	1-10
ClassI	3 (4.8%)
Class II	20 (31.7%)
Class III	27 (42.9%)
Class IV	13 (20.6%)

Initial treatment consisted of total thyroidectomy with or without lymph node dissection in all patients. According to the tumor stage classification (1), 3 patients (4.8%) had Class I tumors (tumor limited to the thyroid gland), 20 (31.7%) had Class II (lymph node metastases), 27 (42.9%) had Class III (tumor extending outside the thyroid gland), and 13 (20.6%) had Class IV (distant metastases). In one patient it was not possible to ascertain the Class.

Post-surgical treatment consisted in all cases of ^{131}I therapy for ablation of any thyroid residue and/or treatment of functioning local or distant metastases and l-T$_4$ suppressive therapy. L-T$_4$ therapy was withdrawn before performing whole body scan (WBS) to obtain a TSH level greater than 30 μU/ml. Two-three mCi (74-111 Mbq) of ^{131}I, were used as tracer dose and diagnostic scan was performed 48 hours later. A patient was considered cured when serum Tg off l-T$_4$ was undetectable and WBS was negative. In the case of residual or metastatic ^{131}I uptake a therapeutic dose was administered (1-2 mCi/Kg of body weight) and a post-therapy scan was performed 3-5 days after treatment. L-T$_4$ suppressive therapy was resumed immediately after radioiodine therapy. This procedure was repeated after 6-18 months. Serum level of Tg and anti-thyroglobulin antibodies (AbTg) were measured before the administration of the tracer dose. Contamination with stable iodine was excluded by measurement of urinary iodine excretion. The following test were performed: TSH (Gamma Coat HTSH IRMA Kit, INCSTAR Corporation-Stilwater, Minnesota), Tg (Sorin Diagnostics s.r.l., Saluggia, Italy), AbTg (BIOCODE s.a., Sclessin, Belgium; IRMA method).

All patients were submitted to neck ultrasound and chest-X ray. Patients with evidence of lung metastases at the WBS were submitted to lung CT scan.

The result of treatment was analyzed according to serum thyroglobulin (Tg) levels and ^{131}I whole body scan (WBS). Eight patients performed only one WBS showing the presence of uptake in the thyroid bed, and were not considered in the subsequent analysis of the outcome.

Results

The clinical status at the moment of the first WBS is shown in Fig. 1, comparing the results of WBS with the level of serum Tg. Detectable Tg concentrations (>3 ng/ml) were found in 10/15 (66.6%), 12/20 (60.0%), 10/12 (83.3%) subjects in the group positive for thyroid residue, lymph node metastases and distant metastases, respectively, at the first WBS.

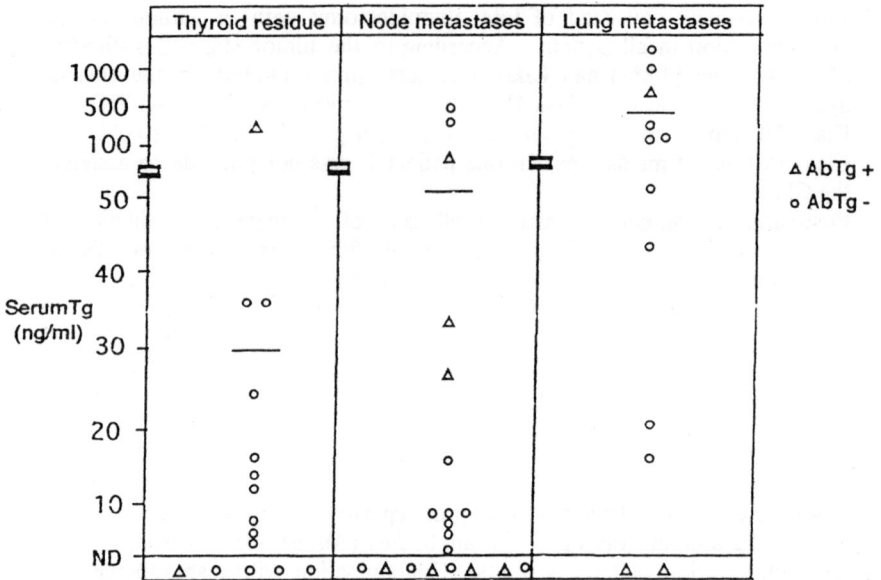

Fig. 1. Serum Tg levels at the time of the first Whole Body Scan

After a mean follow-up of 38.6±25.8 months, 33 (58.9%) patients were free of disease and 23 (41.1%) had persistent disease, including, 14 with lymph node metastases, and 9 with lung metastases.

Mean ^{131}I dose delivered was 101±80 mCi in the first group (cured) and 167±105 mCi in the other group (persistent disease). Complete remission was observed in 100% of Class I, in 57.1% of Class II, in 65.3% of Class III, and in 38.5% of Class IV patients. Furthermore, 7 patients, although not completely cured, obtained an amelioration of the disease. Two patients (one in Class II and one in Class III) developed lung metastases during follow-up (Table 2).

Tab. 2. Outcome at the last evaluation

	N.	Complete Remission N. (%)	Persistent Disease N. (%)	Progression N. (%)
Class I	3	3 (100)	0	0
Class II	14	8 (57.1)	5 (35.7)	1 (7.1)
Class III	26	17 (65.3)	8 (30.7)	1 (3.8)
Class IV	13	5 (38.5)	8 (61.5)	0
Total	56	33 (58.9)	21 (37.5)	2 (3.5)

The changes of serum Tg are showed in Fig. 2. Serum Tg, at the last control, became undetectable in 27 (48.2%), decreased with respect to post-surgical levels in 7 (12.5%), was unchanged in 9 (16.1%) and was not reliable because of positive anti-Tg antibodies in 12 (21.2%).

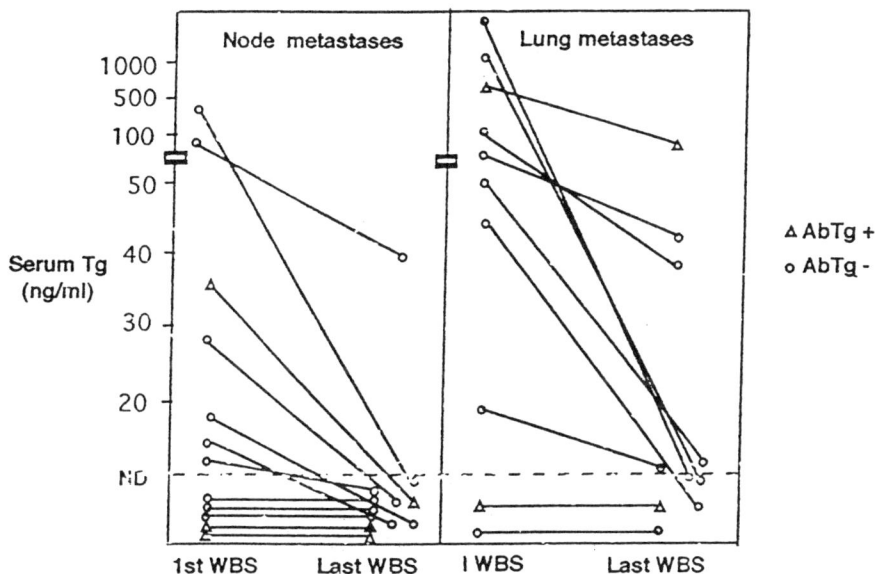

Fig. 2. Serum Tg levels at the time of the first Whole Body Scan

Conclusion

The results of this study, although limited by the short period of follow-up, indicate that young patients with radiation-induced papillary thyroid carcinoma have advanced tumors and frequent metastatic involvement at initial evaluation. Total thyroidectomy, radioiodine treatment and thyroid suppressive therapy, represent an effective combination of treatments for this disease and allow a good quality of life, not different from that observed in age-matched series of patients with naturally-occurring papillary thyroid carcinoma. Serum Tg determination should be a routine part of the follow-up because it is the most sensitive marker for residual disease or relapse (7).

References

1) DeGroot LJ, Kaplan EL, McCormick M, Straus FH. Natural history, treatment, and course of papillary thyroid carcinoma. *J Clin Endocrinol Metab* 1990; **71**: 414 - 424.
2) Ceccarelli C, Pacini F, Lippi F. et al. Thyroid cancer in children and adolescents. *Surgery* 1988; **104**: 1143-1148.
3) Winship T, Rosvoll RV. Thyroid carcinoma in childhood: final report on a 20-year study. *Clin Proc Children's Hosp Washington DC* 1970; **26**: 327-334.
4) Kazakov US, Demidchik EP, Astakhova LN. Thyroid cancer after Chernobyl. *Nature* 1992; **359**: 21.
5) Baverstock K, Egloff B, Pinchera A, Ruchti C, Williams D. Thyroid cancer after Chernobyl. *Nature* 1992; **359**: 21-22.
6) Pacini F, Vorontsova T, Demidchik E.P. et al. Post-Chernobyl thyroid carcinoma in Belarus children and adolescents: comparison with naturally occurring thyroid carcinoma in Italy and France. *J Clin Endocrinol Metab* 1997; **82**: 3563-3569.
7) Pacini F, Lari R, Mazzeo S, Grasso L, Taddei D, Pinchera A. Diagnostic value of a single serum thyroglobulin determination on and off thyroid suppressive therapy in the follow-up of patients with differentiated thyroid cancer. *Clin Endocrinol.* 1985; **23**: 405-411.

CHARACTERISTICS OF DIFFERENTIATED
CHILDHOOD THYROID CANCER FROM BELARUS

J. FARAHATI, J. BIKO AND CHR. REINERS
Clinic and Policlinic for Nuclear Medicine, University of Würzburg,
Josef-Schneider St. 2, D-97080-Würzburg, Germany
e-mail: farahati@nuklearmedizin.uni-wuerzburg.de

E.P. DEMIDCHIK
Center for Thyroid Cancer, Skorina Av. 54, 220600 Minsk, Belarus

The current investigation was undertaken to assess the characteristics of differentiated childhood thyroid carcinoma (DTC) with respect to age, gender, and histology in 503 children and adolescents from Belarus.

Characteristics of 305 females and 198 males less than 15 years of age from Belarus who have been diagnosed with DTC following the Chernobyl nuclear reactor accident since 1986 at the center for thyroid cancer in Minsk was evaluated and the influence of age, sex, histology, tumor stage, and lymph node involvement on distant metastases was tested.

The overall incidence of DTC in females was in all age-groups slightly higher than in males (ratio: female/male: 1.6). Irrespective of sex, age at diagnosis correlated with age at accident significantly (r=0.67, P<0.001). Papillary thyroid carcinoma PTC (n.s), male sex (P=0.03) and lymph node involvement (P=0.001) were associated with more distant metastases, however, multivariate analysis revealed younger age and advanced tumorstage to be the only powerful factors influencing the risk for distant mestastes in this malignancy.

Younger age at accident and advanced tumor stage pT4 seems to be the most important prognostic factors in children with radiation induced childhood thyroid cancer. In children follicular thyroid cancer appears to be less agressive than papillary type.

1 Introduction

Higher incidence of childhood thyroid cancer in areas exposed to fallout from the Chernobyl nuclear reactor accident has drawn attention to the need for a better understanding of the relationship between radiation exposure and the risk for thyroid cancer as well as the clinical features of this malignancy. Based on the temporal and geographical distribution, the increased incidence of childhood thyroid carcinoma in Belarus is believed to be due to radiation exposure from the Chernobyl nuclear reactor accident on April 26th 1986.

The current investigation was undertaken to assess the characteristics of this malignancy with respect to age, gender, and histology in 503 children and adolescents with differentiated thyroid cancer from Belarus.

2 Patients and Methods

Only children with differentiated thyroid carcinoma from Belarus were included in this analysis, because the most reliable epidemiological data regarding radiation induced thyroid carcinoma after the Chernobyl accident are reported to be available in this country (1,2). A total of 503 children with differentiated thyroid carcinoma were treated and followed between June 1986 and December 1996 at the center for thyroid cancer in Minsk. Characteristics of the 305 females and 198 males with a follow-up time of at least 1 year (all children under 15 years of age at diagnosis) was evaluated and the influence of age, sex, histology, tumor stage, and lymph node involvement on distant metastases was tested using multivariate discriminant analysis.

Comparison between groups was performed using the Student`s t test and chi-square test. Correlation between age at accident and age at diagnosis was assessed by linear regression analysis.

Multivariate discriminant analysis was performed to examine the effect of age at accident, sex, histology, tumor-stage and lymph node involvement on the frequency of distant metastasis.

3 Results

The overall incidence of DTC in females was in all age-groups slightly higher than in males (ratio: female/male: 1.6). Irrespective of sex, age at diagnosis correlated with age at accident significantly (r=0.67, P<0.001). FTC (n.s), male sex (P=0.03) and lymph node involvement (P=0.001) were associated with more distant metastases, however, multivariate analysis (Table 1) revealed younger age at accident (P<0.001) and advanced loco-regional tumor extension (P<0.001) to be the only powerful factors influencing the risk for distant metastases in this malignancy.

4 Discussion

Distant metastasis is reported to be the only prognostic factor in childhood thyroid carcinoma. Reiners et al. treated 158 children with differentiated childhood thyroid carcinoma form Belarus mostly with advanced disease. The only powerful factor influencing the time to complete remission in a multivariate analysis was the distant metastasis (P<0.001), whereas age at accident (P=0.42), sex (P=0.87), histology (0.30), tumor stage (P=0.52) and lymph node involvement (P=0.91) revealed no significant prognostic effect (Reiners et al. unpublished data). Thus, we performed multivariate discriminant analysis to clarify the effect of different factors on the frequency of distant metastasis as the most important prognostic indicator. Multivariate discriminant analysis revealed younger age at accident and extra thyroidal tumor invasion to be the most powerful factors affecting the frequency of distant metastasis in this cohort.

In accordance with radiation induced thyroid carcinoma, in 114 children with non-radiation induced thyroid carcinoma from Germany (3), loco-regional tumor extension was demonstrated by multivariate discriminant analysis to be the only powerful factor influencing the prognosis adversely. Younger age at diagnosis tend to associate with more advanced disease, however, statistical analysis failed just to reach the significant level (P=0.08).

It can be concluded that the younger age at accident and advanced tumor stage pT4 are the most important prognostic factors in children with radiation induced childhood thyroid cancer. In adition, in children FTC appears to be less agressive than PTC.

Table 1. Influence of Age at Accident, Sex, Histology, Tumor Stage, and Lymph Node Involvement (N-Status) on Frequency of Metastases at Staging in 503 Children with Differentiated Thyroid Carcinoma from Belarus (Multivariate discriminant analysis).

		Patients (n)	M1	P
Age at accident		503	35	<0,001
Sex	female	305	15	
	male	198	20	=0,58
Histology	pap.	478	35	=0,13
	foll.	18	0	
Tumorstage	pT1-3	242	2	
	pT4	249	33	=0,001
N-Status	N0	164	2	
	N1	328	33	=0,06

References

(1) Demidchik EP, Kazakov VS, Astakhova LN, Okeanov AE, Demidchik YE. Thyroid cancer in children after Chernobyl accident: clinical and epidemiological evaluation of 251 cases in the Republik of Belarus. In: Nagataki S, ed. Nagasaki Symp., Chernobyl: Update and future. Amsterdam: Excerpta Medica, Elsevier Press 1994;21-30.

(2) Sobolev B, Likhtarev I, Kairo I, Tronko N, Oleynik V, Bogdanova T. Radiation risk assessment of the thyroid cancer in Ukrainian children exposed due to Chernobyl. In: European Commission and the Belarus, Russian and Ukrainian Ministries on Chernobyl Affairs, Emergency Situations and Health: The Radiological Consequences of the Chernobyl Accident. Karaoglou A, Desmet G, Kelly GN, Menzel HG eds. European Commission, Brussels 1996; 741-748.

(3) Farahati J, Bucsky P, Parlowsky T, Mader U, Reiners C. Characteristics of differentiated thyroid carcinoma in children and adolescents with respect to age, gender, and histology. Cancer 1997;80:2156-2162.

COMPARATIVE THYROID CANCER RISK OF CHILDHOOD AND ADULT RADIATION EXPOSURE AND ESTIMATION OF LIFETIME RISK

ROY E. SHORE AND XIAONAN XUE

Dept. of Environmental Medicine, New York University Medical School, 550 First Ave., New York NY 10016, USA

E-mail: shorer01@gcrc.med.nyu.edu

The degree to which other studies confirm that recent risk estimate from a pooled analysis of five large studies of thyroid cancer from childhood irradiation is of interest; other available studies provide a risk estimate very similar to the pooled analysis. In addition, a number of studies agree that the risk from irradiation in adulthood is much smaller than in childhood.

The lifetime risk of thyroid cancer from irradiation in childhood was estimated using several dose-response models. Both a constant excess relative risk model and a constant excess absolute risk model gave similar estimates, namely, that the lifetime excess risk of thyroid cancer from 1 Gy of radiation at ages 0-4 is about 50-55 per 1,000 white females or 18-20 per 1,000 white males. However, an excess relative risk model that allows risk to vary by time since exposure yielded smaller lifetime risk estimates than the constant-risk models. This highlights gaps in our knowledge and the potential importance of considering various modifying factors in estimating thyroid cancer risk from radiation exposure.

1 INTRODUCTION

This paper will attempt to summarize information on two facets of radiation that have not been widely reported: studies of thyroid cancer risk following radiation exposure in childhood and adulthood that have been less widely used in estimating risk, and lifetime risk estimates for radiation-induced thyroid cancer.

2 EXTERNAL IRRADIATION IN CHILDHOOD AND ADULTHOOD

The current standard for risk estimates of radiation-induced thyroid cancer is the pooled analysis of five cohort studies of childhood exposure by Ron et al.[18] However, risk estimates have been derived from several other studies that can serve as a further comparison with the pooled analysis results.

In Stockholm, Sweden a cohort of 14,351 infants was treated (mostly) with [226]Ra for skin hemangiomas and followed up for an average of 39 years using the Swedish tumor registry.[10] The dose ranged from <0.01 Gy to 4.3 Gy with a mean of 0.26 Gy. There was an elevated risk of thyroid cancer (SIR = 2.28, 95% CI= 1.3-3.7). The thyroid cancer excess persisted at least 40 years after exposure.

A study was conducted in Gothenburg, Sweden of 11,807 infants treated with [226]Ra for hemangiomas of the skin and followed up for an average of 31 years via the Swedish tumor registry.[8] The mean estimated thyroid dose was about 0.12 Gy. They found an excess of thyroid cancer (SIR= 1.88, CI= 1.05-3.1) based on 15 thyroid cancers. The results of these studies are shown in Table 1.

Table 1. Thyroid Cancer: Relative Risk (RR) at 1 Gy and Excess Absolute Risk (EAR) for Cohort Studies with Acute, External Irradiation before Age 20

Study [Reference]	Mean Dose (cGy)	Observ. / Expected Cancers	RR at 1 Gy (95% CI)	EAR/ 10⁴ Person-Year Gy
Skin hemangioma [10]	26	17/7.5	5.9 (2.3,11)	0.9
Skin hemangioma [8]	12	15/8.0	8.5 (1.4,19)	1.6
Tinea capitis [20]	6	2/1.3	10 (<1,69)	1.5
Thymus/cervical adenitis [11]	290	16/1.3	4.9 (1.4,26)	1.1
Combined			6.3 (2.6,10)	1.1

The New York tinea capitis study [19, 20] has sometimes been cited as suggesting that the results of the Israeli tinea capitis study represent an outlier because there was no statistically significant excess in the former (Table 1). Actually, the results of the two studies are marginally compatible (p=0.07 for the difference between them). In addition, if the risk estimate in the New York study were as large as in the Israeli study there still would be only about 4-5 thyroid cancers rather than two, so the evidence for incompatibility is weak.

Maxon et al [11] conducted a mean 36-year follow-up of 1,266 patients who had received external radiotherapy for benign diseases in childhood and 958 unirradiated persons matched on age, sex and race. The mean thyroid dose was estimated to be 0.29 Gy. Sixteen thyroid cancers were found in the irradiated group but only one among controls.

The results of these studies can be compared to the studies that were analyzed in the pooled analysis by Ron et al.[18] As shown at the bottom of Table 1, the weighted average relative risk at 1 Gy was 6.3 (95% confidence interval (CI) = 2.6, 10) (where weighting was by the inverse variance of the excess relative risk estimates). This is similar to and statistically compatible with the value of 8.7 from Ron's pooled analysis.

The few studies that have analyzed thyroid cancer risk by age at radiation exposure have all shown that risk is high when exposure occurs before five years of age and declines for older ages at exposure. The atomic bomb survivor study, the only study with a wide age span, shows little thyroid cancer risk from radiation exposure after age 20.[22] It is therefore of interest to examine other studies of risk following acute, external radiation exposure to the thyroid gland in adulthood. Table 2 summarizes the largest of the available studies. The only study that

Table 2. Thyroid Cancer: Relative Risk (RR) at One Gray and Excess Absolute Risk (EAR) for Cohort Studies with Acute, External Irradiation in Adulthood

Study Group Reference	Mean Dose (cSv)	Observ./ Expected Cancers	Relative Risk at 1 Sv (95% CI)	EAR/ 10⁴ Person-Yr Sv
A-bomb survivors (Age ≥20 y) 22	26	73/70.9	1.1 (<1, 1.8)[a]	0.2[a]
Cervical cancer therapy [1]	11	43/18.3	13.3 (<1, 78)[a]	6.9[a]
Hodgkins disease therapy [3]	~3400	6/0.4	1.4 (1.1, 1.9)	0.1
X-ray for tuberculous adenitis[4]	850	8/0.1	10.3 (5.3, 19)	1.6
X-ray for cervical adenitis [2]	730	25/4.4	1.6 (1.4, 2.0)	1.6
Chinese medical x-ray workers 23	~70	8/4.8	2.0 (<1, 6.3)	0.1
UK Radiation Workers [7]	3.4	9/4.2[b]	2.0 (<1, 13)[a]	0.1
Combined (except A-bomb)			1.6 (1.1, 2.0)	0.4

[a] Risk estimate based on the dose-response relation.
[b] Based on mortality only.

apparently showed a substantial radiation effect, the study of tuberculous adenitis treatment by Hanford,[4] may well have been subject to surveillance bias, since the irradiated group was being compared to expected rates in the general population. The other studies besides the Japanese atomic bomb study have a weighted average relative risk at 1 Gy of 1.6 (95% CI= 1.1, 2.0). This contrasts with relative risk estimates for the combined series with childhood irradiation which are on the order of 6- to 9-fold at 1 Gy. It is clear that there is a substantial agreement between the atomic bomb study and other studies in affirming that adult irradiation confers little risk to the thyroid gland.

3   LIFETIME RISK FROM CHILDHOOD RADIATION EXPOSURE

Projections of risk by radiation protection organizations and other official bodies on radiation risks have traditionally used either a constant excess absolute risk model (EAR) [12] or, more recently, a constant excess relative risk (ERR) model [6, 13, 17] to project risk estimates over a lifetime. The term "constant" indicates that the EAR or ERR under consideration does not vary according to time since exposure; however, the EAR or ERR coefficients can vary according to age at exposure. Constant EAR or ERR models have been used to project thyroid cancer risk as well. The monograph on thyroid cancer risk by the U.S. National Council on Radiation Protection and Measurements in 1985 [16] used a constant EAR model for lifetime risk projection, while the recent estimates of risk to the U.S. population from ^{131}I fallout from the Nevada atomic bomb tests used a constant ERR model.[15]

Lubin and Ron [9] recently explored the fits of the constant ERR and EAR models for the five combined studies they had previously analyzed [18] compared to models that varied by time since exposure or by attained age (subsequent to exposure). With their permission, we have used the results to model lifetime risk. The models for lifetime risk (to age 90) used the age-, gender-, race-specific thyroid cancer rates from the U.S. SEER registry for 1983-87,[5] and the U.S. all-cause mortality rates for 1995 [14] to take into account concurrent mortality. To implement appropriate methodology for lifetime risk estimation [21], the mortality from the radiation-induced thyroid cancers had to be modeled; we made the assumption that the thyroid-cancer survival curve was exponential and reached 10% mortality by 40 years after diagnosis. Monte Carlo methods were used to estimate confidence intervals on lifetime risk estimates.

For 1 Gy of acute, external radiation to the thyroid gland at ages 0-4, the constant excess relative risk (ERR) model showed a lifetime risk of 50 (95% CI= 32, 69) excess thyroid cancers per 1,000 white (Caucasian) females irradiated (Table 3). The estimate for the constant excess absolute risk (EAR) model was very similar, namely, 55 (95% CI= 44, 67) excess cancers per 1,000. These estimates compare to a lifetime risk of thyroid cancer absent irradiation of about 5 per thousand for white females.

Table 3. Lifetime Excess Risk of Thyroid Cancer (Number of Cases per 1,000 Irradiated) from a 1 Gy Dose at Ages 0-4 Years, Estimates Derived from Various Models According to Gender and Race

Race & Gender	Constant Excess Relative Risk Model[a]	Excess Relative Risk Model, Varying by TSE[a]	Constant Excess Absolute Risk Model[a]
White Female	50	31	55
White Male	20	8	18
Black Female	24	9	52
Black Male	8	2	16

[a] The TSE model of Lubin & Ron[9] has varying risk by Time Since Exposure: ERR-TSE = $0.063 \cdot d \cdot r \cdot t^{3.24} \cdot e^{-0.2t}$ (where r= age-, sex-, race-specific baseline thyroid cancer rate, t= time (years) since exposure, and e is an exponential term). The constant ERR model has a dose coefficient of 7.7 (ERR/Gy), and the constant EAR model has a dose coefficient of 3.1 excess cancers per 10^4 person-year Gy for males and 8.0 for females.

Lubin and Ron [9] also examined whether models that allowed for variation in risk according to time since exposure improved the fit of the model to the data from their five pooled studies. They modeled the time-since-exposure variation in risk estimates in two ways: using a continuous function or using discrete 5-year (or 10-year) time intervals. Although the discrete intervals provided a better fit by statistical criteria, the temporal risk coefficients were fairly irregular, so we chose to use the continuous temporal function that smoothed the irregularities. In all cases, terms for time-since-exposure (TSE) were statistically significant, i.e., they improved the fit of the models. However, because the TSE-EAR model seemed rather implausible (it predicted that risk increased sharply across the life-span) and we disagreed with one of its technical assumptions that had an impact on the results, we did not consider it further.

Incorporating TSE into the lifetime risk model made a considerable difference in the temporal pattern of radiation-induced thyroid cancer for the ERR model, as shown in Figure 1. Note that the area under the curve is smaller for the TSE-ERR model than for the constant ERR model, which indicates that projected total lifetime risk is smaller if one takes into account TSE. Specifically, the lifetime risk for the TSE-ERR model, as compared with the constant ERR model, was about 35-40% smaller for white females and about 60% smaller for white males (Table 3). The smaller relative difference between the constant and TSE models for females than for males is because the ERR models multiply the baseline rates of thyroid cancer, and, whereas the female baseline rates tend to level off and even decrease at older ages, the male rates continued to increase through most of the life-span.

As expected, age at irradiation made a large difference in the lifetime thyroid cancer risk projection using either the constant ERR model or the TSE-ERR model. Irradiation before five years of age was estimated to confer about five times as much lifetime risk as irradiation in the age range of 10-14 years under the ERR models. However, the constant EAR model derived by Lubin and Ron [9] did not indicate a significant effect of age-at-irradiation; hence, the lifetime risks using this model are very similar for ages 0-4 and 10-14 at irradiation.

Gender and ethnicity also make a difference in lifetime thyroid-cancer risk projections. For example, Table 3 shows that lifetime risk estimates are 2.5, 3.8 and 3.0 times as high in white females as in white males for the constant ERR, TSE-ERR and constant EAR models respectively. The elevated ratios are mostly because of the higher baseline rates of thyroid cancer among females, but some fraction is attributable to the greater longevity of females. The lifetime risk estimates are 2.1 to 3.7 times as high among whites as blacks for the ERR models. For the EAR model there is little difference by ethnicity since the only factor that differs between races in this model was the total mortality rates.

The discrepancies between the lifetime risk predictions of the several models highlight the gaps in our knowledge about thyroid risk. For example, there are no data on radiation-induced thyroid cancer in blacks with which to evaluate the discrepant predictions made by the constant ERR and EAR models. The temporal projections are also problematic. As the main irradiated groups are followed up for longer periods of time, it will be increasingly possible to narrow the range of predictions made by the several models and perhaps determine which is the most appropriate model.

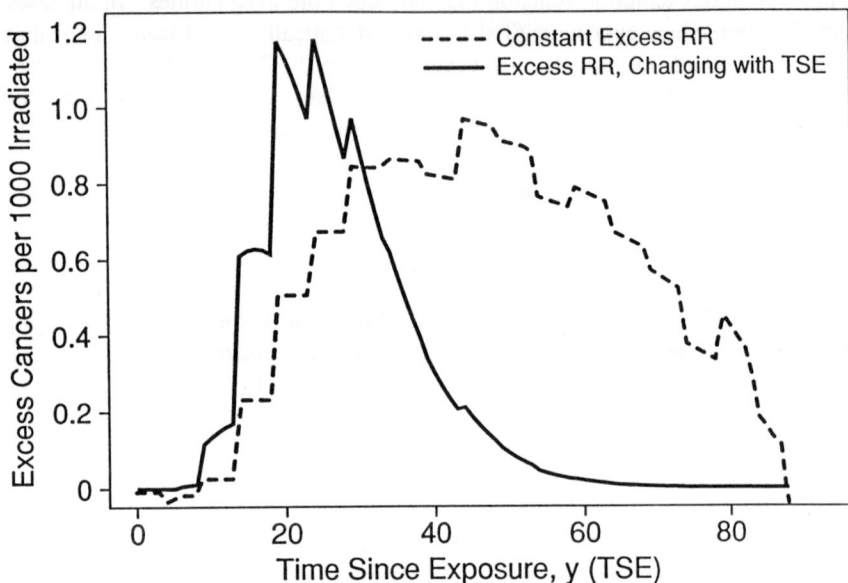

Figure 1. Excess thyroid cancers in white females after 1 Gy exposure at age 2, according to constant and time-varying excess relative risk models

Acknowledgments

Drs. Jay Lubin and Elaine Ron graciously granted permission for us to use their unpublished risk models and supplied additional details needed for calculations of lifetime risk. This work was supported in part by the Kaplan Comprehensive Cancer Center NCI Grant CA16087 and the NIEHS Center Grant ES-00260 to New York University.

References

1. Boice JD, Engholm G, Kleinerman R *et al.* Radiation dose and second cancer risk in patients treated for cancer of the cervix. *Radiat Res* 1988; **116**: 3-55.

2. Fjalling M, Tisell L, Carlsson S, Hansson G, Lundberg L, Oden A. Benign and malignant thyroid nodules after neck irradiation. *Cancer* 1986; **58**: 1219-1224.

3. Hancock SL, Cox R, McDougall I. Thyroid diseases after treatment of Hodgkin's disease. *New Engl J Med* 1991; **325**: 599-605.

4. Hanford JM, Quimby E, Frantz V. Cancer arising many years after radiation therapy. *J Am Med Assoc* 1962; **181**: 132-138.

5. IARC. *Cancer Incidence in Five Continents, 1986-1989.* Lyon, France: International Agency for Research on Cancer (WHO) & International Association of Cancer Registries, 1992.

6. ICRP. 1990 Recommendations of the International Commission on Radiological Protection. *Ann ICRP* 1991; **21 (Publication 60)**: 1-201.

7. Kendall GM, Muirhead C, MacGibbon B *et al.* Mortality and occupational exposure to radiation: first analysis of the National Registry for Radiation Workers. *Br Med J* 1992; **304**: 220-225.

8. Lindberg S, Karlsson P, Arvidsson B, Holmberg E, Lundberg L, Wallgren A. Cancer incidence after radiotherapy for skin haemangioma during infancy. *Acta Oncologica* 1995; **34**: 735-740.

9. Lubin J, Ron E. Excess relative risk and excess absolute risk estimates for pooled analysis of thyroid cancer following exposure to external radiation. National Cancer Inst., Rockville, MD, 1998.

10. Lundell M, Hakulinen T, Lindell B, Holm L-E. Thyroid cancer after radiotherapy for skin hemangioma in infancy. *Radiat Res* 1994; **140**: 334-339.

11. Maxon H, Saenger E, Thomas S *et al.* Clinically important radiation-associated thyroid disease. *J Am Med Assoc* 1980; **244**: 1802-1805.

12. NAS/NRC (BEIR I Committee). *The Effects on Populations of Exposure to Low Levels of Ionizing Radiation.* Washington, DC, 217 pp.: National Academy of Sciences - National Research Council, 1972.

13. NAS/NRC (BEIR III Committee). *The effects on populations of exposure to low levels of ionizing radiation.* National Academy of Sciences - National Research Council, National Academy Press, 1980.

14. NCHS. Death rates from 72 selected causes by 5-year age groups, race, and sex: U.S., 1979-95. Division of vital statistics, National Center for Health Statistics, CDC, Washington, DC, 1998.

15. NCI. Estimated exposures and thyroid doses received by the American people from iodine-131 in fallout following Nevada atmospheric nuclear bomb tests.

Volume 1. National Cancer Institute, US National Institutes of Health, Bethesda, MD, 1997.

16. NCRP. *Induction of Thyroid Cancer by Ionizing Radiation, Report No. 80.* Bethesda, MD: National Council on Radiation Protection and Measurements, 1985.

17. NCRP. *Risk Estimates for Radiation Protection.* Bethesda, MD: National Council on Radiation Protection, 1993.

18. Ron E, Lubin J, Shore R *et al.* Thyroid cancer after exposure to external radiation: a pooled analysis of seven studies. *Radiat Res* 1995; **141**: 259-277.

19. Shore R, Albert R, Pasternack B. Follow-up of patients treated by x-ray epilation for tinea capitis. *Arch Environ Health* 1976; **31**: 21-28.

20. Shore RE, Hildreth N, Moseson M. Studies of skin cancer and thyroid tumors after irradiation of the head and neck. *Intl. Conf. on Radiation Effects and Protection.* Japan Atomic Energy Res. Inst., Mito, Japan, 1992; 77-79.

21. Thomas D, Darby S, Fagnani F, Hubert P, Vaeth M, Weiss K. Definition and estimation of lifetime detriment from radiation exposures: principles and methods. *Health Phys* 1992; **63**: 259-272.

22. Thompson D, Mabuchi K, Ron E *et al.* Cancer incidence in atomic bomb survivors. Part II: Solid tumors, 1958-1987. *Radiat Res* 1994; **137**: S17-S67.

23. Wang JX, Inskip P, Boice J, Jr., Li B. Cancer incidence among medical diagnostic X-ray workers in China, 1950 to 1985. *Int J Cancer* 1990; **45**: 889-895.

FUTURE ISSUES: AN ICRP PERSPECTIVE

R. H. CLARKE,

Chairman, ICRP
NRPB, Chilton, Didcot, Oxon OX11 ORQ, UK
E-mail: roger.clarke@nrpb.org.uk

The principal health effect of chronic exposure to low levels of ionising radiation is the risk, some time after exposure, of the appearance of a small excess of cancers in the irradiated population. Studies of irradiated human populations are available from which estimates of the probability of cancer induction can be derived. This paper summarises the ICRP conclusions on the lifetime probability of fatal radiation-induced cancer and the biological issues that ICRP is addressing, with particular regard to the thyroid. The ICRP philosophy for intervention is then outlined and its implementation in emergency planning discussed for a range of countermeasures including stable iodine administration.

1 INTRODUCTION

The major effect of occupational or public exposure to radiation appears to be the appearance, at long times after exposure, of a small excess of cancers in any irradiated population. It is not possible to distinguish a radiation-induced cancer from one arising naturally, so that any estimate of the risk has to be made from a statistical analysis of the long-term health of irradiated populations. Although there are several population groups who were exposed in the past to high doses of radiation and from which estimates of cancer risk can be made, including patients treated for ankylosing spondylitis and other medical conditions, or those exposed at work, the single most important source of information is from the survivors of the Hiroshima and Nagasaki atomic bombs.

While an estimate of the risk of whole body exposure is made from the Japanese survivors, there is insufficient evidence for the quantification of risks to some organs and tissues. Notable amongst these are the thyroid, liver, bone surfaces and skin. the risk factors for these tissues are taken from other epidemiological studies (ICRP, 1991). The resulting fatal cancer risk estimate for whole body exposure is 5% Sv^{-1}. Doses to different organs or tissues need to be combined in a way that correlates with the effect of total body irradiation. This is done by use of weighting factors representing the relative contributions of the different organs to whole body risk and they are shown in Table 1. The tissue weighting factor, w_T, represents the relative contribution of the tissue, T, to the total risk of whole body irradiation in the protection quantity effective dose, E. The use of effective dose means that the risk of irradiation can be expressed in the same terms whether the whole body or only part of the body is irradiated. It can be seen from Table 1 that the thyroid is responsible for 5% of the total risk. The remainder tissues, which contribute in total the residual 5% of the risk, include, adrenals, brain, muscle, small intestine, kidneys, pancreas, spleen, thymus, uterus and extrathoracic airways.

1.1. Table 1

Tissue weighting factors

Organ	w_T	Organ	w_T	Organ	w_T	Organ	w_T
Skin	0.01	Bladder	0.05	Bone marrow	0.12	Gonads	0.2
Bone surface		Breast		Colon			
		Liver		Lung			
		Oesophagus		Stomach			
		Thyroid					
		Remainder					
Total (1.00)	0.02		0.30		0.48		0.20

In this paper a broad perspective on the carcinogenic risks of exposure to ionising radiation is given and the issues for the future identified, with some indication of those that are particularly relevant to the thyroid. The paper then proceeds to discuss the concept of intervention, again in the broad context, and to consider the implications for emergency planning with particular emphasis on countermeasures applicable when the thyroid is liable to be exposed.

2 CURRENT BIOLOGICAL ISSUES

Committee 1 of the International Commission on Radiological Protection has the responsibility for maintaining under review the biological effects of ionising radiation and developing documents that relate such effects to the needs of radiological protection. During the present four-year period of Committee 1, from 1997-2001, there are three task groups each reviewing a broad topic that includes a range of biological, biophysical and epidemiological issues.

This programme of work that has been agreed by the Commission will include the preparation of reports by the three task groups on:

- A review of epidemiological evidence of radiation-induced cancer at low doses and characterisation of the dose-response relationship;
- Radiation effects on the developing embryo/fetus to include judgements on the risks of cancer, neurological dysfunction and other deterministic effects;
- Evaluation of RBEs in respect of deterministic and stochastic effects.

In support of these task groups the Committee will continue to review epidemiological studies published each year and to survey developments in cell and molecular biology relevant to the effects of ionising radiation. In addition it will also continue to identify cells at risk, to provide evidence of dose and dose-rate effects from animal studies and to advise on genetics risks in relation to both mendelian and multifactorial disorders. The evidence of synergism or additivity between the effects of ionising radiation and chemical carcinogens on cells and tissues is also kept under review.

In the particular context of the thyroid the questions that will be addressed begin with whether the current risk factors for cancer incidence and fatality continue to be the most appropriate ones for use, especially at the low doses and dose-rates that prevail in normal situations. This will involve the need to consider the evidence for the differing effects of external versus internal irradiation of the thyroid. There is also the issue of age dependence of the risk, when the current system of protection uses single values of risk averaged over a lifetime. Finally there are questions of whether there is any genetic predisposition to the carcinogenic effects of ionising radiation with sensitive subgroups. All of these aspects of the effects of exposure will need to be considered by ICRP, not only for the thyroid but also for all the organs and tissues at risk, in establishing the next generation of recommendations.

3 INTERVENTION

The intervention situation differs from that of the practice in that action is being taken to **reduce** the level of exposure as much as reasonable, whereas with the practice the objective is to restrict added exposures and the risk of being exposed. The two situations normally quoted for intervention are radon in buildings and countermeasures for the public after a nuclear accident. In both cases, protection measures taken are designed to lower the dose and hence **dose limits do not apply**. The question is by how much to reduce the dose and therefore the risk?

Intervention cannot usually be applied at the source and has to apply to the environment or people. Countermeasures forming the intervention have disadvantages, so that they must be justified as doing more good than harm. Their scale should be optimised to maximise the benefit. Since there is some harm to the affected individuals from the disruption and risk from the execution of a countermeasure, the philosophy is to maximise the difference between the risk averted by the reduction of dose and the risk added by the countermeasure. In this scenario, there is no equivalent to the unacceptable level of risk used to establish dose limits for practices, although there will normally be a level of risk when the dose to the individual is high enough that intervention is bound to be justified.

The system of radiological protection recommended by the Commission for intervention is thus based on the following general principles:

(a) any intervention must do more good than harm so the reduction in radiation detriment must exceed the harm and social cost of the intervention.

(b) the scale and duration of the intervention should be optimised such that the net benefit of the reduction in dose, i.e. the benefit of the reduction in radiation detriment less the detriment associated with the intervention, should be maximised.

Principles (a) and (b) will lead to intervention levels which are appropriate for the circumstances. However, there will be some level of projected dose above which, because of serious deterministic effects, intervention will almost always be justified.

4 EMERGENCY PLANNING

For most foreseeable accidents that release radioiodines, there will be accompanying releases of other radionuclides. Stable iodine prophylaxis protects against the radiation dose from the radioiodines only and therefore it is important that a countermeasure strategy is prepared that includes sheltering and evacuation in addition to the administration of stable iodine. There is existing international advice from both ICRP (1993) and IAEA (1996) on the establishment of intervention levels for the most common countermeasures. The intervention level represents a judgement on the balance between the benefits, which include dose saved and reassurance, and the social cost and risk of the countermeasure (other risks, disruption, anxiety, costs). In the case of stable iodine the benefits are the dose averted and the reassurance, while the harms would be taken as the health detriment from stable iodine intake (if any), the costs of maintaining the stocks and the costs of distribution. The resulting intervention level is the optimum dose saving by the implementation of the countermeasure.

In general sheltering, which means keeping the population at risk indoors with doors and windows closed for some hours, together with stable iodine administration, are seen as low risk countermeasures. Evacuation of a population for a period of up to a few days is accepted as a countermeasure of medium social cost and risk. However, the serious disruption and break-up of social infrastructure that results from permanent relocation means that it is a high cost countermeasure that would only be undertaken to avert very high doses.

Clearly emergency plans need to be prepared well in advance and rehearsed regularly so that they do not have to be invented on the day an accident occurs. At present stable iodine administration is envisaged as being undertaken in conjunction with the other countermeasures of sheltering or evacuation. The protective action of stable iodine administration should be considered when inhalation of radioiodines is a major exposure pathway. In situations where uncontaminated food supplies are readily available, it is more appropriate to reduce the doses from ingestion by imposing restrictions on the production and consumption of foodstuffs. Another simple option is to feed livestock on stored uncontaminated feed.

The question of the pre-distribution of stable iodine to population groups liable to be affected by a nuclear accident is also relevant. To be effective, stable iodine needs to be taken within a relatively short time of the recognition of an emergency. If it is used in conjunction with an evacuation, it can be distributed as the population is evacuated. However, if sheltering is used there may be advantage in having supplies in homes, schools and offices in anticipation of the accident. The difficulties are that if stable iodine is distributed in advance, will people remember where it is and how much to take and when, in the event. To be useful, adequate stocks and instructions need to be kept up to date and therefore national authorities have to give careful consideration to their policy on this subject.

5 CONCLUSIONS

This paper has reviewed the current risk factors used for setting protection standards and considered future issues that would affect them and emphasised those that are particularly relevant to the thyroid.

The question of stable iodine prophylaxis has been reviewed in the context of a countermeasure strategy involving other interventions that can be taken. At present stable iodine administration is envisaged in conjunction with either sheltering or evacuation. If there is new information on the risks of radioiodines, and risk (or lack thereof) from ingestion of stable iodine, there will be a need to reconsider the balance between benefits and harms that may lead to a revision in the intervention level or a change in countermeasures strategy. The international bodies concerned with giving advice in these areas, ICRP, WHO, and IAEA will need to address this and national authorities will need to reconsider their plans in the context of their own situations.

504

References

International Commission on Radiological Protection (ICRP), 1991. The 1990 Recommendations of the Commission, Publication 60, Annals of the ICRP, 21, 1-3, Pergamon Press, Oxford.

International Commission on Radiological Protection (ICRP), 1993. Protection from potential exposure: a conceptual framework, Publication 63, Annals of the ICRP, 23, 1, Pergamon Press, Oxford.

International Atomic Energy Agency (IAEA), 1996. International Basic Safety Standards for Protection against ionising radiation and the safety of radiation sources, jointly sponsored by FAO, IAEA, ILO, OECD/NEA, PAHO, WHO, Safety Series 115, IAEA, Vienna.

OPEN DISCUSSION, CONCLUSIONS, LESSONS AND ACTIONS

Mediators: L.E. Holm & A.Pinchera
Panel: Session chairmen
5 topics were selected by the mediators for comment from the chairmen and for open discussion: Basic problems: E.D. Williams; Epidemiology aspects: S. Nagataki; Dosimetry: A. Bouville; Clinical problems: J. Robbins; Public health problems: D. Becker

Topic 1: Basic problems

E.D. Williams: The conference has covered 2 areas: 1. General review of what is known of science underlying cancer, and in particular thyroid cancer; 2. Genes and related findings in the post-Chernobyl thyroid cancers. Papillary thyroid cancer is the dominant tumour; the oncogene *ret* has been identified; *ret* rearrangements occur after radiation exposure and there is particularly an increase in *ret* PTC3.
Further work: 1. What is the situation of involvement of *ret* gene with external irradiation? *ret* PTC1 and 3, especially in the cases in Japan; are the changes in the gene age related ?; 2. How does this interact with the other genes, such as *trk* gene?; 3. Is this just gene hunting for the sake of gene hunting?; 4. There is very little hard data on genetic susceptibility; 5. Animal experimentation and epidemiology. There is very little work done in transgenic animals; 6. There is molecular biology work to be done. There must be interaction with morphology and cellular work.

F. Pacini: PTC rearrangements. On which basis are you expecting the involvement of other genes? Having been able to identify one gene able to transform in "vitro", why should we expect the involvement of other genes? For colon cancer I can understand that several genes may be involved, but for the thyroid?

E.D. Williams: G. Vecchio has shown that other genes are involved. One gene is not enough, an additional event is required for a cancer to occur.

H. Rabes: M. Schlumberger has shown that those exposed to external irradiation at <20 years of age show rearrangements in PTC1. So can we say that PTC3 is specific for internal uptake of radioiodine? The *trk* gene is involved only in 4.4% post-Chernobyl childhood thyroid carcinomas, and it is not as much involved as the *ret* gene.

E.D. Williams: We need more studies on the *trk* gene. Maybe PTC3 is involved only in children and not in adults.

K. Baverstock: Is the pursuit of radiation signature the only practical benefit resulting from determining the pattern of gene expression characteristic of the malignant state of the thyroid cells? If so, what are your views on M. Atkinson's paper?

E.D. Williams: Maybe there is not a radiation signature, but we do not know, and therefore we should continue to look for it.

Topic 2: Epidemiology

S. Nagataki: In Session "Radiation and the Incidence of Thyroid Cancer in Man", E. Ron reviewed the effects of external radiation on the thyroid and found that the results of investigation on atomic bomb survivors show that external radiation clearly increases the ERR of thyroid cancer. However, Dr. Holm summarised the effects of ^{131}I on the thyroid and concluded that ^{131}I for diagnostic and therapeutic use does not increase thyroid cancer. In the same session, "US experience" in the Nevada atmospheric nuclear bomb tests calculated precisely the thyroid dose of ^{131}I, but the health consequences of ^{131}I have not been investigated. Experiences in the Marshall Islands have shown that thyroid cancer increased by the radioactive fallout, but it is still not elucidated which of the radioactive iodines (^{131}I, ^{132}I, ^{125}I, etc.) is the cause of thyroid cancer. Panel and proffered papers on the Chernobyl accident showed a clear increase of thyroid cancer after the accident, but the dose response relationship is not shown because the dosimetry in the Chernobyl accident is very variable. In summary, the cause of increased thyroid cancer in Chernobyl still depends on circumstantial evidence, chronological and geographical. ^{131}I may be the cause of thyroid cancer in Chernobyl with other factors such as low iodine intake, young age, genetic factors, etc. However, the Gomel area where thyroid cancer incidence is the highest is not a low iodine area, and it is too early to conclude that ^{131}I is the cause of thyroid cancer, because we have no data of other radioactive iodines nor of external radiation and we do not know the difference of the biological effects between various radioactive iodines and external radiation. We must recognise that investigation of the cause of thyroid cancer is essential in the diagnosis, treatment and prevention of thyroid cancer. In addition to these general comments on the cause of thyroid cancer, I would like to mention the need of animal experiments to compare external and internal radiation and to compare the biological effects of various radioactive iodines. As mentioned by C. Capen, there is only one experiment comparing external and internal radiation. We have to perform more animal experiments under different conditions, but the cost of one experiment will be one million US dollars or more. It is also important to avoid duplication of the study because of the cost. We are planning this kind of animal experiment and would like to propose international collaboration.

L.E. Holm question to E. Cardis: There are 10 sibling parents with thyroid cancer. Is there more information on possible familial predisposition ?

E. Cardis: There are no results as yet, but this is one of the main objectives of the case-control study we have started with support from the EC. To complement what S. Nagataki said, as this is a session on epidemiology: not only are animal experiments needed, but there is also epidemiological work to be done. We need to understand why there are inconsistencies between the results of different studies: the atomic bomb survivors, the Marshall islanders and the Utah studies. Are these linked to differences in the quality of the dosimetry, to different levels of screening, of iodine deficiency or genetic make-up of the populations? It is important that this be resolved and for this we need well-designed studies of the aetiology of thyroid cancer. We also need to continue monitoring the trends of thyroid cancer incidence over time, particularly to assess the efficiency of prevention measures. As Nick Day showed in his presentation, studies of trends in incidence over time can teach us much about the process of disease and can complement studies of aetiology.

K.H. Chadwick: I would like to come back to the question of whether it is radioiodine or not which is causing these post-Chernobyl thyroid cancers. There is in my opinion no doubt it is and there is evidence with the mutations and translocations we see. As to comment on continuing epidemiological studies on these cancers, I have some reservations about whether we will be able to derive good risk estimates from the Chernobyl accident. The question of dose rate will play a role and also how uniformly irradiated the thyroid was. It may be important to obtain some predictions from epidemiology to be used by the public health authorities on how many cancers will be forthcoming in the near future.

G. Burrow: Genetic predisposition. Has there been previous exposure to radiation? Can anybody answer ?

E.P. Demidchik: There is no such direct evidence.

A. Tsyb: In the area where the accident happened there was no previous radiation exposure. Is there other modifying factors? It is a high endemic region for goitre; e.g. in the Bryansk region a lot of people have been operated for thyroid complaints. I would like to point out that we must not only study them but also help them.

E.P. Demidchik: What to do with these children? Their follow up is a very important factor.

N. Tronko: Sh. Nagataki is saying there is no proof. But why can we not take into account a joint effect of ^{131}I and iodine deficiency? Let us study these effects. Analyse the pattern of the cancers check whether there was endemic goitre or not.

S. Nagataki: I believe that the cause is radioactive iodine, but not necessarily the ^{131}I. Maybe other types also should be considered.

J. Robbins: There is still some uncertainty about the contribution of the short-lived ones in the Marshall Islands. There is a paper in press by Beebe et al. on a case control approach to determine cause and effect.

B. Goslings: What animal model to do? C.Capen could answer that maybe.

E.D. Williams: The guinea pig has a papillary tumour which resembles the human situation.

I. Likhtarev: It is impossible to find a radiation factor more important than ^{131}I to explain the large incidence of thyroid cancers among children after the Chernobyl accident. Short-lived radionuclides can give you 30% additional cause but not more. We must harmonise our points of view in epidemiology and dosimetry. I can see that between the genetic molecular and pathology teams there is harmonisation, but not with the epidemiology and dosimetry teams.

Topic 3: Dosimetry

A. Bouville: The task of the dosimetrists is to assess as accurately as possible the thyroid doses received by the populations of Belarus, Russia, and Ukraine, which were most affected by the Chernobyl accident. I agree with I. Likhtarev that ^{131}I appears to be by far the most important contributor to the thyroid dose, especially when the principal pathway of exposure was the ingestion of contaminated milk or other foodstuffs. It is only when the dose was mainly due to inhalation and when the intake of the radioiodines occurred within two days after the accident that ^{132}TE (via its decay product, ^{132}I) and ^{133}I may have contributed up to 30% of the thyroid dose. The initial thyroid dose estimates that have been so far based on the results of the so-called 'direct thyroid measurements', which are measurements of the gamma radiation emitted by the thyroid by means of an instrument placed against the neck of the individual. These initial thyroid dose estimates have been organised in databases in the three republics. The work that needs to be done now is to improve the accuracy of these dose estimates, particularly those that will be used in epidemiological studies. This could be achieved in various ways: 1. in studying carefully the important parameters used in the derivation of the thyroid estimates; 2. in developing model-derived thyroid dose estimates that can be compared with the 'measured' doses, and 3. in assessing the uncertainties attached to the thyroid dose estimates in as objective a manner as possible. The dosimetrists of the three Republics are currently involved in those three tasks. It is important to realise that, with the exception of [129]I, there is no physical measurement of environmental radiation that could be currently done to help in the estimation of the thyroid dose from ^{131}I and shorter-lived radioiodines. In that respect, it would be very helpful if a biological dosimetry technique could be developed to assess thyroid doses received a decade ago.

L.E. Holm: Are the dosimetric methods in the three republics harmonised?

A. Bouville: This is an issue that I should have pointed out. There is a need of exchange of information between the three republics. This is catalysed by the foreigners for the moment. The three republics should get together and derive a single methodology.

E. Cardis: The work that is going on in dosimetry is extremely important. I would like to stress that we need work on reconstruction both of individual and group doses. As an epidemiologist, I must say that, despite what was mentioned during the dosimetry session, what we need in analytical epidemiologic studies is not group doses, but good (accurate and precise) estimates of individual doses. Group doses, on the other hand, are important tools to assess the public health impact of an exposure for prevention and screening.

I. Likhtarev: It is extremely difficult to estimate reliable estimates of individual thyroid dose, especially for the subjects without 'direct thyroid measurements'. It must be realised that only about 10% of the subjects with thyroid cancer were subjected in 1986 to 'direct thyroid measurements'. In order to obtain better estimates of individual thyroid dose, it would be important to develop a single methodology of dose reconstruction that would be used in the three Republics. Today there are 10 dosimetrists and 10 different methods.

A. Brill: I think that I. Likhtarev and A. Bouville and I are in agreement that short lived radionuclides provided a small contribution to the thyroid dose in all but a very few areas where relatively few people could have been exposed. Thus, it is unlikely that the high incidence of thyroid cancer observed in people exposed at multiple separated locations can be attributed to short-lived nuclide exposures. The age distribution points to the high sensitivity of the very young child. A second point is that in regions with iodine deficiency, the uptake in the gland is very irregular. To get a firmer handle on the dose effect correlation, it seems likely that work on biomarkers of radiation dose to the thyroid is an important area of research which could be helpful in adding confidence to our dose predictions.

Topic 4: Clinical aspects

J. Robbins: General: Since thyroid cancer in children was very rare before the accident, it is clear that almost all of the large number of cases occurring after 1990 were caused by the accident. What is not entirely clear, however, is whether the clinical features that have been observed are specific for cancers caused by radiation or whether they are simply a reflection of the young ages at which the cancers occurred. Comparison with childhood thyroid cancer cases in Italy and France indicated that the Chernobyl cases were more aggressive and were less well differentiated histologically. Similar findings were reported by E.D. Williams when comparing Chernobyl cases with cases in the UK, and as reported at a workshop held at the NIH in 1992, in Mayo clinic cases that did or did not have a history exposure to external radiation. The problem with most of these comparisons is that the ages are not exactly matched. In my opinion, the evidence suggests that both the young ages at which the cancers occur and the radiation aetiology are contributing factors to the biological behaviour observed in the cancers after the accident. It is very important to continue these comparisons as the exposed persons reach post pubertal and adult ages when their cancers develop since the difference between radiation exposed and unexposed cases may then be more apparent. In the discussion period it was said that these comparisons are just beginning and there is not yet enough information to answer the question. Careful analysis will be required since the incidence of spontaneously occurring cancers will be higher at the older ages and there is still no way to distinguish between a cancer that has been induced by radiation and one that has not.

There is no argument against surgical excision of the cancer as primary therapeutic procedure although there may be variations in technique and in the extent of the thyroidectomy. This was not discussed but there was some discussion of post surgical radiation therapy with ^{131}I. Much of the earlier ^{131}I therapy was done outside of the Chernobyl region - especially in Germany on Belarussian children as described by Ch. Reiners. Both Ch. Reiners and A. Pinchera advocated routine ^{131}I ablation therapy following removal of the primary tumour, as well as ^{131}I therapy for metastatic disease. The very high incidence of distant metastases reported by Ch. Reiners (74 of 145 cases, most with lung metastases) may be related to his receiving only more advanced cases for treatment in Germany. At present facilities for ^{131}I therapy in Minsk and Kiev have been improved and it is expected that most future therapy will be done in those centres. Ch. Reiners reported that the majority of the cases so treated achieved complete remission. In the future, attention should be paid to the possibility of improving ^{131}I treatment by the application of quantitative dosimetry, as well as the use of agents such as lithium carbonate to enhance retention of ^{131}I in the tumour.

A third aspect briefly discussed was the possibility of employing measures to prevent the development of thyroid cancer in exposed individuals. M. Schlumberger and J. Naumann presented detailed information on the well-established ability to reduce radiation exposure by the timely administration of potassium iodide. S. Yamashita made a case for early detection of cancer by screening the exposed population in order to improve treatment outcome. The most likely method that <u>might</u> prevent cancer from developing, however, is to suppress TSH secretion by giving thyroid hormone. This had been discussed extensively at the NIH workshop in 1992 but it was concluded that the benefits in exposed humans were not well established. It was also felt that an experiment to determine its utility in the Chernobyl population would be exceedingly difficult, and that its widespread use in young children might be hazardous. Now that the exposed population is older, this question should be revisited. Consideration could be given to the wisdom of employing this therapy, and especially, to designing an experiment that could establish whether it would be risk-free and effective.

A. Pinchera: There are difficulties at present setting in the provision of medication. The treatment is done in an adequate way, but in the follow-up it is not known whether other cancers or diseases will develop in those treated.

Ch. Reiners: There is an important question to be dealt with on an international level. There are 1.200 children operated and treated with radioiodine. The remission rate is good, but late recurrences is a considerable risk. If detected early they can be treated better. There are side effects of the treatment on a long-term basis, therefore, protocols for follow-up have to be installed, we must guarantee the follow-up of these protocols and guarantee medication. I, therefore, would like to make recommendations on three aspects of the clinical issues: 1. Screening/Diagnosis: Screening has to be performed further taking into consideration now adolescents and young adults. The priority of different projects which are carried out may benefit from some more co-ordination. 2. Treatment: Protocols for treatment of children with thyroid cancer have been established and evaluated. Structures for the interdisciplinary co-operation between surgeons, nuclear medicine, radiotherapists and endocrinologists have been identified. However, the continuity of treatment and the supply of materials needed for surgery, radioiodine therapy and hormone replacement has to be guaranteed. 3. Follow-up: A standardised protocol for follow-up of children with thyroid cancer is under discussion. It should be set up and approved by the different institutions involved as soon as possible. Central issues for follow-up in the future are: - Treatment of side effects (hypothyroidism, hypoparathyroidism); -Early detection of (late) recurrences or metastases; - Early detection of (late) complications of therapy, i.e., lung fibrosis, leukaemia.

E.P. Demidchik: There are complications that directly affect their quality of life. A clear system for rehabilitating those who have thyroid cancer should be established.

L.E. Holm: How can the international community help?

Ch. Reiners: The European Commission produced a protocol for treatment, however a follow-up is not yet included. We are on the way to produce a second booklet which will include follow-up.

A. Tsyb: We appeal to the International Community for such a protocol.

N. Tronko: Maybe the classification of tumours should be reviewed for children by clinicians and pathologists. I recommend to co-ordinate the pathology and the tissues and accelerate with the international project creating a thyroid tissue bank in the three republics; it is important both for molecular biology and epidemiology and other studies.

A. Pinchera: There is an agreed protocol between the EU and the three republics. This protocol has been distributed in September and will be used in the three countries. The booklet addresses the difficulties for follow-up.

Topic 5: Public health implications - the need for recommendations and regulations

D. Becker: Prevention: Potassium iodide safety concerns can be used effectively. This issue was covered by M. Schlumberger and J. Naumann. R. Clarke pointed out the question of timing: be there at the right time. It depends on predistribution which is difficult to do.

Detection: This issue still remains open as well as how complete this kind of detection is done by ultrasound. This is a major issue with regard to case detection.

No mention was made at the conference about the public. Issues of communication, information and education were not touched upon. The public and the press depend upon us. Centres on the question of educating the public to respond intelligently and not have any kind of hysteria.

K. Baverstock: WHO guidelines on stable iodine prophylaxis were first published in 1989 by the European regional Office. It was envisaged in those guidelines that KI would be distributed to protect against the deterministic effects of exposure to radioiodine. The experience gained after Chernobyl demonstrated that there is now a need for a much more widespread protection against cancer in children. Stable iodine has been demonstrated to be safe for widespread administration to children and is known to be effective in blocking subsequent iodine uptake. The European regional Office has already issued informal advice and WHO is in the process of embodying this advice in revised guidelines prepared in collaboration with IAEA. Personally I am very much in agreement with the view expressed earlier by P. Crane that there is a need for the greater involvement of public health expertise in nuclear emergency preparedness and response and the revised WHO guidelines will be available early next year for the benefit of the ICRP and EURATOM.

E. Cardis: Public health - there are other aspects of public health actions which have not been discussed fully here. One is screening: screening id expensive, particularly in the case of low-level exposures which affect very large populations. It would be useful to make recommendations - based on the cost effectiveness of screening - about when to screen and when not to screen. The other aspect is prevention; not only primary prevention in the event of an accident, but also secondary prevention, i.e., how to reduce thyroid cancer risk among those who have been exposed. Should iodine supplementation be recommended? If iodination is recommended, proper monitoring of its efficiency of such an intervention would be important for the future.

Ch. Reiners: Iodine prophylaxis: Supplementation in diet is mandatory. You can prevent development of nodules. For goitre: it is cheaper to supplement with iodine to reduce goitre frequency than to intervene surgically. Screening is mandatory. Maybe it should be a little bit better co-ordinated.

D. Becker: Thyroid hormone suppression needs to be discussed.

J. Harrison: Education. Public health physicians have very little knowledge. NRPB is working with WHO to upgrade public health issues through the Radiation Emergency Medical Preparedness Advisory Network (REMPAN). This is important because these professionals are responsible for medical contingency planning, such as, the implementation of iodine prophylaxis. It is important therefore for the risk factors for thyroid cancer to be agreed and promulgated so that we can make decisions in case of another nuclear accident. The aftermath of the Chernobyl accident has shown countermeasures against ^{131}I inhalation and ingestion were not effective and that the psycho-social problems were a major problem. Medical practitioners need good information on radiation risks if they are to provide advice to the public and their patients. We hope to run courses on public health issues to increase the knowledge of the public and how the public can be counselled after an accident to avoid psycho-social aspects.

E.D. Williams: Conclusive remarks: During this conference we wanted to put what is happening in Chernobyl in a larger context of the thyroid problem and opened co-ordination for a far better understanding not only for science but for the patients.

List of Participants

Dr Nadeem Abbassi
St Luke's Institute of Cancer
Research
Highfield Road, Rathgar, Dublin
6, Ireland
00 353 1 496 0852
00 353 1 497 4886

Prof Theodor Abelin
Director
Dept of Social and Preventative
Medicine
University of Bern, 3012, Bern,
Switzerland
00 41 31 631 35 11
00 41 31 631 35 10
ABELIN@ISPM.UNIBE.CH

Dr Alexander Abrosimov
4 Kereliev Street
Obninsk 249020,
Kaluga Region, Russia
007 095 956 1439
00 7 095 956 1440
mrrc@obninsk.ru

Dr Zhanat Abylkassimova
PO Box 16
Semipalatinsk City
490049, Republic of Kazakstan
00 7 322 264 5649
00 7 322 266 2915
zhanata@yahoo.com

Dr M. Atkinson
GSF, Postfach 1129,
Ingolstadter Landstrasse 1,
D-85758 Oberschleissheim,
Germany

Dr S Bauer
Federal Office for Radiation
Protection
Institute for Radiation Hygiene
Ingolstaeter Landstrasse 1
D-85762 Obershleissheim,
Germany
00 49 89 316 03184
sbauer@bfs.de

Dr Keith Baverstock
WHO
ECEH, Rome Division
Via Francesco Crispi, 10
I - 00187, Rome, Italy
00 39 6 487751
00 39 6 4877599
kba@who.it

Dr David V Becker
Research Effects Branch,
National Cancer Institute,
6130 Executive Blvd,
EPN/530
Rockville MD 20852, USA
00 1 301 496 1224

Dr Vladimir Berkovski
Head, Radiation Safety of
NPP Lab
Radiation Protection Institute
Melnikova Str 53
Kiev 50, Ukraine
00 380 44 213 7208
00 380 44 213 7192
or 219 4900
vlad@rpi.kiev.ua

Dr Johannes Biko
Department of Nuclear
Medicine
Josef-Schneider Stre 2,
D-97080, Wurzberg,
Germany
00 49 931 201 5368
00 49 931 201 2247

Dr Tania Bogdanova
Institute of Endocrinology
and Metabolism
Vyshgorodskaya str 69,
254114, Kiev, Ukraine
00 380 44 432 8644
00 380 44 430 3718
tb@viaduk.net

Dr Andre Bouville
NCI, 6130 Executive Blvd,
EPN/ 530, Bethesda, MD
20852, USA
00 1 301 496 9326
00 1 301 496 1224
bouvilla@epndce.nci.gov

Professor Aaron Brill
Vanderbelt Univeristy,
Radiology Department
MCN R1302, Nashville, TN
37232-2675, USA
00 1 615 322 3190
00 1 615 322 3764

Dr David Brown
Institute of Naval Medicine
Alverstoke, Gosport, Hants,
SO24 0DR
01705 768 074
01705 504 823
ye30@dialpipex.com

Prof Gerard Burrow
Yale University School of
Medicine
333 Cedar Street,
SHM L220, Newhaven, CT
06520-8085, USA
00 1 203 785 7691
00 1 203 785 7693
gerard.burrow@yale.èdu

Professor Charles Capen
Department of Veterinary
Biosciences
The Ohio State Univ.
1925 Coffey Road,
Columbus, OH 43210, USA
00 1 614 7292 4489
00 1 614 292 6473
capen.s@osu.edu

Dr Elizabeth Cardis
IARC
150 Cours Albert Thomas,
69372, Lyon, France
00 33 4 72 73 85 05
00 33 472 73 85 75
cardis@iarc.fr

Dr Claudia Ceccarelli
Institute of Endocrinology
Di Cisanello Hospital
Pisa, Italy
00 39 50 955 034
00 39 50 57 8772
claudiac@endoc.med.unipi.it

Dr Ken Chadwick
European Commission
DG XII F6 (MO75, 4/15),
200 Rue de la Loi, 1049
Brussels, Belgium
00 32 2 295 4334
00 32 2 296 6256
kenneth.chadwick@dg12.cec.be

Prof Evgeny Cherstvoy
Institute of Pathology,
Pr Dzerzhinski 83
Minsk 220116, Belarus
00 375 172 787814
00 375 172 787814

Dr Gennaro Chiappetta
Oncologia Sperimentale "D"
Instituto Nazionale dei
Tumori
Fondazione Sen, Pascale,
Napoli, Italy
00 81 590 3517
00 81 590 3817

Dr Elizabeth Chua
University of Sydney
Department of
Endocrinology
Sydney, NSW Australia
2066
00 612 9515 6150
00 612 9516 1273
echua@earth.endocrin.usyd.edu.au

Dr Roger Clarke
NRPB
Chilton, Didcot, Oxford
OX11 0RQ
01235 831 600
01235 833 891

Dr Vincenzo Covelli
ENEA,
Via Anguilla rese 301
00060 S Maria di Galeria,
Roma, Italy
00 39 6 3048 3401
00 39 6 3045 4270
covelli@casaccia.enea.it

Mr Peter Crane
Counsel for Special Projects
US Nuclear Regulartory
Commission 4809
Drummond Avenue, Chevy
Chase, MD 20815, USA
001 301 656 3998
001 301 415 3200
pgcrane@erols.com

Professor Scott Davis
Hanford Thyroid Disease
Study
Fred Hutchinson Cancer
Research Centre
1124 Columbia Street, Mail
stop, MP 425, Seattle,
98104, Washington,
00 1 206 667 2683
00 1 206 667 5733
sdavis@fhcrc.org

Prof Nick Day
Department of Community
Medicine
Institute of Public Health
University of Forvie Site,
Robinson Way
Cambridge, CB2 2SR

Dr Giuseppe De Luca
ANPA
Va Vitaliano Brancati 48
00144, Rome, Italy
00 39 65 00 72 009
00 39 65 00 72 941

Dr Florent de Vathaire
Unite 351 INSERM
Institut Gustave Roussy, Rue
Camille Desmoulins 94805,
Villejuif, France
00 33 1 42 11 54 57
00 33 1 42 11 53 15
fdv@igr.fr

Prof E P Demidchik
Minsk State Medical
Institute
F Skorina Ave 64
220600 Minsk, Belarus
00 375 172 269 360

Dr Yu Demidchik
Minsk State Medical
Institute
F Skorina Ave 64
220600 Minsk
Belarus
00 375 172 269 360

Ms Angelique Dreijer
Genzyme,
Gooimeer 3-30
1411 DC Naarden
The Netherlands
0031 35 699 1200
0033 1 35 694 3214

Dr V M Drozd
Research Institute of
Radiation
Medicine and Endocrinology
Pritytsky Str 38, Apt 86,
220082, Minsk
Belarus
00 375 172 321 344

Prof Jacques Dumont
Faculte De Medicine, ULB.
Campus Hop. Erasme, Route
De Lennik 808, 1070
Brussels, Belgium
00 32 2 555 4134
00 32 2 555 4655
jedumont@ulb.ac.be

Dr Christie Eheman
Centre for Diseases, Control
and Prevention
MSF-35, 4770, Burford
Highway, Atlanta, Georgia
30341, USA
00 1 770 488 7618
00 1 770 488 7044
crel@cdc.gov

Prof. Ovsei Epshtein
Institute of Endocrin.
Vyshgorodskaya 69
Kiev, Ukraine
00380 432 85 77

Dr Farahati
Klinik and Polyklinik for
Nuclear Medicine
University of Wurzburg
Roentgenring 11,
D-9707 Wurzburg, Germany
00 49 931 565 37

Dr M Ferdeghini
Depart. of Oncology
Div. of Nuclear Medic.
University of Pisa, Italy
00 39 050 555259
00 39 050 552100
mferdigh@nucl.ned.unipi.it

Dr Christine Frenzel
Strahlenbiologisches
Institute, Ludwig
Maximillians Univ.
Schillerstrase 42,
D-80336, Munich
Germany
00 89 5996 833
00 89 5996 840
Lengfelder@Irz.unimuenchen.de

Dr Juergen Froehlich
Brahms Diagn. GmbH
Komturstr 19 - 20
D - 12099
Berlin, Germany
00 49 30 750 12789
00 49 30 750 12640

Prof. Keisei Fujimori
2nd Dep. of Surgery
Univ. School of Medic.
Seiryo-Machi 1-1 Aobaku
Sendai, Japan
00 81 22 717 7214
00 81 22 717 7217
fujimori@gonryo.med.tohoku.ac.jp

Dr S Gazal
Conseil General De Tarn Et
Garonne
Hotel Du Department
bvd Hubert Gouze GP 783
F82013, Montauban, France
00 33 5 63 91 82 00
00 33 5 63 03 28 52

Prof Maciej Gembicki
School of Medicine
Dep. of Endocrinology
Przybyszewskiego 49
60-355, Poznan, Poland
00 48 61 867 3083
00 48 61 869 1682

Prof Eystein Glattre
Cancer Research Registry
Montebello, N-0310 0310,
Norway
00 47 22 45 1334
00 47 22 45 13 70

Dr Bernard Goslings
Endocrinologist
Dep. of Endocrinology,
University Hospital, PO Box
g600, 2300 RC Leiden, The
Netherlands
00 33 71 52 62 645
00 31 71 52 48 136

Dr Guennadi Goulko
GSF Forchungszeutrum
Ingolstyadter Laudstr 1, D-
85764,Neuherberg, Germany
00 49 89 3187 2225
00 49 89 31 87 3363
goulko@gsf.de

Dr Patrick Gourmelon
Institut De Protection et De
Surete Nucleaire
IPSN BP 6
F 92265, Fontenay-Aux-
Rose, France
00 33 1 46 54 70 80
00 33 1 46 54 46 10
gourmelon@ipsn.fr

Dr Tom Hamilton
Fred Hutchinson Cancer
Research Centre
1100 Fairview Avenue
North, MP-425 PO Box
19024, Seattle, Washington
98109-1024, USA
00 1 206 667 5733
00 1 206 667 2683
tehamilton@aol.com

Dr H Ruben Harach
Department of
Histopathology
St Bartholomew's Hospital,
West Smithfield, London
EC1A 7BE
0171 601 8533
0171 601 8543

Dr John Harrison
NRPB
Chilton, Didcot
Oxon, OX11 0RQ
01235 822 612
01235 822 630
johnr.harrison@nrpb.org.uk

Dr F Hawkins
Office of International
Health Programs,
Department of Energy,
EH-63 270CC,
19901 Germantown Road,
Germantown
MD 20874
001 301 903 1757
001 301 903 1413

Dr Wolfgang Heidenreich
GSF ISS, D-85758
Neuherberg, Germany
00 49 89 3187 3032
00 49 89 3187 3363
heidenreich@gsf.de

Dr Ludwig Hieber
Inst. of Radiobiology
GSF, Ingolstadter Landst 1,
85758
Neuherberg, Germany
00 49 89 31 87 4118
00 49 89 31 87 3381
ludwig.hieber@gsf.de

Ass Prof Colin Hill
USS SCH of Medicine,
Department of Radiation,
CRL BLDG 209, 1303, N
Mission Road, Los Angeles,
CA 90033, USA
00 1 323 224 7783
00 1 323 255 2557
ckhill@hsc.asc.edu

518

Dr Cuong Hoang-Vu
Experimentelle and
Chirurgisce Onkologie
Klinik
feurAllgemeinchirurgie
Martin-Luther Univers.,
Magdeburger st 18
06097 Halle/S,Germany
00 49 345 557 1366
00 49 345 557 1232
mjont@mlucom6.urz.uni-
halle.de

Dr Lars Holm
Swedish Radiation
Protection Institution
SE - 17116,
Stockholm
Sweden
00 46 8729 7110
00 46 8729 7108
lars.erik.holm@ssi.se

Mr Hasan Hoser
Genzyme,
Gooimeer 3-30
1411 DC Naarden
The Netherlands
0031 35 699 1200
0033 1 35 694 3214

Ms Nezahat Hunter
Univers. of Birmingham
School of Physics,
Edgbaston, Birmingham
B15 2TT
0121 414 4695
0121 414 4725
n.hunter@bham.ac.uk

Professor Masahiro Ito
Atomic Bomb Disease
Institute
Nagasaki University School
of Medicine
1-12-4 Sakamoto,
Nagasaki,
Japan
00 81 95 849 7106
00 81 95 849 7108
m-ito@net.nagasaki-u.ac.jp

Dr V Ivanov
Medical Radiology Centre
Russian Academy of
Medical Sciences
Korolov Str 4,
249020 Obninsk,
Kaluga Obl, Russia
00 7 095 956 9412
00 7 095 956 1440
mrrc@obninsk.ru

Dr Peter Jacob
GSF National Research
Centre
D-8574 Oberschleibheim,
00 49 89 3187 4008
00 49 85 3187 3363
Jacob@gsf.de

Dr Barbara Jarzab
Department of Nuclear
Medicine and Oncological
Endocrinology
M Sklodowskiej-Curie
Institute of Oncology
Gliwice, Poland
00 48 3231 3512

Prof. Guillermo Juvenal
Atomic Energy Commission
Avda del Liberatador 8250
1429 Buenos Aires,
Argentina
00 54 1 754 7121
juvenal@cnea.edu.ar

Dr Anna Karaoglou
European Commission,
DGXII F-6 (MO75 4/14)
200 rue de Loi,
B 1049 Brussels
Belgium
0032 2 296 5415
0032 2 296 6256
anna.karaoglou@dg12.cec.be

Ms Julie Kelly
Genzyme,
Gooimeer 3-30
1411 DC Naarden
The Netherlands
0031 35 699 1200
0033 1 35 694 3214

Dr J Kenigsberg
Radiation Medicine and
Endocrinology
Masherov Ave 23
220600
Minsk, Belarus

Dr Ausra Kesminiene
IARC
150 Cours Albert-Thomas
69372 Lyon Cedex 08
France
00 33 4 72 73 88 35
00 33 4 72 73 83 61
kesminiene@iarc.fr

Dr Andreas Kofler
Department of Social and
Preventive Medicine,
University of Bern, 3012,
Bern, Switzerland
00 41 31 631 3867
00 41 31 631 4861
KOFLER @ ISPM.UNIBE.CH

Dr Olexandr Komov
IFRC, 14 Ulitsa
Mayakovskogo,
220006 Minsk,
Belarus
00 375 172 21 72 37
00 375 172 21 90 60
komov@ifrc.minsk.by

Dr Y O Konstantinov
Institite of Radiation
Hygiene
Mira Str 8
197101, St Petersburg,
Russia
Fax - 00 7 812 315 8897

Dr Jeannine Lallemand
Electricite De France
Radioprotection Service
3 rue de Messine,
75384, Paris,
France
00 44 85 17 82 or 17 87
00 44 95 17 90

Dr Michael Lassmann
Department of Nuclear
Medicine
Josef-Schneider Stre 2,
D-97080,
Wurzberg,
Germany
00 49 931 201 5368
00 49 931 201 2247

Prof Edmund Lengfelder
Strahlenbiologisches
Institute
Ludwig Maximillians
University
Schillerstrase 42
D 80336
Munich,
Germany
00 89 5996 834
00 89 5996 840
Lengfelder@irz.uni-muenchen.de

Prof Ilya Likhtarev
Radiation Medicine Centre
53 Melnkiova Str,
Kiev 253050
Kiev, Ukraine
00 380 44 213 7192
00 380 44 213 7192
likh@rpi.kiev.ua

Dr Rolf Lipecky
BRAHMS Diagnostica
GmbH
Komturstr 19 - 2
D -12099 Berlin
Germany
00 49 30 750 12639
00 49 30 750 12640

Dr Craig Lipman
Mid-South Imaging Inc
Therapeutics
c/o 10229 Poston Oak Circle
Collierville,
TN, 38017, USA
00 1 901 854 0496
00 1 901 853 1675
craigl@hotmail.com

Dr Jay Litvin
Medical Liaison, Chadbad's
Children of Chernobyl, PO
Box 14, Kfar Chabad,
72915, Israel
00 972 3 9607 588
00 972 3 9606 169
tzachhg@trendline.co.il

Professor Virginia Livolsi
University of Pennsylvania
Medical Centre
3400 Spruce St/F6042
USA
00 1 215 662 6544
00 1 215 349 5910

Dr Marie Lundell
Karolinska Hospital
Department of Hospital
Physics
S-171, 76 Stockholm
Sweden
00 46 8 517 73634
00 46 8 736 6280
mariel@asf.ks.se

Prof Eugeny Lushnikov
MRRC RAMS
4 Kereliev Street, Obninsk
249020, Kaluga Region
Russia
00 7 095 956 1439
00 7 095 956 1440
mrrc@obninsk.ru

Mrs H Maki
Sasakawa Memorial Health
Foundation
Senpaku Shinko Bldg
1-15-16, Toranomon,
Minatoku
Tokyo, 105-0001, Japan
00 81 3 3508 2201
00 81 3 3508 2204

Dr Daniel Meire
Leopoldlaan 17 A
B-9900 Eeklo Belgium
00 32 9 378 4757
00 32 9 378 0768
rxmeire@unicall.be

Dr C Miller
Chief, Emergency
Preparedness
Radition Protection Branch
Office of Nuclear Regulatory
Commission,
Washington DC
20555, USA
00 1 301 415 1086
001 301 415 2968
clm1@nrc.gov

Prof. Baruch Modan
Chaim Sheba Medical Centre
Tel-Aviv University
Sackier School of Medicine
Tel - Hashomer
52621, Israel
00 972 3 5303262
00 972 3 534 8369
bmodan@ccsg.tau.ac.il

Prof A G Mrotchek
Research and Clinical
Institute
Radiation Medicine and
Endocrinology
Masherov Ave 23, 220600
Minsk Belarus
00 375 172 269 360
risk@rcirme

Dr Brian Mullen
Department of Nuclear
Medicine, Mayo Clinic
200 First Street SW
Rochester, MN, 55905, USA
00 1 507 284 8095
00 1 507 266 4461

Dr Ritta Mustonen
Radiation Laboratory,
STUK-Radiation and
Nuclear Safety Authority,
PO Box 14, FIN-00881,
Helsinki, Finland
00 358 9 7598 8553
00 358 9 7598 8556
riitta.mustonen@stuk.fi

520

Prof Shigenobu Nagataki
Chairman, RERF
5 - 2 Hijiyama Park
Minami-Ku
Hiroshima, Japan
00 81 82 263 7279

Dr Mykola Nagonyy
IFRC, 14 Ulitsa,
Maykovskogo
220006 Minsk, Belarus
00 375 172 21723
00 375 172 219060
nagornyt@ifrc.minsk.by

Dr Noriaki Nakashima
2nd Depart. of Surgery
Tohoku University
School of Medicine, Seiryo-
machi
1-1 Aoba-ku Sendai, Japan
00 81 22 7177 214
00 81 22 717 7217
norinaka@mail.cc.tohoku.ac.jp

Dr Anna Christina
Nascimento
Inst De Radioprotecae e
Dosimetria
IRD/CNEN
Av Salvador Allende 5,
Recreio dos Bandeirantes,
Rio De Janiero, Brazil
00 55 21 442 9639
00 55 21 442 2405
acris@ird.gov.br

Dr J Nauman
Dep. of Endocrinology
Medical Centre for
Postgraduate Research
Marymoncka 99
PL - 01813, Poland
00 48 22 629 1040

Dr Tatjana Nedveckaite
Institute of Physics
Savanoriu 231 Lt 2028
Vilnius, Lithuania
00 370 2 641336
00 370 2 235182
Vitfil@julius.KTL.mii.lt

Dr A Nerovnya
Institute of Pathology,
Pr Dzerzhinski 83
Minsk 220116
Belarus
00 375 172 787814
00 375 172 787814

Dr Ruth Neta
Office of International
Health Programs
Department of Energy,
EH-63 270CC,
19901 Germantown Road,
Germantown MD 20874
001 301 903 1757
001 301 903 1413
ruth neta@eh.doe.gov

Prof. Valeriy Oliynyk
Instit. of Endocrinology
Vyshgorrodskaya 69
Kiev, Ukraine
00380 432 79 06

Dr Furio Pacini
Inst. of Endocrinology
Casanello Hospital
Via Paradisa 2, Cisanello
56/24 Pisa, Italy
00 39 50 544 723
00 39 50 578 772
fpacini@endoc.med.unipi.i

Dr Wendla Paile
STUK Radiation and
Nuclear Safety Auth
Laippatie 4 (PO Box 14)
FIN-00881
Helsinki, Finland
00 358 9 7598 8480
00 358 9 7598 8498
wendla.paile@stuk.fi

Dr Galina Panashuk
Gomel Specialised Medical
Dispensary
Bratyev Lizyukovich 5
Gomel, 246029, Belarus
00 375 232 48 7120
00 375 232 53 1903

Dr Herwig Paretzke
GSF - Institut fur
Strahlenschutz
Ingolstadter Landstr 1
D-85764
Neuherberg, Germany
00 49 89 3187 3323
00 49 89 3187 4006
paretzke@gsf.de

Prof Aldo Pinchera
Instit. of Endocrinology
Cisanello Hospital,
Via Paradisa 2
Cisanello,
56/24 Pisa, Italy
00 39 50 54 4723
00 39 50 57 8772
a.pinchera@endoc.med.unipi.it

Dr Tatiana Poliakova
Institute of Pathology
Minsk State Medical
Institute, Minsk, Belarus
00375 172 787814

Dr Veronika Pozcharskaya
Institute of Pathology
Pr Dzerzhinski 83
Minsk 220116, Belarus
00 375 172 787814
00 375 172 787814

Prof. Hartmut Rabes
Experim. Pathologist
Institute of Pathology
University of Munich
D 80337, Germany
00 49 89 5160 4081
00 49 89 5160 4083

Prof Albey M Reiner
Univ. of Massachusetts at
Amherst
203 Morrill Science Centre,
Amherst,
MA 01003, USA
00 1 413 545 2051
00 1 413 545 1578

Dr Ch Reiners
Clinic for Nuclear Medicine
University of Wurzberg
Josef-Schneider Str 2,
D-97080, Wurzberg
Germany
00 49 931 201 5868
00 49 931 201 2247
reiners@nuklearmedizin.uni-
wuerzburg.de

Dr Andrew Riches
University of St Andrews
Bute Medical Building
St Andrews,
Scotland
KY16 9TS
01334 463603
01334 463600
acr1@st-andrews.ac.uk

Dr Jacob Robbins
National Institute of Health
Genetics and Biochemistry
Branch
Bldg 10, Room MSC, 201A,
10 Centre Drive, MSC 1587,
Bethseda MD, 20892-1587
00 1 301 496 5761
00 1 301 480 0406
jacobr@bdg10.niddk.nih.gov

Dr Elaine Ron
National Cancer Institute,
NIH, EPN-408, Bethesda,
MD 20892 USA
00 1 301 496 6600
00 1 301 402 0207
rone@epndce.nci.nih.gov

Dr Henry Royal
Washington University
School of Medicine
510 South Kingshighway
Boulevard St Louis,
Missouri
63110-1076
00 1 314 362 2809
00 1 314 362 2806
royal@mirlink.wustl.edu

Dr Charles Ruchti
Institute of Pathology
University of Bern
Murtenstr 31
CH-3010,
Bern, Switzerland
00 41 31 632 88 75
00 41 31 632 99 38

Dr Siegal Sadetzki
Chaim Sheba Medical Centre
Tel-Aviv University
Sackier School of Medicine
Tel - Hashomer 52621,
Israel
00 972 3 5303 262
00 972 3 534 8369
epid15@post.tau.ac.il

Prof Atsuhiko Sakamoto
Department of Pathology,
Kyorin University School of
Medicine,
6-20-2 Shinkawa, Mitaka,
Tokto 181-8811
Japan
0081 422 47 5511
0081 422 40 7093

Dr Aki Salo
STUK - Radiation and
Nuclear Safety Auth
Lab. of Radiobiology,
PO Box 14 ,
Fin-00881, Helsinki, Finland
00 358 9 7598 8546
00 358 9 759 88556
AKI.SALO@STUK.FI

Prof. MJ Schlumberger
Chef d'unite
Service De Medicine
Nucleaire
Unite Hospitalisation Haute
De Seine
39 Rue Camille Desmoulins,
94805 Villejuif, France
00 33 1 42 11 44 96
00 33 1 42 11 52 23

Dr Cornelia Schmutzler
Medizinislhe Poliklinik
Universitaet Wuerzburg
Roentgenring 11
97070, Wurezberg, Germany
00 531 201 7103
00 531 201 7102
c.schmutzler@mail.uni.wurzberg.de

Dr Minouk Schoemaker
Cancer and Public Health
Department of Epidemiology
and Public Health,
London School of Hygiene
and Tropic Medicine,
Keppel Str,
London
0171 927 2301
0171 436 4230
minouk.schoemaker@lshtm.ac.uk

Dr Christian Seidel
Medipan Diagnostica GMBH
Rotberger Str 18,
D-15831, Selchow
Germany
00 33 79 38304
00 33 79 383 08

Dr Vladimir Shakhtarin
Medical Radiological
Research Centre
Russian Academy of
Medical Sciences
Koroliov Str 4
Obninsk, russia
00 7 095 956 1440

Dr Yakov Shoikhet
IRMEP,
PO Box 4663
126 Papanintsev Str, Barnaul
656043,
Russia
00 7 3852 229 027
00 7 3852 260 735
vik@biomed.altai.su

Prof Roy Shore
New York University
Medical School
341 E 25th Street, New
York, NY 10010-2598, USA
00 1 212 263 6498
00 1 212 263 8570
shorer01@gcrc.med.nyu.med

Dr Kenneth Silver
Boston University School of
Public Health
Box 2977, Santa Fe,
NM 87507 USA
00 1 505 820 1143
00 1 505 820 6642
ksilver@bu.edu

Dr Steven Simon
Radiation Effects Research
2101 Constitution Ave,
NW, Washington DC 20418,
USA
00 1 202 334 2232
00 1 202 334 1639
ssimon@nas.ed

Dr Jaak Sinnaeve
European Commission,
DGXII F-6 MO75,
200 rue de la Laoi,
B1049 Brussels,
Belgium
0032 2 296 6256
jaak.sinnaeve@dg12.cec.be

Dr David Slavin
Royal Navy (MoD)
Office of Naval Nuclear
Technical Safety Panal, Ash
Building, 970, Abbey Wood,
Bristol, BS34 8JN
0117 913 5027
0117 913 5902

Dr Patrick Smeesters
Radiation Protection
Department
Ministry of Public Health,
Cite Administration
B1010, Brussels
00 32 2 210 5978
00 32 2 210 4967
patrick.smeesters@health.gov.be

Dr Jan Smida
Institute of Radiobiology
GSF, Ingolstadter Landst 1,
85758
Neuherberg,
Germany
00 49 89 31 87 2282
00 49 89 31 87 3381
smida@gsf.de

Dr James Smith
US Centre for Disease
Control (MS F-35)
4770 Buford Highway,
Atlanta GA 30341 - 3724,
USA
00 1 770 488 7040
00 1 770 488 7044
jms5@cdc.gov

Prof Guennadi Souchkevitch
WHO, Avenue Appia 20
CH-1211 Geneva 27
Switzerland
00 41 22 791 37 62
00 41 22 791 41 23
souchkevitchg@who.ch

Dr Valery Stepanenko
Medical Radiological
Resarch Centre of RAMS,
Korolev Street 4
249020 Obninsk,
Kaluga Region,
Russia
00 7 095 956 1440
valeri@imr.obninsk.su

Dr Fred Stevenson
Institute for Toxicology,
Brunswiker Str 10
D-24105,
Kiel,
Germany
stevenson@toxi.uni-kiel.de

Prof. Christian Streffer
Univ - Klinikum Essen
D-45122 Essen
Germany
00 49 201 723 4152
00 49 201 723 5966

Dr Eero Suonio
Project Officer
Intern. Thyroid Project
28 Fabriciusa Str, Room 401,
Belarus
00 375 172 220445
00 375 172 204165
itp@un.minsk.by

Ass Prof Tatsuya Takahashi
Dep. of Epidemiology and
Surgery
Nagasaki University
School of Medicine, 1-12-4
Nagasaki
852-8523 Japan
00 81 95 8497063
00 81 95 8497064
t-taka@netnagasaki-M.ac.jp

Dr Gerry Thomas
TCRG,
Univer. of Cambridge,
Strangeways Research
Laboratory,
Wort's Causeway,
Cambridge CB1 4RN
0044 1223 243231
0044 1223 411609
gerry@srl.cam.ac.uk

Dr Margot Tirmarche
Institute for Protection of
Nuclear Safety
BP 6, 92265, Fontenay
Aux Rose France
00 33 1 46 54 71 94
00 33 1 46 57 03 86
tirmarche@mandrake.ipsn.f

Mrs Jocelyn Towson
Royal Prince Alfred
Hospital, Camperdown,
NSW 2050, Australia
00 612 9515 6023
00 612 9515 6381
jtowson@nucmed.roa.cs.nsw.gov.au

Prof Nickolai Tronko
Institute of Endocrinology
and Metabolism
Vyshgorodskaya str 69,
254114, Kiev Ukraine
00 380 44 432 8644
00 380 44 430 3718

Dr Katherine Troshina
Endocrinological Research
Centre
D Ulyanosa Str 11
Moscow, Russia 117036
00 7 095 124 5502
00 7 095 124 3503
kat@home.relline.ru

Dr Klaus Trott
Dep. of Radiat. Biology
St Bartholomew's and the
Royal London School of
Medicine and Dentistry,
Charterhouse Square,
London
0171 982 6106
0171 982 6107
krtrott@mds.gmw.ac.uk

Prof A Tsyb
Med. Radiology Centre
Russian Academy of
Medical Sciences
Korolov Str 4, 249020
Obninsk, Kaluga Obl,
Russia
00 7 095 956 1439
00 7 095 956 1440
mrrc@obninsk.ru

Dr Istvan Turai
International Atomic
Energy Agency
Wagramerstrasse 5,
PO Box 100, A-1400
Vienna,
Austria
00 431 2060 22738
00 431 2060 29653
I.Turai@iaea.org

Dr R Michael Tuttle
Assistant Chief, DCI
Walter Reed Medical Centre,
Endocrine Clinic,
7D, 6800 Georgia Ave,
Washington DC
20302, USA
00 1 202 782 7840
00 1 202 782 3881
rmtuttle@hotmail.com

Prof G Vecchio
Faculty of Medicine and
Surgery, University of
Naples
Via Sergio Pansini 5
80131, Naples, Italy
00 39 81 746 3037

Dr Tatiana Vorontsova
Institute of Radiation
Medicine and
Endocrinology, Masherov
Ave 23, 220600 Minsk,
Belarus
00 375 172 269 360

Dr Bruce Wachholz
National Cancer Inst.
6130 Executive Blvd,
EPN/530
Rockville MD, 20852
USA
00 1 301 496 9326
00 1 301 496 1224
bw36i:nih.gov

Dr Peter Waight
6 Comptons Court
Comptons Lane
Horsham, West Sussex
RH13 6TA

Prof Dillwyn Williams
TCRG
Univ. of Cambridge,
Strangeways Research
Laboratory,
Wort's Causeway,
Cambridge
+44 1223 243231
+44 1223 411609
gat1000@cam.ac.uk

Dr Regina Winkelmann
Epidemiologist
Danish Cancer Society
Strandboulevarden 49, DK-
2100
Copenhagen, Denmark
00 45 35 25 76 25
00 45 35 25 77 31
regina@cancer.dk

Dr Dave Wynford-Thomas
CRC Thyroid Tumour
Research Group
Department of Pathology
University of Wales, College
of Medicine
Heath Park, Cardiff, CF4
4XN
01222 743496
01222 744276

Prof Shunichi Yamashita
Chairman,Department of
Nature Medicine
Atomic Bomb Disease
Institute,
Nagasaki University School
of Medicine, 1 - 12 - 4
Sakamoto, Nagasaki
8528523, Japan
00 81 95 849 7114
00 81 95 849 7117
shun@net.nagasaki-u.ac.jp

Dr Evgeny Zaitsev
IRMEP, PO Box 4663
126 Papanintsev Str, Barnaul
656043
Russia
00 7 3852 229027
00 7 3852 260735
vik@blomed.altai.su

Dr Lyuda Zurnagdhy
Institute of Endocrinology
and Metabolism
Vyshgorodskaya str 69,
254114, Kiev,
Ukraine
00 380 44 432 8644
00 380 44 432 3718
tb@viaduk.net

Dr Irina Zvonova
Leading Scientist
Institute of Radiation
Hygiene
Mira Str 8
197101, St Petersburg,
Russia
00 7 812 233 4147
00 7 812 230 6319
Ira@katia.stud.pu.ru